Medline +

The Art of Medical Interpretation® Third Edition

Contents

PO Box 2308, Woburn, MA 01888-0508, **p:** 781-729-3736, **www.EmbracingCulture.com**
PO Box 6401, Manchester, NH 03108, **p:** 1-888-678-CCCS

Introduction

The Art of Medical Interpretation®, First Edition was completed in March 2002. In June 2004, the Second Edition was published.

The Art of Medical Interpretation®, Third Edition was completed in September 2009. This 14-lesson comprehensive manual for foreign language interpreters is a result of seven years of teaching, consulting and collecting feedback from users of our two previous editions. This edition is unique and innovative, but it still maintains the "Paulo Freire" approach to teaching adults upon which we have based all of our instructional and supplementary materials.

The manual was designed to first elicit the student's own knowledge by encouraging self-reflection through individual and group exercises. It then guides students through an incredible learning experience that builds upon this base knowledge and enables the student to develop key strengths as an interpreter that include a deep understanding of the practical, cultural, and ethical variants of real-life triadic encounters.

The manual accommodates many different learning styles, and new information is introduced in a seamless way from lesson to lesson. Each of the 14 lessons can be thoroughly taught in four to six hours. Thus, instructors have the choice to adapt the manual for 40-hour to 80-hour trainings. Colleges that use this manual as a primary textbook can also borrow from its supplementary sections and bibliography for course enrichment.

The Art of Medical Interpretation®, 3rd edition covers basic interpreting skills, ethics for professional interpreters, anatomy and pathology and many of the main body systems, and common medical procedures. In addition to reading assignments, critical thinking exercises, group activities and topics for discussion, there are over 90 true-to-life role-plays for consecutive interpreting practice. Each role-play tells a story through which the interpreter will learn about medicine and medical terminology, and several of these role-plays allow for practice in ethical decision-making, an important skill for medical interpreters.

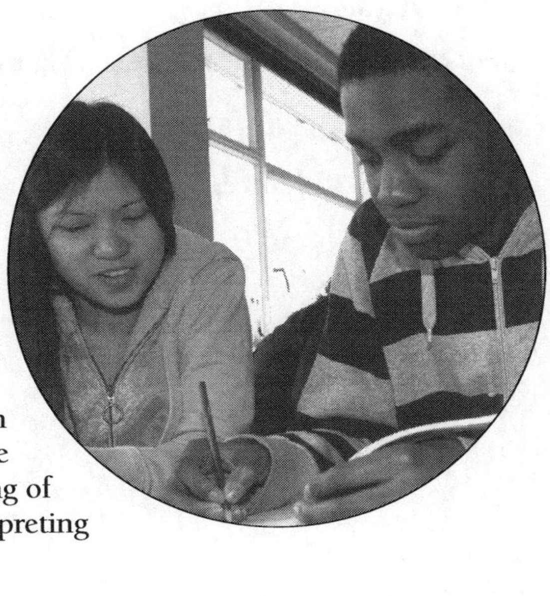

As in our first two editions, we introduce the student to the Samurai! Technique, an easy-to-learn method of breaking down complex medical terminology into prefixes, roots and suffixes for quick comprehension. We have also added two wonderful lessons: "Introduction to Mental Health" and "The Professional Interpreter." The former provides the interpreter with a basic understanding of clinical insight and practice in the most appropriate interpreting

PO Box 2308, Woburn, MA 01888-0508, **p:** 781-729-3736, **www.EmbracingCulture.com**
PO Box 6401, Manchester, NH 03108, **p:** 1-888-678-CCCS

modes for various common mental health settings; while the latter addresses concrete marketing skills for new interpreters, including building one's resume, schedule management, and dressing for the job.

Out of consideration for the environment, we have kept the spirit of our famous pre- and post- quizzes, but each quiz will appear in print just once. The quizzes should be completed by the student at the beginning of each lesson and reviewed in class prior to the start of the next lesson.

The last section of this manual is a compilation of the main vocabulary terms taken from the publication's role-plays and glossaries. The vocabulary section is divided into the following topics:

1. Body Parts and Organs
2. Pathology / Symptoms / Conditions
3. Laboratory Tests and Diagnostic procedures
4. Idiomatic Expressions
5. Treatment Procedures
6. Medications
7. Medical Supplies
8. Other

This manual is a true collaboration between active interpreters, students, faculty, providers, managers and our incredibly dedicated staff at CCCS, Inc.™. It embraces current market needs by training interpreters as generalists and giving students a solid understanding of the professional, ethical, cultural considerations in navigating a complex health care system. The manual sends a message, loud and clear, that an introductory training is not enough to carry an interpreter throughout his/her career and that all professionals need to continuously further their education.

For those who will be teaching from this manual, CCCS, Inc.™ has developed a complementary short guide on how to best use the manual in a classroom setting. Please inquire about information and workshops for prospective trainers by contacting info@embracingculture.com.

Visit Media Resources for additional materials you can purchase to teach this course. **(page 891)**

Dedication

I have to thank so many individuals and groups of people: my family, our colleagues and our LEP patients for their work, support, inspiration and partnership in this social justice initiative of training qualified bilingual individuals as professional medical interpreters. It takes a team to build a future!

On a personal note:

Seven years ago, I dedicated our first edition to my family. All these years later, my husband and three wonderful daughters are still keeping me on track as a human being!

I remember when my youngest daughter was little and her sisters told her that I was an "alien". She cried, thinking that I was an alien from outer space, not understanding what it meant to be an alien resident in the United States. Truthfully, in my experience as an immigrant, I have often felt like a real alien, both in this country and in my country of birth. This business of being a new immigrant does not always go smoothly for everyone. But it has changed me as a person and perhaps my passion and dedication to the cause of medical interpretation is a way of perpetuating the hope that I will someday heal from the immigrant experience.

My passion in this work and my dedication of many hours towards the professionalization of interpreters has brought me many joys, but it has also "separated" me from my daughters at important times in their development as amazing young women. My husband Rick was often both "poppy" and "mommy," and I want to thank him for being so wonderful for so long! Rick has been a great life and work partner for over 30 years, and he continues to dedicate time as a medical advisor and instructor at CCCS, Inc.™

Seven years ago, when writing our first edition, I was challenged by the death of the two most important women in my life. My mother, Maria Celestino Almendro de Araújo, passed away in June 2002. Known to all as "Tininha," she had been a nurse in Santa Maria Island, Azores, Portugal. She showed compassion, care and great technical skill while working at the Airport Hospital and throughout her nursing career as she cared for passengers from all over the world and from diverse ethnic backgrounds.

As a child, I was lucky to keep my mother company at work. Often, she would call me into the emergency room so that I could help entertain tearful, frightened children with head injuries or broken limbs. I would tell them stories to make them laugh or I would share my toys with them.

I also accompanied her when visiting many patients who were too ill to come to the hospital. She passed on to me her belief that patients would get better if nurtured and cared for. She always did her best, though at times she could not speak the languages of some of her international patients. She would quickly get dictionaries and call my father or anyone

PO Box 2308, Woburn, MA 01888-0508, **p:** 781-729-3736, **www.EmbracingCulture.com**
PO Box 6401, Manchester, NH 03108, **p:** 1-888-678-CCCS

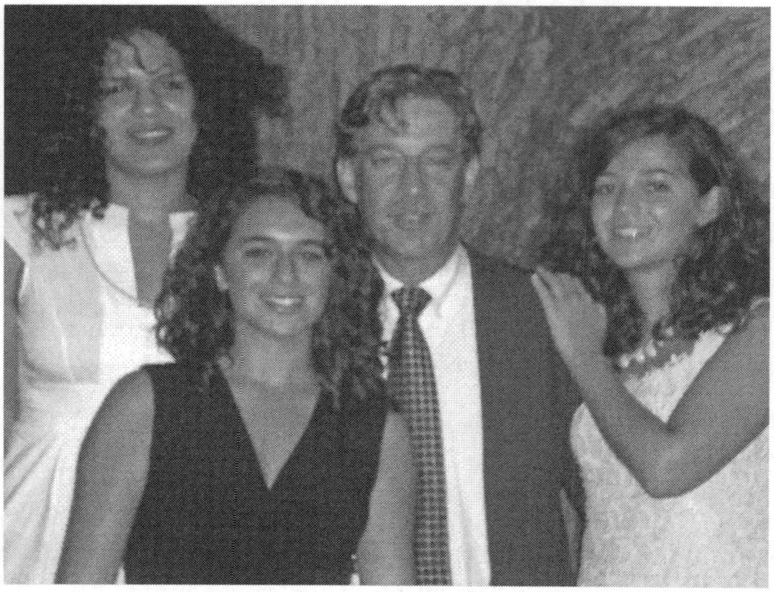

who could communicate in the patient's language. It was evident that she took her job seriously and loved being a nurse.

As I visited her in the intensive care at a hospital in Portugal, I grieved the sudden death of her sister, Virginia Neves, my favorite aunt who was also a nurse and who passed away a few days before my mother. I want to thank them both for teaching me to be caring and compassionate towards people in general and especially toward patients.

As I continue to grieve their loss, I feel stronger in a way, because I now understand a bit more about the circle of life. Knowledge gets passed on from generation to generation, a bit by actions, a bit by reading, and a bit through life experiences.

Acknowledgements

To My Colleagues:

First Edition: The conceptualization of this manual started with Power Point presentations developed for CCCS, Inc.™ trainings nationwide. At the time, Dr. Richard Lane, Ben Ready and Vonessa Phillips were our main contributors, and Luis Torres was our graphic designer. We spent sleepless nights and endless weekends working together in creating one of the country's first medical interpreter training manuals.

Second Edition: Vonessa Phillips and I collaborated in preparing the second edition of this manual and we are very thankful to Megasystems for allowing CCCS, Inc.™ to use their anatomical graphics.

Third Edition: Vera Duarte Outeiro, a friend and an extremely dynamic High School teacher with a Masters degree in Applied Linguistics, was the main force in redesigning the manual in a way that invites the student to be an active part of the learning process. Vera carefully directed, dissected, and rearranged the raw materials that I call my "intellectual babies" – a painful process, but well worth it!

Dr. Ana Filomena (Mena) Macedo, a dear friend and faithful source of guidance for over 30 years, graciously undertook the responsibility of co-editor in this fine endeavor. She accepted this major task of reviewing the final round of edits with her usual warmth and calm approach; which contributed to the completion within a very short deadline. Mena holds a Masters in Business Administration from Simmons College and a Ph.D. in Sociology from Brandeis University. Her educational background, coupled with her intellectual abilities were very appreciated throughout the process of revamping this manual. Never one to back away from hard work, she labored alongside Vera Outeiro as they entered into a "zone" in July of 2009 and rapidly accomplished the work!

Mena has encouraged and supported my efforts from the beginning when I started one of the first interpreter programs in the USA in 1978. I am forever thankful for her invaluable contribution to yet another undertaking.

Esther Phillips, a long-time colleague and teacher at CCCS, Inc.™, is the primary text co- editor of the entire manual – not an easy task when writers are bursting with ideas and at times need help reorganizing them. Esther, thanks for your friendship, humor and great collaborative spirit.

Vonessa Phillips Costa, a friend, long-time colleague, and former student when I taught at Bentley College, has worked very closely with me in developing key theories such as CIFE, the Six W's, and the interpreter as a butterfly. We have worked hard for many years and have enjoyed each and every minute of our collaboration. Most of the text used in this manual was developed and edited by us together. Vonessa has recently opened her professional wings to a different job and we miss her and wish her well in her new career at a local hospital. Life is an amazing circle – Vonessa is now managing a division of an interpreter program that I started 30 years ago!

Tania West was the primary quiz developer and she assisted Vera Outeiro on the compilation of the main vocabulary at the end of this manual. Tania has a Masters degree in international business, a law degree from Nicaragua, and is a court certified interpreter. She is a friend, a former CCCI student and a great teacher of medical interpretation at our Institute. Thanks, Tania, for keeping up with all the teaching and with the deadlines for this manual.

Dr. Richard Lane, mentioned in the dedication, has been the best possible partner (and a pretty good doctor too!) We met 30 years ago and together we fought for the hiring of professional interpreters, developed round-the-clock coverage, and trained interpreters at the hospital where we worked. Rick was a bilingual teacher in Chicago before he went to medical school, and he still applies his teaching ability to the training of medical interpreters in the Samurai! Technique. His medical knowledge and noteworthy ability to build bridges with other professions is a great gift to our students. Rick, thank you for meeting all the last minute deadlines where you wrote or reviewed the medical components of our manual.

Aida Cases, who has an educational background in bilingual education, is a dear friend and CCCS, Inc.™ supporter. Aida brings to the organization the perspective of being a family member and community organizer. She has represented CCCS, Inc.™ and CCCI nationwide, and contributed a few pieces to this manual.

PO Box 2308, Woburn, MA 01888-0508, **p:** 781-729-3736, **www.EmbracingCulture.com**
PO Box 6401, Manchester, NH 03108, **p:** 1-888-678-CCCS

Amanda Duross, a great friend and colleague in charge of critical incidents in our interpreter program, is a co-teacher with CCCS, Inc.™. Her stories and her perspective on the interpreter's struggles were integrated throughout this manual. I want to thank her for always lifting our spirits with a great smile and positive outlook.

Debbie Eccles has directed the Interpreter Dispatch Department at CCCS, Inc.™ for almost ten years. Debbie is an incredibly caring, hard working supervisor, and a wonderful human being. Although she is not bilingual, she understands the language of interpreting. Debbie has passed along many stories shared with her by our interpreter pool, and some of these stories have been developed into talking points for our workshops and trainings.

Andrew Jerger for his insight and great eye for detail as we asked him to review this manual one more time with a very short deadline. He brought to our team, the insight of being a former Medical Interpreter student, the experience of being an active new interpreter and we are so happy that he has joined our faculty.

I want to thank **Mandy Lau, Daniel de Oliveira, Amy Lau** and **Karla Rebello** for showing us how well an interpreting business can be run. To all our staff at CCCS, Inc.™, **Gail Marinaccio, Lily Tam, Mariana de Paula, Linda Demmons,** and **Alejandra Lloveras**, thank you for directly or indirectly contributing to the manual. Some of you were typists, others made sure our equipment was working properly, and all of you put up with me and helped to calm my anxieties throughout the production process.

We have had many contributors of articles and role-plays, and we would like to especially thank **Dr. Dan Teplin**, a psychiatrist working in the Boston area, for his role-plays on substance abuse and mental health, and **Susan Spang**, a Nurse Practitioner, for her role-plays on birth control. We also thank **Bruce L. Adelson, Esq.** of Federal Compliance Consulting, LLC, and **Mara Youdelman**, Project Director for the National Language Access Advocacy Project at the National Health Law Program, for allowing us to print their articles in this manual.

We also thank interpreter associations and related multidisciplinary organizations such as the **IMIA, ATA, CHIA,** and the **NCIHC** for their efforts in making sure that interpreters and LEP patients have a voice in healthcare and health law. Thanks for allowing CCCS, Inc.™ representatives to present at almost every conference for the past ten years. It has been a great learning experience and we hope to continue to participate in all major industry events.

Many thanks to all **LEP patients** and to the **providers** who treat them for making interpreters feel that their studies and efforts toward self-improvement and professionalization are making a difference in the delivery of equal access to health care for all. This movement towards the professionalization of health care interpreters is a reminder of the need to listen to the patient's voice.

Last but not least, **Lisa Ordway**, our wonderful graphics designer, has been an incredible team player in times of chaos and last-minute changes. Thank you Lisa for your excellent work!

Zarita Araujo-Lane, LICSW

Biographies

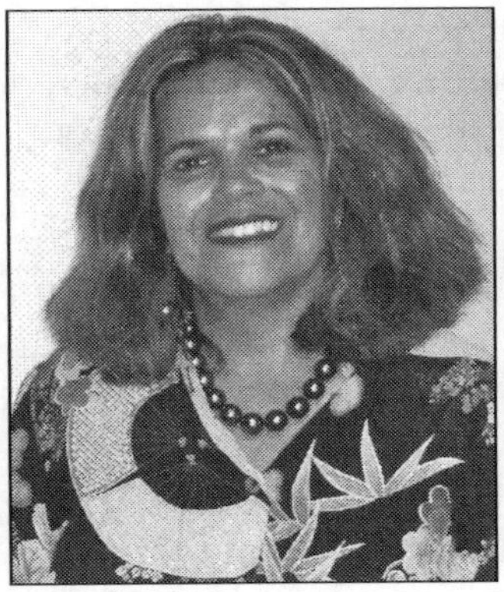

Zarita Araújo-Lane, LICSW, the main author of this manual, holds a Masters degree from Simmons College, School of Social work since 1985 and a Bachelor's degree from the University of Massachusetts in Human Services. In 1977, she started one of the first Interpreter Programs in the country at Cambridge Health Alliance, Cambridge, Massachusetts.

Zarita is the president of Cross Cultural Communication Systems, Inc.™ She has over 25 years experience working with cross cultural populations in medical and mental health organizations. She was the director of a mental health cross cultural team for over ten years at Health and Education Services in the North Shore area. She has published articles in Cross Cultural Management including a chapter written in 1996 and 2005 on "**Portuguese Families**" for the book, *Ethnicity and Family Therapy* by Monica McGoldrick second and third edition. She has authored multiple articles for the American Translation Association on Medical Interpretation and she is the main writer for a column on the ATA Medical Division Newsletter called *Interpreters at Work*.

Zarita created two main cultural competency models called: *Immigration as a Grieving Process* and the *Four Character Values* which have been used nationwide in her cultural competency and diversity trainings for healthcare and human services providers, administrators and staff members.

Zarita has a long history of designing, implementing, supervising and training Interpreter Programs in the Cambridge and North Shore areas and nationwide. She taught a course on Cultural Competency for Medical Interpreters at Cambridge College and for several years taught Portuguese Medical Interpretation at Bentley College.

Zarita is the main writer of this manual, along with a team she organized in developing the manual. She has written several other manuals on medical interpretation as well as other educational materials such as, videos and role-plays for her company.

She is a member of the National Council on Interpreting in Health Care (NCIHC) National Association of Judiciary Interpreters and Translators (NAJIT), the International Medical Interpreters Association (IMIA), the American Translators Association (ATA), California Health Care Interpreter Association (CHIA), The Association of Language Companies (ALC), the New England Translators Association (NETA) and the National Social Workers Association (NASW).

Zarita is a native of Portugal and speaks Portuguese and French. She is an interpreter and translator for the Portuguese language. Most of all, she is a Portuguese immigrant raising an interracial and interfaith family and has three wonderful daughters.

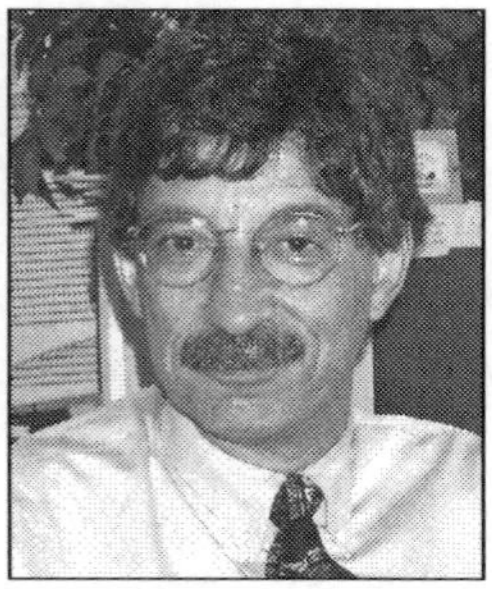

Dr. Richard S. Lane, an Internist in the Extended Care Facility Program at Harvard Vanguard Medical Associates of Boston, Massachusetts. He is a bilingual educator, fluent in Spanish. Dr. Lane's interests are the doctor/patient relationship, teaching interview skills to medical students and residents, cross-cultural communication in medicine, care of elderly patients in rehabilitation and sub-acute units and palliative medicine and hospice care at end of life. Dr. Lane became board certified in Palliative Care and Hospice Medicine in 2005. He is the main writer of the many role-plays in this manual.

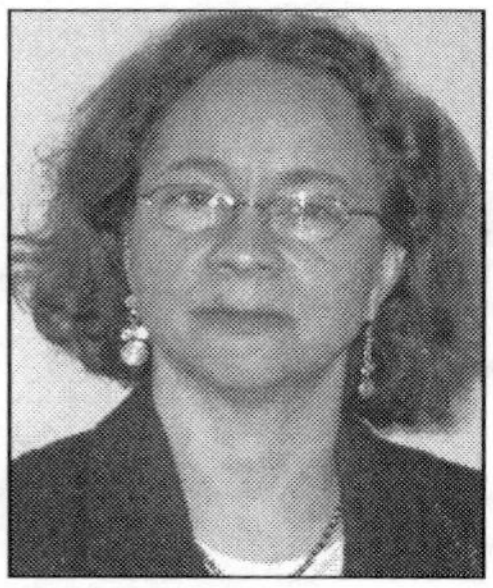

Dr. Ana Filomena (Mena) Macedo, holds a Masters in Business Administration from Simmons College and a Ph.D. in Sociology from Brandeis University. For the past 15 years she has worked as the Director of Research and Planning at Blue Cross Blue Shield of Massachusetts. Prior to that she worked as a bilingual social worker at The Dana Farber Cancer Institute. She is a native speaker of Portuguese and Cape Verdean Creole. She also speaks Spanish and French fluently. She is the co-editor and assisted with manual content.

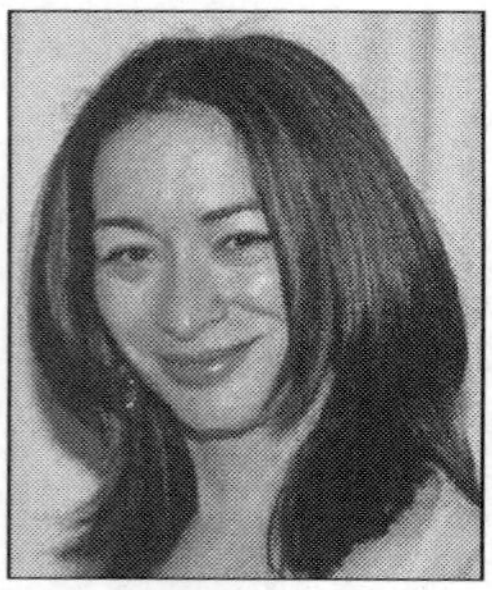

Vera Duarte Outeiro, Primary Medical Interpretation Instructor at CCCS, Inc.™, holds a BA and MA in Foreign Language Education from Portugal and a MA in Applied Linguistics from the University of Massachusetts. Vera is certified by the Massachusetts Department of Education to teach ESL to grades 5-12. She currently teaches a course that addresses issues of minority students and academic achievement. She also teaches ESL, World Literature, and Medical Interpretation at Cambridge Rindge and Latin School in Cambridge, MA. She is a native speaker of Portuguese. She also speaks Spanish and French fluently. She is the main force behind the manual, revamping, organizing and reviewing and updating information in this manual.

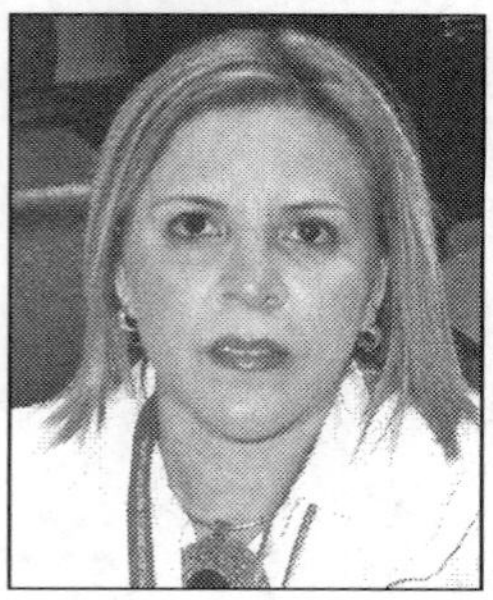

Tania V. West is a Certified Court Interpreter and for almost five years, she has been an active Spanish freelance interpreter in the Greater Area of Boston. She also travels throughout the U.S. as an interpreter's trainer and language coach with the Cross Cultural Communication Institute.

She is an attorney in Nicaragua and holds a MA in Law and Diplomacy from the Fletcher School (Tufts University, administered with the cooperation of Harvard University). Tania has participated in different trainings in the fields of Legal, Medical, and Court Interpreting from recognized institutions such as Boston University, The Cross Cultural Communication Institute at CCCS, Inc.™, University of Massachusetts, and University of Arizona. She has also received intensive training in English as a Second Language from the Harvard Extension School.

Tania is a member of the National Association of Judiciary Interpreters and Translators (NAJIT), the International Medical Interpreters Association (IMIA), the American Translators Association (ATA), and the New England Translators Association (NETA).

She was the main quiz and vocabulary developer for this manual.

Lesson One:
Medical Interpretation as a Profession

Understanding Goals

Students will be able to:

- define the profession of Medical Interpretation
- learn about the Standards of Practice
- set the stage in the triadic encounter
- understand the structure of a medical encounter
- become familiar with interpreting jargon

Key Concepts

- Interpreter vs. Translator
- Professional interpreter
- Standards of Practice
- Triadic Encounter
- Setting the stage
- CIFE
- Pre-Session and Session
- Accuracy
- Register
- Different interpreting modes (Simultaneous vs. Consecutive)

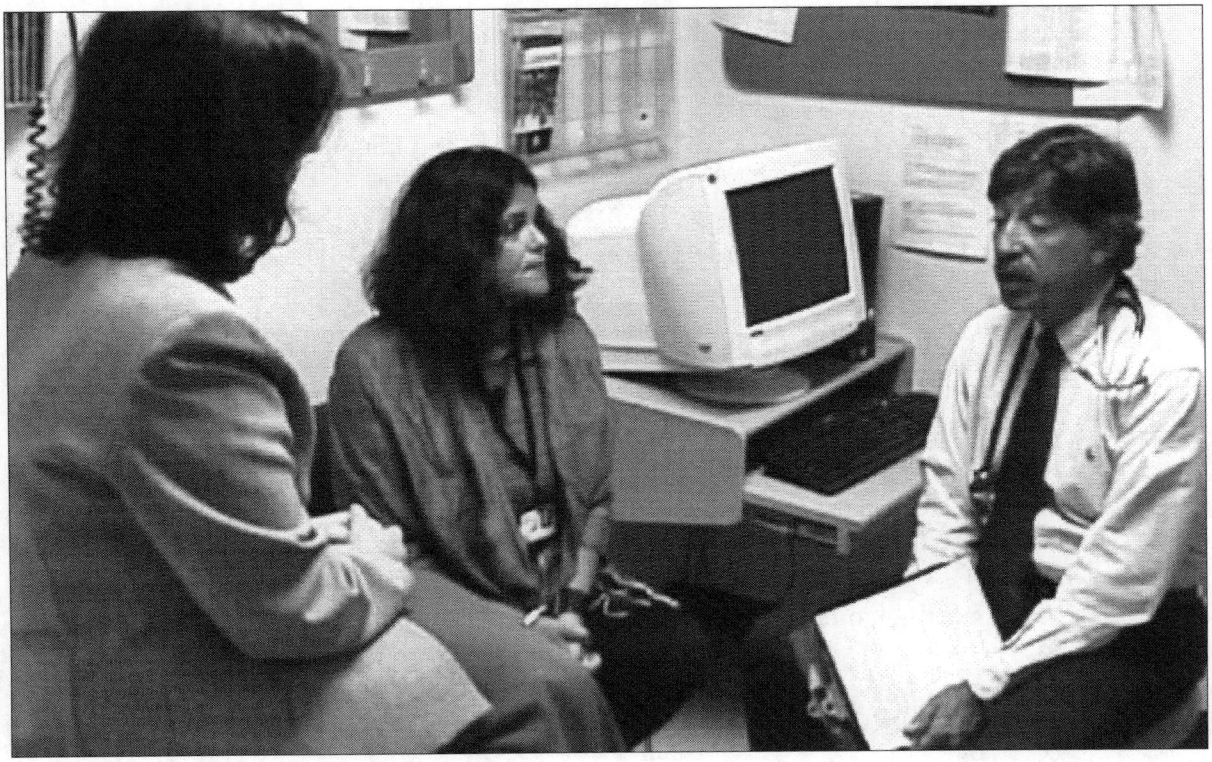

PO Box 2308, Woburn, MA 01888-0508, **p:** 781-729-3736, **www.EmbracingCulture.com**
PO Box 6401, Manchester, NH 03108, **p:** 1-888-678-CCCS

Quiz

THE ART OF MEDICAL INTERPRETATION®

Lesson One: Quiz
Medical Interpretation as a Profession

Mark each item "True" or "False."

1. A professional interpreter is one who speaks without an accent.
   ○ True ⊗ False
2. A translator converts the message in the written form.
   ⊗ True ○ False
3. An interpreter converts the message in the written form.
   ○ True ⊗ False
4. Interpreters need to set the stage in order to facilitate communication between the provider and patient in the medical encounter.
   ⊗ True ○ False
5. The three participants of the triadic encounter are: the provider, the patient, and the interpreter.
   ⊗ True ○ False
6. CIFE is the tool created by CCCS to help interpreters set the stage.
   ⊗ True ○ False
7. In CIFE, "C" stands for communication. Confidenciality
   ⊗ True ⊗ False
8. Accuracy implies a faithful representation of meaning.
   ⊗ True ○ False
9. Interpreters always need to bring the words to a level where the patient can understand them.
   ⊗ True ⊗ False
10. It's OK to interpret the word "acne" into the target language as "pimples."
    ○ True ⊗ False
11. The IMIA Standards of Practice refer to consecutive interpreting as the mode of choice for most medical interpreting sessions.
    ⊗ True ○ False
12. *"Break it down,"* it's a simple short sentence that serves as a great tool for the interpreter and the patient when the information being shared is ambiguous.
    ⊗ True ○ False
13. In the following example of an interpretation dialogue, the interpreter maintained the register:
    Patient: Doctor, when my husband and I do it, I feel a lot of pain down there.
    Interpreter: I am getting pelvic pain from having intercourse with my husband.
    ○ True ⊗ False
14. Seating arrangements can play a significant part in keeping balance in a session.
    ⊗ True ○ False
15. When the interpreter does not understand something said by the provider, he/she should ask for clarification.
    ⊗ True ○ False

Lesson One: Class Activities
Medical Interpretation as a Profession

What makes an interpreter a professional interpreter?

What comes to your mind when you hear the word "interpreter"? Use the graphic organizer below to brainstorm words that you associate with the making of a professional interpreter.

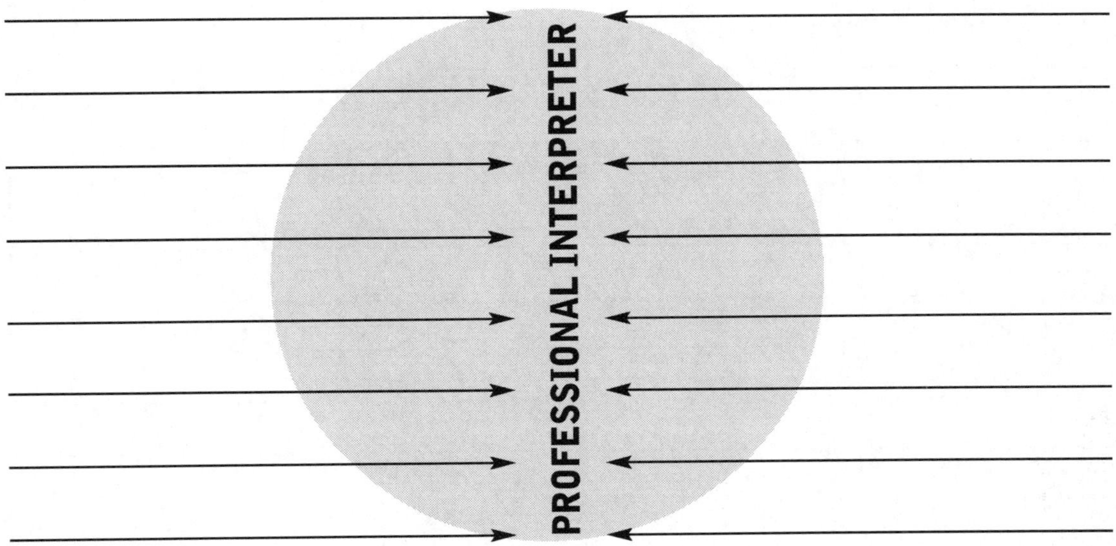

What is the difference between an Interpreter and a Translator?

According to Danica Seleskovitch (1994), a translator converts the message in the written form and the interpreter does it by using the oral form. The ASL interpreters use the gesture form.

I have met many great translators at professional conferences who could write fluently in five languages but could only converse in two. Clearly, the skills for oral and written conversation are different. Seleskovitch states that interpreters need to convey the message at a much higher speed than that of the translators, at least 30 times greater.

PO Box 2308, Woburn, MA 01888-0508, **p:** 781-729-3736, **www.EmbracingCulture.com**
PO Box 6401, Manchester, NH 03108, **p:** 1-888-678-CCCS

Watch the video "The Professional Interpreter." Be prepared to discuss it afterwards. Use the space below to take notes on what you see or what you found interesting.

Apply Critical Thinking:

1. What went right? What went wrong? Organize your notes in the following table.

+	-

Whole-Group Discussion

How do you grade the interpreting skills? What tool do we use to assess the interpreting skills?

PO Box 2308, Woburn, MA 01888-0508, **p:** 781-729-3736, **www.EmbracingCulture.com**
PO Box 6401, Manchester, NH 03108, **p:** 1-888-678-CCCS

The Triadic Relationship

An environment needs to be created in which there is equal balance between the provider, the patient and the interpreter; this means not favoring one side over the other. Because the interpreter shares a common language with the patient and a different common language with the provider there is a tendency for the interpreter to become the center of the triangle. To promote better communication between patient and provider, this should be avoided.

According to the standards of practice, interpreters need to set the stage in order to facilitate communication between the provider and patient in the medical encounter.

I PRE-SESSION

Setting the Stage

THINK: How would you “set the stage” in order to facilitate communication between provider and patient in the medical encounter?

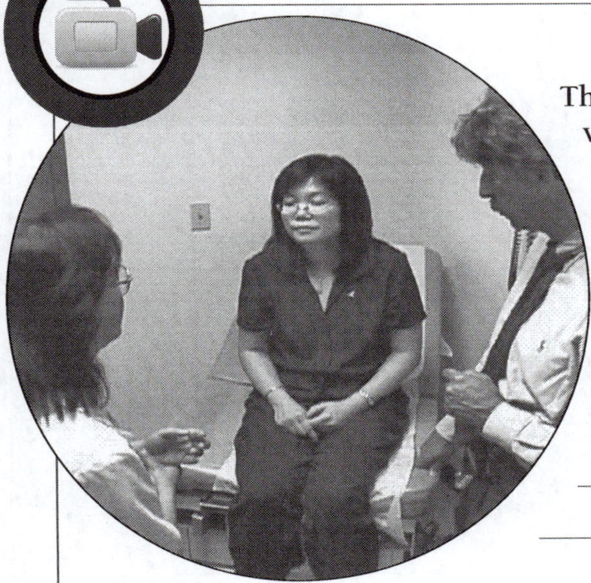

The standards of practice provide you with a variety of guidelines.

Watch the video *The Healthcare Interpreter's Tools for Successful Communication in the Triadic Encounter* to learn how to successfully set the stage in the triadic encounter. Take notes and be prepared to discuss your thoughts afterwards.

1. What is the primary goal of a healthcare interpreter?

2. According to the video, what are the two skills a professional interpreter must develop?

3. How do interpreters set the stage?

4. What is the tool created by CCCS, Inc™ to help you "set the stage"?

PO Box 2308, Woburn, MA 01888-0508, **p:** 781-729-3736, **www.EmbracingCulture.com**
PO Box 6401, Manchester, NH 03108, **p:** 1-888-678-CCCS

5. What does CIFE stand for?

C ONFIDENTIALITY

I USE FIRST PERSON

F LOW

E VERYTHING WILL BE INTERPRETED

6. What is the purpose of CIFE as mentioned in the video?

7. In what ways can you customize CIFE?

Interpreters set the stage by:

Pre-session

- Being on time (means arriving at least 15 minutes earlier)
- Wearing a ID badge
- Introducing themselves
- Stating the language they will be interpreting
- Verifying the name of the patient
- Using CIFE

By properly setting the stage an interpreter can avoid potential complications that could interfere with the triadic relationship or even cause a misinterpretation. In the mental health visit, the equivalent of setting the stage is called making an initial contract. There are certain fears and expectations that a patient/client may already have of a provider. When the interpreter, a third party, is introduced, these feelings and expectations are naturally magnified.

Remember to mention at least 4 points as you set the stage in the triadic encounter:

C onfidentiality (see federal and state laws)
I use the first person
F low
E verything you say will be interpreted

Avoid being alone in the same room with the patient.

Check policy with the hiring or contracting institution regarding interpreters being alone with patients. There are legal and clinical reasons why interpreters should not be left alone in the room with a patient.

Think and Write:

Clinical Reasons	Legal Reasons

PRACTICE

1. Form two lines facing each other. Take turns practicing *CIFE* in English.
2. Create two lines facing each other. Make sure that the person facing you shares the same Target Language. Take turns practicing *CIFE* in your TL.

Now you have completed one major component of the triadic encounter, the pre-session. According to the IMIA standards, the triadic encounter has three major components:

1. **Pre-Session**
2. **Session**
3. **Post-Session or Follow-up**

PO Box 2308, Woburn, MA 01888-0508, **p:** 781-729-3736, **www.EmbracingCulture.com**
PO Box 6401, Manchester, NH 03108, **p:** 1-888-678-CCCS

II SESSION

The Standards state that the primary goal of an interpreter is to make possible communication between a healthcare provider and a patient who do not speak the same language. The Standards define two types of skills, linguistic and interpreting. Linguistic proficiency is the ability of an interpreter to accurately comprehend and understand the content of the information being shared between two languages. Medical interpreters owe it to themselves, to patients, to providers and to their communities to be accurate in their interpretation.

THINK: What is **accuracy**? How do you define it?

Look at the following example:

Provider: *Provera works by preventing ovulation. It also makes the mucus in a woman's cervix thick so that sperm can not pass in the uterus to reach the egg. Depo Provera also thins the lining of a woman's uterus so that an egg cannot attach and develop pregnancy.*

Interpreter: *This shot will keep your body from allowing the egg to enter your feminine organs inside by making things difficult for the sperm to go in.*

1. Was the interpreter **accurate**? Why or why not?

No. Missing some information - not as specific
Vague (feminin organs)!

In addition to accuracy, **register** is also important.

THINK: What is **register**?

____

____

Look at the following example:

Provider: *You have told me that you have been constipated for the past four weeks, and your stools have changed shape and color. I will perform a rectal exam. First I will touch your rectum. When you feel my glove touch the rectum, bear down, then relax. This will allow me to examine you without so much discomfort. I will examine your rectum and do a hemocult of your stool.*

Interpreter: *I heard you are having difficulty going to the bathroom in the past four weeks, and your poop changed shape and coloring. I am going to examine you through your anus. When you feel the finger, push down, then relax. This will let me examine you without pain. I will check your behind and check your poop for blood.*

What words were changed? Use the following table:

High Register (HR)	Low Register (LR)
constipated	difficulties going to bathroom
stool	poop
rectum	anus
hemocult of your stool	check poop for blood

Complete the definitions:

High Register is ____

____

Low Register is ____

____

Remember to be prepared for the different interpreting sessions that may require an interpreter to use different registers. Changing the register is dangerous and does not present an accurate picture of the educational level of the speaker. We hope that providers adjust their register to the needs of the patient and, by you conveying an accurate register the provider will naturally do so.

PO Box 2308, Woburn, MA 01888-0508, **p:** 781-729-3736, **www.EmbracingCulture.com**
PO Box 6401, Manchester, NH 03108, **p:** 1-888-678-CCCS

PRACTICE

Match the HR words in column A to its equivalent LR words in column B.

Column A

d 1. abdominal
e 2. vomit
c 3. intravenous
f 4. acne
a 5. androgens
g 6. puberty
b 7. side effects

Column B

a. hormones
b. consequences
c. liquids
d. stomach
e. throw up
f. pimples
g. teenage years

In addition to accuracy and register, how the message is delivered is also important. According to the IMIA and the NCIHC standards, medical interpreters should use the **consecutive mode** of interpretation.

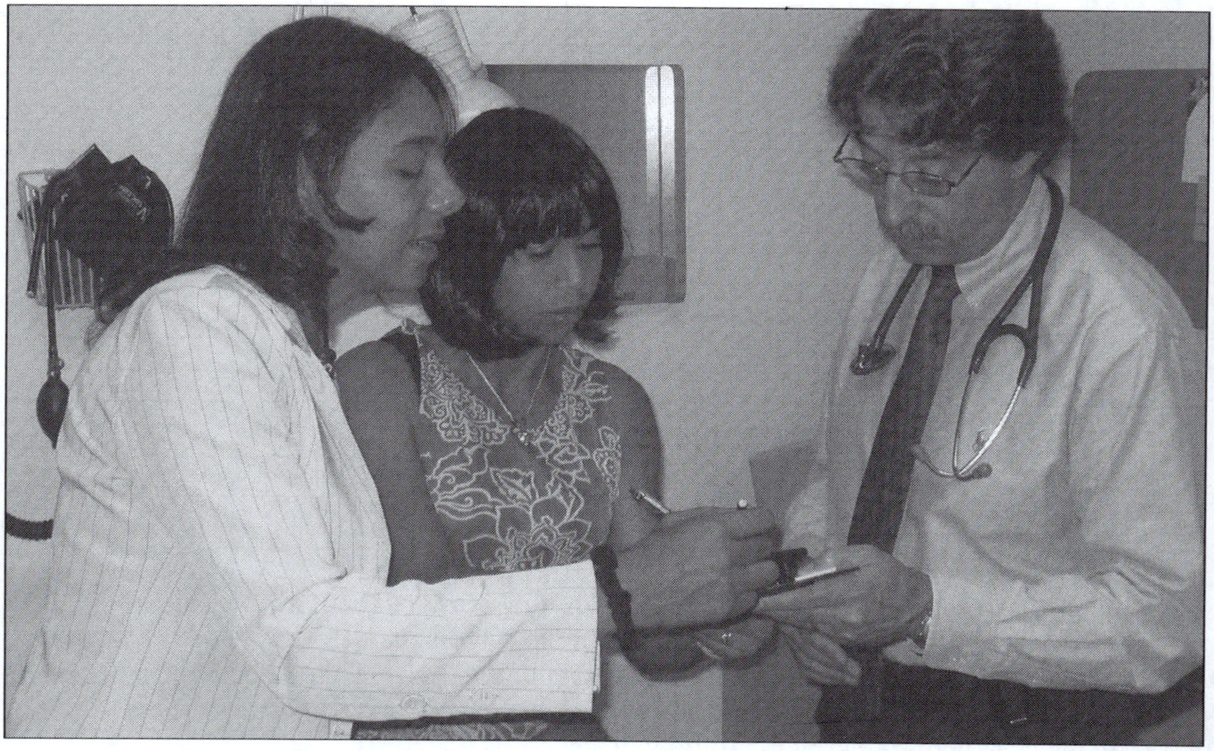

INTERPRETATION MODES

1. **Consecutive:** Understanding the meaning and relaying a message from one language to another in an organized manner only after the speaker has completed a thought.
2. **Simultaneous:** The interpreter speaks at the same time as the speaker with minimal pauses.
3. **Sight Interpretation:** The interpreter reads a document, understands it and provides an oral interpretation from the written source language into the oral target language.
4. **Relay:** When there is a need for more than one interpreter. For example, a patient may need an ASL interpreter and a family member may only speak another foreign language. So, there is a need to have two interpreters in the room, the ASL interpreter who converts American Sign Language to English, and the foreign language interpreter will convey the message from English to the target language, and vice-versa.
5. **Summary:** The interpreter summarizes the main points of the speaker. This mode may create major problems related to the completeness and accuracy of the interpretation. In this mode an interpreter arbitrarily omits/filters out what he/she believes to be irrelevant information. The problem, of course, is that the information the interpreter chooses to omit could prove to be very significant to the speaker.
6. **Remote:** When an interpreter is conveying a message via telephone or videoconference. Most of the time, the consecutive mode is also used.

THINK

Which interpretation mode(s) would you feel more comfortable using? Which one(s) would be a challenge to you? Explain.

PO Box 2308, Woburn, MA 01888-0508, **p:** 781-729-3736, **www.EmbracingCulture.com**
PO Box 6401, Manchester, NH 03108, **p:** 1-888-678-CCCS

PRACTICE

Take out the NCIHC standards. Think about everything we learned in class today to best assess your understanding of the key concepts we discussed. According to the standards, did the interpreter do his or her job appropriately in the following vignettes? Use the standard numbers and appropriately match them with the vignettes. You may use more than one standard for each vignette.

	Vignettes	NCIHC Standards
1	**Provider:** Provera works by preventing ovulation. It also makes the mucus in a woman's cervix thick, so that sperm cannot pass through the uterus to reach the egg. Depo Provera also thins the lining of a woman's uterus so that an egg cannot attach and develop pregnancy. **Interpreter:** This shot will keep your body from allowing the egg to enter your feminine organs inside by making things difficult for the sperm to go in.	Accuracy diff. (registry)
2	**Provider:** I was thinking of your situation. You seem to have a lifestyle where the diaphragm may work well, but (pause) remember that this method of birth control is not permanent. If you do not use the diaphragm properly and consistently, you may get pregnant. Let me examine you and size your cervix. So, just a reminder, one in five women gets pregnant using this method. Are you okay with that? **Interpreter:** I think I can trust you and that you will be doing well with the diaphragm. But this is not the best birth control method because 20 women out of every 100 get pregnant. The doctor will get you the right size diaphragm after examining you.	Accuracy ~~Rote~~ Bound. Impartiality
3	The interpreter is assisting the patient with the medical history form. The patient does not know what cardiovascular illness is. The interpreter circles the word and asks the patient to ask the provider when they get to the room. The patient is young and shy and she does not ask the question. The interpreter reminds the patient and the patient asks the interpreter to ask the provider to explain what these big words are all about.	

	Vignettes	NCIHC Standards
4	**Provider:** Good morning. Let me review your chart. Um… (To the interpreter: "Multiple partners and she wants the diaphragm? What a risk! But don't tell her that yet.") To the patient: "I am just reviewing the chart and your birth control counselor has informed you that there are better birth control methods for you."	Accuracy Respect Professionalism Advocacy
5	**Interpreter:** I am looking at your chart and our birth control counselor has informed you that there are better birth control methods for you. The interpreter says to the doctor, "But isn't the EC a way to terminate a pregnancy?"	Role Boundaries Impartiality Accuracy
6	The interpreter is approached by the provider about the need to be very clear with the patient about her understanding of her pregnancy and her options. The provider says that he wants to talk to the patient alone, without the presence of family members. The interpreter does not agree, but understands the concept of patient autonomy. The provider and interpreter enter the exam room and begin to speak with the patient. The patient starts to cry and says that she wants her husband to be present, since he is the one that makes these types of decisions with her.	Confidenciality Respect Cultural Awareness ~~Boundaries~~ Advocacy
7	**Provider:** I understand that because of religious beliefs you only want to use a birth control method that is not post coital so the IUD is not going to work for you. (Provider's beeper goes off and she asks the interpreter to finish explaining about the IUD while she answers the call). IntraUterineDevice	Role boundaries Professionalism
8	**Provider:** The IUD does not protect you from HIV and other sexually STD transmitted diseases, and it may cause changes in your periods like bleeding or spotting between periods. **Interpreter:** The IUD does not protect you from HIV and other contagious diseases…excuse me...sexually transmitted diseases, and it may cause changes in your periods such as bleeding or spotting.	
9	**Patient:** Doctor, when my husband and I do it, I feel a lot of pain down there. **Interpreter:** I am getting pelvic pain from having intercourse with my husband.	Accuracy

PO Box 2308, Woburn, MA 01888-0508, **p:** 781-729-3736, **www.EmbracingCulture.com**
PO Box 6401, Manchester, NH 03108, **p:** 1-888-678-CCCS

	Vignettes	NCIHC Standards
10	**Provider:** The EC works by preventing or delaying ovulation. **Interpreter:** EC? Can you break it down? **Provider:** Emergency Contraception. So side effects include nausea, vomiting, breast pain or breast tenderness, feeling tired, headache… **Interpreter:** Breast tenderness and...? **Provider:** Fatigue, headache. (Interpreter switches to simultaneous mode) Dizziness, early or late menstrual period, spotting before your period…	
11	A **young woman** dressed in a hijab waits quietly for the interpreter to enter the exam room. The clinical assistant had previously given her a johnny and asked her to leave it open in the front. When the **interpreter** enters the room, the provider is frustrated. The patient is sitting in a chair, fully dressed. The provider had tried to encourage her to get undressed by using gestures to communicate the idea. The **patient** tells the interpreter that she does not want to take off her clothes. The interpreter encourages the patient to share her feelings with the provider and assures her that she will interpret the message. The provider answers, "When we get to the pelvic exam, you'll have to take off your underwear." The **interpreter** does not interpret this piece and says to the patient, "The provider and I need to step outside the room for a moment. We'll be right back."	

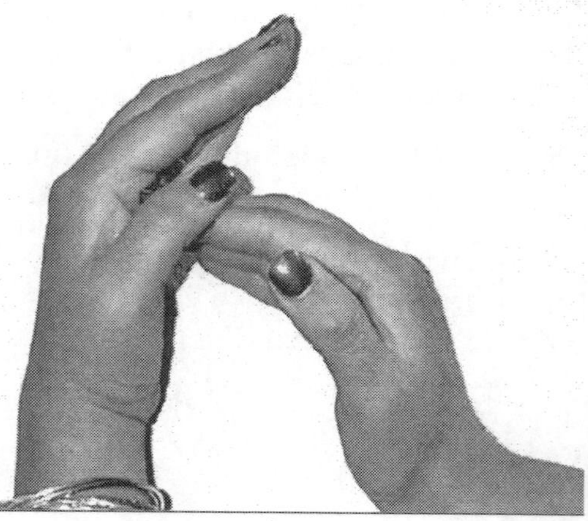

Lesson One: Homework
Medical Interpretation as a Profession

1. Go over your notes for today's class and read section "Additional Resources."
2. Read NCIHC and IMIA (formerly MMIA) Standards of Practice.
3. Write two paragraphs about a standard of practice that was most interesting to you. Answer the following questions:
   a. Which standard did you find the most interesting and why?
   b. How do you plan to apply this standard in your future work as an interpreter?
   c. What might make it difficult to apply this standard?
4. Browse bookstores and internet for bilingual medical dictionaries. You need to bring a dictionary to all classes.
5. Read and practice ALL role plays for this lesson and begin to develop your glossary.

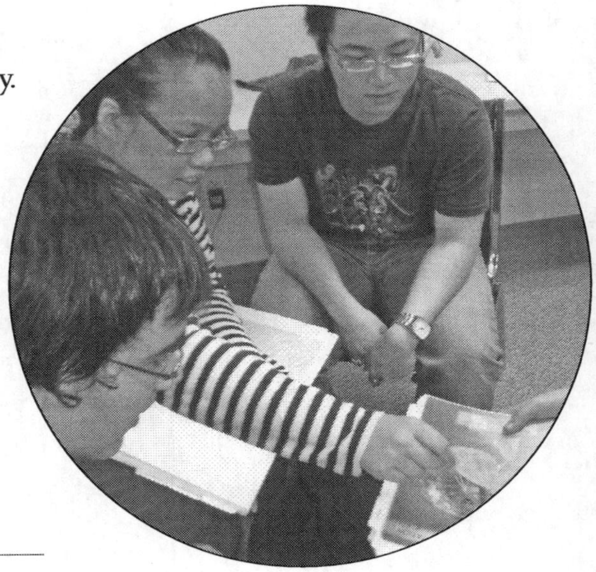

Comments? Questions? Reflections?

PO Box 2308, Woburn, MA 01888-0508, **p:** 781-729-3736, **www.EmbracingCulture.com**
PO Box 6401, Manchester, NH 03108, **p:** 1-888-678-CCCS

Lesson One: Role-Plays
Medical Interpretation as a Profession

Work individually at first:

- Read the entire role-play
- Get a general sense of its meaning
- Circle the most challenging medical terms
- Apply the Samurai! technique to those terms
- Read the role-play again for a deeper understanding
- Find an accurate equivalent in the target language

Work in a language-specific group of friends, fellow students or colleagues:

- Share your doubts
- Ask for other ways of expressing the same meaning
- Develop a glossary
- Check the dictionary
- Practice the role-plays – remember to do CIFE for all your role-plays
- Have your colleagues observe you and provide feedback on your accuracy and register.
- These colleagues can keep track of any omissions, additions, mistakes or distortions in your interpreting and point these out to you in a follow-up discussion.

Student Interpreter Evaluation

Student Name ____________________ Date ________

Language ____________________

Mode of Interpreting (check one): ☐ Consecutive ☐ Simultaneous

Role-Play/System ____________________

Areas Observed ____________________

Accuracy

Register ____________________

Omissions ____________________

Additions ____________________

Distortions ____________________

Pronunciation ____________________

Speaker's emotions conveyed? ____________________

Explain ____________________

Technique

General flow ____________________

Flow when requesting clarification ____________________

Speed ____________________

Eye Contact ____________________

Distracting Habits ____________________

Ethical Issues

Answered questions for patient? ____________________

Advised patient? ____________________

Vocabulary Expansion Recommendations

____

____

Other Recommendations

____

____

Language Coach Signature ____________________ Date ________

Role-Play 1: Acne

		Pronunciation	Additions	Omissions	Mistakes
MD:	How was your summer?				
PT:	I worked at Target for most of the summer. But whenever I had a chance, I took the train to Revere Beach. I'm worried, though, because my face looks horrible! School is starting in a few days. Can you give me some medication to make this go away?				
MD:	The good news is that most likely, your acne will get better. This acne is probably due to hormonal changes.				
PT:	What do you mean?				
MD:	Acne can be caused by the following three different factors: hormones, hereditary and plugged oil ducts. In your case, you have no family history of acne and your oil ducts have always looked clear.				
PT:	So do you think that this has to do with the fact that I got my period so early?				
MD:	Girls aren't the only ones that get acne. In fact, you see many boys with the same skin problems. During puberty, hormones called androgens seem to increase in both girls and boys. This increase may cause oil ducts to get plugged causing redness, swelling and pimples.				
PT:	I hate pimples! I can't control myself. I feel like popping them.				
MD:	I guess that the pinching and the squeezing of pimples is not just a teenage thing. However, if you want to get better and you do not want scars, you could try a lotion or gel. It could take several weeks until you notice an improvement, but if you are patient and follow the instructions on the medication, you should notice an improvement.				
	Let's go over what you might want to avoid, so that your acne can improve.				
PT:	I know that I shouldn't pop the pimples or eat fatty foods.				
MD:	Actually, food is not an issue, but you are right about the popping. In severe cases, I have seen some mothers have their teenage daughters temporary wear artificial nails, so that they can't pop the pimples.				

continued

PO Box 2308, Woburn, MA 01888-0508, **p:** 781-729-3736, **www.EmbracingCulture.com**
PO Box 6401, Manchester, NH 03108, **p:** 1-888-678-CCCS

Role-Play 1 *continued*

	Pronunciation	Additions	Omissions	Mistakes
PT: What do you mean?				
MD: I guess that you and your mother will need to decide what is best for you and what you can do to stop yourself from squeezing the pimples. You know that by squeezing them you can cause an infection or even leave a permanent skin mark.				
PT: So, how do you think I got these pimples? Could it be from my boyfriend?				
MD: No, this is one thing that you cannot get from your boyfriend. Acne is not contagious. But wearing makeup doesn't help, since certain cosmetics can block the oil ducts and make the acne worse.				
PT: I can't go to school without some makeup. I look absolutely terrible!				
MD: You look fine, but I understand that you are not happy with your pimples and that it is quite difficult for you to stop behaviors that you have maintained for so long. This is not just a teenage thing; even adults have a hard time stopping bad habits. So, I guess you have to believe that you want to do something about your pimples. When you are ready, here is what you may want to try: you may want to try this lotion called Topical Benzol Peroxide. This will help you kill any skin bacteria, unplug the oil ducts and heal acne pimples.				
(silence)				
This is how you will apply the lotion: 1. Start slowly with the lotion, once every day before bedtime. Do this for one week. 2. Increase to twice a day after the second week, perhaps once in the morning and once at bedtime. 3. When applying the lotion, avoid the skin around your eyes, mouth and the corner of your nose. These are delicate areas. 4. Apply the lotion in the area with the pimples.				
PT: That's a lot to remember. Can you tell my mom what I have to do?				
Mother: I have heard of a medication that works wonders on pimples. Can you prescribe her the pills instead of cream? She'll never remember to follow all those steps, you know how teenagers are!				

continued

Role-Play 1 *continued*

	Pronunciation	Additions	Omissions	Mistakes
MD: Actually the miracle drug that you are talking about is called Accutane or Isotretinion. They are very strong chemicals and should be used only for severe cases of acne. Your daughter's acne is really not that severe. The side effects of Accutane or Isotretinion are so dangerous that patients taking these medications require close medical supervision.				
PT: What do you mean?				
MD: Although you are too young for childbearing, you should know that this medication is known to cause birth defects. Before we even consider such a drastic route, let's complete my explanation about the Benzoyl Peroxide lotion. It takes 3-6 weeks to see any improvement. You need to be consistent with the treatment regimen, by never interrupting it. Do not mix this treatment with other treatments. Stay with the one treatment until you've completed it. And don't overdo it; two applications a day are more than enough. The words you need to remember are patience, stick to it, and don't overdo it!				
PT: I will try, but this is pretty hard to remember.				
Mother to daughter: I will help you with the treatment at home, honey.				
MD: Actually, you are very lucky that your mother is willing to help you through this difficult time. Most parents are too busy nowadays. Perhaps you want to reward her for her positive behaviors.				
Mother: When should we return? Two weeks?				
MD: If this lotion does not work, we have other treatments. So don't get discouraged. Just remember: this is a lengthy process. You will not see results right away. That's probably the hardest part. Everyone wants instant results!				
Break It Down	☐	☐	☐	☐

☐ **CIFE with patient** ☐ **CIFE with provider** ☐ **FLOW** ☐ **REGISTER**

Role-Play 1: Glossary

______________ ______________ ______________

______________ ______________ ______________

______________ ______________ ______________

continued

PO Box 2308, Woburn, MA 01888-0508, **p:** 781-729-3736, **www.EmbracingCulture.com**
PO Box 6401, Manchester, NH 03108, **p:** 1-888-678-CCCS

1. Pathology (diseases, conditions)

2. Laboratory Tests and Diagnostic Procedures

3. Treatment Procedures

4. Idiomatic Expressions (if any)

5. Other (vocabulary in this particular role-play that you feel is important/relevant or that you anticipate problems with)

Role-Play 2: Diarrhea

		Pronunciation	Additions	Omissions	Mistakes
MD:	How can I help you?				
PT:	I just got back from Mexico yesterday and for the last four days I've been having diarrhea. If it weren't for the Imodium, I wouldn't have been able to make the flight home.				
MD:	Did you have a fever?				
PT:	Yeah, a little the first day.				
MD:	Do you have abdominal cramps?				
PT:	When the diarrhea comes, it's crampy and explosive.				
MD:	Did you vomit?				
PT:	Yeah, for the first two days.				
MD:	Anyone else sick?				
PT:	Well there was this woman friend that I went out with the night before I got sick. She said she had the *turistas* a year before.				
MD:	But not this time?				
PT:	No, not this time. I tell you, I've been to Mexico before and I have never had diarrhea this long. I really need something to stop this. I can't take much more of it.				
MD:	OK, let me examine you and see what I can come up with.				
	(Examines patient)				
MD:	Well, you are tender, but it's superficial, like muscle pain from vomiting. I took a sample of your stool when I did the rectal exam and I did a wet prep that allowed me to see if you had pus.				
PT:	Am I okay?				
MD:	You didn't have pus. I don't think this diarrhea is bad enough to be called dysentery, but it is lasting a bit too long. Do you have any allergies?				
PT:	No.				
MD:	Well, here is the antibiotic Levoquin. You take this every morning for the next five days. Drink lots of fluids and rest for the week. Call me in two days if you are still not feeling better.				

continued

PO Box 2308, Woburn, MA 01888-0508, **p:** 781-729-3736, **www.EmbracingCulture.com**
PO Box 6401, Manchester, NH 03108, **p:** 1-888-678-CCCS

Role-Play 2 *continued*

	Pronunciation	Additions	Omissions	Mistakes
(Two days later. A phone call from doctor to the patient.)				
MD: I just got the stool culture back. It's a simple e.coli, the usual kind that causes Traveler's Diarrhea. You'll do well. By the way, when you're done with the antibiotic, you can go back to eating solid foods. Stick with rice, bread and apple sauce.				
PT: Fine. I wish I were still in Mexico.				
MD: Why?				
PT: In Mexico, I was sick, but at least I had a tan!				
Break It Down	☐	☐	☐	☐

☐ **CIFE with patient** ☐ **CIFE with provider** ☐ **FLOW** ☐ **REGISTER**

Role-Play 2: Glossary

continued

1. Pathology (diseases, conditions)

2. Laboratory Tests and Diagnostic Procedures

3. Treatment Procedures

4. Idiomatic Expressions (if any)

5. Other (vocabulary in this particular role-play that you feel is important/relevant or that you anticipate problems with)

PO Box 2308, Woburn, MA 01888-0508, **p:** 781-729-3736, **www.EmbracingCulture.com**
PO Box 6401, Manchester, NH 03108, **p:** 1-888-678-CCCS

Role-Play 3: Salmonella

		Pronunciation	Additions	Omissions	Mistakes
MD:	How can I help you?				
PT:	I have been very sick for three days. I have a headache, fever and the worse abdominal cramps and diarrhea you've ever seen.				
MD:	Do you have blood in your stool?				
PT:	No, but they are watery.				
MD:	Have you had nausea or vomiting?				
PT:	Yup, last night I was in the bathroom and I was sick from both ends. What a nightmare!				
MD:	Have you done any traveling?				
PT:	No.				
MD:	Have you eaten anything in the past week that could have made you sick or made a friend sick?				
PT:	Well, four days ago, I went to the gym and afterwards my friends and I ate raw eggs in a power drink. Now that you mention it, my lifting partner is sick too, but he didn't get it like I did. He hasn't missed work.				
MD:	Where did you buy the eggs?				
PT:	From a corner store in my neighborhood.				
MD:	You didn't buy them from a farmer's market?				
PT:	No.				
MD:	Do you have a fever?				
PT:	Not now.				
MD:	Let's examine you.				
	(MD examines patient)				
MD:	Well, your exam is good but your blood pressure is very low. I think you have become dehydrated. I am going to give you some fluids in an IV over the next few hours and I think you will feel a lot better. The nurse will come in and draw your blood, then put an IV in.				
PT:	Do you think I really need it?				

continued

Role-Play 3 *continued*

		Pronunciation	Additions	Omissions	Mistakes
MD:	Well, don't you feel a little dizzy when you stand?				
PT:	Well, yes.				
MD:	That means you are dehydrated. You will feel much better after the IV.				
PT:	Are you going to give me some medicine for this?				
MD:	I don't think so. I think you'll do fine if you drink clear liquids and stay away from dairy. Do you think you could go to the bathroom and give me a stool sample for a culture?				
PT:	Absolutely.				
MD:	Good. I think you may have gotten salmonella. It is a bacterial diarrheal illness that can be found in poultry, meat and eggs. I won't need to give you an antibiotic unless the culture shows something of concern.				
PT:	What about the diarrhea? It is really a pain.				
MD:	Well, at night you can take 2mg of Imodium so you can get some sleep. During the day you can drink clear liquids and move your bowels as much as you need to as long as you are getting fluids. Let's get started. After the IV, you are going to feel much better.				
	Break It Down	☐	☐	☐	☐

☐ **CIFE with patient** ☐ **CIFE with provider** ☐ **FLOW** ☐ **REGISTER**

Role-Play 3: Glossary

PO Box 2308, Woburn, MA 01888-0508, **p:** 781-729-3736, **www.EmbracingCulture.com**
PO Box 6401, Manchester, NH 03108, **p:** 1-888-678-CCCS

1. Pathology (diseases, conditions)

2. Laboratory Tests and Diagnostic Procedures

3. Treatment Procedures

4. Idiomatic Expressions (if any)

5. Other (vocabulary in this particular role-play that you feel is important/relevant or that you anticipate problems with)

Lesson One: Additional Resources
Medical Interpretation as a Profession

I PRE-SESSION

The Triadic Relationship

In essence, the interpreter must take into consideration the dynamic between the provider and the patient, understand messages and convey them accurately in two languages (source and target), act impartially, and maintain the flow of communication at a manageable level. Being in a group of three people there is always one member that may feel left out. The interpreter most likely will feel the pressure of being in the middle. S/he speaks both the target and the source language, so both the patient and the provider are looking and are speaking towards the interpreter.

Interpreters must be aware of this pull and they should do their best to manage this triadic dynamic by setting the tone with the spatial configuration.

Wow!! We are asking interpreters to simultaneously exercise the sensitivity of an artist, the objectivity of a scientist, and the compassion of a therapist. An environment needs to be created in which there is equal balance among the provider, the patient and the interpreter. Understanding the dynamics of a triadic relationship means not favoring one side over the other.

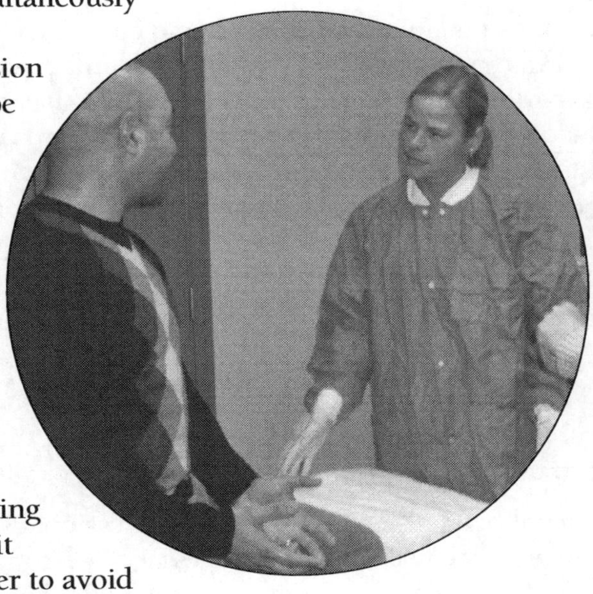

Seating Arrangements

Seating arrangements can play a significant part in keeping balance in a session. Years ago, many interpreter training materials suggested that the interpreter sit behind the patient or the provider in order to avoid becoming the center of all attention. This concept of having an interpreter as invisible as possible is a positive one, but the reality is that many of us do not feel safe having someone behind our backs. Therefore the

PO Box 2308, Woburn, MA 01888-0508, p: 781-729-3736, www.EmbracingCulture.com
PO Box 6401, Manchester, NH 03108, p: 1-888-678-CCCS

interpreter is left with the task and skill of trying to get the best seating arrangement so that ideally all parties should sit in a perfect triangle; thus facilitating appropriate eye contact between the patient, provider and interpreter preventing from leaving one of the parties out.

However, the reality is that most sites and rooms lack the space or the chairs so that one can create a perfect triangle. At times, exam rooms are so tight that only the patient can sit, while the provider and interpreter go through the session standing up. Remember though, whatever the situation, an interpreter should never sit on the examination table, or hold a child on his or her lap.

As the session progresses, the provider and patient may have the tendency to look only at the interpreter because s/he is able to share a different language with each party – English with the provider and the target language with the patient. Instead of literally instructing the parties to look at each other, the interpreter may quietly move his or her chair (or standing position) so as to encourage more eye contact between the parties to the session.

Can you think of other discreet ways of encouraging provider/patient contact?

Another possibility for managing eye contact is for the interpreter to quickly look down to the floor and at the same time as conveying the message, gently gesture a semi-circle and look towards the party where eye contact should be addressed.

When eye contact is not appropriate due to culture, religious issues or topic being discussed and the patient is looking down, not making eye contact; create an imaginary curtain when a provider is performing a physical or other exams that involve the checking of genitals. You may want to look towards the wall with your back towards the patient and explain to the patient that you are listening attentively and not watching the examination. Another option may be to ask if patient and provider want you to step outside the room and through a crack open in the door you may interpret for the exam. When the patient and the provider only look at the interpreter, the interpreter may want to break the fact that s/he becomes the center of attention, by looking down or gently moving the chair so that it stays in a position where the patient and the provider are looking at each other.

According to the interpreter standards it is not wrong to remind the patient during the pre-session or throughout the session to look directly at the provider and vice versa, although, one may want to use caution with tone of voice when expressing instructions.

The dynamic of being the messenger of a professional standard during, or in the beginning, of a medical encounter may create an unnecessary interruption and cause unnecessary tension. We have several reports from interpreters in the field where providers seemed to have resented being told what to do when they were already feeling overwhelmed by the powerlessness of not speaking the patient's foreign language. If allowed, during the pre-session, an interpreter might want to encourage eye contact with the provider. Interpreters need to help form the natural alliance which, through body language or words, enhances the fluidity of the dynamic between the provider and the patient.

CIFE and the Pre-session

Interpreters set the stage by introducing themselves, encouraging appropriate eye contact between the provider and the patient/client, explaining how the interpreting sessions may flow, keeping the client's language register in mind, arranging the spatial configuration of the session and explaining their need to keep information confidential, complete and accurate.

C-Confidentiality: The interpreter must explain to the patient and provider that all information shared in the session will stay among the parties in that session. A session starts with the first contact between interpreter and patient. Often, this happens in the waiting room of a clinic or hospital.

I-Use the First Person: The interpreter will be using the first person during most interpreting sessions. Therefore, when a patient or provider says "I have", the interpreter will say, "I have" not "he has/she has" or "the patient/the provider has."

Many interpreters have been working for years with little or no recognized training. Often these interpreters interpret in the third person rather than the first. In general, interpreting in the third person results in a longer and less direct form of communication, leaving patients and providers with the feeling that the interpreter is untrained and unprofessional.

F-Flow: The flow of a session is crucial to its success. Often, it may be necessary for an interpreter to ask either a provider or a patient to slow down or to pace their speech. During the pre-session, the interpreter may negotiate the use of an acceptable "stop sign" or hand signal to indicate the need for a speaker to slow down.

E-Everything You Say Will Be Interpreted: Everything, including the information shared in the waiting room, during a session, and after a session, must be interpreted. Interpreters are not allowed to keep secrets from patients or providers. You need to agree with the institution when the interpreting session starts; at the moment you meet the patient or only when the provider is present?

CIFE is guaranteed to anchor a session if the interpreter makes sure that all parties understand its purpose. Both patient and provider should be included in the explanation of CIFE. The waiting room is usually the best place to explain the workings of CIFE to a patient, while the provider might be given a concise explanation just prior to a session.

Interpreters have sometimes observed that providers seem too busy to hear about CIFE. Some providers have even been known to occasionally walk right into a session and begin the medical interview without bothering to meet or greet the interpreter. In such extreme cases, the interpreter might simultaneously interpret the first few words the provider says, then quickly interrupt the provider's flow by saying something to the effect of, "Hello. My name is ___, and I'm the (language) interpreter for (patient's name). Let me take a moment to explain how an interpretation session works." The whole explanation of CIFE can take no more than 40 seconds if a provider is in a hurry.

II SESSION

Challenges in Interpreting

Accuracy and completeness are crucial elements for professional interpreters.

Accuracy consists in comprehending the message, with its full meaning, and conveying that message in the same register used by the person for whom you are interpreting. Accuracy does not imply word for word transliteration but rather a faithful representation of the meaning. This is accomplished by staying as close as possible to what was spoken without changing the register of the person speaking.

If an interpreter only interpreted word for word, the meaning of the message most likely would be lost. We would have interpreters so worried about finding the exact word and not paying attention to the meaning, that soon, interpreters would become like broken machines, losing the ability to be complete and accurate in their interpretation. Relying solely on the words, messages may be misunderstood and, in turn, misrepresented. The best and most accurate interpretation of a message is not necessarily a word-by-word mirror-image reproduction, but a deep understanding and careful transformation of that message. The more an interpreter preoccupies himself/herself with the search for words, the more he/she becomes mentally distracted. With the interpreter's mind thus distracted, the integrity of a message is compromised.

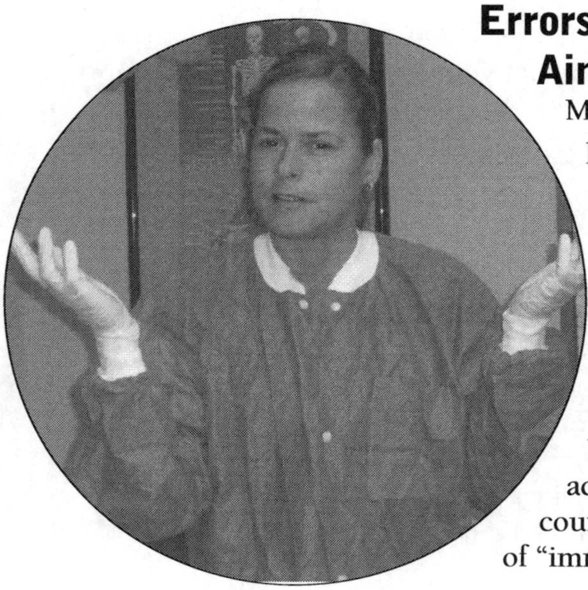

Errors in Interpretation: Aiming for 100% Accuracy

Medical interpreters owe it to themselves, to patients, to providers and to their communities to be accurate in their interpretation. Accuracy in consecutive interpretation is not an easy skill to master. In their struggle for accuracy, interpreters are not only paying attention to an immediate word conversion from one language to another, but their words must also be transmitted in a way that preserves the speaker's original meaning.

Interpreters who might be considered fluent in both English and target languages may still face challenges in accuracy. For example, an interpreter who has lived in this country for over five years will have gained an understanding of "immigrant" life and vocabulary crucial to accurate interpretation. On the other hand, this same interpreter may render a variety of common words and phrases in an incorrect manner. This phenomenon has been described as "false fluency."

False fluency occurs primarily when an interpreter converts words into a language that does not exist in any textbook. I call it the "immigrant language." For example, I often catch myself saying in Portuguese that the *"tráfico"* (traffic) is pretty bad today. In reality though, the word *"tráfico"* means a type of business exchange, not a multitude of cars! The correct word for "traffic" is *"trânsito."* Never has a fellow Portuguese immigrant corrected me; only family visiting from Portugal seem to notice my mistake!

Other examples of immigrant language are the words "appointment" and "follow-up" or "check-up." It is quite common for interpreters to transpose these words into their target languages, changing not the term, but merely the accent with which it is uttered! While a patient who has a background similar to that of the interpreter may easily understand these Anglicism's, they are rarely comprehensible to a newly arrived immigrant. Interpreters must always take care to avoid "Americanizing" their target language usage and to keep their interpretation of any message faithful to its original meaning.

Recently, in an area interpreting class, a student did a great job with her first role-play. The only inaccuracy occurred when the patient stated that he had a "funny voice" and a sore throat. The student rendered the term "funny" in a manner that implied comedy, like the "funny" of a joke or comic strip. In reality, though, the patient had said that his voice was changed, that it did not sound normal, that it was strange. But the student, a new interpreter nervous about role-plays, was so concerned with word conversion that she completely distorted the real meaning of the spoken term.

Another potential interpreting error is the conversion of idiomatic expressions specific to a particular country or region. Idiomatic expressions can be ambiguous and require that an interpreter ask for a clarification from the speaker to ascertain meaning and guarantee accuracy. The following cases illustrate what can happen if an interpreter is not familiar with idiomatic expressions.

An adolescent boy, in a session with his mother, screams "**get off my back.**" The interpreter converts this message literally and misses the intended meaning "do not bother me" or "**leave me alone.**" The same boy refers to the fact that his teacher is a "pain in the neck." Again, the interpreter converts this message literally, giving it an anatomical spin, while completely missing the correct meaning, "this teacher is always bothering me."

In the Emergency Room, an agitated young woman whose family member has died in a car crash says to the attending physician, "I have paid my dues. I do not deserve this now!" The interpreter renders the message "I have paid the money," rather than "I have asked for forgiveness" or "I have more than made up for my wrong."

PO Box 2308, Woburn, MA 01888-0508, **p:** 781-729-3736, **www.EmbracingCulture.com**
PO Box 6401, Manchester, NH 03108, **p:** 1-888-678-CCCS

A provider, frustrated with a patient's continuous demand for the completion of an insurance questionnaire says, "I have bent over backwards for you, and still you're not satisfied! You can't expect me to bear the brunt of your insurance not wanting to pay for treatment." The interpreter distorts the message, blurring the intended meaning by using literal terms for "bending over" and "carrying" rather than interpreting "I have done all that I can" and "I cannot take responsibility."

In addition to familiarity with idiomatic expressions, interpreters must also cultivate their understanding of human anatomy and common illnesses. For example, a common interpretation error is the inversion of the terms *gall bladder* and *bladder*; *spleen* and *liver*; and *angina*, which is a type of chest pain, and *heart attack*. Interpreters might also refer to *strep throat* as a mere *infection*, when in fact, strep, if not treated with antibiotics, can cause health problems such as rheumatic fever, which are far more serious than those generally caused by an average throat infection.

Do patients always hear the correct message from their interpreters? Glenn Flores et. al., in the article, *"Errors in Medical Interpretation and their Potential Clinical Consequences in Pediatric Encounters,"* documented research to determine the frequency, categories and potential clinical consequences of errors in medical interpretation.

The research turned up an average of 31 errors per session. More than half (60%) of these errors carried a potential for serious medical consequences. Despite the fact that the study lumped professional interpreters together with bilingual providers, who the study treated as interpreters, the number of errors is alarming. The most common errors charted were omission, false fluency, substitution, editorialization and addition.

In *The Art of Medical Interpretation* training programs for medical interpreters at The Cross Cultural Communication Institute at CCCS, Inc.™, we present a segment on consecutive interpreting skills in which interpreters have an opportunity to learn more about three main impediments to memory: *emotional, mechanical and physical blockers*.

Let's consider a brief example of each of these potential memory blocks. Imagine interpreting for a young child with a knee laceration. The child is bleeding and crying out in pain. How easy it could be for an interpreter to become emotionally absorbed in the child's pain to the point of pausing or halting the interpretation! The flow of communication thus obstructed, the provider may have to repeat a word or phrase. Hence, emotional blockers can prevent an interpreter from doing a good job. Fortunately, the provider in this particular case was aware of the interpreter's silence, for it is much less likely that a provider would notice omissions that occur as an interpreter is speaking.

When an interpreter, for one reason or other, misfiles or accesses and retrieves the wrong information, this mechanical blocker will automatically result in an inaccurate interpretation. In a classic case, an interpreter, when taking notes in a medical training, might wrongly assume that the bladder and the gallbladder are essentially the same organ. In a subsequent interpreting session, that interpreter will use both terms interchangeably, with the potential for tragic consequences.

Physical blockers are also common in medical interpretation. For example, an interpreter might suffer from severe allergies and need to take antihistamines, which might result in drowsiness and impaired thinking ability. In a session with an alcoholic patient, the provider might inquire as to how often that patient drinks. While the patient might answer "only one glass per meal," the interpreter might repeat "one glass a day." In this case, a physical blocker caused the interpreter to unwittingly omit important medical information (the word "only") and wrongly substitute the term "meal" with "day."

In short, interpreters are extremely powerful and their interpretations can have incredible ramifications, both in the lives of their patients and in their own professional paths. We urge all medical interpreters to attend on-going trainings and stay up-to-date with the latest in techniques for mastery. Aim for 100% accuracy!

Note: For more information on false fluency, see the article, *"Errors in Medical Interpretation and their Potential Clinical Consequences in Pediatric Encounters"* by Glenn Flores et. al.

Should an Interpreter Instruct a Provider to Look Directly at the Patient?

Location: A teaching hospital in New England
Scene: The physician turns her back on the patient while sitting at a small desk. Throughout the examination, she directs her questions to the interpreter without ever making eye contact with the patient. The interpreter asks the physician to look directly at the patient when speaking.

Result: Having asked, "Would you please make eye contact with the patient," the interpreter immediately noticed a change in the provider's affect. Tension grew as the provider snarled, "I work with a lot of interpreters and I don't see what the big deal is."

The interpreter kept interpreting the session and when the patient left, she kindly approached the provider and offered her the opportunity to comment on the interaction using a Service Verification Form (interpreter agency time and comment sheet). Brushing the interpreter off, the provider replied, "No, everything's fine."

Immediately after the session, the interpreter called her supervisor and discussed a number of concerns and questions regarding her "duty" to make sure that providers maintain eye contact with patients. She questioned if she had done the right thing by instructing the provider to look at the patient. She asked if in the future she should wait for the end of the session to let the provider know of her "duty" as a professional interpreter. She wondered out loud if her intervention had made it worse for the patient, since the ensuing tension between provider and patient had been obvious to all.

Comments: A lot of pressure is placed on the trained interpreter to set the physical stage for direct communication in the interpreting session. Section A-2 of the IMIA Standards of Practice (1995), under the heading *Manage the spatial configuration of patient-provider – interpreter to maximize ease and directness*, states that the masterful interpreter "is able to hear and see both patient and provider," "can be seen and heard by both parties," and works to "arrange spatial configuration to support direct communication between provider and patient." In this case, the interpreter could not see the provider while her back was turned. Also, the provider could not see the patient or the interpreter. The interpreter was right to be concerned.

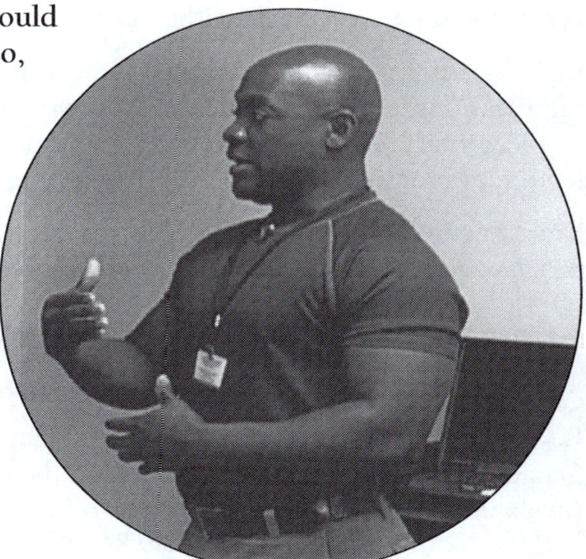

Section A-7 of the IMIA Standards of Practice states that the masterful interpreter "suggests that patient and provider address each other directly." During the examination, the provider was not addressing comments to the patient. Again, the interpreter's concern is justified, but the issue is timing. When and how should the interpreter encourage direct communication between patient and provider?

Three cheers for the interpreter who chose to transform this painful experience into an opportunity for personal and professional growth! The "easy way out" would have been to label the provider as arrogant and uninformed. "What a jerk!" the interpreter could have said to herself, before moving on to the next assignment. But this interpreter is special, and chose the more noble path of introspection. She asked questions, and with her supervisor, took a closer look at variables such as the size of the room, the gender and ethnicity of the provider and patient, and both parties' previous experiences with interpreting.

A good question to start from is "was this intervention good for the patient?" The provider's behavior changed from the point of intervention, but only for the worse. Tension grew, and this may have made the patient nervous. Another question is "Did I do the right thing by intervening?" Well, no one likes to be told what do. How would the interpreter have felt if the provider had told her how to do her job? This intervention became such an issue, perhaps because the provider was not properly trained to work with interpreters.

We know that only a select few providers have had the opportunity to be trained in working with interpreters. Most are not familiar with the Standards of Practice for Medical Interpreters. A true working partnership between providers and interpreters is still in its embryonic stages. With this in mind, should the interpreter succumb to passive silence, hoping that he/she never again has to work with an "arrogant" provider? Or is there a safe way to address the issues?

The best way of dealing with such a situation depends on where the interpreter works. In some healthcare organizations and contracting agencies, there are specific steps outlined in an employee "Guidelines and Policies" handbook. However, in the absence of a set procedure for conflict resolution, the issue of how to best address the situation at hand is generally left to the judgment of the interpreter.

Some interpreters would choose to wait until the end of the session to share their concerns regarding the lack of eye contact, presenting these as "technical" observations. However, there are other possibilities in this type of interaction. The interpreter might have chosen to look briefly at the floor, thus "forcing" the provider to look at the patient. Or the interpreter could have discreetly moved her chair closer to the patient so that they would both be in the provider's line of vision. These simple, silent actions could do much to break the cycle of poor communication without creating unnecessary tension. But by verbally giving instructions or suggestions at times when life does not hang in the balance, the interpreter not only fails to break that cycle, but also often makes it worse!

Unfortunately, there are real power differentials in the medical field, and it will likely be years before providers as a group begin to view interpreters as colleagues with authority to request change. Wherever intervention is met with negativity, interpreters need to be able to voice their concerns and to partner with other professionals in conflict resolution. Interpreters should report to a direct supervisor and discuss the dynamics of any critical interaction. Until the system changes, making one's supervisor aware of the situation before discussing it directly with the provider is a wise course of action.

PO Box 2308, Woburn, MA 01888-0508, **p:** 781-729-3736, **www.EmbracingCulture.com**
PO Box 6401, Manchester, NH 03108, **p:** 1-888-678-CCCS

Modes of Interpretation

Simultaneous or consecutive mode?

The consecutive mode is the most recommended one for healthcare interpreters, although interpreters who are anxious sometimes resort to the simultaneous mode of interpretation in medical sessions. This makes the session flow quickly, and providers are often left with the impression that the interpretation was successful. However, much of the meaning of the messages interpreted can be lost, and the result can be damaging to the triadic relationship.

The IMIA Standards of Practice refer to consecutive interpreting as the mode of choice for most medical interpreting sessions. The consecutive mode is when an interpreter listens to a message, understands the message, and after the speaker has paused, accurately conveys the message from source to target language or vice versa.

For example, a provider may come into a session and say, " I am sorry that you had to wait this long, but I have good news; your MRI was great! Congratulations!" The interpreter must be able to register three main points, "sorry for the delay," " good news," and "MRI." Soon after the provider completes the thought, the interpreter is able to say, in the target language," I am sorry that you had to wait this long, but I have good news: your MRI was great! Congratulations!" In this interaction, the interpreter did not speak at the same time as the provider and did not summarize the information.

If the interpreter had chosen to interpret simultaneously. The spirit of the message, as conveyed in the details, might have been lost. A simultaneous conversion of the message would have not represented the voice of the speaker with the completeness it deserves.

Recently, I trained a group of medical interpreters who appeared resistant to the idea of using the consecutive mode in their role play practice. All of these interpreters were trained in a college-level interpreting program, and their teacher instructed them that it does not matter whether an interpreter uses the simultaneous or consecutive mode. Some of these interpreters felt strongly that the simultaneous mode is best, largely due to its speed.

Indeed, it is not easy for an interpreter to use the consecutive mode in the triadic medical encounter. There are so many potential distractions, or "blockers." Some are caused by the interpersonal dynamics of the patient-provider relationship; others are caused by the interpreter's own emotional responses to the messages being conveyed. Then there are the environmental work hazards: sudden or sustained noise, foul smells, interruption by third parties, and challenges to the flow of communication posed by multiple speakers. Consecutive interpretation requires a special level of concentration and a developed skill.

And yet, with each role play performed by the group of trained interpreters mentioned above, there were marked flaws in the interpreters' simultaneous interpreting performances. In each case, sizable units of meaning were completely missing in the converted message. Afterward, whenever the interpreters were asked what they remembered from the interpretation in question, they would hesitate, struggling to find the meaning of the messages they so recently interpreted. Why is this so?

Take the example of a parent reading a storybook to his child for the hundredth time. The parent can do it well, even imitating the voices of the different characters. But after some time, the reading becomes rote. Afterwards, does the parent even know what he read? Probably not. The scientific explanation for this phenomenon involves the differences between immediate and short-term memory. When a reader (or an interpreter) works primarily with immediate memory (as occurs in simultaneous interpretation), there is little time to process and sort information.

Any meaningful retention of the source message is improbable. While simultaneous interpreters will remember very little of a message post-session, the interpreter who uses the consecutive mode, which exercises short-term memory, is more likely to recall the general topic and main points of the message conveyed. The consecutive mode allows the interpreter to listen to complete units of meaning (generally consisting of up to five to seven items) before conveying the message in a target language. Danica Seleskovitch, in her book *Interpreting for International Conferences*, comments, "In consecutive interpretation the interpreter has the advantage of knowing the line of argument before he interprets." This is beneficial, not only for the interpreter, but also for the patient.

How does the patient benefit from consecutive interpretation? Claudia Angelelli, in her book *Medical Interpreting and Cross-Cultural Communication*, explores the essence of the provider-patient relationship. She quotes experts who assert that in terms of outcomes, the provider's relationship with the patient is more important than the actual delivery of medical care. This is because patients who are comfortable in their relationships with providers are more likely to follow through with treatment and to stick with the same providers throughout the course of the treatment, while less likely to worry about their illnesses. Yes, healthy provider-patient relationships, characterized by the patient's sense that a provider is caring, respectful and compassionate, are natural stress-relievers.

All patients, even those who speak the same language as their providers, at times experience feelings of powerlessness and anxiety. For the LEP patient, there is the added anxiety of not being able to communicate with the provider, and the stress of having a third person, the interpreter, in the room. As a result of these emotions, a patient's ability to make sense of meaning is often somewhat impaired. In sessions where simultaneous interpreting technique is used, there is the compounding factor of two persons speaking at the same time. The patient is left a bit confused, half listening to the provider and half to the interpretation, with trouble making sense of the rapid ping-pong of words exchanged in the session.

Does this mean that interpreters should never use the simultaneous mode in the medical encounter? Of course not! The simultaneous mode is recommended for commands and directions in the medical encounter, such as; "Follow my finger with your eyes" "Grab my arm and do not let it go" "Push up when I press down." When using these commands, the provider needs to be able to judge the patient's reaction and timing. Furthermore, the simultaneous mode is recommended when the parties to a session are unable to slow their speech or take turns speaking. It is also best when the speaker is not making sense, as often occurs with patients who are distraught or who suffer from certain mental disorders. Another situation in which the simultaneous mode might be implemented is when an interpreter gets distracted or blocked and needs to temporarily shift modes until he or she can concentrate more fully.

Simultaneous interpreting may be love at first sight for some interpreters and trainers, but upon closer inspection, we find flaws. If the medical encounter were only about words and speed and making providers happy, then simultaneous interpreting would be the first choice for all interpreters. But the reality is that the medical encounter is more about trust, understanding, and a healthy provider-patient relationship. These are feelings best conveyed in the consecutive mode.

Interpreting Mode for Groups

Few interpreters have received specialized training in group therapy. As a result, there are many different opinions regarding the "best" interpreting mode and arrangement for foreign language interpreters working in group settings.

When it comes to setting the stage for the interpreted group interaction, one view is that remote interpretation, with the LEP group participant listening in with headphones, is best. In this manner, some argue, the interpreter's voice does not interfere with the group dynamic.

In contrast, others have experienced successful group interactions in which the interpreter is physically present and no electronic equipment is used. These individuals comment that if the group leader openly discusses the possible discomfort resulting from the unfamiliar sounds of chuchotage (*"whisper"* interpretation), the group will begin to accept the interpreter and with time the sounds of chuchotage will "fade" from the collective consciousness of the group until the interpreter is barely noticed. (Note that such interactions generally involve groups in which there is just one foreign language represented by a single interpreter.)

There are also conflicting opinions in regard to choosing a mode of interpretation for group therapy. One view is that the interpreter should exclusively practice the simultaneous mode. Others feel that a group is best served when the interpreter is able to navigate between modes, applying both simultaneous and consecutive techniques, and in some cases, a summarization of thought while preserving key points of meaning.

A closer look at the basic principles of group therapy can help the interpreter make an informed decision regarding the appropriate mode and arrangement for each type of group interaction. Although there are many different types of groups, most share similar development stages, regardless of whether they are monolingual or multilingual. According to experts James Garland, et al. (1973), there are five main stages through which a group will progress:

1. Pre-Affiliation
2. Power and Control
3. Intimacy
4. Differentiation
5. Separation

Pre-Affiliation is the beginning stage of any group. This is when group members introduce themselves and begin the process of connecting with other group members and with the group leader. In Pre-Affiliation, members will limit intimacy with a view to protecting themselves from misunderstanding and attack. Often, individual members will compare the current group leader to leaders of past groups in which they had participated and there is some ambivalence in the decision to continue with (or leave) the present group.

In Pre-Affiliation, the group leader is key to creating an environment in which members can maintain some distance while beginning to develop a level of trust. The development of trust occurs primarily through dialogue in which group dynamics are explored, expectations revealed and cooperative planning encouraged. In multilingual groups, it is crucial that the group leader use this time to introduce the interpreter and to acknowledge the possibility of discomfort among some group members in regard to chuchotage and the presence of the interpreter.

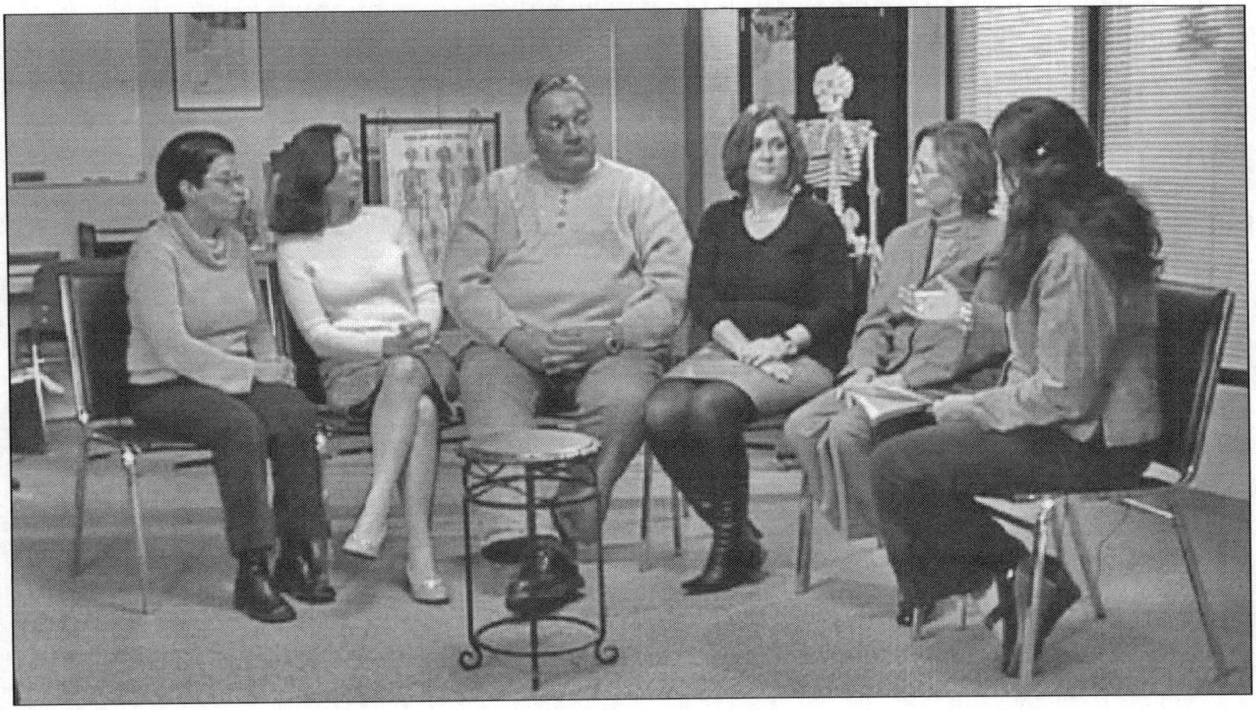

PO Box 2308, Woburn, MA 01888-0508, **p:** 781-729-3736, **www.EmbracingCulture.com**
PO Box 6401, Manchester, NH 03108, **p:** 1-888-678-CCCS

Many clinicians invite the interpreter to explain his/her role during the first session of a new group. At this point, the group leader may want to refer to the purpose of the group while stating that, although group members may experience an initial awareness of a language barrier, they will soon realize that they share similar issues and concerns.

The second stage of most groups can be called "Power and Control." This occurs when the group loses its initial reserve and members begin to express a range of emotions. Members will take opposing positions on the issues in discussion, and there is a tendency to develop "cliques" in which certain members form alliances against other allied members.

Group leaders and interpreters need to be aware of this struggle for power and control. It is in this stage that members may complain that the presence of the interpreter is an impediment to forging a real intimacy with the LEP participant. The group leader and interpreter may want to rethink the logistics of the interpreting environment. Should seating arrangements be altered? Might the interpreter experiment with switching from the simultaneous mode to summarization when it is important that a group member not be interrupted? Would it be helpful if the LEP participant were specifically invited to express his/her fears to the group?

Often the LEP patient's expression of being misunderstood by society in general (and by the group in question) does much towards stimulating the other members to connect around the issues that brought them together in the first place. This can lead to Intimacy, a stage in which group members begin to feel safer about sharing personal information. During Intimacy, participants may begin to believe that their openness as individuals will bring some resolution to the group as a whole. There is a growing awareness of the importance of the group as a functioning unit.

At this point, the therapist will often begin to implement a more confrontational form of questioning. The interpreter must be careful to mirror the group leader's tone and intent, and to resist the "pull" of the group for the interpreter to "participate" as if he/she were a true group member.

The next stage is Differentiation, a time in which group members, while recognizing the importance of the group as a functioning unit, begin to appreciate each other as individuals. A mutual respect is present when differences arise, and participants begin to develop relationships outside the group.

At some point in the Differentiation process, the group leader will facilitate a clarification of group identity, echoing the participants' reflections on how the group evolved and how it impacted the lives of its members. This is a good time in which to revisit the presence of the interpreter throughout the treatment process.

If the group leader and interpreter expertly manage the steps listed above, the general group feeling regarding exposure to interpreter services will likely be quite positive. Not only has the interpreter facilitated the experience of one LEP participant, he/she has also played a role in preparing each group member for the realities of daily life in a multilingual society, imbuing them with a new appreciation for the fact that with each difference, there are also commonalities that will join them to any individual in the world.

The final stage, Separation, is often characterized by a general regression in which members become distant and may display signs of anger, in many cases reliving some of the initial issues of power and control. The group leader will echo these feelings, elicit clarification and make empathic statements regarding the different ways in which individuals experience endings. The leader will reaffirm the group's readiness for separation and will encourage members to share their growing involvement with the community. At this point, the group leader may allow the interpreter to address the participants directly with an expression of thanks for their individual and collective efforts towards making the group a safe area in which to practice the profession.

The physical presence of the interpreter and the practice of chuchotage, if expertly managed, will not prevent the group from experiencing the five stages of progressive group therapy. In fact, as time goes by and participants move deeper into the group experience, the interpreter will naturally "fade" into the background and participants will at times forget that the LEP participant is indeed speaking in a different language.

Over the course of treatment, a competent group leader will address many things that make individual group members different from each other. These may include race, gender, class, ethnicity, age, profession, and so on. From a therapist's viewpoint, language is just one of the many facets of a patient's individuality. And as long as linguistic differences are properly acknowledged, and the interpreter is given time to explain the mechanics of our craft, a multilingual group can be a great success.

III FOLLOW-UP – Challenges in Interpreting

Ethical issues that can hamper best practices in the post-session and follow-up.

CCCS has made a distinction between post-session and follow-up. The post–session occurs after the interpreter stops interpreting for the clinical session. The interpreter or the provider may need clarification about the technicality of the interpreting session, such as eye contact, register used or cultural issues that could have enhanced the patient-provider relationship.

Interpreters through their own life experiences are often used to managing various aspects of a bilingual-bicultural world and after being professionally trained they are able to recognize that the unspoken language of a session can speak as clearly as words. The interpreter understands that expressions like a frown, rolling of the eyes, shaking of the head when a certain treatment is mentioned, wringing one's hands, pulling on clothing, etc., can be telltale signs that some part of the session still may not be clearly understood. Are these just nervous twitches or do they have a deeper meaning? The interpreter encourages this 'check-in' with provider and possibly the patient, to make sure that all the loose ends are neatly wrapped up in a successful session.

PO Box 2308, Woburn, MA 01888-0508, **p:** 781-729-3736, **www.EmbracingCulture.com**
PO Box 6401, Manchester, NH 03108, **p:** 1-888-678-CCCS

The interpreter recognizes that issues with accuracy due to patient's lack of logic or inability to understand questions or difficulty with flow from provider or patient's part are just a few of the challenges that may need further clarification. It may be advantageous to explain why a certain mode of interpretation was chosen. The Post-session is enriched with the quality of a true team approach between two or more professionals who are trying to enhance their understanding on how to work with each other, and thereby, strengthen the patient/ provider relationship.

This dialogue or check-in may happen at times with the patient present, but most likely it will take place between the provider and the interpreter after the clinical session. An interpreter could say to the patient: "I am sorry that I interrupted you so many times but I was trying not to miss any information and I wanted to represent your voice as accurately as possible." Or an interpreter may ask for a specific linguistic issue that needed some clarification due to regionalism in the target language. A provider was abusive to the patient and the interpreter may want to contact a supervisor who could follow the proper channels of the institution so as to assist the patient if needed.

Closely related to the post-session is the follow-up. This includes activities related to the session that don't necessarily take place in the provider's presence. Did the provider leave certain instructions to be followed immediately after the clinical encounter? Will assistance be needed to schedule future appointments? Does the patient need help in obtaining information (brochures, fact sheets, etc) about his health that the provider indicated he could receive from the receptionist? Are there arrangements for transportation? Interpreters need to be on hand for the specifics of immediate and long-term follow-up.

When the interpreter helps to schedule the next appointment, walks to the lab or the pharmacy where further interpretation will be needed, the interpreter needs to exercise caution since unwanted information may be shared by the patient or even a patient's family member. This important follow-up can become like an obstacle course, tricky to maneuver, due to the potential for ethical issues to creep in by allowing an environment where boundaries are not as regulated. That short walk to the lab may begin to feel like a mile for the interpreter who has perhaps permitted additional conversation about an abusive relationship or who has broken confidentiality when chatting about the patient's condition with someone who was not part of the treating team. Keep the conversation to the business at hand and you will leave feeling satisfied with your work, knowing that all the loose ends were neatly tied together.

Sight Translation or Sight Interpretation Mode

Sight translation is an interpreting mode that should be used with caution. Interpreters may want to update their understanding with the most recent policies of the interpreting associations and the NCIHC.

CCCS, Inc.™ abides by the National Council on Interpreting in Healthcare's Standard #22, which states, "The interpreter avoids sight translation, especially of complex or critical documents, if he or she lacks sight translation skills. For example, when asked to sight translate a surgery consent form, an interpreter instead asks the provider to explain its content and then interprets the explanation."

Thus, CCCS, Inc.™ encourages its interpreters to request providers to designate a healthcare professional to explain the form to the patient. The interpreter should then interpret that professional's explanation, careful to always request clarification for any unfamiliar or highly technical medical terms.

This does not mean that the CCCS, Inc.™ interpreters should avoid sight translation altogether. There are many situations in which strong sight translation skills are a must, such as when interpreters assist patients in filling out medical history questionnaires or other necessary documentation, usually in a waiting area prior to the consult.

When doing sight translation of a medical history form or other documentation, the interpreter might perceive that the patient does not clearly understand the meaning of a question or term. If this is the case, and a provider is not immediately available to answer the question, the interpreter should circle the question or term and request clarification from the provider at the start of the medical interview.

Even if you think you can explain the meaning of the question or term, we recommend that you seek clarification from the provider. There are two good reasons to take this course of action. First, by seeking clarification from a medical professional, the interpreter avoids any potential for miscommunication around a medical explanation; thus protects him/herself from future legal action on the part of the patient or patient's family. Second, by allowing the provider to explain medical terms, the interpreter fosters the therapeutic alliance (patient-provider relationship), which, in turn, promotes greater trust and healing.

Let's consider the word "hepatitis," a common medical term not easily understood by patients with limited education. Imagine that you, the interpreter, decide to explain the meaning of "hepatitis" to a patient while filling out a medical history form. Later in this patient's treatment, it is discovered that the patient has an inaccurate understanding of this disease. The patient then tells the provider, "But this is how the interpreter explained my disease to me." Whether your explanation was precise or not, it is the patient's word against yours. How would this matter be defended in a court of law? Well, if you were widely known for never having crossed professional boundaries, and if there were doctors who could testify to your consistency in requesting clarification, you might have a chance at winning the case. However, if you are

PO Box 2308, Woburn, MA 01888-0508, **p:** 781-729-3736, **www.EmbracingCulture.com**
PO Box 6401, Manchester, NH 03108, **p:** 1-888-678-CCCS

known as someone who "explains" medical terms to patients, your chances of preserving your reputation and protecting your assets are minimal. Truly then, sticking to the standards of practice is the best policy for any interpreter, whether staff or freelance.

How can you improve your sight translation skills? For some expert advice, go to http://www.acebo.com/sitintro.htm. There you will find tips from The Interpreter's Edge, an excellent self-training manual that includes 24 lessons in Sight Translation.

The Making of a Professional Interpreter

Besides understanding and complying with the National Standards of Practice for Medical Interpreters (NCIHC) and the hiring institution policies, interpreters must become familiar with their own state interpreter association standards along with state and federal laws pertinent to the healthcare industry.

Interpreter Code of Ethics

Governing principle: The interpreter will use all available knowledge, skills and techniques to provide an accurate interpretation of all communications (verbal, non-verbal, contextual and cultural) between the provider, the patient and other individuals involved in the care and treatment of patients.

1) Confidentiality: All patient information of any kind is confidential and privileged and may not be divulged to anyone (except supervisory staff, to achieve the best possible patient care).
2) All written documents related to patients are confidential and should be treated as such.
3) The above provisions apply both during and after working hours and continue beyond the end of the interpreter's tenure with contracting organization.
4) Any questions regarding the appropriateness of sharing patient information with a particular person should be addressed immediately, while the interpreter is still at the site, to supervisory clinical staff, before the information is shared, except where the information is needed in a medical emergency. In case supervisory staff are not accessible, contact the provider or the department supervisor for guidance on how to best proceed with the situation.

ACCURACY: Interpreting the true meaning of what is being said without editing or deleting anything and with an awareness of educational, cultural, and regional variations; explaining cultural differences or practices to healthcare providers and patients, as appropriate.

LACK OF BIAS: Recognizing and eliminating the interpreter's own opinions and values from the interpreting interaction.

IMPARTIALITY: Remaining committed to the communication between the healthcare provider and patient; not taking the side of either party; refraining from interpreting when impartiality is compromised.

DISCRETION: Making sound judgments in all situations so that no individual is put in jeopardy, and so the professional appropriateness of the interpreter is never in question. This includes acknowledgment of the interpreter's limits in language, in interpreting skills, knowledge of the subject, and cultural mediating.

PROFESSIONALISM: Behaving and presenting one's self in a professional manner at all times, regardless of the familiarity or unfamiliarity with the individuals involved; asking questions to clarify unfamiliar medical terms or idioms of speech; openly asking for clarification when uncertain about something. Interpreters are not allowed to initiate any telephone contact with patients/customers unless advised to do so by the supervisory staff.

HUMANITARIANISM: Maintaining a humane and unprejudiced treatment of individuals; communicating any special needs of the patient to the provider.

CCCS, Inc.™ Code of Ethics Interpreter Agreement

CCCS, INC.™ INFORMATION DISCLOSURE POLICIES

1. All patient/client information is confidential and privileged and may not be divulged to anyone except as provided in this form.
2. All information gained while interpreting is considered confidential.
3. All written documents related to interpreting cases are confidential and should be treated as such.
4. Cases must not be commented on or discussed with anyone other than the staff or interpreting representatives, unless otherwise permitted by the patient and the treating provider.
5. The above provisions apply both during and after working hours and continue beyond the interpreter's tenure with the contracting organization.
6. When providing services via telephone, no other person will be present within hearing distance of the interpreter.
7. Contact patients/clients only when requested by your contracting organization. Always comply with HIPAA regulations. When calling a patient/client at home, be discreet. Do not leave messages with individuals other than the patient/client.
8. Do not leave messages on answering machines or voice mail unless requested by the contracting organization or healthcare institution and always in compliance with HIPAA regulations. If you leave a message on the answering machine/voice mail, please state your first name and inform of time of appointment and general area, i.e: "This is Maria calling Mr. Fontes confirming an appointment on March 3rd in Boston." Do not mention exact, identifying information such as street location, department or type of appointment.

PO Box 2308, Woburn, MA 01888-0508, **p:** 781-729-3736, **www.EmbracingCulture.com**
PO Box 6401, Manchester, NH 03108, **p:** 1-888-678-CCCS

The Making of a Professional Medical Interpreter

Be Prepared:

- Beforehand, develop a glossary with assignment-specific terms
- Build a glossary every time you complete an assignment
- Check web sites for accurate glossaries, use monolingual and bilingual dictionaries and resources
- Attend on-going trainings on different healthcare topics and interpreting skills
- Check appointments the day before
- If you are a freelance interpreter be familiar with directions and location of assignment; you will arrive early and ready to interpret
- Get familiar with Emergency and Public Health Codes for each health institution

Know How to Handle a Conflict:

- Acknowledge perceived conflict
- Ask for clarification
- Work together with the person on facts
- Agree to disagree
- Compromise
- Find appropriate setting
- Use the "I" person
- Not a personal issue but reframe conflict as how to best deliver promised services

Professional Attitude:

- Project yourself well
- Wear appropriate professional attire
- Follow business etiquette with polite, cordial greeting
- Pay attention to tone of voice
- Decline inappropriate requests and offer an alternative
- Be humble, ask if you do not understand words or meaning –Ask for: "Break it down"
- Have a respectful approach: "It seems to me," "It appears," " I have noticed"
- The session is for the patient-provider and not about the interpreter. Do not become a burden
- Have a dictionary with you on-site so to consult after session
- Be on time (15 minutes earlier)
- Follow policies and standards and the Law

Professional standards that have shaped the healthcare interpreting profession

In the past twenty-two years, three major sets of standards for medical interpreters were developed. It started with the MMIA (Massachusetts Medical Interpreters Association), now called IMIA (International Medical Interpreters Association), which later on led to an adaptation and expansion of the standards by the CHIA (California Healthcare Interpreting Association), and, more recently, the NCIHC (National Council on Interpreting and Healthcare) that consolidated both versions of the standards by engaging different interpreter focus groups, nationally, in a dialogue around the standards.

IMIA

The IMIA Standards of Practice was created by a committee of dedicated interpreter coordinators in the Boston, Massachusetts, area in 1986. The Standards states that the primary goal of an interpreter is to "make possible communication between a healthcare provider and a patient who do not speak the same language."

The *Standards* are organized into three major task areas:

(1) interpretation
(2) cultural interface
(3) ethical behavior

Each of these three areas have multiple subdivisions and they have been used as a model for interpreting practice nationwide. The *Standards* can be ordered at **http://www.imiaweb.org/**

CHIA

http://chiaonline.org/

The California Healthcare Interpreters Association (CHIA) has published a set of ethical principles, protocols and guidance on roles and intervention for healthcare interpreters.

The CHIA Standards and Certification Committee began its work in January 2001 by reviewing existing standards of the day; then, collaborating and refining the process until the first edition came to production. Page 20 of the standards states: "The guiding purpose of these standards of practice is to support the health and well-being of the patient. This document includes three main sections that guide interpreters through the complex tasks of healthcare interpreting."

The main sections cover:

(1) Ethical principles
(2) Standardized protocols
(3) Guidance on interpreter roles and interventions

One highlight of the CHIA standards is the practical process outlined for ethical decision-making. These 6 actions help the interpreter to develop critical thinking and reasoning.

PO Box 2308, Woburn, MA 01888-0508, **p:** 781-729-3736, **www.EmbracingCulture.com**
PO Box 6401, Manchester, NH 03108, **p:** 1-888-678-CCCS

NCIHC

In addition, the *Code of Ethics for Interpreters in Health Care*, published by the National Council on Interpreting in Health Care (NCIHC) in July 2004, is available for download at **www.ncihc.org**. CCCS encourages all of its interpreters to familiarize themselves with all sets of guidelines.

The NCIHC *Code of Ethics for Interpreters in Health Care* has gained nationwide acceptance, and many healthcare institutions and interpreting agencies openly declare that their interpreters follow these guidelines.

The NCIHC *Code* can be summarized in the following nine principles:

- The interpreter treats as confidential, within the treating team, all information learned in the performance of professional duties, while observing relevant requirements regarding disclosure.
- The interpreter strives to render the message accurately, conveying the content, spirit, and cultural context of the original message.
- The interpreter strives to maintain impartiality and refrains from counseling, advising or projecting personal biases or beliefs.
- The interpreter maintains the boundaries of the professional role, refraining from personal involvement.
- The interpreter continuously strives to develop awareness of his/her own and other (including biomedical) cultures encountered in the performance of their professional duties.
- The interpreter treats all parties with respect.
- When the patient's health, well-being, or dignity is at risk, the interpreter may be justified in acting as an advocate. Advocacy must only be undertaken after careful and thoughtful analysis of the situation.
- The interpreter strives to continually further his/her knowledge and skills.
- The interpreter must at all times act in a professional and ethical manner.

Federal Law and Medical Interpretation. Title VI of the Civil Rights Act of 1964

By Bruce L. Adelson, Esq.

With one stroke of the pen on July 2, 1964, President Lyndon Johnson signed the Civil Rights Act of 1964 into law, enacting perhaps the most sweeping civil rights legislation in American history. Title VI of this landmark law prohibits race, color, and national origin (or language-based) discrimination by any organization receiving federal funds. It requires federally subsidized healthcare providers to give non-English language assistance to limited English proficient ("LEP") people. The U.S. Census Bureau defines an LEP person as someone who speaks English "less than very well," "not well" or "not at all."

In 2000, President Clinton took Title VI a step further. He signed Executive Order 13166, which requires all federal agencies to adopt regulations and guidance for their financial assistance recipients regarding the provision of services to LEP individuals. In 2002, the U.S. Department of Justice ("DOJ"), the federal agency charged with enforcing Title VI and providing guidance to other federal agencies, issued its LEP regulations. Other federal agencies modeled their regulations on DOJ's and most issued them subsequently.

Today, with tens of millions of LEP people living in this country and billions of federal dollars distributed across all states, the reach of Title VI is tremendous. This article outlines Title VI's basic legal requirements and describes several scenarios that medical interpreters and translators may face that concern Title VI.

Title VI's prohibition against discrimination applies only to agencies, organizations, hospitals, clinics, state and local governments that receive federal financial assistance. This law has no minimum amount for it to apply. A healthcare provider's receipt of the smallest amount of federal funds brings the provider's entire organization under Title VI.

Title VI requires all recipients of federal aid to provide LEP individuals with "meaningful access" to their federally subsidized services by using, for example, competent, trained, proficient interpreters for communications between LEP patients and medical professionals and "vital documents" accurately translated into the relevant languages. Failure to do so would likely violate federal law.

By law, each federal aid recipient should decide which of its documents are "vital." For example, the law considers an informed consent form used by a hospital to be "vital." Therefore, it must be translated into other languages. The languages the form should be translated into will vary depending upon the community served by the provider, the languages spoken in the community, and the size of each non-English speaking population.

If a complaint alleging a Title VI violation by a federally subsidized hospital is made to the federal government, that hospital could lose its federal funds, be subject to an intrusive federal audit called a compliance review, and have its operations supervised by the federal government. The federal government can also file lawsuits to enforce Title VI. Private individuals, such as patients, have the right to sue for money damages if they believe their Title VI rights have been violated.

Medical interpreters and translators encounter Title VI every day. Here are some scenarios you may encounter in the healthcare industry.

Each LEP individual has the right to language assistance. However, an individual may choose to use a friend or relative to interpret for them instead of the interpreter offered by the provider. In this case, the LEP person can use his/her own interpreter ONLY after the provider has one of its trained interpreters explain Title VI and the federal right to language assistance in the patient's own language.

Then, the provider may also ask the patient to sign a waiver of rights. This waiver might say the patient understands his right to language assistance from the provider but chooses to use his own interpreter. This waiver form would be considered a "vital" document by law and should be translated into the patient's language. The waiver should also be explained to the patient by the provider's trained interpreter.

The provider may use a telephone language line and have in-person interpreters available for language assistance. A telephone language service is often most helpful where a patient speaks a rare language that is not spoken by anyone on the provider's staff. However, while telephone services are helpful, providers should not rely on them to provide all kinds of language assistance in all cases. The U.S. Department of Justice recommends that using an in-person interpreter remains preferable in most situations. Providers are required by law to determine the types of services and personnel they need to provide legally required language assistance.

Providers should not ask minor children to act as interpreters. It is thought that minors are not capable of providing accurate language assistance, especially if their parents or relatives are patients. Federal law permits providers to use children as interpreters in emergency situations, such as when a parent or guardian is unconscious and the child is the only person available to give needed information to medical professionals. Federal law states that other third persons, such as friends or relatives, should also not be asked to act as interpreters. The only exceptions would be in emergencies and if the LEP patient chose to use a particular person instead of the provider's interpreter.

Providers can use bilingual staff to offer certain information to LEP patients in non-English languages. Interpreters and bilingual staff both fulfill important functions but **they are not interchangeable**. For example, an employee who is not fluent in a given language, who is unfamiliar with medical terminology, and not trained as an interpreter should not interpret a doctor's instructions for an LEP patient. Using untrained and unqualified people to provide language assistance could be illegal by not giving LEP people the "meaningful access" that the law mandates.

While bilingual staff should not typically provide interpretation between doctor and patient, they can fulfill other key roles as part of a federally subsidized entity's Title VI compliance. For example, they can staff a facility's information desk and provide important information to LEP people about how to access various services.

The United States' LEP population continues to grow. With this growth comes an increased need for LEP services as well as greater awareness by LEP people of their rights. Healthcare providers have a federal obligation under Title VI to ensure that their LEP patients have meaningful access to the providers' federally subsidized services by having trained, proficient interpreters and accurately translated documents available for their patients' use.

Interpreter Evaluation Tool based on the IMIA standards.

Name:______________________________Target Language:_____________Date: ___/___/___

OBSERVATION

1 PRE SESSION

Client/patient	Yes	No
1. Introduction?		
2. Interpreter helped client with registration?		
3. Interpreter explained the usage of the first person?		
4. Interpreter informed client of confidentiality policy?		
5. Interpreter informed client that everything said during the session will be interpreted?		
6. Did the interpreter handle the waiting period appropriately?		
7. Did the interpreter appropriately acknowledge similarities and differences?		

Provider	Yes	No
8. Introduction?		
9. Interpreter explained the usage of the first person?		
10. Interpreter informed the provider that everything said during the session will be interpreted?		

2 THE TRIADIC RELATIONSHIP

Interpreter/provider and client	Yes	No
1. Did the interpreter appropriately arrange seating?		
2 Did the interpreter show appropriate eye contact?		
3 Did the interpreter appropriately handle the comments from client or provider?		
4 Did the interpreter stay in the room alone with client?		
5 Did the interpreter help with medical procedures?		

6 Who makes the decision of when to stay behind the curtain?
○ Interpreter ○ Client ○ Provider

PO Box 2308, Woburn, MA 01888-0508, **p:** 781-729-3736, **www.EmbracingCulture.com**
PO Box 6401, Manchester, NH 03108, **p:** 1-888-678-CCCS

3 INTERPRETATION TECHNIQUE

Interpreter	Yes	No
1. Usage of First Person?		
2. Omissions?		
3. Additions?		
4. Meaning/Accuracy?		
5. Meaning/Completeness?		
6. Keeps appropriate flow?		
7. Asks for clarification?		
8. Checks with client if he/she understood everything?		
9. Mode of interpretation: consecutive, simultaneous, sight, and summary?		
10. Memorization techniques: note-taking, echoing key words, and finger counting?		

4 KNOWLEDGE OF MEDICAL TERMINOLOGY

Strengths:

Weaknesses:

Areas for growth:

5 FOLLOW-UP

5 FOLLOW-UP	Yes	No
1. Interpreter helps client with follow-up visits?		
2. Interpreter helps client getting home?		
3. Interpreter does not provide advice when asked for his or her opinion?		
4. Interpreter handled a distraught client appropriately?		

6 CULTURAL KNOWLEDGE/CLARIFICATION

6 CULTURAL KNOWLEDGE/CLARIFICATION	Yes	No
1. Interpreter clarified cultural meaning by checking with appropriate party?		
2. Interpreter understood vocabulary used by both, provider and client?		
3. Interpreter understands client's immigration history?		
4. Interpreter shows how to best address client by showing respect?		
5. Interpreter asks permission to become a cultural coach when appropriate?		
6. Interpreter showed respect for client's own individuality?		
7. Interpreter understands provider and client's communication styles?		
8. Interpreter understands USA medical system and that of client's native country?		

SELF-OBSERVATION:

7 ETHICS

7 ETHICS	Yes	No
1. Do you accept gifts?		
2. Do you share your opinion regarding controversial beliefs?		
3. Do you ask questions to clients/personal/clinical?		
4. Do you provide your telephone number?		
5. Do you give your opinion when asked by the clients?		
6. Do you deliberately delete information for political/religious/personal beliefs?		
7. Do you call clients at home when not asked by provider to do so?		
8. Do you drive clients to places?		
9. Do you give money to clients?		
10. Do you make remarks that are pejorative against anyone?		
11. Do you use power of knowledge for personal gain?		
12. Do you discuss prior sessions with different providers?		
13. Do you tell clients what to say in the session?		
14. Do you discuss the sessions and identify clients/providers?		

PO Box 2308, Woburn, MA 01888-0508, **p:** 781-729-3736, **www.EmbracingCulture.com**
PO Box 6401, Manchester, NH 03108, **p:** 1-888-678-CCCS

Notes

Lesson Two:
The Different Roles of the Interpreter

Understanding Goals

Students will be able to:

- understand the different roles of the Medical Interpreter
- review the Standards of Practice
- apply proper consecutive interpreting practice in immunization role-plays

Key Concepts

- Conduit
- Culture Broker/Coach
- Clarifier
- Advocate
- Facilitator
- Transparency
- Impartiality
- The Interpreter as a Butterfly
- HIPAA
- The Joint Commission
- Six "W(s)"

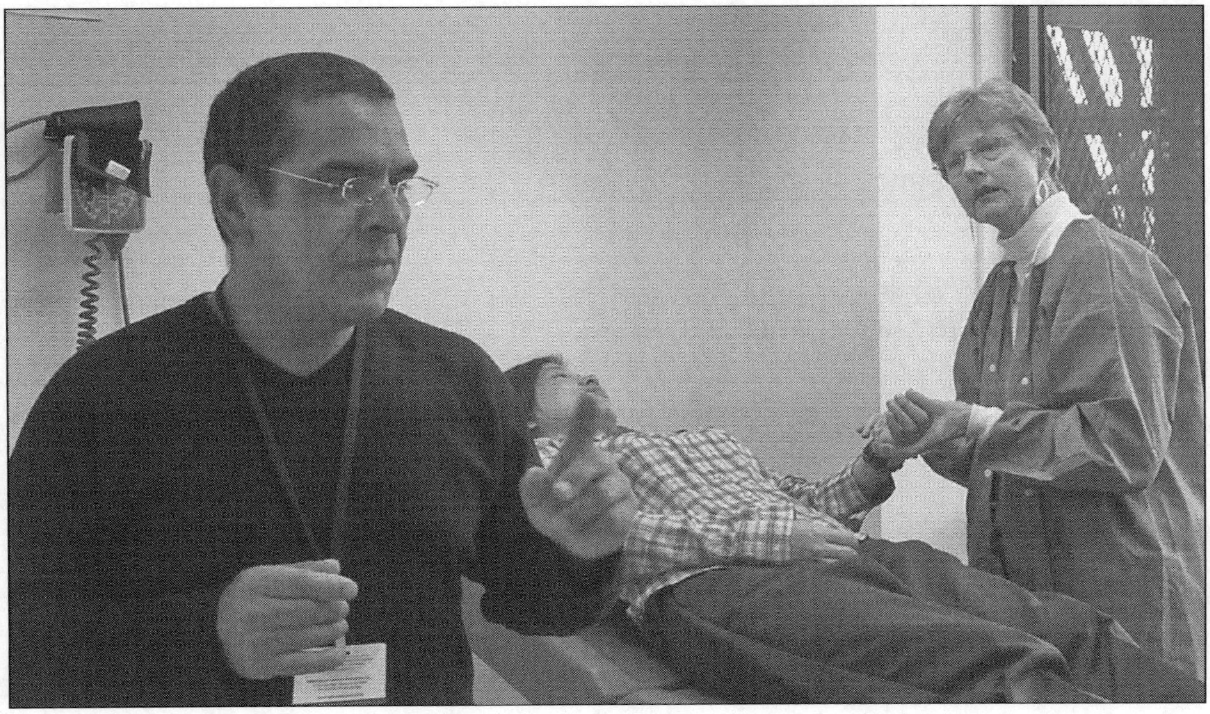

Lesson Two: Quiz
The Different Roles of the Interpreter

Mark each item or items that best complete each sentence.

1. A good triadic encounter should include the following pieces (Circle all that apply):
   A. Pre-session with provider.
   B. Pre-session with patient.
   C. Post-session to schedule follow-up appointments.
   D. Exchanging phone numbers and addresses with the patient.

2. The interpreter should arrive:
   A. 15 minutes after the scheduled appointment time.
   B. 15 minutes prior to the scheduled appointment time.
   C. An hour before the scheduled appointment time.
   D. At the exact appointment time.

Mark each item "True" or False."

3. The ethical interpreter will respect patient confidentiality by keeping secrets from the provider and not interpreting all the information the patient shares.
   O True O False

4. In the medical session, the interpreter should not inform the provider what is occurring when taking time out to clarify meaning with the patient.
   O True O False

5. The role a professional interpreter plays most of the time is to be an advocate.
   O True O False

6. Being a CONDUIT means that the interpreter plays the role of a bridge, communicating by sticking to the spoken content and words.
   O True O False

7. When acting as a cultural coach the interpreter tries to assist the provider in finding common ground in order for a dialogue to occur between the provider and the patient.
   O True O False

8. A medical interpreter could be an effective culture broker or coach while maintaining neutrality in the triadic encounter.
   O True O False

9. A transparent interpreter, when facing a perceived cultural conflict, has a private conversation with the provider and then collaborates in the provider's search for healthy alternatives.
   O True O False

10. The impartiality clause was instituted to teach interpreters that they cannot take sides or impose their own ideas in a session, even if they personally believe they are doing something good.
   - ○ True ○ False

11. In CIFE, "Everything will be interpreted" does not cover matters discussed prior to the doctor's arrival in the room.
   - ○ True ○ False

12. When an interpreter foresees that a patient from a certain ethnic or religious group will storm out of a session as soon as the word "abortion" is uttered, he/she should not interpret the provider's suggestion of abortion in order to maintain harmony in the session.
   - ○ True ○ False

13. The following example is not an interpreter's violation of HIPAA, since the interpreter is acting out of culture consideration and respect: The interpreter goes to the waiting room and tells a relative; "I just checked and your sister/daughter is doing well, do not worry!"
   - ○ True ○ False

14. HIPAA stands for Health Insurance Portability and Accountability Act.
   - ○ True ○ False

15. According to JCAHO guidelines, interpreters are not required to be knowledgeable in emergency codes for the organization, wear their badges, and follow codes for contagious disease, as well as other policies.
   - ○ True ○ False

16. As an interpreter you must always check disclosure policies from each institution contracting with you, also keeping in mind the existence of State and Federal laws.
   - ○ True ○ False

17. In some US states, medical interpreters are considered mandatory reporters for any kind of child, elderly, and person with a psychiatric illness and/or suffering from a physical challenge abuse or mistreatment that they became aware of through the interpretation session.
   - ○ True ○ False

18. Interpreters should follow HIPAA and JCAHO confidentiality policies only during working hours and they are not bound to respect them beyond the interpreter's tenure with the contracting organization.
   - ○ True ○ False

19. Since a contracting organization requests the interpreter to call the patient to remind his/her of an appointment with the oncologist, if the patient is not home it is alright for the interpreter to leave a message with an individual other than the patient or on the answering machine.
   - ○ True ○ False

PO Box 2308, Woburn, MA 01888-0508, **p:** 781-729-3736, **www.EmbracingCulture.com**

PO Box 6401, Manchester, NH 03108, **p:** 1-888-678-CCCS

Lesson Two: Class Activities
The Different Roles of the Interpreter

1. *Bridging the Gap*, a training manual for medical interpreters by the Cross Cultural Healthcare Program, visually depicts the various roles of an interpreter in a diagram. Imagine a pyramid with several layers. From its base up to almost the middle of the pyramid, the interpreter works as the conduit of information. The increasingly smaller layers represent the roles of clarifier, culture broker, and, at the peak of the pyramid, advocate.

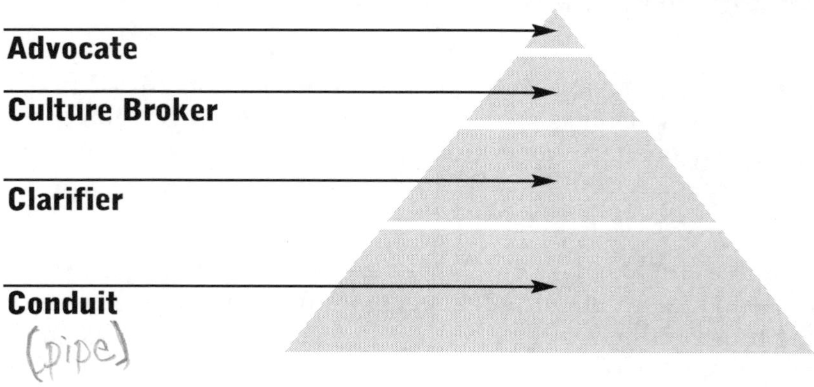

What is the role that the interpreter plays most of the time?

____

____

____

____

____

____

What is the difference between the roles?

____

____

____

____

____

____

CONDUIT

This is the most recommended role for medical interpreters. The interpreter listens to the speaker, understands the information and immediately conveys the information as close to the speaker's register as possible. In this case, the interpreter plays the role of a bridge, communicating by sticking to the spoken content and words. Imagine yourself carrying a big bag full of information that does not belong to you. You are only the messenger or transporter. On one side of the bridge you collect all the information (content and words), and close the bag. When you cross to the opposite side, you just open the bag and let the information roll out in the appropriate target language. Remember that you do not open the bag on the way over and you do not add or delete information. The information should be kept as pure as possible.

CLARIFIER

The second most common role of the interpreter is that of clarifier, one who is ever-ready to adjust to any spoken register in order to produce a linguistic equivalent, and asks questions to ascertain the true meaning of a speaker's ambiguous term or phrase. For example, in the US, the use of the term Special Education can be a description replete with cultural implications. Although interpreters may find the transliteration of the words "Special" and "Education," they may have a harder time rendering the term's true meaning. When this happens, the interpreter must inform both parties of the need for clarification, so that an accurate meaning of this term can be precisely rendered.

CULTURE BROKER

This is the role an interpreter takes when he or she becomes aware of possible misunderstandings in the communication between a patient and provider. For example, during a mental status examination, (to determine if the patient is oriented in time, place and person), a patient may be asked where he/she lives. The patient may answer, "In a blue house near the old tire factory." Unless the interpreter steps in, there is a possibility that the provider will immediately assume that this patient is not oriented in place. In this case, the interpreter needs to inform the provider if this is a common description coming from a person of a given age and immigrant group. The interpreter could suggest another method the provider might use in order to determine if the person is oriented in place. Of course, in any culture brokering, the interpreter must be sure to never present a personal opinion as a fact and should always preface any coaching with a tactful comment such as, "It may not be the case in this particular situation, but in my experience (this type of reaction) is common among members of (a certain) community, but perhaps you can check in with the patient on this issue." You might want to initiate your statement by using "It seems to me" or "I have noticed."

PO Box 2308, Woburn, MA 01888-0508, **p:** 781-729-3736, **www.EmbracingCulture.com**
PO Box 6401, Manchester, NH 03108, **p:** 1-888-678-CCCS

THE ADVOCATE

In this role the interpreter will take a side and speak on behalf of another person, usually the patient. This role is more problematic for the interpreter. He or she may take on this role but should first consult with the hiring institution's policies. Some organizations do call on their interpreters to act as patient advocates, so remember: You can fight for a cause without causing a fight! Be professional! Fortunately, in most cases, medical interpreters are not expected to serve as advocates, but rather to share their concerns with a supervisor who has the authority to make any change, if necessary.

The feeling of frustration and inadequacy resulting from an inability to implement a change (on the spot, so to speak) is one of the most difficult pills to swallow. The positive aspect is that, being removed from this awkward position, allows the interpreter to concentrate solely on the information spoken, thus permitting a more faithful rendition. Clearly then, it is better for interpreters to stay within their role as conduits, only occasionally crossing into the roles of clarifier and culture broker.

> Wow!! We are asking interpreters to simultaneously exercise the sensitivity of an artist, the objectivity of a scientist, and the compassion of a therapist, while at the same time, maintaining an equal balance among provider, patient and interpreter triad.

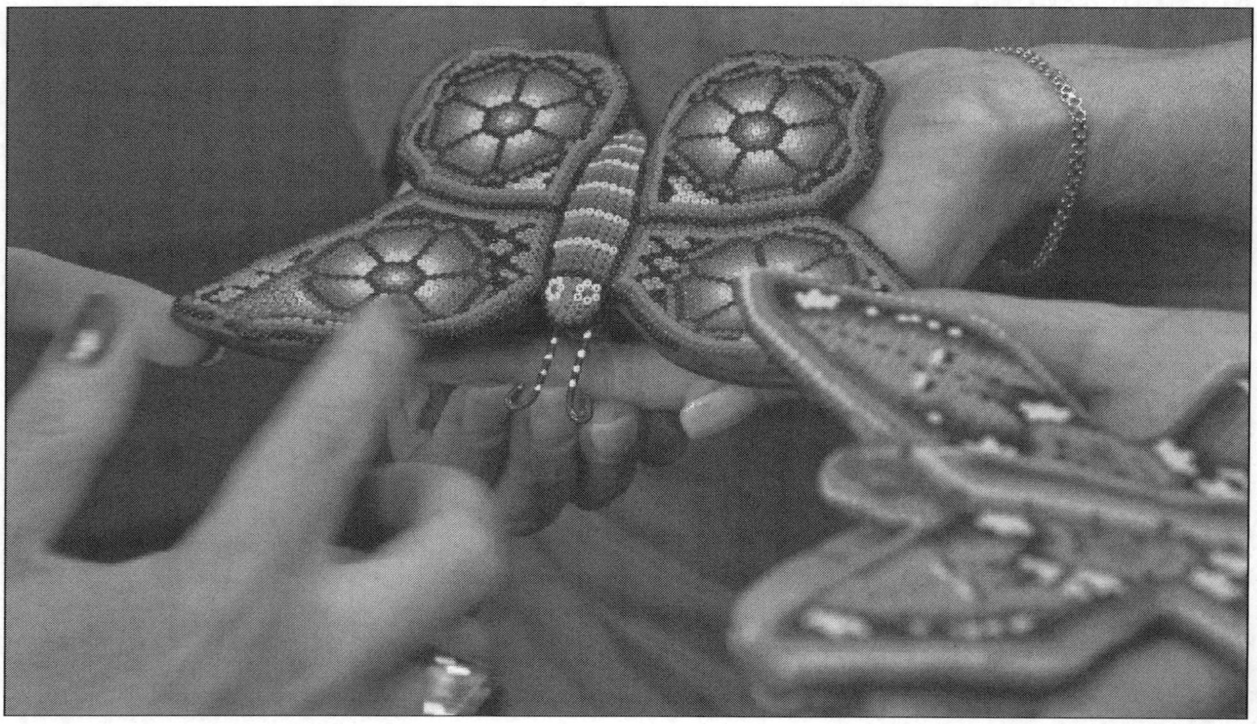

2. Watch vignettes from the video "Mental Health Interpreting: A Mentored Curriculum"

Video Vignette #2

1. What went wrong in this session?

Not speak in 1st person / Start with a pre-session with patient CIFE

2. What role(s) did the interpreter play?

3. What is your assessment of the interpreter's performance?

not so well

4. Was there something the interpreter could have done in order to prevent that embarrassing situation?

CIFE

PO Box 2308, Woburn, MA 01888-0508, **p:** 781-729-3736, **www.EmbracingCulture.com**
PO Box 6401, Manchester, NH 03108, **p:** 1-888-678-CCCS

Video Vignette #3: Cultural Attitudes toward Mental Illness (Part 1)

1. What was the problem?

2. What role(s) did the interpreter play in the session?

3. Comment on the way the interpreter handled the situation.

4. What did the interpreter ask the doctor for at the end?

(Part 2)

5. Why is the post-session important?

____

____

____

6. What did the interpreter suggest in order to help the doctor bridge the cultural gap?

____

____

____

Video Vignette #4: I Can't Do Your Job for You

1. What did the doctor ask the interpreter for?

____

____

____

2. What was the interpreter's reaction? How do you feel about it?

____

____

____

PO Box 2308, Woburn, MA 01888-0508, **p:** 781-729-3736, **www.EmbracingCulture.com**
PO Box 6401, Manchester, NH 03108, **p:** 1-888-678-CCCS

THE INTERPRETER AS A BUTTERFLY:

Imagine the interpreter as a beautiful butterfly with a great strong body, full of linguistic and cultural knowledge. On the body of this butterfly rest two sets of wings. One wing is the provider and the other wing, the client. Beneath each of these upper wings are two lower wings.

The two lower wings are the wings that store information regarding the policies, ethics and guidelines the interpreter is expected to follow.

The client guidelines and policies, located on the lower left wing inform you about how to proceed professionally with the client. The provider guidelines, on the lower right wing, inform you about how to proceed as a professional when working with the provider.

The body or center of the butterfly serves to connect the two wings. Without the body neither wing can exist, and without the wings the body has no meaning.

But when the body unites the two wings, a beautiful creature comes to life. An interpreter is a bridge between the two wings. And what these two wings have in common is the need for the interpreter (body). An interpreter treasures and honors his /her uniting role by maintaining grace, strength and balance, and by showing both wings the respect that leads to trust, which in turn leads to greater communication, and ultimately to healing.

What happens if you cut the wing of the provider?

What happens if you cut the wing of the patient?

What happens if the provider or patient cut the body of the butterfly, the interpreter?

PO Box 2308, Woburn, MA 01888-0508, **p:** 781-729-3736, **www.EmbracingCulture.com**
PO Box 6401, Manchester, NH 03108, **p:** 1-888-678-CCCS

Creating this incredible balance of accurately representing the voices spoken by not adding, distorting or omitting information is a skill that takes practice and a good understanding of one's values. Interpreters cannot control the information being shared, but they can manage their own feelings as they get triggered by both or one of the triadic members.

The interpreter is in some fashion the mailperson who delivers the mail even if the person at the receiving end is not nice or the sender mailed an ugly post card. The job of the mailperson is to deliver the mail on time to the right address undamaged, unopened and uncensored!

IMPARTIALITY AND TRANSPARENCY

What is the difference between impartiality and transparency?

side — not to hide
opinion — anything
judgement — not to omitt

How difficult is it to remain impartial? What situations might be challenging for you to remain impartial?

Lost of respect / stereotype
Domestic abuse
Alcohol Abuse

A fundamental rule in all the interpreter handbooks we have seen is that interpreters must be impartial. Likely, the impartiality clause was instituted to teach interpreters that they cannot take sides or impose their own ideas in a session, even if they personally believe they are doing a good deed. But the concept of impartiality has often been taken to extremes. Some interpreters argue that culture brokering or coaching is, in itself, a violation of impartiality, since the culture broker imposes a personal observation on the triadic encounter.

Do you agree? Is it possible to be an effective culture broker or coach while maintaining neutrality in the triadic encounter?

Yes - be professional

It is noteworthy that even professionals with many years of experience struggle with impartiality. The act of acknowledging this struggle, together with the ability to manage personal discomfort, is called transparency. In transparency, the interpreter must be careful not to let transference issues (unconscious feelings related to the ways in which the interpreter's own relationships with family and connection to culture influence his or her behavior as a culture broker), interfere with the triadic relationship.

A transparent interpreter, rather than omitting information for whatever reason, would first acknowledge a perceived cultural conflict in a private conversation with the provider and then collaborate in the provider's search for healthy alternatives. Interpreters have feelings about situations and people, but they cannot impose nor act on those feelings and then become the center of attention. The session is about the patient, not the interpreter. Interpreters should understand themselves and "find their center" so that their values are not imposed (become the center of attention) in a session.

How is transference a problem in the triadic encounter?

How would you handle triadic encounters where YOUR taboos are challenged?

PO Box 2308, Woburn, MA 01888-0508, **p:** 781-729-3736, **www.EmbracingCulture.com**
PO Box 6401, Manchester, NH 03108, **p:** 1-888-678-CCCS

REFLECT:

What would you do if you hadto interpret for potential taboo situations?
Write down your first feeling when you read the following:

substance abuse?	Anihilate yourself?
abortion?	My deassion
birth control?	Absolutely
sexual orientation issues?	Totally necessary
battered women?	Unacceptable
sexual abuse?	Crime
other? Euthanasia	Right to decide for your life

You can only manage yourself and not others. Creating a balance in the triadic relationship makes sense for most professional interpreters, but in the real world of interpreting it is not always easy. No matter how many trainings an interpreter has on the importance of being impartial, this is not an easy undertaking. We know that as human beings we bring into our interpreting our own understanding of human behavior, choices and how one handles an illness.

Let's consider alcoholism. What comes to your mind when you hear the word "alcoholism"?

THINK:

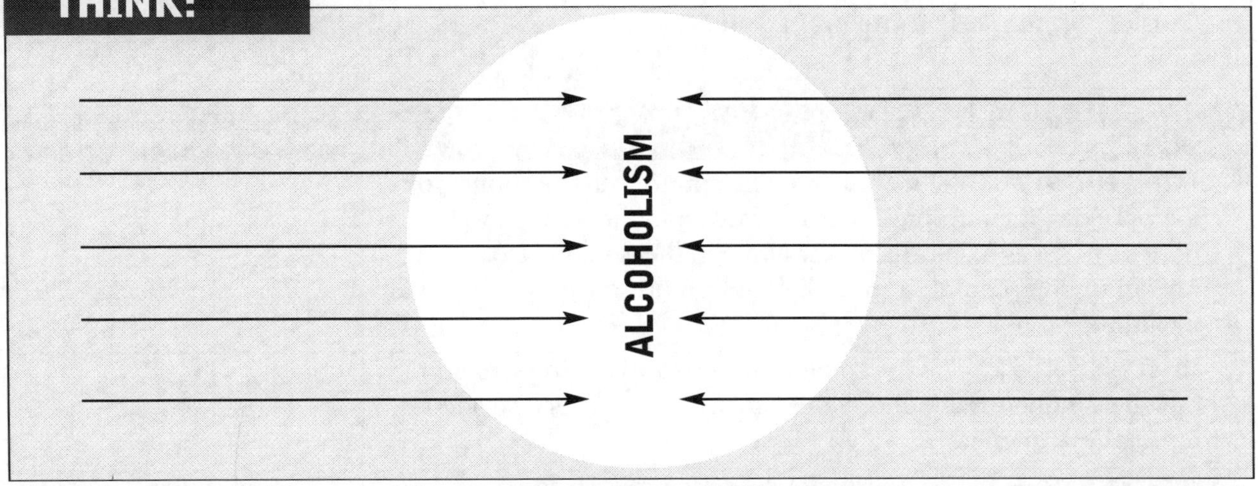

Alcoholism is probably one of the most misunderstood illnesses by interpreters for cultural and religious reasons. Part of this illness and many other chronic illnesses is the denial of having it. Providers, although caring, are very straightforward about asking questions. This behavior can be perceived as "distant" by the interpreter.

Also, alcoholism is one of the most prevalent illnesses among us and our families. Often it carries a stigma and it is perceived as a character issue.

Part of alcoholism is the denial of having it. Interpreters who do not understand this dynamic may feel pulled to act as culture brokers leading to an unhealthy dynamic by creating an alliance between the patient and the interpreter. In order to assess the potential alcoholism, providers ask four main questions called CAGE.

Case: CAGE Assessment

This is a tense session between the provider and the patient. Read the following case and review which interventions you may take as a professional interpreter.

NP:	Mr. Colombaro, have you ever felt like you could cut down on your drinking?
PT:	I do not need to; I only drink at my meals.
NP:	I understand but can you not drink for the next four weeks?
PT:	*(Patient crosses his arms and gets a bit agitated)* OK doctor!
NP:	You seemed a bit annoyed when I asked you to cut down?
PT:	What do you want me to say, I am a good man! My wife is the one… and I love my kids!
NP:	Did you ever feel guilty about your drinking?
PT:	Only when my kids beg me not to drink…. my wife is putting things in their heads!
NP:	Do you need an eye-opener in the morning?
PT:	No.

PO Box 2308, Woburn, MA 01888-0508, **p:** 781-729-3736, **www.EmbracingCulture.com**
PO Box 6401, Manchester, NH 03108, **p:** 1-888-678-CCCS

CRITICAL THINKING:

Now that you understand the CAGE assessment tool, note which intervention you may consider appropriate or inappropriate.

	Appropriate	Inappropriate
Intervention #1. Before finishing interpreting all questions from the provider, the interpreter senses tension in the session and decides to act as a culture broker while in the session "Doctor, in my culture it is common for individuals to drink a glass of wine at mealtime."		✓
Intervention #2. The interpreter interprets all the information but she is not clear about the meaning of "eye opener", so she repeats "eye opener".		✓
Intervention #3. The interpreter asks the provider for clarification of the word "eye-opener" and states: "Doctor I do not believe that the patient understands the term 'eye-opener'."		✓
Intervention #4. The interpreter literally interprets "eye-opener" without the correct meaning. The patient seems nervous but does not ask for clarification and the session continues.		✓
Intervention #5. The Interpreter takes it on her own to explain "eye-opener" to the patient, without informing the doctor of what is being said.		✓
Intervention #6. The interpreter leaves the session and the patient's wife is looking concerned and worried in the waiting room. Tearfully she comes to the interpreter and asks if everything is ok with her husband; she is concerned with his drinking. The interpreter shrugs her shoulders and states "your husband is fine, he answered "no" to all the CAGE questions."		✓

Be aware that your willingness to act outside the conduit role might be based on your perceived feelings about an illness or situation as opposed to the dynamic of the patient and provider relationship. It is important that you assess your own feelings and biases as those may interfere with your ability to remain impartial.

The following six cases require that you take different roles as an interpreter. You may find some challenging words, dynamics and misunderstandings.

APPLY CRITICAL THINKING:

In small groups, read the following cases and note the different roles the interpreter may have. Be ready to share it with the whole class. As an interpreter, which of the roles should you be taking?

Case #1
A visit to the Nurse Practitioner

NP: Good morning. I will be your Nurse Practitioner today. I see that you were referred to the eye doctor. Did you have any luck with this follow-up?

Patient: Yes, the doctor gave me a special cream to cut down the itching and I am feeling better.

NP: I am glad you saw the eye doctor. Your reaction looked a bit more serious than just a simple reaction to hay fever.

Patient: I know, thank my doctor for the referral.

NP: Anyway I just want to make sure that you are washing your hands frequently and well, to prevent any further infection by the nasty germs that got into your eye.

Patient: You are so nice. I live with a friend who is having trouble with her drinking, Can I ask her to see you?

NP: Sure, what is your friend's name?

Case #2:
Angelica, 7-month-old baby

You are called to the ER to interpret for Luz, a young mother in her early twenties. She insists that her 7-month-old baby, Angelica, suffers from "caída de la mollera" or "fallen fontanelle." Yesterday, Angelica was breast-feeding when the doorbell rang. Luz quickly withdrew her nipple from the infant's mouth and ran to answer the door. The next morning, she noticed a "soft spot" where the fontanelle of the frontal bone of the cranium fell. Later, as the baby breathed, the spot would sometimes vibrate.

Luz is worried, because her mother had told her that the "caída" resulted in a downward projection of the palate, which inhibits an infant's ability to ingest food. Further complicating her situation is the fact that the baby hasn't breastfed since, and has cried incessantly. Luz feels guilty that she withdrew her nipple so quickly and says that perhaps, if she had given Angelica enough time to feed, this never would have happened.

When asked what she had done to treat the baby's symptoms, Luz explained that she had placed her thumb inside the baby's mouth and applied upward pressure on the distended palate. At the same time, she had applied an external "pull technique" by exerting a sucking pressure on the fontanelle with her mouth. A neighbor had also instructed her to hold Angelica upside down and brusquely shake her body toward the head. They had tried this twice and applied a poultice of fresh soap shavings to the depression of the head, which she removed only when dressing the baby to come to the ER.

The nurse practitioner is indignant and sneers, "Has it ever occurred to you that maybe the kid cries because you're shaking the daylights out of her? Don't you know you're hurting the baby?" Luz looks confused and hurt. "I'm a good mother," she says.

Case #3:
Sabrina is 5 years old.

For about two weeks, Sabrina has been unable to sleep soundly. Night after night, she wakes her mother with screams. Her mother, Consuelo, rushes to console her, but she shakes and weeps uncontrollably. Consuelo is convinced that her daughter suffers from "mal ojo" or "evil eye." Several days ago, she took Sabrina to a local curandero (folk healer), who recommended several herbal remedies. When these didn't work, the curandero tried "sweeping" or passing an egg over the contours of Sabrina's body while chanting magical-religious ritual phrases. After this, Sabrina's condition worsened. Consuelo believes that perhaps the curandero's spirit is not as strong as the spirit of the person who, through "mal ojo," introduced this disorder in her daughter's life.

The medical assistant steps out of the room momentarily, and you follow. He turns to you and says, "Well, NO WONDER the girl has nightmares! That voodoo is enough to scare anybody!"

* Cultural - Broker *
→ Conduit
* Clarifier -

→ Perfect case to do a Pre-sesion w. the Provider (+ M. Assistant) if possible before the Provider comes in.

PO Box 2308, Woburn, MA 01888-0508, **p:** 781-729-3736, **www.EmbracingCulture.com**
PO Box 6401, Manchester, NH 03108, **p:** 1-888-678-CCCS

Case #4:
Manuela has recently immigrated to this country.

She brought her baby in for his 1-year check-up. He's a hefty baby, and you think he's just adorable! But the pediatrician weighs him and he's several pounds overweight. He suggests that Manuela put the baby on a diet. She looks shocked. The doctor explains that by over-feeding the baby, Manuela could actually harm him. Tears well up in her eyes and she says to you, "I love my baby! How can he say I'm a bad mother?" Later, during the post-session, the doctor comments, "I just can't understand why these people insist on over-feeding their babies!" You, as an interpreter, know that in Manuela's culture, a robust or "well-fleshed" body, defines a healthy person.

Case #5:
TB case worker who is also the interpreter

After her last visit to Haiti, Ms. Joseph started losing weight and coughing. After a few weeks, her cough resolved. However, the Doctor found a large spot of pneumonia in the right upper lobe of her lung. He did tests on some sputum and found proof that Ms. Joseph had TB. Tuberculosi

She is waiting in the waiting room to find out which medicine she will have to take. She hopes it is not the medicine that bothers her.

The only Haitian interpreter at the clinic is Mr. St. Louis. He is well known for helping many people in the Haitian Creole-speaking community.

Ms. Joseph knows Mr. St. Louis; he had interpreted when many of her friends were forced to take medicine for TB even when they were not sick.

Mr. St. Louis also interpreted for Ms. Joseph when the school wanted to hold back her son in 6th grade. "It will give him more exposure to English," he had said.

Ms. Joseph was worried. Which side is Mr. St. Louis on? Was he helping abuse his own people like the doctors did in Haiti or was he really trying to help?

Ms. J: Hello Mr. St. Louis.

Mr. S: How are you, Ms. Joseph? Before we go in, I want to remind you to go to register for citizenship class tomorrow. We need to have more of our people become citizens so we can vote and get more services from the politicians.

Ms. J: I will do it.

Doctor: Ms. Joseph, will you come in? Hello Mr. Saint Louis. It's good to see you again!

Mr. S: It's good to see you too, Doctor.

Doctor: Ms. Joseph, I got all the tests back and your pneumonia is actually TB.

Ms. J: I can't believe a little cough could be TB.

Doctor: You will have to have your children checked and most likely they will need to take a medicine as well.

Ms. J: I will do that.

Doctor: Ms. Joseph, you have active TB. You'll need to take three medicines for the next 6 months. You will not be able to work in the nursing home until you have three sputum samples examined and you are free of TB bugs upon examination.

Ms. J: (Starts to cry, speaks to Mr. S. in Creole.) This is all your fault. You help them keep our children back and keep us from being able to work.

Doctor: What did she say?

PO Box 2308, Woburn, MA 01888-0508, **p:** 781-729-3736, **www.EmbracingCulture.com**
PO Box 6401, Manchester, NH 03108, **p:** 1-888-678-CCCS

Case #6
Wrong toes!

A patient is having his right toes amputated due to gangrene caused by poor circulation and uncontrolled diabetes.

At the operating room the interpreter becomes aware that there is a misunderstanding. The surgeon keeps referring to the patients' left toes but looks at his right toes.

The interpreter at first interprets as the provider states "left toes," the patient seems nervous and unaware of the misunderstanding , the interpreter nicely informs the provider that it appears that there is some confusion about which toes are going to be amputated. As soon as the interpreter states his concern, he conveys the message to the patient.

The patient right away corrects the provider and states: "oh, no, it is my right toes!"

These are just a few examples of situations that you will likely encounter in your career as a medical interpreter. Further discussing these case scenarios and others more relevant to the population you work with will broaden your horizons and better equip you in how to best apply your interpreter roles. Remember to check the standards of practice and the institution's policies in regards to your roles.

Interpreting Glossary Matching Exercise

Exercise II	
1. Clarifier	a. Interpreter provides the necessary cultural framework for understanding the message being interpreted
2. Conduit	b. Rendering in one language what has been said in another: no additions, omissions, editing or polishing
3. Culture Broker	c. Interpreter adjusts the level of verbal and cultural expression of the patient, explains or makes word pictures of terms that have no linguistic equivalent and checks for understanding
4. Culture Coach	d. The interpreter, with permission from his/her sponsoring organization, takes a direct and active role in assisting patients in dealing with problems such as discrimination and financial matters
5. Patient Advocate	e. Interpreter provides the necessary cultural framework to the provider by encouraging him/her to further explore the patient's cultural belief system

Exercise II	
1. Accuracy	a. Interpreter asks provider or patient to break down meaning of information for an accurate interpretation
2. Clarification	b. Interpreter must encourage both patient and provider to address each other directly, both verbally and nonverbally, to avoid the tendency both parties have to want to form an alliance with the interpreter
3. Completeness	c. Exact to the meaning; conveying the spirit and content of what is being said
4. Explanation	d. Everything said by either provider or patient will be transmitted. Interpreter waits for speaker to complete thought before starting the interpretation
5. Interpretation	e. In the pre-session, interpreter sets clear expectations of his/her role, stressing the elements of accuracy, completeness, and confidentiality. Interpreter also considers the seating arrangement
6. Managing the triadic relationship	f. Conversion of a message from a source language into an equivalent message in the target language
7. Note-taking	g. Interpreter checks whether listener clearly understands what is being said and looks for linguistic/cultural idiosyncracies to give an accurate interpretation
8. Repetition	h. Interpreter should ask for repetition if message is not heard or understood, always clarifying that the request is due to the interpreter's own need

PO Box 2308, Woburn, MA 01888-0508, **p:** 781-729-3736, **www.EmbracingCulture.com**
PO Box 6401, Manchester, NH 03108, **p:** 1-888-678-CCCS

Matching Exercise continued:

	9. Setting the stage	i. A tool that helps the interpreter retain information and be accurate
	10. Visualization	j. Mental pictures
Exercise III		
	1. Cultural interface	a. Definition; significance
	2. Ethical behavior	b. Level of comprehension and depth of expression on the part of the interpreter which can be expanded through clarification and management of the flow of communication
	3. Evaluation tool	c. Interpreter interprets message at the same linguistic level in which it was originally spoken
	4. Interpreting skills	d. Interpreter has to be accurate, non-judgmental, refrain from conveying own thoughts, avoid being arbitrary, and respect the confidential nature of the provider/patient relationship
	5. Linguistic proficiency	e. Level of vocabulary and ability to speak fluently and write in source and target languages
	6. Meaning	f. "Catch words" or verbal triggers
	7. Message	g. Language is an expression of culture. Interpreter has to know the words that are being used and understand the cultural context in which they are spoken
	8. Non-verbal clues	h. Body language and cultural innuendos
	9. Register	i. Standards of practice which can be used to determine whether or not an interpreter has achieved mastery of the required skills
	10. Verbal clues	j. Communicated information

Lesson Two: Homework
The Different Roles of the Interpreter

1. Go over your notes for today's class and read section "Additional Resources"
2. Go over CAGE interpreter interventions. Answer the following questions:
   a) Which intervention did you find most appropriate and why?
   b) Look for a standard of practice that supports your position.
   c) Which intervention did you find least appropriate and why?
   d) Look for a standard of practice that supports your position.
3. Read and practice ALL role-plays for this lesson and continue to develop your glossary.
4. Complete pain table.

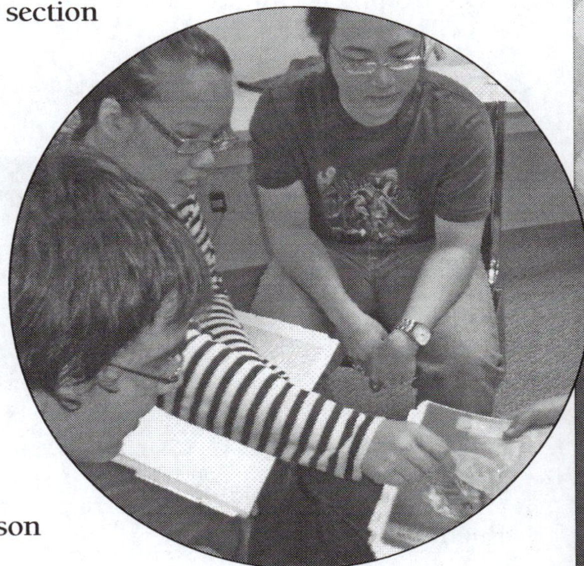

Different Types of Pain

English	Target Language
1. Ache	dolor / dolor persistente
2. Lancinanting	punzante
3. Throbbing	dolor pulsátil (con cada latido del corazón)
4. Dull	embotado
5. Band-like	presionante (?)
6. Sharp	dolor agudo / punzante
7. Needle-like	dolor como 1 pinchazo
8. Pressure	presión
9. Tearing or Searing	Desgarro
10. Grabbing	arrebatador (?) agarrado (?)
11. Burning	ardor / escozor / quemazón
12. Knife-like	punzante
13. Piercing	~~punzante~~ / perforación

Stiffness — Rigidez (muscular)
Rigidity / cramp → calambre

PO Box 2308, Woburn, MA 01888-0508, **p:** 781-729-3736, **www.EmbracingCulture.com**
PO Box 6401, Manchester, NH 03108, **p:** 1-888-678-CCCS

5. Complete Immunization table in your Target Language.

Know Your Immunizations

ENGLISH	TARGET LANGUAGE
Diphtheria	Difteria
Haemophilus Influenzae Type B (HIB)	Same
Hepatitis B	Hepatitis B
Measles	Sarampión
Mumps	Paperas
Pertussis	Tos Ferina
Pneumococcal	Neumocócica (Neumonía)
Polio	Polio / Poliomelitis
Rubella / German Measles	Rubéola
Small Pox	Viruela
Tetanus	Tétano
Varicella (Chicken Pox)	Varicela

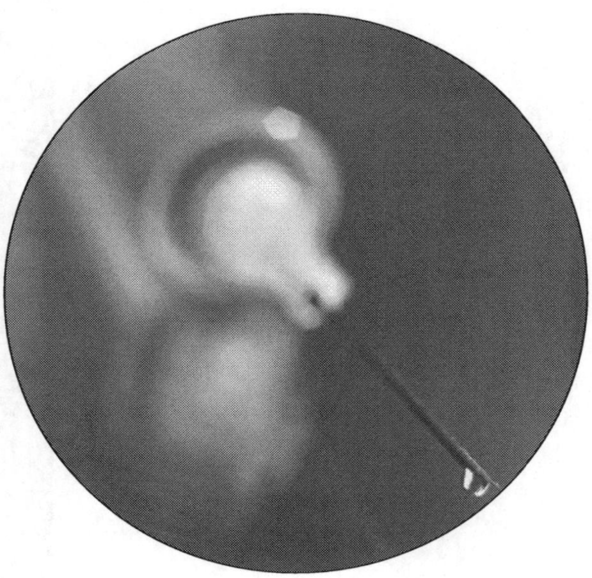

6. The following is a health report for a 15-year old female.

   Translate the immunization history.

Health Report for Schools, Camps, and Employers

Name: Muluken Gebru **Gender:** Female **Date of birth:** 12/6/93

Immunization History:

Name	Date(s) Administered
• DTP Vaccine	02/04/1994, 05/06/1994, 07/08/1994, 03/24/1995
• DTaP Vaccine	03/01/1995
• HPV Vaccine (6, 11, 16, 18)	07/03/2007, 07/07/2008, 07/01/2009
• Hep A Vaccine Pedi/Adol-2 Does Sched	10/17/2001, 07/08/2003
• Hep B Vaccine (Recombinant)	12/06/1993,02/04/94, 09/16/1994
• Hflu b conj (HbOC)	02/04/1994, 05/06/1994, 07/08/1994, 01/31/1995
• MMR Vaccine	01/31/1995, 07/28/1997
• Meningoc IM (Menactra) Vaccine	05/27/2005
• Polio Vaccine (Oral,Trivalent)	02/04/1994, 05/06/1994, 03/24/1995, 03/01/1999
• TB Test	01/31/1995
• Td Vaccine (Adult)	05/27/2005
• TdaP	07/07/2008
• Vacricella Vaccine	01/29/1997, 07/01/2009

Immunizations are up to date.
Allergies: Review of patient's allergies indicates no active TB
TB Risk Assessment: Low
Current Health Issues: No significant health issues
Medications: None
Physical Exam: **Date:** 07/1/2009 **Provider:** Richard S. Lane

BP 108/60/ Ht 5'4" (1.626 m) / W 131 lb 6.4 oz (59.603 kg) Body mass index is 22. 55 kg/(m^2). 74.35% of growth percentile based on BMI-for-age.
Physical exam was normal.

Restrictions: No restrictions. May participate fully in competitive sports.

PPD Result/Lab results:	HGB	12.4	1/29/1997
	HGT	35.6	1/29/1997

Hearing/Vision Screen: (Done by school RN)

Richard Lane, MD Date: 7/1/2009

PO Box 2308, Woburn, MA 01888-0508, **p:** 781-729-3736, **www.EmbracingCulture.com**
PO Box 6401, Manchester, NH 03108, **p:** 1-888-678-CCCS

Role-Plays

THE ART OF MEDICAL INTERPRETATION®

Lesson Two: Role-Plays
The Different Roles of the Interpreter

Work individually at first:

- Read the entire role-play
- Get a general sense of its meaning
- Circle the most challenging medical terms
- Apply the Samurai! technique to those terms
- Read the role-play again for a deeper understanding
- Find an accurate equivalent in the target language

Work in a language-specific group of friends, fellow students or colleagues:

- Share your doubts
- Ask for other ways of expressing the same meaning
- Develop a glossary
- Check the dictionary
- Practice the role-plays – remember to do CIFE for all your role-plays
- Have your colleagues observe you and provide feedback on your accuracy and register.
- These colleagues can keep track of any omissions, additions, mistakes or distortions in your interpreting and point these out to you in a follow-up discussion.

Student Interpreter Evaluation

Student Name ____________________ Date ________

Language ____________________

Mode of Interpreting (check one): ☐ Consecutive ☐ Simultaneous

Role-Play/System ____________________

Areas Observed ____________________

Accuracy

Register ____________________

Omissions ____________________

Additions ____________________

Distortions ____________________

Pronunciation ____________________

Speaker's emotions conveyed? ____________________

Explain ____________________

Technique

General flow ____________________

Flow when requesting clarification ____________________

Speed ____________________

Eye Contact ____________________

Distracting Habits ____________________

Ethical Issues

Answered questions for patient? ____________________

Advised patient? ____________________

Vocabulary Expansion Recommendations

____

____

Other Recommendations

____

____

Language Coach Signature ____________________ Date ________

Role-Play 4: Do I Need Vaccines?

	Pronunciation	Additions	Omissions	Mistakes
Mother: Doctor, I am not sure if I should let my kids have the vaccines you are recommending.				
Doctor: I understand your feelings and we now hear such bad press about the vaccines; but the shots will produce antibodies that will protect your child and the public from the presence of antigens that can do a lot of harm to anyone's health.				
Mother: Antibodies?				
Doctor: Antibodies are proteins produced by the body to neutralize or eliminate toxins or disease-carrying organisms for specific diseases.				
Mother: So, does it mean that you will be injecting the antibodies?				
Doctor: Yes. In some ways there are two types of immunity: active and passive. The active immunity is long-lasting.				
Mother: I am very confused; so we have the virus inside us?				
Doctor: Interesting... active immunity may be a result to the exposure to a disease organism that triggers the immune system to produce antibodies to that disease. This exposure through infection with the actual disease may result in a natural immunity.				
Mother: OK, so I get the antibody when I get the disease?				
Doctor: As you get sick and your body has survived the disease, you will develop a natural protection against the disease. It is like the body recognizes the infection and built in protection.				
Mother: So what doesn't kill you makes you stronger!				
Doctor: Yes, but not everyone has a positive outcome, so we created vaccines!				
Mother: So this is the passive immunity that you mentioned earlier?				
Doctor: Good question! The MMR vaccine will contain just enough antibodies that are weak enough not to give you the full blown disease, but possibly giving you some minor side effects; such as in the case of rubella, you may get the following reaction when vaccinated: Burning or stinging at the injection site, cough, diarrhea, dizziness, feeling ill, fever, headache, nausea, painful or swollen joints, sore throat, vomiting.				

continued

PO Box 2308, Woburn, MA 01888-0508, **p:** 781-729-3736, **www.EmbracingCulture.com**
PO Box 6401, Manchester, NH 03108, **p:** 1-888-678-CCCS

Role-Play 4 *(continued)*

	Pronunciation	Additions	Omissions	Mistakes
Mother: So, my daughter if not vaccinated when pregnant and if exposed to Rubella during her pregnancy could give birth to a baby with birth defects?				
Doctor: Yes, it all could happen and it starts with contact with an infected person, through coughing and sneezing and there is a 20% possibility that her baby could suffer from deafness, cataracts, heart defects, mental retardation, and liver and spleen damage. The Rubella vaccine is given in 2 doses with the MMR vaccine: • The first dose at 12-15 months of age • The second dose at 4-6 years of age These are the recommended ages; but children can get the second dose at any age, as long as it is at least 28 days after the first dose.				
Mother: But according to the literature the MMR vaccine is not recommended for everybody. There are severe side effects such as allergic reactions like rash, hives, itching, difficulty breathing, tightness in the chest, swelling of the mouth, face, lips, or tongue, pain, redness, or swelling at the injection site; swelling of the glands in the jaw; swelling of the testicles.				
Doctor: One needs to weigh the pros and cons. There is a very small percentage of those who get such severe side effects from the vaccine. For the most part the side effects are minor (for example, a sore arm or low-grade fever) and go away within a few days. **Mother:** You sold me, the vaccine for Measles, Mumps and Rubella!				
Doctor: Good!				
Break It Down	☐	☐	☐	☐

☐ **CIFE with patient** ☐ **CIFE with provider** ☐ **FLOW** ☐ **REGISTER**

Role-Play 4: Glossary

continued

1. Pathology (diseases, conditions)

2. Laboratory Tests and Diagnostic Procedures

3. Treatment Procedures

4. Idiomatic Expressions (if any)

5. Other (vocabulary in this particular role-play that you feel is important/relevant or that you anticipate problems with)

PO Box 2308, Woburn, MA 01888-0508, **p:** 781-729-3736, **www.EmbracingCulture.com**
PO Box 6401, Manchester, NH 03108, **p:** 1-888-678-CCCS

Role-Play 5: Chicken Pox

	Pronunciation	Additions	Omissions	Mistakes
Mother: Doctor do you think my son has chicken pox? He has rash like blisters all over his body.				
MD: *(Looking towards son)* So, you're not feeling so hot?				
Patient: I got up this morning and I had all these red spots on my face! It was so gross!				
MD: How were you feeling before the spots appeared?				
Patient: Really yucky! I had a runny nose and a cough. I thought it was just a cold, but my mom said today that it's chicken pox. That's a really weird name.				
MD: Chicken pox got its name from a vegetable. People used to think that the red bumps looked like chickpeas on skin. And a long time ago, the word "pox" meant bad luck. Getting chicken pox might seem like bad luck to you, but the word "pox" now refers to skin eruptions like the ones on your face and body.				
Patient: My friend Tommy had chicken pox. My mother says I got it from him. But when I was playing with Tommy, he didn't have any spots. Do you think I got it from him?				
MD: Well, I don't know. Chicken pox is most contagious during the first 2 to 5 days that you are sick, before the rash shows up. So if it was your friend Tommy who gave it to you, he probably didn't even know he had it yet!				
Patient: But how do you get it?				
MD: The virus travels in tiny droplets that are too small for us to see. The first sign is something like a cold, and a person who is infected with chicken pox can easily pass it along when he coughs or sneezes.				
Patient: That's gross! I get this urge to scratch my face, but my mother told me that I was going to get marked forever!				
MD: A bath with oatmeal is very soothing and will help with the itching, but if you pop one of the blisters yourself most likely you will get a scar, so be careful!				
PT: But do I really need a Varicella vaccine?				
NP: Let me see.. (looking into medical records) … uhm, I do not have your immunization history.				
PT: I was born in another country and I got the chicken pox when I was a kid... my mother isolated me from everyone. I remember it very well and it was not fun.				

continued

Role-Play 5 *(continued)*

		Pronunciation	Additions	Omissions	Mistakes
NP:	The Varicella vaccine can prevent this disease. Currently, two doses of vaccine are recommended for children, adolescents, and adults. But if you got the disease as a child then you are ok. Let's just do a few blood tests.				
PT:	OK, my boss was insisting that I get the vaccine so her kids do not get exposed to varicella and I told her I got it as a child, so am I all set?				
	Break It Down	☐	☐	☐	☐

☐ **CIFE with patient** ☐ **CIFE with provider** ☐ **FLOW** ☐ **REGISTER**

Role-Play 5: Glossary

PO Box 2308, Woburn, MA 01888-0508, **p:** 781-729-3736, **www.EmbracingCulture.com**
PO Box 6401, Manchester, NH 03108, **p:** 1-888-678-CCCS

1. Pathology (diseases, conditions)

2. Laboratory Tests and Diagnostic Procedures

3. Treatment Procedures

4. Idiomatic Expressions (if any)

5. Other (vocabulary in this particular role-play that you feel is important/relevant or that you anticipate problems with)

Role-Play 6: D.P.T. Shot

	Pronunciation	Additions	Omissions	Mistakes
MD: It's nice to see you again. Today's visit is an important one, since Junior will be getting his first D.P.T. shot.				
Patient's father: What will this shot do to him?				
MD: Today's shot will protect him against diphtheria, whooping cough and tetanus. For full protection, your child will need three injections.				
Patient's father: What is diphtheria?				
MD: Diphtheria causes a thick covering in the back of the throat. It can lead to breathing problems, paralysis, heart failure, and even death. There are several combination vaccines used to prevent diphtheria: DTaP, Tdap, DT, and Td.				
Patient's father: Wow, that is very scary!				
MD: There are four combination vaccines used to prevent diphtheria, tetanus and pertussis: DTaP, Tdap, DT, and Td. Two of these (DTaP and DT) are given to children younger than 7 years of age, and two (Tdap and Td) are given to older children and adults.				
Patient's father: OK. I understand.				
MD: Children should get 5 doses of DTaP, one dose at each of the following ages: 2, 4, 6, and 15-18 months and 4-6 years.				
MD: DT does not contain pertussis, and is used as a substitute for DTaP for children who cannot tolerate pertussis vaccine.				
Patient's father: So my infant will be getting his first shot today?				
MD: Yes				
Patient's father: In my country, there are a lot of diseases. I didn't think there were so many diseases in America.				
MD: Vaccines give protection against many dangerous diseases, most of which are rare in the US. But one of the main reasons such diseases are uncommon in this country is the nationwide push for vaccination.				
Patient's father: How do you remember all these abbreviations Td and Tdap?				
MD: Td is a tetanus-diphtheria vaccine given to adolescents and adults as a booster shot every 10 years, or after an exposure to tetanus under some circumstances.				
Patient's father: and Tdap?				

continued

PO Box 2308, Woburn, MA 01888-0508, **p:** 781-729-3736, **www.EmbracingCulture.com**
PO Box 6401, Manchester, NH 03108, **p:** 1-888-678-CCCS

Role-Play 6 *(continued)*

	Pronunciation	Additions	Omissions	Mistakes
MD: Tdap is similar to Td but also contains protection against pertussis. A single dose of Tdap is recommended for adolescents 11 or 12 years of age, or in place of one Td booster in older adolescents and adults age 19 through 64.				
Patient's father: I got it....Are there any other vaccines my baby needs? What about those drops you gave him last time?				
MD: Yes, here are the shots your child will need to take until High School age:				
Tetanus-Diptheria-Pertussis vaccine Meningococcal vaccine HPV vaccine series Hepatitis B vaccine series Polio vaccine series Measles-Mumps-Rubella (MMR) vaccine series Varicella (chickenpox) vaccine series Influenza vaccine Pneumococcal polysaccharid (PPV) vaccine Hepatitis A vaccine series				
Patient's father: OK, I guess we have to grow a thick skin each time we drive to the clinic. This is harder when it is your kid getting the shots.				
MD: Ah, the polio vaccine! Yes, your baby received the drops by mouth at birth, and at his one-month check-up. He'll need two more doses: one today with the D.P.T. vaccine and another next month. The polio vaccine helps prevent infantile paralysis.				
Patient's father: What about the cholera vaccine? I had to get that before I could leave my country. Does the baby need it too?				
MD: Not unless you will be traveling into areas of the world with cholera!				
Break It Down	☐	☐	☐	☐

☐ **CIFE with patient** ☐ **CIFE with provider** ☐ **FLOW** ☐ **REGISTER**

Role-Play 6: Glossary

______ ______ ______

______ ______ ______

______ ______ ______

continued

1. Pathology (diseases, conditions)

2. Laboratory Tests and Diagnostic Procedures

3. Treatment Procedures

4. Idiomatic Expressions (if any)

5. Other (vocabulary in this particular role-play that you feel is important/relevant or that you anticipate problems with)

Role-Play 7: Rabies

	Pronunciation	Additions	Omissions	Mistakes
MD: Yikes! That's a nasty bite you have there!				
Patient: (crying) I was playing hide-and-seek in the park and I hid in the bushes. The skunk chased me and bit me.				
MD: The skunk was in the bushes? In the daytime?				
Patient: Yes, at first it didn't move but when I came near, it chased me and bit me.				
MD: Well, let's clean this up a bit (He begins to disinfect the cut). This may sting a little. You know, from your description, it seems like the skunk that bit you may have had rabies. To be on the safe side, I'd like you to get the rabies vaccine.				
Patient: Vaccine or shots?				
MD: The Rabies vaccine is given through a series of shots with an active immunizing agent used to prevent infection caused by the rabies virus. The vaccine works because it causes your body to produce its own protection (antibodies) against the rabies virus. Have you ever had the rabies vaccine before?				
Patient: No.				
MD: Well, it's an injection for adults and children given in several doses. You'll have one dose today; another by days three, seven, fourteen, and twenty-eight. A total of five doses. On the first day, you will also receive an injection of another medicine (rabies immune globulin).				
Patient: You mean I have to come back again? I hate shots! Am I getting it on my buttocks or on my belly?				
MD: Nowadays the vaccine is injected into the muscle of the upper arm and you may feel some tenderness.				
Patient: What if I decide not to go ahead with the shots? I hate them with a passion!				
MD: Unfortunately, this is a public health issue and we have to report it to the department of Public Health. If left untreated, you could die.				
Break It Down	☐	☐	☐	☐

☐ CIFE with patient ☐ CIFE with provider ☐ FLOW ☐ REGISTER

Role-Play 7: Glossary

______ ______ ______

______ ______ ______

continued

1. Pathology (diseases, conditions)

2. Laboratory Tests and Diagnostic Procedures

3. Treatment Procedures

4. Idiomatic Expressions (if any)

5. Other (vocabulary in this particular role-play that you feel is important/relevant or that you anticipate problems with)

Role-Play 8: BCG

	Pronunciation	Additions	Omissions	Mistakes
Mother: I want to enroll my children in school, but the school secretary told me they must first be vaccinated against tuberculosis. My children have already been vaccinated against the disease! It's a common procedure in our country.				
MD: It's possible that your children received the BCG vaccine, which is a vaccine for TB. This vaccine, however, is not widely used in the United States, but is often given to infants and small children in other countries where TB is common.				
Mother: So I am all set with the TB vaccine?				
MD: The BCG vaccine does not always protect people from TB. (Pause) The school department requires foreign-born students to have a certificate on file verifying that they are free from communicable tuberculosis.				
Mother: The school does not let my children go to school unless they have a test that starts with a P…				
MD: Yes. The PPD skin test and this initial screening must be finished before the child is allowed to attend school but if your children were vaccinated with BCG, they may have a positive reaction to a TB skin test. This reaction may be due to the BCG vaccine itself or to a latent TB infection.				
Mother: So, what do we do if they test positive?				
MD: If they have a positive reaction to the skin test, we'll do other tests to see if they have the disease. These tests usually include a chest x-ray and a test of the phlegm they cough up. Because the TB bacteria may be found in places other than the lungs, we may check your children's blood or urine, or do other tests. If they do have TB disease, they'll need to take medicine to cure it.				
Break It Down	☐	☐	☐	☐

☐ CIFE with patient ☐ CIFE with provider ☐ FLOW ☐ REGISTER

Role-Play 8: Glossary

continued

1. Pathology (diseases, conditions)

2. Laboratory Tests and Diagnostic Procedures

3. Treatment Procedures

4. Idiomatic Expressions (if any)

5. Other (vocabulary in this particular role-play that you feel is important/relevant or that you anticipate problems with)

PO Box 2308, Woburn, MA 01888-0508, **p:** 781-729-3736, **www.EmbracingCulture.com**
PO Box 6401, Manchester, NH 03108, **p:** 1-888-678-CCCS

Role-Play 9: Tetanus

	Pronunciation	Additions	Omissions	Mistakes
Patient: I was playing in the playground when I felt this sharp pain and I realized that I had stepped on a rusty nail.				
MD: (looking at the wound): Wow. The nail went through your shoe. How are you doing?				
Patient: I don't know. It was a big nail, and it looked old.				
MD: Yes, did it have rust on it?				
Patient: Yes, the nail looked pretty rusty to me, old and rusty. My foot hurts a lot. Do they have to give me one of those painful shots?				
MD: I'm sorry it hurts so much, but I will have the nurse come in and clean the cut for you. We will place a new dressing on it and the other nurse will stop by to give you the first of a series of 3 tetanus shots.				
Patient: Three!!! Why not just one?				
MD: Well, because we are uncertain if you've already been given tetanus shots. I'll ask the nurse to give you one shot now, one in a month, and the last one a year from now. I know it sounds scary, but the nurse who'll be giving the shots is the best in the clinic.				
The mother to the child: The nurse will ask you to take a deep breath, you'll feel a pinch for just a second, and then it will be all over.				
MD: (To the mother) A few patients report pain and tenderness around the area of the shot, and at times it may cause a slight fever. If she feels some pain in the arm, you're welcome to give her one Tylenol every four hours. If she gets a rash, redness or a fever with the Tylenol, please call the clinic right away.				
Patient: Do I have to go back to school today?				
MD: You may go back, but ask your mom, she might have other plans for you.				
Mother: Thank you, doctor.				
MD: You are welcome!				
MD to Mother: Mom, do not forget to make sure that her wound stays clean, and any signs of infection contact us right away and you may schedule her shots with the clinical assistant at the front desk.				
Break It Down	☐	☐	☐	☐

☐ **CIFE with patient** ☐ **CIFE with provider** ☐ **FLOW** ☐ **REGISTER**

continued

Role-Play 9: Glossary

1. Pathology (diseases, conditions)

2. Laboratory Tests and Diagnostic Procedures

3. Treatment Procedures

4. Idiomatic Expressions (if any)

5. Other (vocabulary in this particular role-play that you feel is important/relevant or that you anticipate problems with)

PO Box 2308, Woburn, MA 01888-0508, **p:** 781-729-3736, **www.EmbracingCulture.com**
PO Box 6401, Manchester, NH 03108, **p:** 1-888-678-CCCS

Role-Play 10: Mumps

	Pronunciation	Additions	Omissions	Mistakes
MD: You must be in a lot of pain. How long have you had the swelling?				
Patient: I've had the swelling in my throat for about a week. It started slowly on the left side, but got worse. Then I started feeling it on the right. After a few days, I could barely swallow or talk. Once, I tried to drink some orange juice, but the pain was so sharp I thought I was going to die!				
MD: Yes, I can feel the inflammation. The parotid salivary glands, which produce saliva for the mouth, are found toward the back of each cheek, in the area between the ear and jaw. Sometimes, when a patient has mumps, one or both sides begin to swell. You have a temperature of 103°. Why didn't you come to the clinic when the swelling began?				
Patient: I thought it was the flu, or strep throat, or something like that. I had no idea it would get this bad.				
MD: Well, it's not strep, but even if it were, you would need medical attention. A lot of sicknesses, when treated early on, don't progress to this point. Do you have swelling anywhere else?				
Patient: No, just in my throat.				
MD: That's a good thing. You know, mumps in young adult males sometimes leads to the development of orchitis, an inflammation of the testicles, a condition that can ultimately lead to a decreased sperm count.				
Patient: So, can you make me better?				
Break It Down	☐	☐	☐	☐

☐ **CIFE with patient** ☐ **CIFE with provider** ☐ **FLOW** ☐ **REGISTER**

Role-Play 10: Glossary

continued

1. Pathology (diseases, conditions)

2. Laboratory Tests and Diagnostic Procedures

3. Treatment Procedures

4. Idiomatic Expressions (if any)

5. Other (vocabulary in this particular role-play that you feel is important/relevant or that you anticipate problems with)

PO Box 2308, Woburn, MA 01888-0508, **p:** 781-729-3736, **www.EmbracingCulture.com**
PO Box 6401, Manchester, NH 03108, **p:** 1-888-678-CCCS

Role-Play 11: Malaria

	Pronunciation	Additions	Omissions	Mistakes
MD: I wish you a great vacation but before you leave let's make sure that you are well informed on how to prevent yourself from getting malaria.				
Patient: Oh, I don't think malaria is a problem where I'm going. Isn't it just a jungle disease? I'm going to stay in the city.				
MD: Actually, malaria occurs in over 100 countries and territories. In fact, more than 40% of the people in the world are at risk for malaria.				
Patient: What are the symptoms of malaria?				
MD: We get malaria from the bite of a malaria-infected mosquito and the symptoms are fever and flu-like illness, including shaking chills, headache, muscle aches, and tiredness. But nausea, vomiting, and diarrhea may also occur. Malaria may even cause anemia and jaundice (yellow coloring of the skin and eyes) because of the loss of red blood cells. These symptoms usually appear 10 to 15 days after a person is infected. If not treated promptly with effective medicines, malaria can cause severe illness and is often fatal.				
Patient: So it is like having a bad case of Flu. Is there a way to prevent it?				
MD: Malaria is caused by a parasite of the plasmodium species. This infectious disease is considered a public health issue, many people die from malaria.				
Patient: Can one keep from getting it?				
MD: We can write you a prescription for an anti-malarial drug called Malarone, which you should take exactly on schedule without missing doses. Malarone is taken once daily with food or milk, starting two days before entering a malaria risk area and continuing daily until seven days after leaving the area of malaria risk. This is a medication with few side effects; it may cause a few gastro intestinal (GI) problems and headaches. Although it's a bit expensive, around $100.00 or a bit less.				
Patient: Should I still wear long pants and sleeves just like we do for the Lyme disease tick?				
MD: Yes, wearing protective clothes is very important. You can also prevent mosquito and other insect bites by using DEET insect repellent on exposed skin and insect spray in the room where you sleep.				

continued

Role-Play 11 *(continued)*

	Pronunciation	Additions	Omissions	Mistakes
Patient: OK.				
MD: Wear long pants and long-sleeved shirts, especially from dusk to dawn. This is the time when mosquitoes that spread malaria bite. And remember to sleep under a mosquito bed net if you are not living in screened or air-conditioned housing.				
Patient: Thanks for the tips. And if I get malaria is this irreversible?				
MD: See, once we are infected by a mosquito bite, some of its saliva, which contains spores of the parasite, is injected into the bloodstream. Once inside the body, Plasmodium infects liver cells and then red blood cells, and within 48 to 72 hours the parasites create large amounts of toxins into our bloodstream causing you to have the chills, fever and more symptoms. The cycle does not stop. Once you are infected a mosquito bite may pass on the virus to another human being by carrying the virus from you and biting a new person!				
Patient: Is there a vaccine you can give me for malaria?				
MD: Unfortunately not yet, but the medications and wearing the right protective gear and avoiding swamps or very wet areas with a lot of mosquitoes are all things you can do to protect yourself against malaria.				
Break It Down	☐	☐	☐	☐

☐ **CIFE with patient** ☐ **CIFE with provider** ☐ **FLOW** ☐ **REGISTER**

Role-Play 11: Glossary

continued

PO Box 2308, Woburn, MA 01888-0508, **p:** 781-729-3736, **www.EmbracingCulture.com**
PO Box 6401, Manchester, NH 03108, **p:** 1-888-678-CCCS

1. Pathology (diseases, conditions)

2. Laboratory Tests and Diagnostic Procedures

3. Treatment Procedures

4. Idiomatic Expressions (if any)

5. Other (vocabulary in this particular role-play that you feel is important/relevant or that you anticipate problems with)

Vacuna Polio

Role-Play 12: IPV

	Pronunciation	Additions	Omissions	Mistakes
Nurse: Today you are receiving your third inactivated polio vaccine (IPV).				
PT: Does it hurt a lot?				
Nurse: Just a sting.				
Mother: You do not remember all the past three shots, you got them at 2 months, 4 months and 6-18 months ... you were so cute and you only had one quick cry!				
PT: I do not like shots, is there a pill I can take?				
Nurse: You know, in the past kids took this vaccine by mouth, (OPV) but right before you were born, we began to give this shot. When my uncle was a child like you he got very sick with poliomyelitis or polio.				
Mother: It is a very nasty virus that invades the nervous system and can make one very sick with fever, fatigue, nausea, headache, flu-like symptoms, stiffness in the neck and back, and pain in the limbs which often resolves completely.				
PT: But I feel like I get it all the time with the flu!				
Nurse: Some kids only get the flu symptoms but unfortunately a few can get very sick and become paralyzed.				
Break It Down	☐	☐	☐	☐

☐ CIFE with patient ☐ CIFE with provider ☐ FLOW ☐ REGISTER

Role-Play 12: Glossary

continued

PO Box 2308, Woburn, MA 01888-0508, **p:** 781-729-3736, **www.EmbracingCulture.com**
PO Box 6401, Manchester, NH 03108, **p:** 1-888-678-CCCS

1. Pathology (diseases, conditions)

2. Laboratory Tests and Diagnostic Procedures

3. Treatment Procedures

4. Idiomatic Expressions (if any)

5. Other (vocabulary in this particular role-play that you feel is important/relevant or that you anticipate problems with)

Lesson Two: Additional Resources
The Different Roles of the Interpreter

Interpreter's Modes and Roles. The Importance of Setting the Stage with CIFE

The publication of the IMIA Medical Interpreting Standards of Practice in 1996 raised the bar of professionalism in medical interpreting at a nationwide level. As a result of their widespread adoption, the Standards now exercise pervasive influence in the behavior of a multitude of trained medical interpreters.

For example, well-trained interpreters familiar with the Standards will refuse tips or gifts of value offered in conjunction with the triadic encounter. They do not offer opinions on treatment and do not comment on a provider's qualifications. They respect patient confidentiality by not sharing confidential information with community members, family or friends. They strive to be complete and accurate in their interpretation and to stick to the speaker's language register so that all information is conveyed in its purest form. Additionally, they are committed to self-monitoring their interpreting performance and making appropriate corrections.

However, even well-trained interpreters struggle with the ethics of moving among the varied roles of the medical interpreter: conduit, clarifier, cultural broker and patient advocate. Navigating the interpreter's roles is even more challenging when ground rules have not been established through an effective pre-session, or mini-contract, with both the provider and the patient.

CIFE in the Pre-Session

In the belief that an ounce of prevention is better than a pound of cure, Cross Cultural Communication Systems, Inc. created the simple acronym CIFE as a pre-session check-list for interpreters. CIFE was designed for use prior to every medical interpreting session and stands for:

C onfidentiality
I use the 1st person
F low
E verything said will be interpreted

Confidentiality: The Interpreter explains to the patient and provider that all information shared during the session will stay among the parties to that session. A session starts with the first contact between interpreter and patient. Often, this happens in the waiting room of a clinic or hospital.

I-Use the First Person: Interpreter will be using the first person. Therefore when the patient (or provider) says, "I have" the interpreter will say, "I have" not "he has/she has" or "the patient has."

PO Box 2308, Woburn, MA 01888-0508, **p:** 781-729-3736, **www.EmbracingCulture.com**
PO Box 6401, Manchester, NH 03108, **p:** 1-888-678-CCCS

F-low: (interpreter may manage the flow of the session): The flow of a session is crucial to accuracy and there are times when the interpreter may ask both the provider and patient to slow down or to pace their speech. During the pre-session, the interpreter may negotiate the use of an acceptable hand signal to indicate when either party needs to slow down.

Everything You Say Will Be Interpreted: Everything shared in the waiting room, in the session, and after the session, will be interpreted. Interpreters are not allowed to keep secrets from patient or providers.

CIFE only works if all parties involved understand its purpose. The interpreter needs to include both the patient and the provider in the explanation of CIFE, and does so by holding a pre-session with the patient while in the waiting room and reviewing it when the provider joins the session.

But is a pre-session really that important? How does the interpreter benefit from initiating such a discussion? And what could happen if a pre-session is not held? Consider the following vignettes.

The Interpreter-Conduit

A single, young, Muslim woman goes for her first medical appointment in the United States. The provider, who is male, begins to question her about her sexual history. The patient, insulted, abruptly leaves the room. The interpreter runs after the patient and attempts to coax her back to the session. Later, the interpreter apologizes to the provider for the patient's behavior.

In this case, the interpreter initially acted as a conduit by accurately interpreting all of the provider's questions. This backfired when the patient began to feel that her honor and integrity were under attack. Upon seeing that the session was unsuccessful, the interpreter felt ashamed. This shame then led her to apologize to the provider.

The ethical question here is: Should the interpreter have informed the provider of the possibility of a culture clash before the session started? We ask this because, due to a cultural barrier that no one took the initiative to address, this patient, who had previously attempted to seek medical help, will now likely refuse it. And, as we all know, one unhappy patient will probably produce several more, as news of this stressful event spreads to family, friends, and other community members.

Another ethical issue is the abrupt end of the session, where the patient walks out and the interpreter tries to bring her back. Where was the provider in this interaction and is it really the duty of the interpreter to bring the patient back?

Had a pre-session occurred in this case, the interpreter would likely have empowered the provider with the cultural tools needed to deal with a potentially explosive reaction. If the interpreter was aware that a young, unmarried Muslim female would probably feel uncomfortable answering a male provider's questions about sexual activity, she would have done well to share that information with the provider in the pre-session, well before the interpretating began. Such a course of action is supported by section B-2 of the Standards, which states, as an indicator of mastery, that the professional interpreter's duty is to share cultural information that may be relevant and may help clarify the problem. The interpreter should then preface any cultural coaching with a tactful comment such as, "It may not be the case in this particular situation, but in my experience this (...) reaction is common among members of (...) community."

If a pre-session were held and the provider still felt that questions related to sexual activity were crucial to the quality of healthcare delivery, then perhaps the provider could acknowledge the intent of the question and allow the patient to respond in a different fashion. The interpreter in this situation could act as a culture broker by introducing the provider to an explanatory model. Where a provider feels more comfortable with western-style, close-ended, to-the-point questioning, he or she might first ask the patient's permission to use this form of questioning. All of these factors could be negotiated in a pre-session between interpreter and provider.

When Does a Session Begin? When does it End?

Interpreters, although striving to be ethical, are often confused by the concept of patient confidentiality. It is widely maintained that all information shared in the triadic encounter must be accurately and completely interpreted to all parties. In the triadic encounter, there are no secrets!

But the Standards, although establishing excellent directives on what to do within the confines of the traditional interpreting session (patient-provider-interpreter), are not explicit when it comes to dealing with unsolicited information shared by patients outside the triadic confines, thus leaving interpreters to use their best judgment when handling such situations.

While there exists conflicting opinions as to when a session begins, it often happens that while yet in the waiting room, patients are so happy to see an interpreter that they begin discussing issues only a provider can attend to.

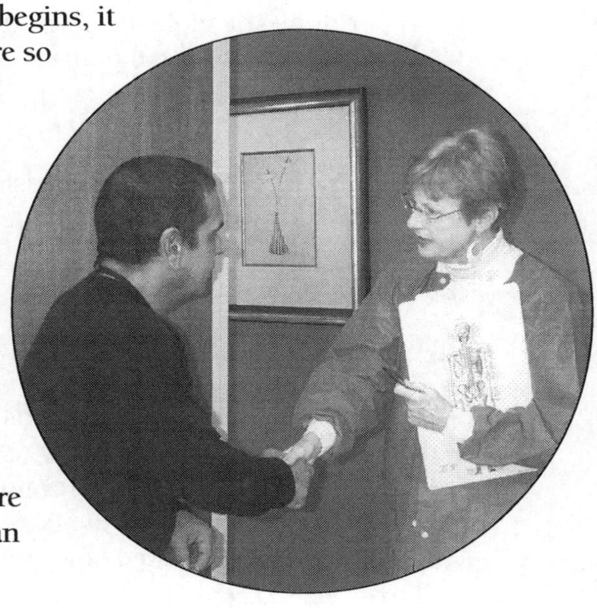

Interpreters usually greet patients in a warm manner. This can do much to dispel a patient's anxiety about the upcoming medical session and to open the channels of communication. Often though, the patient then volunteers a monologue, and the interpreter, out of politeness, becomes a passive listener. The interpreter knows not to ask personal questions, but even the simple act of listening can be misleading to a patient. Before long, the friendly greeting has led to a patient's divulging of medical information, followed by the plea, "Please don't share this with the doctor." What an uncomfortable situation for an interpreter to be in!

PO Box 2308, Woburn, MA 01888-0508, **p:** 781-729-3736, **www.EmbracingCulture.com**
PO Box 6401, Manchester, NH 03108, **p:** 1-888-678-CCCS

However, if a patient is forewarned that the interpreting session has already begun with the first waiting-room greeting, and that all information shared from that point on must be interpreted, he or she will be less likely to divulge "secret" information or to bring medical issues to the interpreter's attention.

Likewise, interpreters often work with patients who are not completely trusting of a provider's medical expertise. In a spirit of "professional conspiracy," interpreters are indirectly asked to collaborate in a game of trust. The following vignette illustrates a relatively common situation among substance abusers who "test" both interpreters and providers by sharing unsolicited information outside of the triadic encounter:

An older Portuguese man is seen by his primary care physician and is told that he has to stop smoking if he wants to live. During the next visit, the patient tells the provider that he no longer smokes. The physician smiles, congratulates the patient, and informs him that his lungs are now clear. After the triadic encounter, as the interpreter walks with the patient to schedule a follow-up appointment, the patient comments on how American doctors are much too easy to please. "Really," he says, "the truth is that I still smoke as much as ever!" The interpreter smiles and goes on to schedule a follow-up appointment at the front desk.

In the vignette above, the patient shared information with the interpreter while walking from the exam room to the front desk. The patient's time with the provider was over. Thus, the interpreter might erroneously believe that he or she is not responsible for the information. It is common to hear interpreters say, "As long the matter isn't life-threatening, I don't have to disclose it."

In fact, some interpreters may cite the Standards as a basis for their silence. Section C-1 states that a medical interpreter, if privy to information regarding suicidal/homicidal intent, child abuse, or domestic violence, should act on the obligation to transmit such information in keeping with institutional policies and code of ethics, and the law. It could appear, then, that anything less than life-threatening is inconsequential. And yet, is it really ethical to keep anything back?

We ask now: If everything in a session must be interpreted, when does a session end? Should we leave the disclosure of unsolicited post-triadic communication up to the judgment of an interpreter who is not trained as a provider to handle that information? Who should decide if information is worth sharing?

Again, a good pre-session will set the expectations for information sharing before, during, and after the triadic encounter. The patient will then know that a session begins with the first interpreter-patient contact and ends with the last "good-bye." Conversations in waiting rooms, walks to the lab, chats with x-ray technicians, tidbits shared on the stairwell, in the elevator, and walking out the door are all relevant, and all medical information must be shared with the provider. In this manner, if the patient knows exactly what to expect from the interpreter, "secrets" will not be shared, and the "game" of trust will not become an uncomfortable reality.

Interpreter-Patient Advocate

Many interpreters have expressed a desire to coach patients in their understanding of the American medical system. They argue that to be a cultural broker with the provider is to be a "provider advocate" and that being the case, it is also part of their job to act as "patient advocates." The question raised is: Should an interpreter act on behalf of a patient without the involvement of the provider? Before you answer, consider the following cases:

A young Latino man, recently diagnosed with AIDS, is in the emergency room. His interpreter instructs him to tell the emergency room physician about his recent case of thrush, as this may result in an additional diagnosis. After all, he explains, he has seen three similar cases in the last two weeks. The patient quietly agrees. The interpreter feels good about his coaching; he may be saving a life.

A veteran Portuguese-speaking interpreter tells patients that in the United States doctors are too busy to listen to long stories. She tells them to say "Yes" and "No" to the questions asked and to avoid bringing up details that are not directly related to the questions. Some of these patients have complained to subsequent interpreters that this interpreter made them feel uneasy.

A Haitian Jehovah's Witness arrives at an emergency room after a bad car crash, bleeding profusely. A blood transfusion is recommended. The patient refuses the transfusion, and the interpreter, familiar with the patient's beliefs, attempts to talk him into accepting the recommended treatment.

In the above-mentioned cases, the interpreters stepped outside the boundaries of their profession and became, for just a moment, medical providers. By practicing cultural coaching with patients, without the presence and orientation of a provider, they run the risk of creating an unequal balance of power and subsequently breaking trust in the triadic relationship.

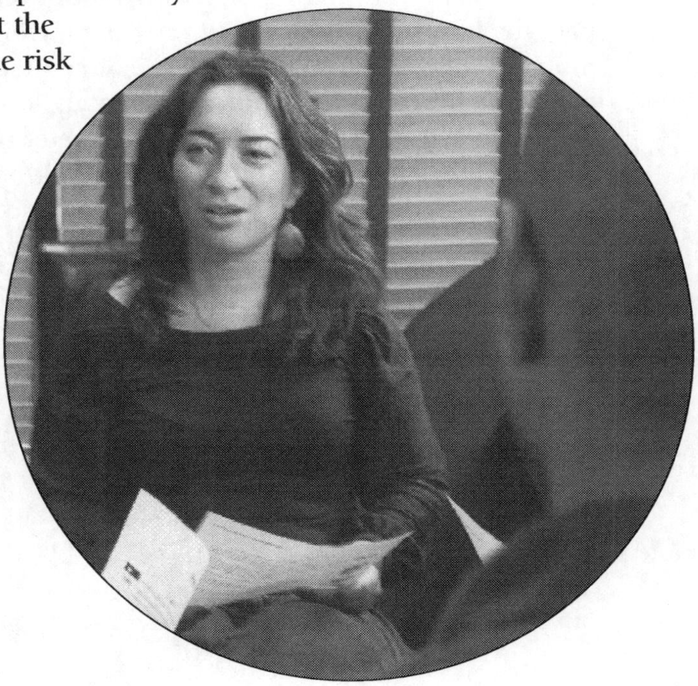

Do interpreters really have "power" over patients? Well, to the patient, the interpreter is the one that speaks the same language, often comes from the same country, and can even share the same physical traits. "The interpreter is like me," the patient reasons, "the interpreter is my friend." And understandably, patients may initially relish the thought of having a friend, or ally, in the triadic encounter, but this can be both confusing and scary.

PO Box 2308, Woburn, MA 01888-0508, **p:** 781-729-3736, **www.EmbracingCulture.com**
PO Box 6401, Manchester, NH 03108, **p:** 1-888-678-CCCS

It is up to the interpreter, then, to balance the distribution of power in a medical session. In the above-mentioned cases, the interpreter would have done well to hold a pre-session with the provider, or at the very least, pull the provider aside to discuss the cultural and/or religious issues that could potentially influence the session. The provider could then take the initiative to address the issue with the patient. After all, the ultimate goal of an interpreting session is that patient and provider develop a therapeutic alliance. A large part of the healing process stems from a patient's trust in a provider. (For more information on the therapeutic alliance, see the bibliography list of essential articles and books by renowned authors.)

The Conclusion: Until recently, the pre-session was perceived solely as a tool for getting a sense of the overall linguistic register of the patient and perhaps a general understanding of the possible clinical path from the provider. Although this understanding is not wrong, it falls short of the full potential of a pre-session and it leaves each interpreter to decide what information shared outside the confines of the triadic encounter is of clinical significance and how much of it should be reported to the provider.

This is why Cross Cultural Communication Systems, Inc. encourages interpreters to limit waiting room conversation with patients to very safe, short topics and to use the bulk of the time before the triadic encounter to tactfully explain CIFE and its relation to the role of the medical interpreter. By thus setting the tone before a session, the interpreter virtually eliminates the potential for confusion of roles and the misplacement of loyalties in the medical session.

Some interpreters find it easier to initiate a pre-session with patients than with providers. Perhaps this is due to the fact that many providers immediately launch into the interview process without introduction and without even acknowledging the presence of the interpreter. If you, the interpreter, work with providers who are not aware of the pre-session concept, seize the moment to briefly introduce CIFE. Some interpreters have found it effective to interpret the provider's first comment, and immediately follow it up with, "Excuse me; I did not have a chance to introduce myself." The interpreter then briefly performs an introduction and mentions the concepts of CIFE. This should take no more than one minute.

Once all parties involved understand the interpreter's role, the interpreter may concentrate on the content of the session, keeping an eye on accuracy and completeness. But undoubtedly, the act of explaining CIFE in the pre-session lays the foundation for a solid interpreting performance.

Finding your "center" is not always easy when you are a medical interpreter!

In trainings, we remind interpreters of the need to avoid "becoming" a patient or a provider while interpreting. We ask them to be transparent, and in some cases, impartial. Interpreters are also asked to strive for accuracy and completeness while interpreting in a medical encounter, thus acting as effective language mediators between patient and provider.

At a **cognitive level**, most trained interpreters agree with and understand the logic of **acting as facilitators** of communication between patients and providers. However, in the heat of a session, interpreters are often challenged by the unconscious awakening of personal feelings. Something in the provider or patient's behavior unexpectedly triggers in the interpreter an immediate adverse reaction and he or she stops being a mediator or facilitator, and for a quick second acts as a provider.

The following case well illustrates how for two fleeting moments, a qualified interpreter, who has attended multiple interpreter training programs, **lost her center**, a misstep which resulted in a threat of legal action:

A patient who had lost some fingers while operating a machine was being seen by a surgeon in a follow-up consult to remove stitches. Halfway into the session, the surgeon stepped out of the examining room to check on another matter, and the interpreter stayed with the patient. While alone in the examining room, the patient began to cry over the loss of her fingers. She asked if the interpreter would give her a plastic bag, so that she, the patient, would not have to look at her hand. The interpreter replied that she, as an interpreter, could not supply a bag. The patient continued to cry, and the interpreter reassured her that the surgeon was on his way.

Later, while the stitches were being removed, the patient became very loud, and her sobbing could be heard throughout the clinic. The interpreter, in a spirit of helpfulness and worried about the other patients in the clinic, quickly asked the emotional patient to please calm down.

Some time after the session, the patient's lawyer called the agency responsible for interpreter services to inform it of pending legal action. The patient had accused the interpreter of suggesting that the injuries were the patient's own fault.

When confronted with these serious allegations, the interpreter immediately denied making any such comment to the patient. When asked by the contracting agency if she had had private communication or side conversations with the patient, she revealed that indeed she had stayed alone with the patient in the exam room when the provider stepped out.

PO Box 2308, Woburn, MA 01888-0508, **p:** 781-729-3736, **www.EmbracingCulture.com**
PO Box 6401, Manchester, NH 03108, **p:** 1-888-678-CCCS

In the course of the interview, it became evident that the interpreter had been accurate and complete in her representation of the patient and provider's voices. How, then, did she err? By adding her own voice! The one additional comment, "please calm down," which she believed was for the good of everyone, set in motion a chain of events that could potentially cost this interpreter her job.

While trying to figure out what motivated the patient to make a formal complaint, the interpreter and her supervisor thoroughly reviewed the case and came up with the following guidelines to be observed in all interpreting sessions:

1. **Interpreters should never stay alone in examining rooms with patients.**
2. **Interpreters should not be owners of a patient's decisions.** (When the patient asked for a bag to cover her fingers, the interpreter should have **given her the option** of either waiting for the provider or having the interpreter go find the provider. Instead, the interpreter had said, " I can't give you a bag. I am only here to interpret for you and the doctor.")
3. **Interpreters should not interfere when patients cry, no matter how much noise they make.** This is the provider's job, not the interpreter's! However, if the crying interferes with the interpreter's ability to hear either the provider or the patient, the interpreter may gently inform both parties, "I'm sorry, the interpreter cannot hear."

Conclusion:

There is no doubt that this patient truly believes the interpreter blamed her for causing her own injuries. On the other hand, the interpreter did not actually state that the patient was at fault. However, the interpreter's two moments of weakness gave cause to the misunderstanding.

The first moment of weakness occurred when the patient asked for a bag. The interpreter, although right in not supplying the bag, responded to the request in a rigid manner. This may have been perceived by the patient as cold-heartedness. So, when denying a request for action, interpreters need to be both caring and diplomatic. In addition, a request should never stop with an interpreter's refusal to comply. All requests for action need to be related back to the provider so that he or she can make an informed decision. In this case, a more appropriate response would have been: "I am so sorry I can not provide you with a bag, I would not want to harm you. Would you like me to call the provider right away or would you like to wait until he gets back?"

The second moment of weakness was when the interpreter's unconscious feelings towards how patients should behave in public flared up and manifested in her impulsive request for the patient to calm down. In this case, the interpreter acted as if she was a provider, and by imposing her values on the patient, she lost both her center and her transparency. This misguided action broke trust between the interpreter and the patient, and caused irreparable damage to the triadic encounter.

As the interpreter and her supervisor discussed the allegations, they took time to discuss background information such as immigration history. In this particular case, both the interpreter and the patient had come to the United States as refugees, likely enduring terrible losses. What had helped the interpreter to survive wartime and immigration trauma was self-control. But for the patient, the loss of her fingers was just too much to bear, emotionally and physically. Understandably, at that moment, self-control and decorum were the last things on her mind.

Like butterflies struggling to manage heavy wings, interpreters work hard to achieve balance as healthcare professionals. They want to support their wings by being helpful to the providers and patients that they serve. Yet, they realize that there are times when they must decline an action or refuse a request. And it is noteworthy that not only patients, but also providers, make unreasonable demands on interpreters.

In the above-mentioned case, the surgeon had left the interpreter alone with the patient. It is common for providers, nurses, and other medical staff to specifically ask an interpreter to stay alone with a patient "to keep the patient company" or "to explain this form."

The interpreter in question did not want to be rude. She also felt bad for the patient and didn't want her to feel isolated. So she consented to stay alone with the patient, and by so doing, risked potential legal action. Now, it is only the word of the patient against that of the interpreter, a classic case of "she said/she said" with no witnesses to support either side!

CCCS, Inc. has created the image of a butterfly, where the interpreter is the body, or center, always busy managing the provider and patient's wings. In this image, we have attempted to artfully represent the dynamics and intricacies of the triadic encounter. And we want you to remember that if even one party to the encounter is neglected, the interpretation will not fly!

PO Box 2308, Woburn, MA 01888-0508, **p:** 781-729-3736, **www.EmbracingCulture.com**
PO Box 6401, Manchester, NH 03108, **p:** 1-888-678-CCCS

The role of the clarifier

Often interpreters are faced with linguistic challenges. Interpreters who cannot find one exact word in both English and/or target languages may resort to an explanation on their own. But should interpreters be the ones explaining or just the ones making both parties aware of a need of an explanation?

It is appropriate for an interpreter to ask for clarification by asking the provider to **break down a word** especially when interpreters are faced with linguistic challenges due to a lack of linguistic equivalency for medical terms and concepts.

Without losing its original meaning, Can you literally interpret the words?

Germs	Interpretation
1. Hay fever	
2. Partner	
3. Provider	
4. Follow-up	
5. Nurse practitioner	
6. Eye-opener	
7. I feel the blues	
8. Special Education	

When and With Whom Should the Interpreter Act as a Clarifier in the Triadic Encounter?

The cultural-clarifier role goes beyond clarification to include a range of actions that typically relate to an interpreter's ultimate purpose of facilitating communication between parties not sharing a common culture. Interpreters are alert to cultural words or concepts that might lead to a misunderstanding triggering a shift to the cultural clarifier role. Section A-8, which states that the interpreter must "ensure that the listener understands the message." *Professional Standards, CHIA Pages 43 & 44.*

When there is evidence that all of the parties, including the interpreter, may be confused by cultural differences, interpreters need to interrupt the communication process with a word, comment, or a gesture, as appropriate, for example, using a hand signal for clarification; Or may alert both parties to potential miscommunication or misunderstanding (interpreters may say, for example, "As an interpreter, I think that there may be potential danger for miscommunication/ misunderstanding...."); Or suggest cultural concerns that could be impeding mutual understanding, for example, relating/discussing private details with someone outside the family circle; Or assist the patient in explaining the cultural concept to the provider, or the provider in explaining the biomedical concept.

When requested, interpreters also need to explain the cultural custom, health belief or practice of the patient to the provider, or educate the patient on the biomedical concept. For example, interpreters might say: "It's been my experience when working with (demographic group) that the word '____' may trigger a negative reaction," or "It is my understanding that a 'handshake' would not be permissible in the patient's culture." *Professional Standards, CHIA Pages 43 & 44.*

Again, although the standards allow for culture brokering from the interpreter to the patient and to the provider, CCCS cautions interpreters and recommends that culture coaching is done through the provider so as to allow patient-provider alliance.

The NCIHC Interpreter Standards of Practice objective is "to facilitate communication across cultural differences. Related ethical principle: Interpreters strive to develop awareness of the cultures encountered in the performance of interpreting duties." *NCIHC Standards of Practice (14).*

The interpreter strives to understand the cultures associated with the languages in which he or she interprets, including the biomedical culture. Ex: an interpreter learns about the traditional remedies some patients may use.

The interpreter alerts all parties to any significant cultural misunderstanding that arises. *The NCIHC Standards of Practice (15)* Ex: If a provider asks a patient who is fasting for religious reasons to take an oral medication, an interpreter may call attention to the potential conflict. Ex: A parent pins an amulet for good luck to a baby's undershirt and the pediatrician perceives this as a danger because of the safety pin. Ex: A patient's culture may consider it disrespectful to look directly at a person of authority, like a provider.

The Standards of Practice by CHIA, IMIA AND NCIHC only complement the cultural clinical constructs: "Through diagnostic activities and labeling, healthcare providers negotiate with patients' medical realities that become the object of medical attention and therapeutics" Dr. Kleinman (1978). The interpreter is the facilitator in this communication process.

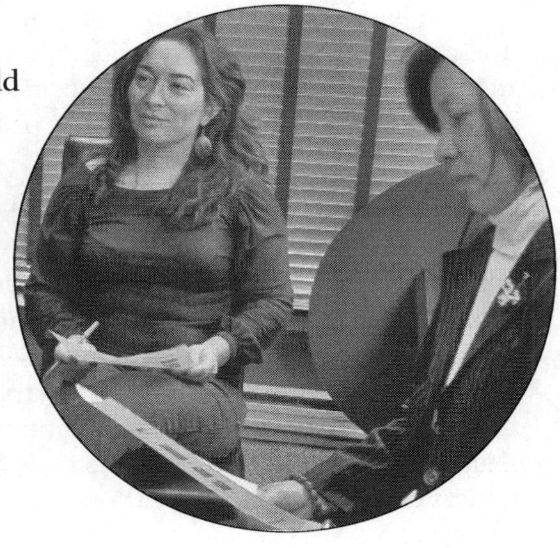

Interpreters need to become aware that the session should flow as smoothly as possible and asking for a **break down** cannot serve as an anchor for a language fluency issue but it **should be used only** when the interpreter **identifies a linguistic or a cultural "red flag,"** or when the interpreter perceives that the patient is likely not getting the correct meaning.
Here are some quick solutions to shorten the amount of time in the session. In the session,

- Ask the provider to "break down" meaning
- Echo the word in question back to the provider
- Ask for clarification

PO Box 2308, Woburn, MA 01888-0508, **p:** 781-729-3736, **www.EmbracingCulture.com**
PO Box 6401, Manchester, NH 03108, **p:** 1-888-678-CCCS

Should an Interpreter use the Interpreting Session to be a Culture Coach?

During my many years of interpreting and teaching interpretation, I have struggled with the question: How can an interpreter be a culture coach and not interfere with the patient-provider rapport?

For example, I have often encountered patients who put the provider right up there with "God." They feel that providers carry indisputable power and truth. These patients may feel uncomfortable when witnessing an intervention by an interpreter who does not view providers as ultimate authority figures, but rather, as partners, and the intervention as a collaborative dynamic between two professionals. This clash of viewpoints can lead to mistrust in the triadic encounter.

A patient once expressed to me her fear that an interpreter may have made a provider mad by telling the provider "how our people think." The patient was worried that, as a result, the provider would treat her differently, perhaps not with the same level of care as before the interpreter's interference. This patient understood that providers in America have a different way of doing things. The last thing she wanted was to disrespect the provider. This statement made me rethink if interpreters who coach providers in the middle of a session are being truly helpful. And are they really representing the patient's wishes?

Let's consider another example. An interpreter working with a provider about to disclose a diagnosis of terminal illness interrupts the session in the presence of the dying patient to inform the provider that in this patient's culture, truth telling may not be the best approach. The interpreter suggests that perhaps the provider might involve the patient's family in the discussion of the diagnosis before disclosing the information to the patient.

On one hand, we do know of some cultures in which patients made aware of a terminal illness are more likely to commit suicide. From this perspective, an immediate intervention by the interpreter-culture broker might seem like the right thing at the moment. But should we also consider this situation from another perspective?

According to D. Robert Buckman in his book *How to Break Bad News*, providers have gone through drastic changes regarding truth telling. In 1950, ninety percent of providers avoided telling the truth to patients suffering from a serious or terminal illness. In 1970, however, ninety percent of providers were telling the truth to patients. Apparently, this progression in addressing terminal illness was a direct result of the Patients' Rights movement. When it comes to cultural conflicts with truth telling, it is my belief that providers will not usually change their methods in a split second just because the interpreter suggests that they do so. Some will ignore the interpreter's suggestions and will continue to insist on "straight talk" with the patient. "This is America," they may say, "Patients have the right to know their medical condition. It is my ethical obligation to tell them!"

Back to the session with the terminally ill patient: the interpreter speaks out in the session, addressing the provider in the presence of the patient, and suggests an alternative to straight talk about the illness. This is done in English, and the LEP patient is left out of the communication. The patient, though, knows that there is something wrong. He senses some stress in the facial expressions of both the interpreter and the provider. The patient is worried. Despite being unaware of the content of the interpreter-provider communication, he sees that the interpreter has interrupted the session. The patient does not want the interpreter to create unnecessary tension with the provider, who in his eyes carries a lot of power. In such a case, was the interpreter's intervention necessary? If so, was there a better way to go about it?

As interpreters, we can be made to feel weighed down by cumbersome mandates: the responsibility of being a conduit, interpreting meaning accurately without additions, omissions or mistakes, and the simultaneous obligation to intervene as a culture broker with the purpose of facilitating a provider's understanding of issues that only someone who has lived or worked within the specific patient's ethnic group understands. And yet, each patient is an individual with a set of legal and moral rights. Are we interpreters imposing our views regarding truth telling in the triadic encounter?

Throughout the years, I have tried and experimented with a variety of interventions that at the time I thought were best for the patients involved. In retrospect, I suppose that at the same time, I often "lost" the providers in the interventions. Now that I am growing older, and have had the benefit of experience as a mental health clinician working with interpreters, and also as an interpreter for other clinicians, I am beginning to find my center as a cultural liaison.

When I first sense the "need" to act as a culture coach, I take a deep breath and mentally revisit the "Six Ws" that help me to differentiate between my own opinions and what may actually be best for the patient.

The "Six Ws" is a general tool that serves as a guide to the interpreter debating whether to "help" a clinician or patient by sharing certain information. Ask yourself:

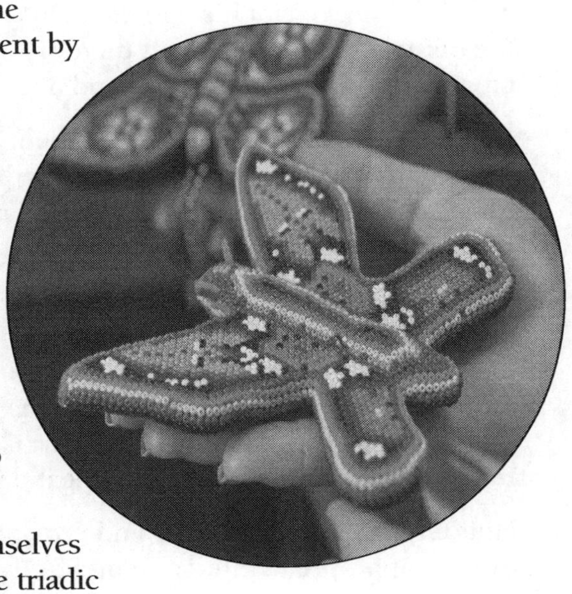

- Who owns the information?
- Whose job is it to share the information?
- With whom can I share it?
- Who is going to be affected by my actions?
- What does the law say?
- Would a professional interpreter association support my action?

Interpreters working through this exercise will likely opt to act as a culture broker after the session or prior to the session, but rarely during a session.

Here are some suggestions for interpreters who see themselves as culture liaisons with a need to be more effective in the triadic communication:

PO Box 2308, Woburn, MA 01888-0508, **p:** 781-729-3736, **www.EmbracingCulture.com**
PO Box 6401, Manchester, NH 03108, **p:** 1-888-678-CCCS

A macroperspective: It will take a long time, but begin to work within the healthcare system to develop a continual dialogue between providers and interpreters. Use the same tools that providers use, such as Grand Rounds, where interpreters and providers can come together to review cases that may have required a culture broker. Suggest that a representative from the Interpreter Services department at your healthcare facility sit on the taskforces and committees that deal with ethical issues. Interpreters should begin to write case studies for the different magazines on ethics in healthcare, and to solicit responses from the medical community. Interpreters can also partner with colleges and universities on research into the issues surrounding cultural liaison work.

A microperspective: Ideally, the interpreter-culture coach should be able to follow a model already existing in healthcare practice: that of the consultant. Interns often call for a consult from a colleague or a superior. Primary care physicians often need to discuss cases with a cardiologist, oncologist or other specialist. The concept of requesting a consult implies an imminent need, and most likely the referring provider will discuss this need with the patient and then proceed to communicate with the consultant. Until this concept of seeking out a consult on cultural and linguistic issues takes flight, interpreters may have to be creative with their interventions.

True, being a culture coach is one of the interpreter's responsibilities. But developing effective coaching techniques is not an easy task. It requires that both sides, interpreters and providers, come to a mutual understanding of the need for professional collaboration and dialogue around the current culture of intervention and on how the behavior of intervention impacts the patient population.

For example, an interpreter who has gone through the Six "W(s)" and decided that the situation at hand is not one of life and death may want to approach the provider privately at the end of the session and mention that there are some tools that the provider can implement to facilitate cross cultural communication and offer to explain them.

In extreme situations where the patient will likely not return to the healthcare facility because the provider has committed a perceived cultural offense, the interpreter may need to take a more immediate action. He or she can ask the provider to step outside. The provider should then inform the patient that the interpreter and provider will be stepping out.

During the intervention, which takes place away from the patient, the interpreter will address the cultural issues with the provider only. The interpreter will preface remarks with, "It seems to me…" "In my experience…" "Often…" and "From what I've observed…" (thus allowing for the individuality of the patient in question), and will end remarks with "…but you may want to check in with the patient to see if this is true" (which encourages the provider to reconnect with the patient through further investigation).

Not only will the interpreter and provider have discussed a potential belief system and gone over an appropriate intervention, but they will also have agreed on an explanation to the patient for the interruption of the session. There should be no secrets in the triadic encounter. Thus, the provider, the one carrying the most power in the patient's eyes, should be the one to explain the interruption by bringing the interpreter in as a consultant. So the session resumes with the provider stating, "Julia (name of interpreter) was concerned with the fact that I may not be aware of a cultural belief that may or may not be true for you. She was so kind as to coach me on this. Let's see if this works for you..."

The intervention of having the interpreter in the role of culture-consultant will allow the patient to continue to deposit trust in the patient-doctor relationship by leaving the provider's role whole and not broken.

In the spirit of promoting a stronger patient-doctor relationship, CCCS believes that cultural coaching may be a better term for interpreters when becoming aware of a culture challenge. A coach assists providers navigate through both their own and the patient's belief system by acknowledging the potential conflict and asking for the patient's assistance on how to best resolve issues.

A culture broker seems to have a more direct action-related behavior by telling the parties involved of the perceived issue and suggesting a way of overcoming the issue. The interpreter appears to be the fixer or the band-aid in order to correct a miscommunication due to a cultural barrier.

See the difference of both culture broker and culture coach in the following case:

An elderly Mandarin speaking patient recently immigrated from China. On the morning of her surgery, she requests to eat an orange before general anesthesia for good luck.

The culture broker could interpret this request and right away inform the patient that in fact eating anything before surgery is not recommended to any patient, not just the Chinese patients and interpreter conveys this statement to the provider.

On the other end, the culture coach interprets patient's requests, and if the provider does not honor the request, and the interpreter believes that this behavior may harm the patient; the interpreter may ask the provider if she can step outside for a short moment informing the patient that they will be right back.

Nicely the interpreter repeats the patient's request and quickly offers to assist the provider by sharing the possibility of the meaning of the orange. For this particular patient and among many of the Chinese speaking patients the orange is perceived as a symbol of good luck. The interpreter understands that depriving the patient of this experience may cause some unnecessary stress before going under general anesthesia.

The interpreter finds common ground with the provider and patient, i.e., the well being of the patient, and suggests a compromise that may not jeopardize the patient's health and the hospital procedures.

PO Box 2308, Woburn, MA 01888-0508, **p:** 781-729-3736, **www.EmbracingCulture.com**
PO Box 6401, Manchester, NH 03108, **p:** 1-888-678-CCCS

One suggestion is that perhaps the provider may want to explain to the patient the thinking behind no food and no fluids, so both the provider and the patient can come to an agreement that will fit both needs.

A possible suggested compromise is to place the orange inside an enclosed sterilized glove, isolating the orange from spreading any unwanted germs; so the patient can have the presence of the orange but not ingest it.

Being a cultural coach may take a few more minutes but the main point is to assist the provider to find common ground so that a dialogue can occur between provider and patient. This intervention is not always welcomed by the providers but if one does it correctly it will promote a healthy dialogue and a path to different thinking.

CULTURAL COACHING

1. Basic guidelines for interpreters:

- Be humble.
- Do not take sides. Go with the facts.
- Be in touch with your own biases.
- Do not act on your own biases.
- You cannot change others.
- You can learn how to manage information in a respectful way.
- Do not become a burden to the other party.

Providers have tools on how to enhance trust between patient-provider. However, when faced with LEP patients, often, untrained providers in cross cultural matters seem to create a clinical void between the patient and themselves. According to the interpreter's standards an interpreter may intervene in a diplomatic and respectful way as a culture coach.

2. Interpreter Culture Competency tools for providers:

- Listen to the story.
- Acknowledge the story by being a good listener: echoing the thinking, uses story telling as a form of externalization.
- Find common ground.
- Build bridges, check assumptions, be flexible.
- Understand patient's relationship with the community and/or the referral source: is the patient a more abstract or more concrete thinker, is the patient more present or past oriented?
- Coach providers in acknowledging loss of present role if patient engages in treatment.
- Understand patient's own immigration history: relationship with authority.
- Understand that patient and family are the best culture coaches.

Managing our "advocate" role as medical interpreters

Over the past few months, in various trainings and from the feedback of active interpreters, I have realized that many medical interpreters share the feeling that although, in theory, the standards of practice created by organizations such as IMIA, CHIA and NCIHC serve a purpose, but in practice each interpreter must do what s/he feels is "best" for the patient.

This belief is prevalent among interpreters who have not received formal training since the publication of these Standards (1997-2005). Many of these "grandfathered" interpreters are extremely proficient when it comes to language fluency and message conversion skills, but they lack an updated outlook on the ethics and role boundaries of our profession. Often, these are the interpreters who take the lead in training newcomers to our profession in community programs and even at the college level.

So many interpreters have dedicated so much of their time and efforts to the reduction of health disparities that, whether consciously or unconsciously, they begin to feel they deserve to make up their own policies regarding "good interpretation" as long as they have the patient's "best interests" in mind. While looking out for a patient's interests can bring positive results, a misdirected advocacy can also do much to harm the patient-provider relationship.

Here are some stories I have heard in recent conversations with active interpreters.

> *"Patients from my cultural group don't understand how things work in America. So after we see the provider, I give the patient the contact information for local social service organizations. Doctors are very busy, and it's not right to take too much of their time when I myself can direct the patient to specific services."*
>
> *"I once interpreted for a poor family that had come to the U.S. for medical treatment. They had very little money and felt quite isolated due to the language barrier. So, I went to church and told their story to my congregation. Soon, the family began to receive visits from church members. I know this helped them feel better during their stay in this country."*
>
> *"If I'm interpreting and I feel that the patient should get a second opinion, I probe the patient to see if this is what s/he wants. After I interpret the provider's diagnosis, I ask the patient (in the target language, of course), 'Do you want to see another doctor?'"*
>
> *"One provider was so rude to my patient, that at the end of the session, I offered to rebook the patient's appointment with a different provider. I never want any of my patients to be seen by that provider!"*

What were your thoughts as you read these interpreters' comments? Was there one statement that bothered you more than another? If so, why?

I did a little research on the term "advocate." Using an Internet language reference, I found, among others, the following definitions:

1. A person who speaks or writes in support or defense of a person, cause, etc.
2. A person who pleads for or in behalf of another intercessor.
3. One who argues for a cause.
4. To push for something.

The concept of the interpreter as an "advocate" is outlined in several current standards of practice. The National Council on Interpreting in Healthcare states, "When the patient's health, well-being or dignity is at risk, an interpreter may be justified in acting as an advocate." Similarly, the California Healthcare Interpreters Association comments, "In this role, interpreters actively support change in the interest of patient health and well-being." Clearly, then, the medical interpreter may need to step into the "advocate" role from time to time. But do the current Standards support any of the above-mentioned interventions?

Current Standards support the concept of the interpreter as one member of a cross-dimensional healthcare team. That team may also include a wide range of professionals, such as physicians, physician assistants, nurses of all levels and specialties, social workers, medical and nursing assistants and other personnel, both clinical and non-clinical. At times, the interpreter may be the first member of this team to become aware of a patient's needs. But does this mean that the interpreter is always the best person to meet those needs? Or, is the interpreter more of a facilitator, bringing the needs of the patient to the attention of the professional best equipped to assist the patient at that moment?

For example, in the case of the patient in need of social services, is the interpreter the best person to decide which organizations would best serve the patient? Or, is there a staff member, a provider or social worker, better equipped to make that decision? The International Medical Interpreters Association requires interpreters to "ensure that concerns raised during or after an interview are addressed and referred to the appropriate resources." As an example, these Standards state that the interpreter should 'encourage the provider to make the appropriate referrals' and that the interpreter who 'takes it upon him/herself to solve the problem' is in fact indicating a lack of mastery (lack of professionalism).

While an interpreter may advocate on behalf of a party or group to correct mistreatment or abuse, is it appropriate to go ahead and reschedule a patient's appointments or to advise the patient to seek a second opinion? The NCIHC standards recommend a different approach to addressing possible mistreatment, "An interpreter may alert his or her supervisor to patterns of disrespect towards patients."

What would happen if the interpreter were to confront the provider directly? CHIA comments, "The healthcare provider or staff member may resent the interpreter's efforts. They might react in a way that actually diminishes quality of care or access for the patient. Lasting resentment may have a long-term impact on the interpreter, resulting in a less effective working relationship. Depending on the type of patient advocacy intervention and whether the action is discussed with the patient, interpreters also risk usurping patient autonomy in determining how their cases are handled."

In the case of the interpreter who alerted her congregation to the plight of a patient's family, do you not feel that she crossed professional role boundaries, the least of which, patient confidentiality? Could it be that the patient's family resented this breach of their private information and the many visits that followed this unsolicited intervention?

In short, professional interpreters must follow professional guidelines. While old habits can be hard to break, keeping pace with the advances in medical interpretation will benefit us as interpreters. It will also promote healthier relationships between the providers and the patients we serve. Before taking action as a patient advocate, take a deep breath and mentally revisit the "Six Ws" that help us to differentiate between our own opinions and what may actually be best for the patient.

It takes humility to acknowledge that we don't always know what is "best" for our patients. Sometimes our perspective is slanted by our own personal biases. But as long as we operate within the parameters set forth in our professional standards, we will be protected in our work as professional medical interpreters.

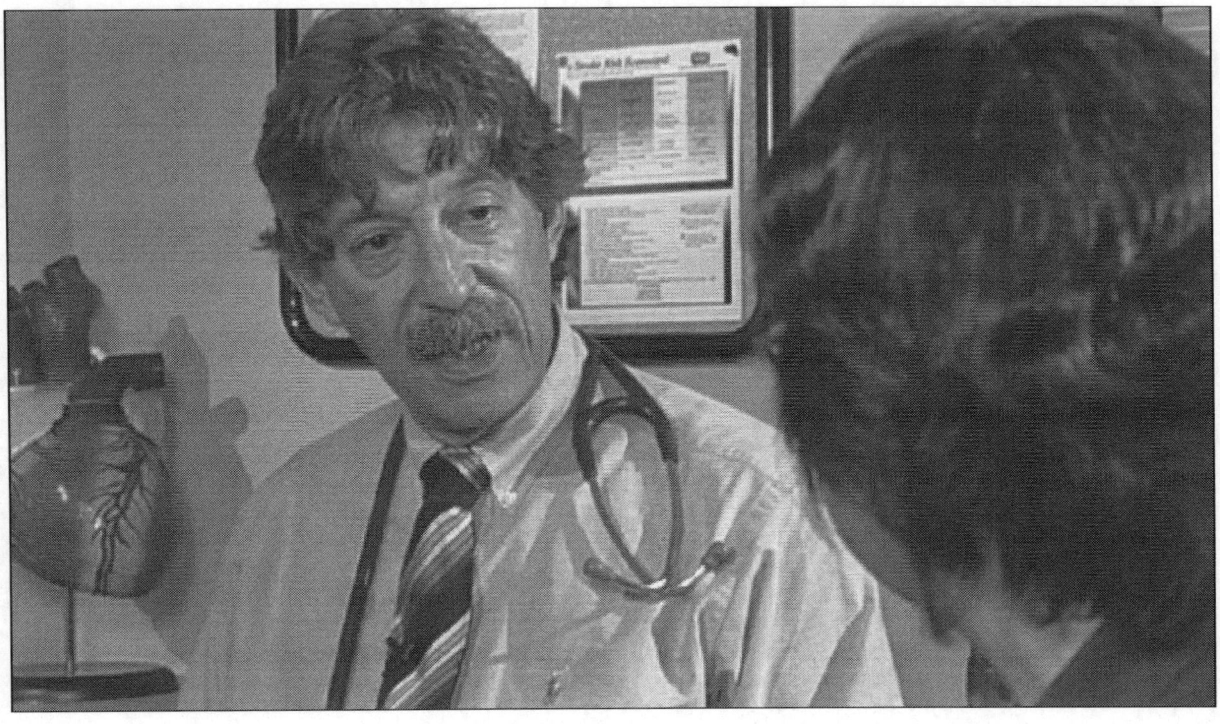

TRANSPARENCY

Interpreters' experiences and values at times may not be the same as the patients'. This might be confusing when one has a lot in common with a patient, and, out of goodness, interpreters wrongly make decisions on how to address personally challenging situations.

A prime example is in cases involving abortion. Abortion is one of several treatment choices commonly offered by providers to pregnant women at high-risk for health complications.

An interpreter may strongly believe that a patient from a certain ethnic or religious group will storm out of a session as soon as the word "abortion" is uttered. Or the interpreter may foresee the patient's failure to return for follow-up treatment after the provider's mention of abortion.

The interpreter, under pressure, might make a quick, but deliberate, decision not to interpret the provider's suggestion of abortion. Clearly, this would be an unprofessional choice and an abuse of power.

So, omitting information due to a perceived culture challenge is not an option but still the interpreter has the challenge to do or not to do anything about it.

The challenge in cultural coaching is that an interpreter must determine whether the perceived conflict stems from the patient, or if it is, in reality, a personal issue. Transparent interpreters are encouraged to identify and work with personal biases that could potentially affect their professional behavior. At the same time, they are trained to discern the potential for cultural misunderstanding in the triadic encounter.

When the interpreter senses a breakdown in cross cultural communication, s/he controls the impulse to "fix" the situation or to act as the provider.

Rather, the interpreter waits for the right moment to coach true providers in their search for culturally appropriate communication techniques. This brief intervention should be done in a non-imposing way, and the interpreter should suggest that the provider explain to the patient that a potentially sensitive topic is about to be discussed. In the above-mentioned example, the interpreter might have suggested to the provider, in a private discussion outside the exam room, the use of a synonym for the term "abortion," such as "terminating the pregnancy." If the provider were to agree, the interpreter would simply interpret and both parties would wait to see the patient's reaction to the clinical recommendations.

The interpreter has the obligation to inform the provider of the possibility that a yes may not mean a yes in the patient's culture. Often a yes is a form of acknowledging that one is listening to the person. In an abortion case, standard close-ended questioning may prove useless to the provider. For example, the provider may inform the patient of her choices and the patient may answer "yes" without really meaning it, which could lead the provider to believe that the patient had agreed to the abortion. Close-ended questioning may not be the best way to approach patients who do not feel comfortable challenging authority.

So, the culture coach, perceiving this miscommunication, may ask the provider to step outside and might privately suggest that the provider uses an explanatory model, in which he or she begins to "explain" the reasons for considering "the ending" or "termination" of the pregnancy, perhaps in a story form. Once, I had a patient who stated yes to all questions even though she did not mean it; yet, her survival depended on her decision to terminate her pregnancy. But her personal belief system forbade her from even mentioning or considering abortion as an option...what would you do in this case?

This quick and complicated series of processes of assumptions and check-ins by the interpreter are necessary so the interpreter does not become an imposition in the triadic encounter. The transparent interpreter's cultural intervention will result, at the very least, in the patient's awareness of her clinical options, and in the provider's greater understanding of that patient's beliefs. Patient and provider will make the ultimate decisions, and the transparent interpreter will leave the session with the freedom that comes from having maintained professional standards of practice.

However, if the interpreter were to act merely as a conduit, interpreting spoken words while ignoring their underlying cultural and religious implications, the patient might leave the session angry or hurt and never request follow-up care, possibly suffering complications and even death. It is clear, then, that by explaining to the provider the possible harmful outcome of the use of the term "abortion," the interpreter is contributing to a positive outcome in a triadic relationship where respect and trust are preserved.

The Interpreter as an Advocate

Should an interpreter stick to the conduit role only when interpreting "bad news" to a patient who does not believe in patient autonomy? How can an interpreter be impartial if s/he only represents the voice of the "provider culture?" Whose "side" is the interpreter on?

We understand that most first generation immigrants and refugee patients do not feel free to assertively inform providers of their "needs." Whose "side" is the interpreter on?

There are patients who believe that making your voice heard when you are dependent on a higher power is not a wise decision. Whose "side" is the interpreter on?

It is ethnocentric to believe that every individual should speak for themselves? Often we find individuals who value not knowing "the truth" about their own health. The open discussion is like bringing a "curse." Whose "side" is the interpreter on?

There are laws that were created to protect the same individuals who now feel unprotected and unheard. Whose "side" is the interpreter on?

There were times in this country where certain ethnic populations were not clearly informed of procedures that could result in major health complications, (IUD, tubal ligation, forced serialization, unnecessary caesarians). Whose "side" is the interpreter on?

PO Box 2308, Woburn, MA 01888-0508, **p:** 781-729-3736, **www.EmbracingCulture.com**
PO Box 6401, Manchester, NH 03108, **p:** 1-888-678-CCCS

There are patients who believe in the right to know "the truth" no matter how great the personal cost. Whose "side" is the interpreter on?

There are family members of patients who resent not having had the opportunity to know "the truth." They did not have a chance to "say goodbye." Whose "side" is the interpreter on?

If an interpreter does not share a possible cultural belief of the patient with the provider, is the interpreter allying with an "ethnocentric" medical system? Or is the interpreter neglecting the rights of a patient or the rights of a family? Whose "side" is the interpreter on?

If an interpreter shares with a provider a possible cultural belief of a patient that contradicts the provider's ethics, is the interpreter interfering with the obligations of a medical system that has clear guidelines regarding patient autonomy?

According to the IMIA standards (1996), "On occasions where the interpreter feels strongly that either party's behavior is affecting access to or quality of service, or compromising either party's dignity, uses effective strategies to address the situation" the interpreter "can explain the boundaries and the meaning of confidentiality, and its implications and consequences." The interpreter "knows and maintains the clinical parameters of information sharing, in keeping with the policies and procedures of the institution and/or team. The interpreter "is able to balance empathy with the boundaries of the interpreter role." The interpreter "monitors own personal agenda and needs, and is aware of transference and countertransference issues."

We believe that patients see interpreters as part of the dominant group. Therefore, interpreters have a very powerful role in patient care. We believe that interpreters often do not feel very powerful and are not aware of their power when they intervene as culture brokers.

Interpreters must understand personal and professional values as medical interpreters. We believe that interpreters should provide proper tools to providers, so that the providers become the ones intervening when there is a need for culture brokerage. We believe that interpreters should encourage as much communication between the provider and the patient as possible and avoid any direct intervention with the patient.

It is essential that the interpreter always has a pre-session with the provider and the patient. This can be a very short pre-session.

Tests have shown that an adequate pre-session in emergency situations can take just 30 seconds.

C onfidentiality
I use the 1st person
F low
E verything said will be interpreted

Other Legal or Hospital accreditation policies and standards also influence the interpreter's ability to manage the different roles:

HIPAA

The Privacy Rule provides federal protections for personal health information held by covered entities and gives patients an array of rights with respect to that information. At the same time, the Privacy Rule is balanced so that it permits the disclosure of personal health information needed for patient care and other important purposes.

Interpreters may be required to successfully complete a HIPAA training. In many countries confidentiality of patient information is non-existent. Interpreters who are newly arrived to this country, out of goodness, violate patient 's confidentiality when, for example, they are asked by a family member if the patient is in the hospital and simply answer "yes" without even discussing any further information. Or by commenting to waiting family members the health status of their dear one, the patient; the interpreter, out of culture consideration and respect naively may say, "I just checked and your sister or daughter is doing well, do not worry!"

The administrative simplification provisions of Health Insurance Portability and Accountability Act of 1996 (HIPAA) require the department of health and human services to establish national standards for electronic healthcare transmissions. It also addresses the security and privacy of health data. The failure to comply with HIPAA guidelines may result in federal prosecution and possible jail time for noncompliant interpreters. The following are a sampling of some of the HIPAA regulations.

1. **Use or Disclosure.** Business Associate agrees to not use or further disclose protected health information created or received by business associate from, or on behalf of. Covered entity ("protected health information") other than as expressly permitted or required by the agreement or as required by law.
2. **Safeguards.** Business Associate agrees to use appropriate safeguards to prevent any use of disclosure of the protected health information other than uses and disclosures expressly provided by this amendment.
3. **Mitigation.** Business Associate agrees to mitigate, to the extent practicable, any harmful effect that is known to Business Associate of a use or disclosure of Protected Health Information by Business Associate in violation of this Amendment of which it becomes aware as soon as reasonably practicable
4. **Reporting.** Business Associate agrees to report to covered entity any use or disclosure of protected health information in violation of this amendment of which it becomes aware as soon as reasonably practicable.
5. **Subcontractors and Agents.** Business Associate agrees to ensure that any agent, including a subcontractor, to whom it provides Protected Health Information received from, or created or received by business associate on behalf of covered entity agrees to the same restrictions and conditions that apply through his Amendment to Business Associate with respect to such information.

6. **Access.** When requested by Covered entity, Business Associate agrees to provide access to protected health information in a designated record set to covered entity or to an individual in order to comply with the requirements under 45C.F.R. & 164.524. Such access shall be provided by Business Associate in the time and manner designated by Covered Entity.

The JCAHO (Joint Commission on Accreditation of Healthcare Organizations) known as the **The Joint Commission** accredits and certifies more than 15,000 healthcare organizations and programs in the United States. This is a non governmental, non-profit, independent organization. The Joint Commission is an esteemed organization and it has been a force behind the creation of standards for linguistic and culturally competent patient-centered care. Hospitals that do not pass an accreditation are placed on a temporary watch, and often, the standards and qualification of medical interpreters are an issue. Interpreters are required to be knowledgeable in emergency codes for the organization, wear their badge, and follow codes for contagious disease, as well as other policies.

Their mission is to "continuously improve the safety and quality of care provided to the public through the provision of healthcare accreditation and related services that support performance improvement in healthcare organizations."

The Joint Commission in 2008 began working and adding to the CLAS (Culturally and Linguistic Appropriate Services Standards).

CCCS. Inc. Information Disclosure Policies:

As an interpreter you must always check disclosure policies for each institution contracting with you. Remember that there are state and federal laws. Check with your state if you are considered a mandatory reporter for any kind of child, elderly abuse or mistreatments of a person with a psychiatric illness and or suffering physical challenge.

All patient/client information is confidential and privileged and may not be divulged to anyone except the provider involved in the case. All information gained while interpreting is considered confidential, unless otherwise specified by a law. All written documents related to interpreting cases are confidential and should be treated as such.

Cases must not be commented on or discussed with anyone other than with staff or interpreting representatives. The above provisions apply to both during and after working hours and continue beyond the interpreter's tenure with the contracting organization. Interpreters do not discuss or disclose seeing or interpreting for patients to other patients and or community members even if there is a naïve question by a another caring community member or patient (such as "Was Jordan here today?"). Interpreters should not be taking pictures of their patients or their babies with their telephones and further more should not be showing them to the general public.

Health Insurance Portability and Accountability

HIPAA AND LANGUAGE SERVICES IN HEALTHCARE[1]

In 1996, the Health Insurance Portability and Accountability Act (HIPAA) became law and began to reshape how patients and healthcare providers think about the privacy of patient information. For interpreters who work in healthcare settings, it is important to understand how the patient privacy requirements of HIPAA affect their work and conduct.

In April, 2003, the regulations outlining health privacy protections became fully operational. The "privacy rule" provides a set of minimum national standards that limit the ways that health plans, pharmacies, hospitals, clinicians, and others (called "covered entities") can use patients' personal medical information. As stated by the Department of Health and Human Services, "A major goal of the Privacy Rule is to assure that individuals' health information is properly protected while allowing the flow of health information needed to provide and promote high quality healthcare and to protect the public's health and well being."[2]

The regulations protect medical records and other individually identifiable health information, whether it is on paper, in computers or communicated orally. The responsibility to abide by HIPAA binds the covered entity not only to ensure that its own staff protect patient privacy but also that anyone who it "controls" (such as volunteers) and with whom it contracts (called "business associates") follows these regulations. Thus interpreters who work in healthcare settings – whether as an employee, independent contractor or volunteer – are generally required to uphold the HIPAA privacy regulations.

The purpose of this memo is to explain HIPAA and its application to interpretation provided in healthcare settings.

1. Who is covered by the HIPAA privacy rule?

HIPAA regulates the conduct of covered entities. The nature and extent of an individual's obligations under HIPAA depend on the person's relationship to the covered entity. An interpreter in a healthcare setting may be:

- a "member of the workforce" of a covered entity;
- a "business associate" of a covered entity; or
- a person approved by the patient – neither of the above but approved by the patient to interpret.

As different situations arise, the nature of the interpreter's relationship to a covered entity becomes increasingly important. While some overlap exists, different HIPAA expectations attach to members of the covered entity's workforce, business associates, and a "person approved by the patient." It is likely that an interpreter may be subject to different rules at different times, varying as the interpreter provides services for a variety of healthcare providers.

Member of the workforce. The HIPAA privacy rule applies directly only to "covered entities."[3] Covered entities include health plans,[4] healthcare clearinghouses,[5] and certain healthcare providers.[6] All members of a covered entity's "workforce" are required to

PO Box 2308, Woburn, MA 01888-0508, **p:** 781-729-3736, **www.EmbracingCulture.com**
PO Box 6401, Manchester, NH 03108, **p:** 1-888-678-CCCS

abide by the HIPAA privacy rule. Being a member of the "workforce" is not limited to employees but also includes volunteers and trainees. Basically, any person whose conduct, when performing work for a covered entity, is under the direct control of the entity is subject to the privacy rule. It does not matter whether a person is actually paid by the covered entity.[7] This would include, for example, interpreters employed (full or part-time) by a hospital or other healthcare provider, volunteer interpreters coordinated through a covered entity's volunteer program, and other interpreters who are under the "control" of the covered entity.

Business Associates. In general, a "business associate" is a person or organization that performs functions for, or provides services to, a covered entity that involve the use or disclosure of individually identifiable health information.[8] The privacy rule requires that the covered entity ensure that its contract or other arrangement[9] with the business associate include specified written safeguards to protect individually identifiable health information used by, or disclosed to, its business associates. In addition, a covered entity may not authorize its business associates to make any use or disclosure of protected health information that would violate the privacy rule. Business associates were recently specifically subjected to the same limitations and penalties regarding use and disclosure of protected health information.[10]

The business associate must ensure that all of its agents, including subcontractors who have access to protected information, agree to implement reasonable and appropriate safeguards to protect it.[11] A business associate would include, for example, both a language agency and an individual interpreter who contracts directly with a covered entity. For the language agency, each of its agents – the interpreters themselves – would be bound to uphold the privacy rule through their relationship with the business associate.

Person approved by the patient. The privacy rule allows other individuals to have access to a patient's health information with the patient's consent. This includes a family member, other relative, or a close personal friend of the individual, or any other person identified by the individual. To these "persons approved by the patient," the covered entity may disclose protected health information directly relevant to the person's involvement with the patient's care or payment related to the patient's healthcare if the covered entity: obtains the individual's agreement; or provides the individual with the opportunity to object to the disclosure and the individual does not express an objection; or reasonably infers from the circumstances, based on the exercise of professional judgment, that the individual does not object to the disclosure.

Thus an interpreter brought by a patient to a clinical visit would be allowed to interpret and have access to a patient's protected health information even if not a member of a covered entity's workforce or acting as a business associate. The "person approved by the patient" category could also include, **but only if the patient consents**, an ad hoc interpreter such as another patient or person in the facility (who is not a member of the workforce or a business associate). Because in this situation the patient has consented and the interpreter is neither a member of the covered entity's workforce nor a business associate, the interpreter is not bound by the privacy rule. But if the patient is concerned about disclosing certain information to an ad hoc interpreter, the patient has the right not to consent. If the patient does not object, the covered entity may reasonably believe consent has been given and disclose the patient's information. The patient may ask the covered entity to provide an interpreter who would be subject to the protections of the HIPAA privacy rule.

2. How do I know if the "member of the workforce" or "business associate" rules apply to me?

It depends on the situation and it can be difficult to determine whether someone is a member of a covered entity's workforce or a business associate. In practical terms, the HIPAA rules must be observed by both members of the workforce (since the rules must be enforced by the covered entity) and business associates (through their contract with the covered entity). The only practical difference relates to HIPAA-required training – a covered entity is responsible for training all members of its workforce about HIPAA requirements. A business associate does not have the same responsibility (unless required by the contract between the covered entity and business associate).

Since payment is not the deciding factor (see definition of "member of the workforce" in Q.1 above), determining whether someone is a member of the workforce depends in part on the nature of the interpreter's work at the covered entity. If the interpreter is under the regular control of the covered entity, then she is a member of the workforce. For example, if a language agency sends the same interpreter to the same covered entity on a regular basis (for example, the same two days each week for the same hours) and the covered entity controls the interpreter's work conditions (e.g. assigning where the interpreter works, when breaks are taken, etc.), the interpreter is more likely to be considered a member of the workforce than if the interpreter worked at a different covered entity each day with hours and responsibilities more closely controlled by the business associate.

It is likely that only a retrospective review would determine that an interpreter should be considered a member of the workforce. This might occur, for example, pursuant to a complaint investigation by HHS' Office for Civil Rights. If OCR determined the interpreter was a member of the workforce, the interpreter should have received training from the covered entity. If no training was provided, the interpreter would not be subject to any penalties but the covered entity might be found in violation of HIPAA.

3. What patient information is protected under HIPAA?

An interpreter who is a member of a covered entity's workforce or a business associate must abide by the privacy rule and not disclose certain protected information about a patient. Generally, the privacy rule protects all "individually identifiable health information" held or transmitted by a covered entity or its business associate. It does not matter what format the information is in – electronic, paper, or oral. "Individually identifiable health information" is information created or received by a covered entity, including demographic data, which identifies the individual (or could reasonably be thought to identify the individual) and relates to:

- the individual's past, present or future physical or mental health or condition;
- the provision of healthcare to the individual; or
- the past, present, or future payment for the provision of healthcare to the individual.[12]

Individually identifiable health information includes many common identifiers such as name, address, birth date, and Social Security Number. This information is protected and may only be disclosed in certain circumstances (see Q. 4 below).

There are no restrictions on the use or disclosure of "de-identified" health information. De-identified health information neither identifies nor provides a reasonable basis for believing it could identify an individual.

In certain circumstances, a person's primary language may constitute individually identifiable health information and be prohibited from disclosure. For example, if there are a relatively small number of foreign language speakers in a community, disclosing a person's language and one other characteristic (such as age) might be sufficient to identify that person and thus disclosure would be prohibited.

4. When can an interpreter disclose protected patient information?
A major purpose of the privacy rule is to define and limit the circumstances in which an individual's protected heath information may be used or disclosed.

Member of the workforce. Interpreters who are members of a covered entity's workforce may not use or disclose protected health information, except:

- as the privacy rule permits or requires; or
- as the individual who is the subject of the information (or the individual's personal representative) authorizes in writing.

A member of the workforce should consult the privacy policy of the covered entity to determine the interpreter's role in disclosing information. While a covered entity must disclose information in certain circumstances, and may disclose information in others, the covered entity may restrict the persons who can make the disclosure. For example, the covered entity may not allow the interpreter to provide the information before obtaining clearance or may only allow certain individuals to disclose this information.

If a covered entity's privacy policy permits the interpreter to disclose this information, these are the rules that apply. A covered entity must disclose protected health information in only two situations:

- to individuals (or their personal representatives) when they request access to, or an accounting of disclosures of, their protected health information; and
- to the federal Department of Health and Human Services when it is undertaking a compliance investigation or review or enforcement action.

A covered entity may – but is not required to – disclose protected health information in the following circumstances:[13]

- in connection with treatment, payment, and healthcare operations;[14]
- if the individual gave "informal permission," that is the individual had an opportunity to object to the disclosure and did not;[15]
- incident to an otherwise permitted use and disclosure – as long as the covered entity has adopted reasonable safeguards as required by the privacy rule, and the information being shared is limited to the "minimum necessary";
- public interest and benefit activities – there are specific recognized activities[16] such as when required by law or for public health activities; and
- providing a limited data set for the purposes of research, public health or healthcare operations – limited protected health information may be provided to researchers without a patient's permission.

If an emergency or an individual's incapacity prevents a patient from agreeing or objecting to the use or disclosure, the covered entity may, in the exercise of professional judgment, determine whether the disclosure is in the best interests of the individual. If so, the entity may disclose only the protected health information that is directly relevant to the person's involvement with the individual's healthcare.

Whenever possible, a patient should be asked prior to disclosing information. But if this is impossible or impractical, whether an interpreter can disclose patient information depends on a number of factors. If the disclosed information is health information, and germane to the person's care, then it can be disclosed (unless the patient said otherwise), assuming the interpreter is viewed as part of the health team (which should be the case). This is allowed under the provision above that allows disclosure "in conjunction with treatment." If the information is not germane to treatment then it should not be disclosed at all. How the information was obtained from or about the client should not matter.

Business Associate. The contract between a covered entity and a business associate may not permit the business associate to disclose any information that a covered entity may not. Thus, a business associate and its agents are subject to the same requirements as a covered entity. This requirement was strengthened in the American Recovery and Reinvestment Act of 2009 which subjects business associates to the same penalties for violations as covered entities.[17] An interpreter should review the covered entity's privacy policy to understand any limits placed on the interpreters' disclosure of information (see above under "member of the workforce" for more information on what must and may be disclosed). The contract between the covered entity and business associate may also impose additional requirements on the business associate, so it may be important for the interpreter to review those requirements as well.

Person approved by the patient. An interpreter who is neither a member of a covered entity's workforce nor working for a business associate is not bound by the privacy rule. However, the interpreter may have independent ethical and confidentiality responsibilities – pursuant to either a Code of Ethics or other governing law or principles – that prohibit an interpreter from disclosing confidential or personal information about a patient.

5. Can an interpreter disclose information the patient discloses related to child/elder abuse or threatened violence to him/herself?
Any time an interpreter learns of this type of information in the course of interpreting, it is the interpreter's responsibility to interpret the information (just as any other information provided by the client would be interpreted). The provider should then address the situation and may be required to report the information pursuant to state mandatory reporting laws. If the interpreter learned of the information outside of the interpreting encounter (for example, while speaking with the client in the waiting room), whether the interpreter must disclose this information to the provider or others depends on state law[18] and the applicable interpreter's code of conduct, regardless of HIPAA.

6. What information should patients receive about the HIPAA privacy rule?
An interpreter may be asked to explain a HIPAA "privacy notice" to a patient. This notice generally explains a covered entity's privacy practices. A covered entity should give it to a patient the first time a patient is seen. If the patient receives healthcare services from an organized healthcare arrangement – such as a managed care organization or group practice – she may receive a single notice of the policies that apply throughout the system.

Member of the workforce. A covered entity that has a "direct treatment relationship" (such as a hospital or individual physician, but not a laboratory) with an individual must make a good faith effort to obtain written acknowledgement from her of receipt of the privacy practices notice. If a translation of the privacy notice is not available, an interpreter who is a member of the workforce likely will be responsible for providing a sight translation of the document and requesting written acknowledgement.

It is questionable whether providing an English privacy notice to an LEP individual would constitute "good faith" on the part of the covered entity. The determination will probably depend on the circumstances, but this would certainly not be a preferred practice.

Business Associate. The business associate does not have a responsibility to distribute a privacy notice to patients. The contract between the covered entity and business associate may require the business associate and its agents to provide a sight translation of a privacy notice to assist the covered entity in meeting its HIPAA obligations.

Person approved by the patient. These interpreters do not have a responsibility to provide any notice but may be asked by the covered entity to provide a sight translation of a privacy notice.

7. Are all interpreters required to attend HIPAA training? If so, who is responsible for providing the training?

Member of the workforce. Yes. The privacy rule requires covered entities to train all workforce members on its privacy policies and procedures, as necessary and appropriate for them to carry out their functions.[19] Because knowledge of what information can and cannot be disclosed is integral to the function of an interpreter, training would be necessary. Thus, for an interpreter who is a member of a covered entity's workforce, the covered entity must provide HIPAA training. If an interpreter does not receive training, the covered entity could be found in violation of HIPAA.

Business Associate. Not by law. The privacy rule does not impose specific requirements on business associates regarding training of its agents. The covered entity could, however, include a provision in its contract with a business associate to require training of the interpreters. Or the business associate could have its own internal policy to train its agents regarding HIPAA since its contract with the covered entity must include written safeguards to protect individually identifiable health information used by, or disclosed to, the business associates.

Person approved by the patient. No requirements exist for a covered entity to train other interpreters. Since the patient had to consent to the other person serving as an interpreter, the covered entity does not have any responsibility to ensure this interpreter maintains the patient's confidentiality according to the privacy rule.

8. What are the implications of the HIPAA privacy rule on the use of interpreters who have not signed an agreement of confidentiality with either the interpreter agency that sent them or the covered entity where they are interpreting?

Member of the workforce. A covered entity may require its staff to sign an agreement of confidentiality or may require compliance with HIPAA as a condition of employment.

Business Associate. A covered entity must sign a contract with a business associate that ensures confidentiality as required by the privacy rule. If the business associate (either an interpreter who has a direct relationship/contract with a covered entity or a language agency) refuses to sign, the covered entity would be violating HIPAA and should not use the interpreter/agency. A business associate may also be required, pursuant to its contract with a covered entity, to have its agents – the interpreters – sign a

PO Box 2308, Woburn, MA 01888-0508, **p:** 781-729-3736, **www.EmbracingCulture.com**
PO Box 6401, Manchester, NH 03108, **p:** 1-888-678-CCCS

confidentiality agreement. If no requirement is included in the contract, the business associate is not required to do so by HIPAA. The business associate may have its own internal requirement for its agents to sign confidentiality and/or other agreements.

Persons approved by the patient. HIPAA does not address these interpreters. Interpreters who provide services through a community based organization or other resource may have independent requirements addressing confidentiality.

9. If an interpreter believes that the privacy rules are being violated, is it the interpreter's responsibility to mention it to the healthcare provider or otherwise report the violation?
An interpreter would only have to report a suspected violation if a specific policy applying to the interpreter requires it. However, an interpreter may affirmatively choose to report a violation to the covered entity and/or the HHS Office for Civil Rights.

Member of the workforce. Reporting would depend on the policies of the covered entity. The interpreter should review the entity's written HIPAA policy and proceed accordingly.

Business Associate. There is no requirement for a business associate to report possible violations (unless the contract with the covered entity requires it). The covered entity must ensure that a business associate does not materially breach its contract. If a material violation does occur, the covered entity must take reasonable steps to cure the breach or terminate the contract with the business associate. The business associate may have its own internal procedures that require reporting.

Person approved by the patient. There is no responsibility to report suspected violations.

10. Often interpreters are asked to call patients to provide information about appointments, medications, or lab results. Is it a HIPAA violation to leave a message on an answering machine or with a family member?
No, it is not a violation of the privacy rule to leave a message on an answering machine or with a family member unless the patient has requested a restriction on the communication of information. Even then, a covered entity does not have to agree to any restriction on the otherwise permissible communication of information. However, if it does agree to a restriction, it cannot violate the restriction except in an emergency where the restricted protected health information is needed to provide emergency treatment. A business associate would be required to uphold any restriction agreed to by the covered entity.

An interpreter who works for a covered entity or business associate should check whether the patient requested a limitation (which should be noted in the patient's record).

11. Does HIPAA require that healthcare providers provide language services or, for larger entities, have a Language Services Department?
No. The requirement to provide language services arises from Title VI of the Civil Rights Act of 1964. However, the privacy rule requires that covered entities distribute a privacy notice to their patients and make a good faith effort to obtain written acknowledgement from patients of receipt of the notice. It is difficult to imagine how a covered entity could meet this requirement without providing a limited English proficient individual with either a translated privacy notice or an oral interpretation of it.

12. Does monitoring of interpreting for quality assurance purposes violate HIPAA?
Generally the answer is no. If the covered entity hires a quality assessor to evaluate either members of its workforce or business associates, it would have to ensure the assessor abides by HIPAA, just like any other business associate. If a covered entity's business associate (such as a language agency or interpreter) conducts its own quality assessment, the business associate must ensure all of its agents as well as secondary business associates uphold its privacy requirements (pursuant to its contract with the covered entity). Thus if the quality assessment monitor is employed by the language agency or working pursuant to a contract with the language agency, the monitor is bound to uphold HIPAA and there is no violation.

The only situation where a violation could occur is if an interpreter who is a business associate of a covered entity submits to quality monitoring requested by a third party (not the covered entity or a business associate) that does not have an obligation to abide by HIPAA. For example, an interpreter may be asked to undergo third party monitoring by a language agency for which the interpreter works part-time. If the entity requesting monitoring does not have its own responsibility to uphold HIPAA, any monitor hired by the language agency would not be subject to HIPAA and could release a patient's protected information. An interpreter should ensure that any monitoring of her work is conducted by a person or entity which is also obligated to keep patient information confidential pursuant to HIPAA.

13. Many interpreters keep detailed appointment books or schedules that include patient information (e.g. patient name, phone number, medical record number, date of birth, physician's name). Is this a HIPAA violation?
No, keeping records does not violate HIPAA. This is allowed because the interpreter – either a member of a covered entity's workforce or a business associate – is collecting this information so that it can perform services on behalf of a covered entity. But the interpreter must be careful to keep the information confidential as required by HIPAA.

PO Box 2308, Woburn, MA 01888-0508, **p:** 781-729-3736, **www.EmbracingCulture.com**
PO Box 6401, Manchester, NH 03108, **p:** 1-888-678-CCCS

14. Some interpreters must report patient information about an interpretation session to obtain payment. However, patients are never told that this information is being collected or reported. Is this practice in compliance with HIPAA?
Yes, this complies with HIPAA because the interpreter is using the information for a management and administrative purpose of receiving payment for her services.[20] However, the covered entity or business associate must obtain reasonable assurances from those processing the information that the information will be kept confidential and will not be further disclosed unless required by law.

15. What if a state's privacy law is different than HIPAA?
In general, state laws that are contrary to the privacy rule are preempted by the federal requirements, which means that the federal requirements will apply.[21] "Contrary" means that it would be impossible for a covered entity to comply with both the state and federal requirements, or that the provision of state law impedes accomplishing the full purpose of HIPAA.[22]

But the privacy rule provides exceptions to the general rule of federal preemption. Thus, contrary state laws remain in effect if they:

- relate to the privacy of individually identifiable health information and provide greater privacy protections or rights with respect to such information;
- provide for the reporting of disease or injury, child abuse, birth, or death, or for public health surveillance, investigation, or intervention; or
- require certain health plan reporting, such as for management or financial audits.

States may also, in certain circumstances, apply to HHS for an exception.[23]

1 *This report was made possible through the generous support of The California Endowment. This report was updated in April 2009.*

2 *HHS Office for Civil Rights, OCR Privacy Brief: Summary of the HIPAA Privacy Rule, at 1, available at http://www.hhs.gov/ocr/privacysummary.pdf.*

3 *45 C.F.R. § 160.103.*

4 *Health plans include: a group health plan as defined in the Public Health Service Act (PHSA) if the plan has 50 or more participants or is administered by an entity other than the employer who established and maintains the plan; a health insurance issuer as defined in the PHSA; a health maintenance organization as defined in the PHSA; Part A or Part B of Medicare and Medicare supplemental policies; Medicaid; a long-term care policy, including most nursing home fixed indemnity policies; an employee welfare benefit plan covering two or more employers; the healthcare program for active military personnel and the Civilian Health and Medical Program of the Uniformed Services; the veterans healthcare program; the Indian Health Service program; and the Federal Employees Health Benefit Plan. 42 U.S.C. § 1171(5), see also 45 C.F.R. § 160.103.*

5 *Healthcare clearinghouses are defined as public or private entities that process or facilitate the processing of nonstandard data elements of health information into standard data elements. 42 U.S.C. § 1320d, Social Security Act (SSA) § 1171, see also 45 C.F.R. § 160.103.*

6 *Healthcare providers are only covered if they electronically transmit health information in connection with certain transactions, like claims. Healthcare providers are defined as including providers of services (hospitals, critical access hospitals, skilled nursing facilities, comprehensive outpatient rehabilitation facilities, home health agencies, hospice programs, or for limited purposes regarding services provided in a teaching facility, a fund), providers of medical or other health services (defined in 42 U.S.C. § 1395x(s), SSA § 1861) and any other person furnishing healthcare services or supplies. See 45 C.F.R. § 160.103.*

7 *45 C.F.R. § 160.103.*

8 *Id.*

9 *The rule requires a covered entity to have a contract or "other arrangement" with a business associate to ensure compliance with the privacy rule. It remains unclear, however, what would constitute an allowable "other arrangement." 45 C.F.R. §§ 164.502, 162.504.*

10 *As part of the American Recovery and Reinvestment Act (P.L. 111-5, sec. 13404, Feb. 17, 2009), the liability provisions applicable to covered entities were extended to business associates.*

11 *Id.*

12 *45 C.F.R. § 160.103.*

13 *The privacy rule contains much more detailed information describing these reasons. See 45 C.F.R. § 164.502(a)(1).*

14 *These terms are defined in the privacy rule.*

15 *Informal permission may be obtained by asking the individual outright, or by circumstances that clearly give the individual the opportunity to agree, acquiesce, or object (where the individual is incapacitated, in an emergency situation, or not available, covered entities generally use their professional judgment to determine if the use and disclosure is in the best interests of the individual). 45 C.F.R. §§ 164.510, 164.512.*

16 *See 45 C.F.R. § 164.512.*

17 *P.L. 111-5, sec. 13404, Feb. 17, 2009.*

18 *For more information on whether interpreters are mandated to report child abuse, see National Health Law Program, Healthcare Interpreters: When Are They Mandated to Report Child Abuse?, available at http://www.healthlaw.org/pubs/200312.interpreter.html. For information on state reporting requirements on domestic violence, see Family Violence Prevention Fund, National Consensus Guidelines on Identifying and Responding to Domestic Violence Victimization in Healthcare Settings, Appendix J, available at http://endabuse.org/programs/healthcare/files/Consensus.pdf.*

19 *45 C.F.R. § 164.530.*

20 *45 C.F.R. §§ 164.501 (defining "payment"), 164.506(c).*

21 *45 C.F.R. § 160.203.*

22 *45 C.F.R. § 160.202.*

23 *45 C.F.R. §§ 160.203-205.*

PO Box 2308, Woburn, MA 01888-0508, **p:** 781-729-3736, **www.EmbracingCulture.com**
PO Box 6401, Manchester, NH 03108, **p:** 1-888-678-CCCS

Interpreter Evaluation Tool based on the IMIA standards.

Name:______________________________Target Language:_____________Date: ___/___/___

OBSERVATION

1 PRE SESSION

Client/patient	Yes	No
1. Introduction?		
2. Interpreter helped client with registration?		
3. Interpreter explained the usage of the first person?		
4. Interpreter informed client of confidentiality policy?		
5. Interpreter informed client that everything said during the session will be interpreted?		
6. Did the interpreter handle the waiting period appropriately?		
7. Did the interpreter appropriately acknowledge similarities and differences?		

Provider	Yes	No
8. Introduction?		
9. Interpreter explained the usage of the first person?		
10. Interpreter informed the provider that everything said during the session will be interpreted?		

2 THE TRIADIC RELATIONSHIP

Interpreter/provider and client	Yes	No
1. Did the interpreter appropriately arrange seating?		
2 Did the interpreter show appropriate eye contact?		
3 Did the interpreter appropriately handle the comments from client or provider?		
4 Did the interpreter stay in the room alone with client?		
5 Did the interpreter help with medical procedures?		

6 Who makes the decision of when to stay behind the curtain?
○ Interpreter ○ Client ○ Provider

3 INTERPRETATION TECHNIQUE

Interpreter	Yes	No
1. Usage of First Person?		
2. Omissions?		
3. Additions?		
4. Meaning/Accuracy?		
5. Meaning/Completeness?		
6. Keeps appropriate flow?		
7. Asks for clarification?		
8. Checks with client if he/she understood everything?		
9. Mode of interpretation: consecutive, simultaneous, sight and summary?		
10. Memorization techniques: note-taking, echoing key words and finger counting?		

4 KNOWLEDGE OF MEDICAL TERMINOLOGY

Strengths:

Weaknesses:

Areas for growth:

PO Box 2308, Woburn, MA 01888-0508, **p:** 781-729-3736, **www.EmbracingCulture.com**
PO Box 6401, Manchester, NH 03108, **p:** 1-888-678-CCCS

5 FOLLOW-UP	Yes	No
1. Interpreter helps client with follow-up visits?		
2. Interpreter helps client getting home?		
3. Interpreter does not provide advice when asked for his or her opinion?		
4. Interpreter handled a distraught client appropriately?		

6 CULTURAL KNOWLEDGE/CLARIFICATION	Yes	No
1. Interpreter clarified cultural meaning by checking with appropriate party?		
2. Interpreter understood vocabulary used by both, provider and client?		
3. Interpreter understands client's immigration history?		
4. Interpreter shows how to best address client by showing respect?		
5. Interpreter asks permission to become a cultural coach when appropriate?		
6. Interpreter showed respect for client's own individuality ?		
7. Interpreter understands provider and client's communication styles?		
8. Interpreter understands USA medical system and that of client's native country?		

SELF- OBSERVATION:

7 ETHICS	Yes	No
1. Do you accept gifts?		
2. Do you share your opinion regarding controversial beliefs?		
3. Do you ask questions to clients/personal/clinical?		
4. Do you provide your telephone number?		
5. Do you give your opinion when asked by the clients?		
6. Do you deliberately delete information for political/ religious /personal beliefs?		
7. Do you call clients at home when not asked by provider to do so?		
8. Do you drive client to places?		
9. Do you give money to clients?		
10. Do you make remarks that are pejorative against anyone?		
11. Do you use power of knowledge for personal gains?		
12. Do you discuss prior sessions with different providers?		
13. Do you tell clients what to say in the session?		
14. Do you discuss the sessions and identify clients/providers?		

Lesson Three:
Memory and Memory Aids

Understanding Goals

Students will be able to:

- learn about short and long-term memory and how it impacts interpreter's performance
- learn and practice memory aids
- identify possible memory blockers

Key Concepts

- Short-term and long-term memory
- Memory aids: visualization, note-taking, mind mapping, finger counting, echoing, anchoring

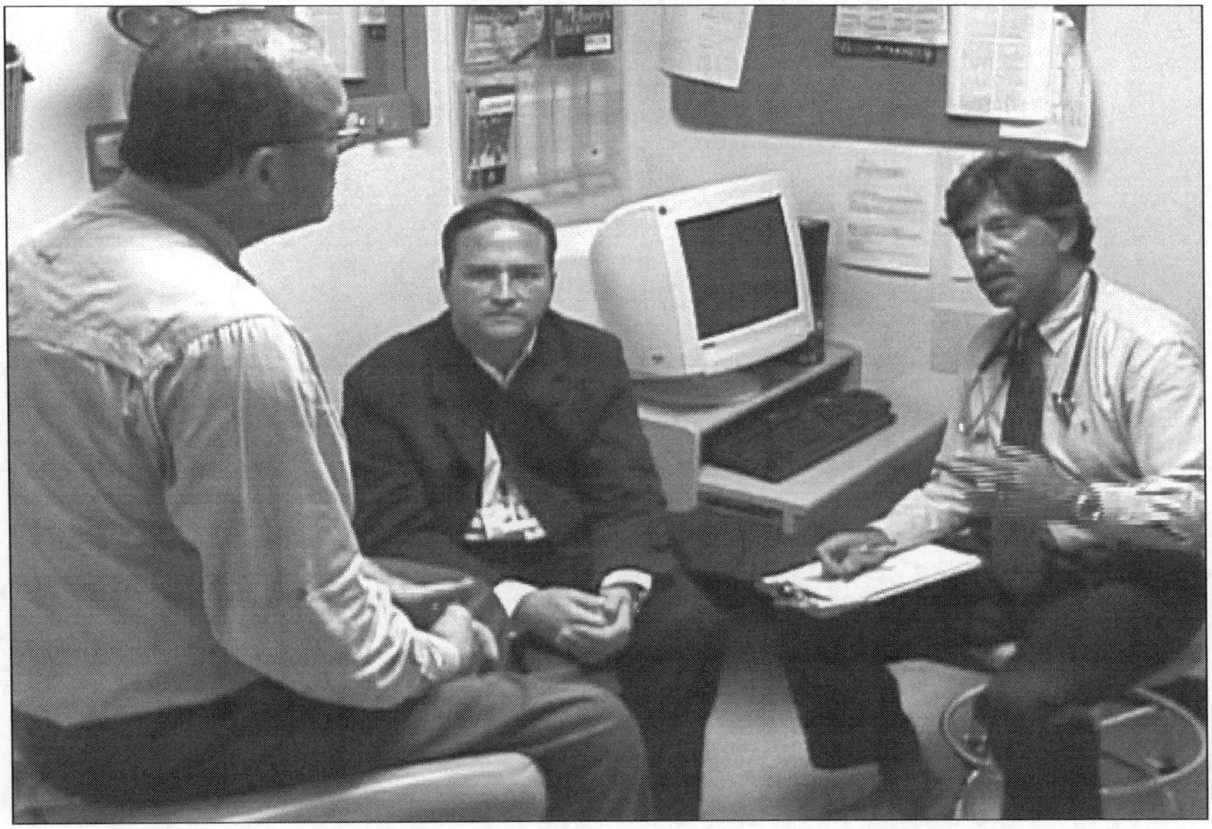

PO Box 2308, Woburn, MA 01888-0508, **p:** 781-729-3736, **www.EmbracingCulture.com**
PO Box 6401, Manchester, NH 03108, **p:** 1-888-678-CCCS

Lesson Three: Quiz
Memory and Memory Aids

Mark the item or items that best complete each sentence.

1. The MMR vaccine combats the following diseases:
   A. Measles, tetanus and mumps
   B. Measles, mumps and diphtheria
   C. Varicella, influenza and chicken pox
   D. Measles, mumps and rubella

2. Tetanus is a disease commonly known as:
   A. German measles
   B. TD
   C. Jaundice
   D. Lockjaw

3. Flu (influenza) can lead to:
   A. Varicella
   B. HIB
   C. Chronic hepatitis
   D. Pneumonia

4. In rare cases, children receiving the measles vaccine suffer:
   A. Brief convulsions
   B. Extensive bruising
   C. Swelling of the glands
   D. Stiffness of the joints

5. Hepatitis B is a viral disease that can damage the:
   A. Brain
   B. Lungs
   C. Spine
   D. Liver

6. In the consecutive mode, interpretation is done word by word.
   ○ True ○ False

7. In consecutive interpretation, the interpreter is working mainly with:
   A. Immediate memory
   B. Long-term memory
   C. Short-term memory
   D. Kinesthetic memory

8. Four major parts of the brain are the: cerebrum, cerebellum, ________ and ________.
   A. brain stem and calpain
   C. calpain and serotonin
   B. register and neurotransmitter
   D. brain stem and diencephalon

9. The cerebellum controls:
   A. Balance
   C. Emotions
   B. Coordination
   D. Involuntary activity

10. The ________ allows humans the ability to consciously change behavior and store logic, language, mathematics and speculation about the future.
   A. Pon
   B. Gray matter
   C. DDAVP
   D. Cortex

11. Recently, scientists have discovered that people have two upper brains, called the:
   A. Left and right memories
   C. Left and right cortices
   B. Left and right neurons
   D. Left and right gestalt

12. Neuron communication is called:
   A. Array
   B. Sequence
   C. Linearity
   D. Synapse

13. If memory is compared to a house, then long-term memory is the:
   A. Basement
   B. Steps
   C. First floor
   D. Attic

PO Box 2308, Woburn, MA 01888-0508, **p:** 781-729-3736, **www.EmbracingCulture.com**
PO Box 6401, Manchester, NH 03108, **p:** 1-888-678-CCCS

Mark each item "True" or False."

1. When faced with an emotional blocker, the interpreter should try to fight it.
   - O True O False
2. Verbal memory is the physical learning aspect of memory.
   - O True O False
3. Lyme disease is easy to diagnose because it has very particular symptoms.
   - O True O False
4. Patients get Lyme disease after being bitten by a deer tick.
   - O True O False
5. The erythema migrans rash is the only trait unique to Lyme disease, nonetheless it is absent in at least 25% of the infected people.
   - O True O False
6. Because some tests do not differentiate Lyme disease antibodies from similar organisms, providers often exercise clinical judgment in order to diagnose infectious disease.
   - O True O False
7. Lyme disease is an asymptomatic illness.
   - O True O False
8. Ticks that transmit Lyme disease are very small and their bites are usually painless.
   - O True O False
9. Immune systems of patients with Lyme disease produce antibodies within hours of being bitten by a tick.
   - O True O False
10. People usually get Lyme disease in late spring and early summer when they are outside more often.
    - O True O False
11. The erythema migrans rash is also known as "bull's-eye."
    - O True O False
12. Most cases of Lyme disease occur when temperatures are very low.
    - O True O False
13. Lyme disease is curable, particularly if caught in the early stages.
    - O True O False
14. Many patients with Lyme disease can be effectively treated with antibiotics, which accelerates the healing of the erythema migrans rash and can prevent future symptomatic complications.
    - O True O False
15. In order for people to avoid being bitten by the tick that transmits Lyme disease, it is advisable to walk often near wooded areas and bordering grasslands.
    - O True O False
16. Wearing dark colored clothing is advisable to detect ticks on a person's body.
    - O True O False

Lesson Three: Class Activities
Memory and Memory Aids

REVIEW

In class take a few minutes and try to match the vaccine names with the matching abbreviations.

	Vaccines	Abbreviations
1	Diphtheria	Hib 4
2	Hepatitis A	PCV
3	H Hepatitis B	DtaP, Td, Tdap 9 7 9, 7
4	H Haemophilus influenza type b	HepA 2
5	sarampion Measles, Mumps, Rubella	Varicella 10
6	Inactivated Poliovirus (Polio)	MMR 5
7	Pertussis	Td 1 tosferina → difteria
8	Pneumococal polysaccharid Vaccine	MCV 12
9	Tetanus, Diphtheria, Pertussis	IPV 6
10	Varicella (chicken pox)	RV 11
11	Rotavirus	PPSV 8
12	Meningococcal	HepB 3
13	Human Papillomavirus	HPV 13

MMR
5 - SPR (in spanish) - Triple viríca

sarampion / paperas / rubeola

pertussis ⇒ tos ferina

RV - (syntoms: diarrea)

PPSV - certain types of pneumonia

HPV

THE ART OF MEDICAL INTERPRETATION®

Class Activities

PO Box 2308, Woburn, MA 01888-0508, p: 781-729-3736, www.EmbracingCulture.com
PO Box 6401, Manchester, NH 03108, p: 1-888-678-CCCS

EXERCISE

Divide into groups of twos.
Think about your favorite food from childhood.
Share it with your colleague.

Keep in mind this image and describe which of your senses you used when reporting on your favorite food from childhood: visual, auditory, olfactory, gustatory and kinesthetic.

Share it with the larger group

How is learning about memory important to you as an interpreter?

____

____

____

Memory is one of the functions or processes of our incredible brain. All of the pieces of information are sorted and decoded in the various sensory areas of the cortex converged in the hippocampus. Afterward, it associates it with other information already filed and then sends the information back where it came from.

What is your first reaction when you think of the word tuberculosis?

____

____

____

By answering this question, we are forcing you to go to your hippocampus which serves as one of the "home bases" for sorting information by comparing it with other already stored information.

So if an interpreter hears the word " tuberculosis," and has studied some medical terminology one would know that "osis" means a condition, "tubercol" means a cluster of tissues called *tuberculum*, "small swelling, pimple," dim. of "*tuber*" lump.

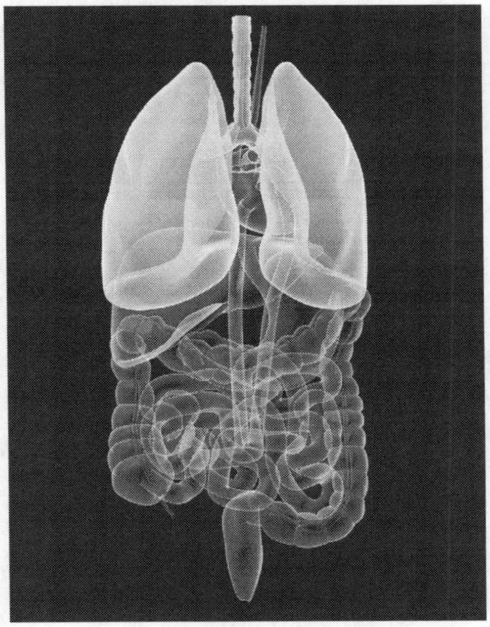

But if the interpreter is not medically trained, the interpreter may recall what tuberculosis is from media reports or from personal experiences such as a need for a TB screening in order to work in a public place or from a family or a friend who had tuberculosis.

Because this word is so publicly known in the U.S.A., one can access the hippocampus and most likely be correct with the associations and descriptions of the meaning of tuberculosis.

PO Box 2308, Woburn, MA 01888-0508, **p:** 781-729-3736, **www.EmbracingCulture.com**
PO Box 6401, Manchester, NH 03108, **p:** 1-888-678-CCCS

Not all of the information we learn as a layperson is correct.
A patient can have tuberculosis in different parts of the body not just the lungs!

For example, several years ago a study was done on two groups of Cambodian refugee settlements in the U.S.A. The interpreters believed that the populations being interviewed by the public health researcher would not understand the word tuberculosis so they described it as the "illness that makes you yellow."

After completing the study, the researchers realized that the Cambodian populations understood that the "illness that makes you yellow" was once a description for liver disease as described by their prior interpreter when they were living in refugee camps in Thailand. So the research became invalid. The patients and the interpreters in the U.S.A. were using the same words but had misfiled the meaning based on wrong associations leading to wrong information.

This is why interpreters need to be humble and start from step one when formally learning medical information; and not base their knowledge only on their experiences as patients or non-trained interpreters.

According to CDC: "Healthcare and correctional facility workers have long been at risk of contracting Tuberculosis(TB)." Cases in healthcare workers constituted 3 percent of all TB cases. TB is a potentially severe contagious disease that is spread from person to person through the air. When a person infected with TB coughs, sneezes, or even speaks, the TB germs can spray into the air; therefore, leaving anyone nearby able to breathe TB germs into their lungs.

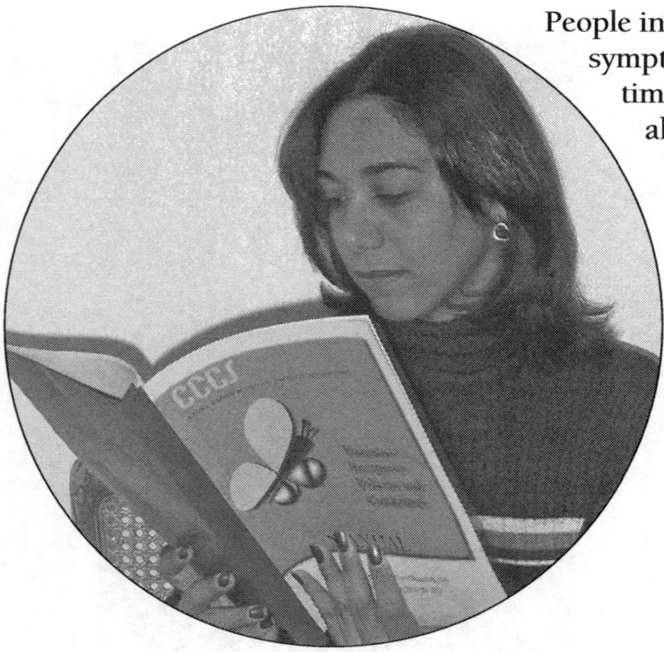

People infected with TB do not feel sick and do not have any symptoms. However, they may develop TB disease at some time in the future. TB usually affects the lungs, but it can also affect other parts of the body, such as the brain, the kidneys, or the spine. Eleanor Roosevelt, wife of Franklin Roosevelt, died from tuberculosis of the bone marrow. The classic symptoms of tuberculosis are a chronic cough with blood-tinged sputum, fever, night sweats, and weight loss. If people have TB disease, they need medical help. If they don't get help, they can die.

I have a feeling that after this exercise you are all going to understand what tuberculosis is.

THINK

Take a few minutes and note what you recall from what you have learned about tuberculosis.

____

____

____

____

____

____

What was old information and what is new information?

OLD	NEW

This exercise, by making you think, write, see pictures is a way to build up your memory so that you remember new facts by repeating them, you are actually passing information through the hippocampus several times. The hippocampus keeps strengthening the associations among these new elements until, after a while, it no longer needs to do so. The cortex will have learned to associate these various properties itself to reconstruct what we call a memory.

PO Box 2308, Woburn, MA 01888-0508, **p:** 781-729-3736, **www.EmbracingCulture.com**
PO Box 6401, Manchester, NH 03108, **p:** 1-888-678-CCCS

THINK

Can you recall a mnemonic that CCCS, Inc.™ developed so as to help you as an interpreter with a pre-session?

____

____

____

The brain is a complex organ that controls body temperature, blood pressure, heart rate and breathing. It not only helps us with our various senses: seeing (visual), hearing (auditory), smelling (olfactory), tasting (gustatory), touching (kinesthetic). It also manages our physical motions such as walking, talking, standing and sitting. It allows us to dream, to use reasoning, and to experience emotions. All these components impact our memory, it is a brain wide process!

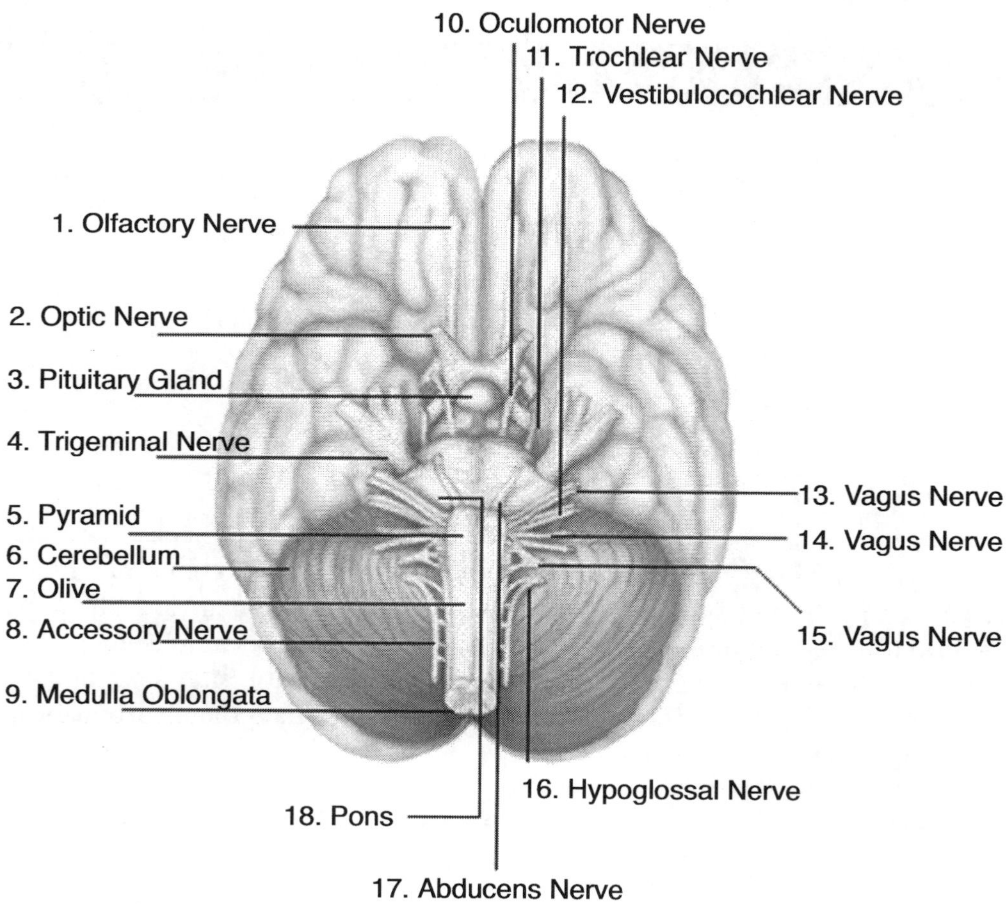

Medical interpreters are asked to listen to a speaker's complete thought, then understand the meaning of the message and convey it accurately while striving to maintain the speaker's language register. In the consecutive mode, the interpretation is not done word by word. Instead, the most important key to a successful interpretation is the understanding and accurate transmission of a message.

In consecutive interpretation, the interpreter is working mainly with the short-term memory, but will still need to have access to both immediate and long-term memory.

We will now discuss general information on how the brain and memory work. It is our hope that you will begin to exercise your memory, thus strengthening your consecutive interpretation skills.

Watch the video ACEBO and answer the questions that follow:

1. According to Holly Mikkelson, why is it important for interpreters to learn about memory?

____

____

2. Give examples of stimuli.

____

____

3. What is the most important stimuli in interpreting?

____

____

4. Why are stimuli rejected by the sensory register?

____

____

5. When does a stimulus get transferred into Short-Term Memory (STM)?

____

____

PO Box 2308, Woburn, MA 01888-0508, **p:** 781-729-3736, **www.EmbracingCulture.com**
PO Box 6401, Manchester, NH 03108, **p:** 1-888-678-CCCS

6. How can interpreters make sure that only relevant stimulus come into STM?

7. STM is limited in two different ways. How?

8. Does Long-Term Memory (LTM) have any limitations? What is the problem with LTM?

9. What do we need to do as interpreters to avoid that problem?

10. How do you personally focus on information?

11. What is your dominant language? Why is that something you should be aware of?

12. When you are processing information in the STM, what might be some examples of interferences that might occur?

13. What could interfere with retrieval from the LTM?

Complete the blanks with information from the video:

Interpreters need to keep the following in mind:

1. We remember what is ________________ .
2. The way we improve our ability to recall information in consecutive interpreting is to know as much as possible about the ________________ (background reading), by paying ________________ , by ________________ with certain types of cases, by making sure we ________________ possible distractions that may interfere, by listening for ________________, and by concentrating on the ________________ .
3. ________________ skills are primary. We listen for ________________, not words. We analyze the message in terms of overall context and we take into consideration all elements of communication.
4. Interpreters should try to avoid being ________________ about the delivery of the information (________________, speech mannerisms, controversial opinions, ________________, ________________)
5. Interpreters should tune out all ________________ and concentrate on the ________________ .
6. ________________ is key.
7. We need to ________________ and act on the information as it comes into short term memory so that we can process it more effectively.
8. The memory skills interpreters need the most are ________________skills. The capacity of short term memory is limited and small. Some propose that it is ________________ items of information, up to ________________ seconds.

PO Box 2308, Woburn, MA 01888-0508, **p:** 781-729-3736, **www.EmbracingCulture.com**
PO Box 6401, Manchester, NH 03108, **p:** 1-888-678-CCCS

Three Stages of Memory

Imagine your memory as a house. There is a set of front steps that lead to the main door.

1. Immediate Memory

These front steps can be called immediate memory. It takes an average of five to seven seconds for a person to climb the stairs of immediate memory, open the first door and enter into short-term memory. Immediate memory is a transient holding of information that declines rapidly and is limited in capacity. Interpreters use a variety of techniques to verify that a message is transferred from the immediate to the short-term memory.

2. Short-term Memory

Short-term memory may span several seconds, hours, or even days. In short-term memory, the interpreter is very active processing information by associating meanings, sorting, organizing, coding and selecting which information gets stored where.

3. Long-Term Memory

Long-term memory can be compared to the attic of the house. The information stored there may span a period of months or years.

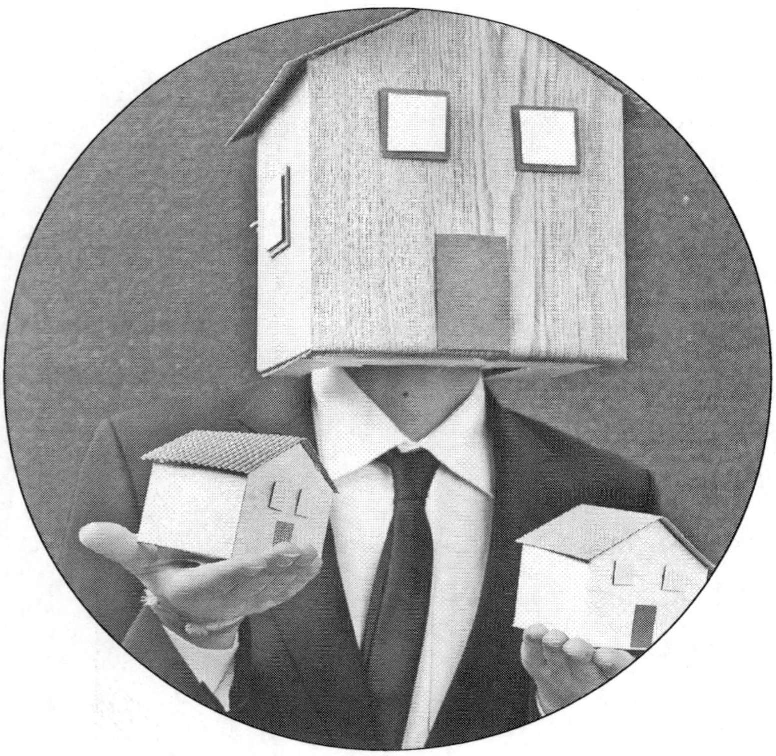

Implications for Interpreters:

Now imagine that each of these three stages of memory can only address a certain number of items (capacity) for a limited amount of time (duration). Immediate memory can only refer to generalities and lasts an average of two seconds. Short-term memory has the capacity for seven things and can last from 30 seconds to 2 days. Long-term memory has an infinite capacity and can last forever.

In order for Interpreters to learn medical terminology, so that it goes into long term memory or the attic of the house one needs to do it not just by memorizing words and converting them from source to target language, but mainly by looking into a story (role-plays) and understanding (making meaning), sorting information(looking into dictionaries using bilingual and monolingual ones), repeating it by using the oral and written form(role-play practice and glossaries).

Knowing terminology saves times and places the interpreter at ease when interpreting. In order to remember information, the interpreter needs to:

- Register
- Retain
- Retrieve the speaker's information

Practice the following memory exercises:

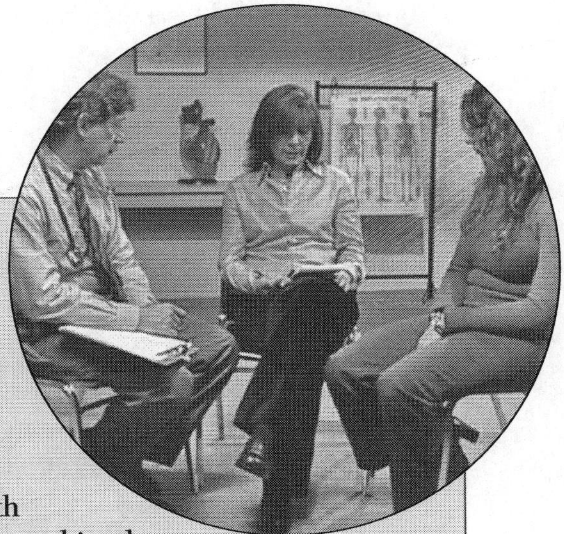

EXERCISE

- Divide into groups of twos
- Have your partner read the entire paragraph without stopping
- Convey it accurately from one language to another

Immunizations: Before there were available vaccines, nearly everyone contracted measles, mumps and rubella while growing up. These diseases can cause serious health problems. Usually, the vaccines for the three diseases are combined and given as one shot called the MMR vaccine. It is usually given two times between the age of 15 months and 6 years old.

Feedback:

____

____

____

____

In the retrieval phase, the interpreter may use two different types of memory: recall and recognition. With recall, the interpreter is going into his/her consciousness and finds the information. With recognition, the interpreter might not identify the origin of the memory at first, but when looking for it, he/she begins to recognize or re-experience it.

EXERCISE

Divide into groups of twos. Take turns interpreting and giving feedback. Read each paragraph in two major sections with a short pause in between, ask your colleagues to repeat it. After the interpretation ask the interpreter how s/he recalled the information.

~~paperas~~ Sarampión

Measles: Measles is serious and easily passed from one person to another. It causes high fever, cough, and rash and lasts for 1 to 2 weeks. One out of ten children who catch measles will also have an ear infection or pneumonia. It can cause an infection of the brain that could lead to convulsions, hearing loss and mental retardation.

Feedback:

____

____

____

____

paperas

Mumps: Mumps causes fever, headache, and swollen glands under the jaw and lasts for several days. It can also cause a mild inflammation of the coverings of the brain and spinal cord, and hearing loss. One out of every four males with mumps will have a painful swelling of the testicles for several days.

Feedback:

____

____

____

____

Memory Blocks

Individuals have a tendency to be hard on themselves when they forget something. A situation, an event, or a person, gets blamed for this inability to remember. We hope that, with this lesson, the interpreter will begin to understand what memory blocks are and how he/she reacts to them.

In her book *Total Recall*, Dr. Joan Minninger explains the following three types of memory blocks: emotional, mechanical, and physical.

1. An **emotional blocker** results from a conflict of an emotional (feelings) nature that might interfere with one's ability to remember. We as human beings have a defensive mechanism that protects us from feelings that can hurt us.

What are some of your emotional blockers?

Join another family for dinner. / experience in London

How do you feel when you forget something?

Embarrassed / Blank

What techniques do you use in your daily life when you feel emotionally blocked?

Think – happy memory w. family / Kids / best friends

It is common for interpreters to have experienced similar life tragedies as patients, especially if both patient and interpreter are refugees. Everyone with some traumatic life experience uses different defense mechanisms to survive and at times make peace with his/her particular painful experience.

Let's imagine a refugee interpreter who is now interpreting for a refugee patient and suddenly gets overloaded with flashbacks of a particular traumatic event that had been put to sleep for many years. The awakening of this trauma can become an emotional blocker and might cause the interpreter to become distracted while trying to handle all these conflicting feelings.

The interpreter could forget to listen to the speaker due to an overload of emotions. Emotional blockers are inevitable; they are part of life and often protect people from additional pain. However, at times they can become obstacles that prevent a medical interpreter from rendering an accurate interpretation.

PO Box 2308, Woburn, MA 01888-0508, **p:** 781-729-3736, **www.EmbracingCulture.com**
PO Box 6401, Manchester, NH 03108, **p:** 1-888-678-CCCS

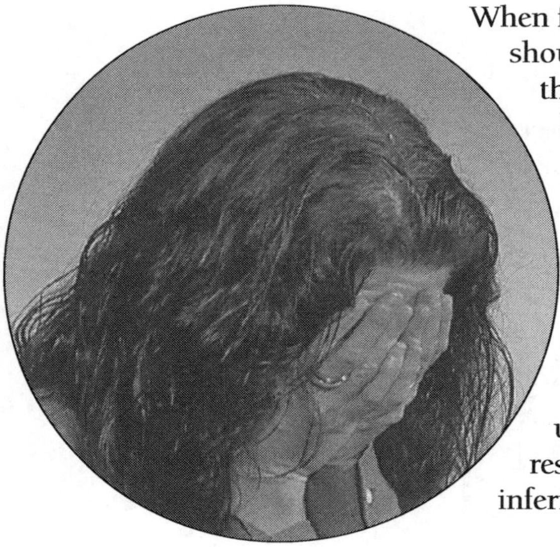

When faced with an emotional blocker, the interpreter should not fight it, but accept the fact that the feeling is there. Try not to get rid of it but instead learn how to live with it and try to develop a coping strategy for the moment. Later on after the session, the emotional blocker will need to be addressed appropriately; otherwise it will come back again.

At times, interpreters who are doing consecutive interpretation, and feel emotionally overloaded, will resort to simultaneous, temporarily, to stay focused. You may want to find a way of coping with unexpected emotional blockers due to feelings of resistance, resentment, guilt, anger, superiority, inferiority towards the patient and/or the provider.

2. **Mechanical Blocks**

These are blocks that, for some reason, have been stored incorrectly; something that we see or hear leading to a misunderstanding of information. This is common also when an individual is still struggling with his or her bilingual skills. So it is important for interpreters to always look into context and not focus on words and meaning. As a native Portuguese speaker I do not sound words that start with "H" like the English words. So, often, I misfiled the word "hair" as "air" because that is the way I hear it. Perhaps because they sound a bit alike, another common mistake among interpreters are the words "ureter" (ureters are muscular ducts that allow urine from the kidneys to the urinary bladder) and "urethra" (the tube that connects the urinary bladder to the outside of the body. Other confusing words are "gallbladder" and "bladder," "nape" and "neck." A mechanical block might originate in the storing process or when accessing and retrieving information. Look into the following words and define them:

Affect: ____________________

Affect: ____________________

Bare: ____________________

Bear: ____________________

Bear: ____________________

Sometimes, the same or similar words may have different meanings in different contexts. If a provider sends you for a "stress test" a person who has lived in the USA for a while knows that it is the test to measure whether or not there are signs of ischemia in your heart when you exercise. It is not related to your emotional type of stress. Any distraction such as noise during any of the following memory stages such as processing, accessing or retrieving may be enough to cause a mechanical block.

3. **Physical Blocks**

Due to a physical situation, information may have not been appropriately delivered to the brain. Illness (atherosclerosis, senility, amnesia, injuries, allergies, drugs), and physical challenges (blindness, deafness) are common physical blockers. Not all these physical blockers are permanent. Interpreters who are not good in taking care of themselves such as eating balanced meals and drinking fluids, or sleeping enough hours may be unable to perform well with their memory skills due to low blood sugar, dehydration and fatigue. As a non-native English speaker I noticed that when I am tired my e-mails often are full of minor spelling errors such as "te" instead of "the."

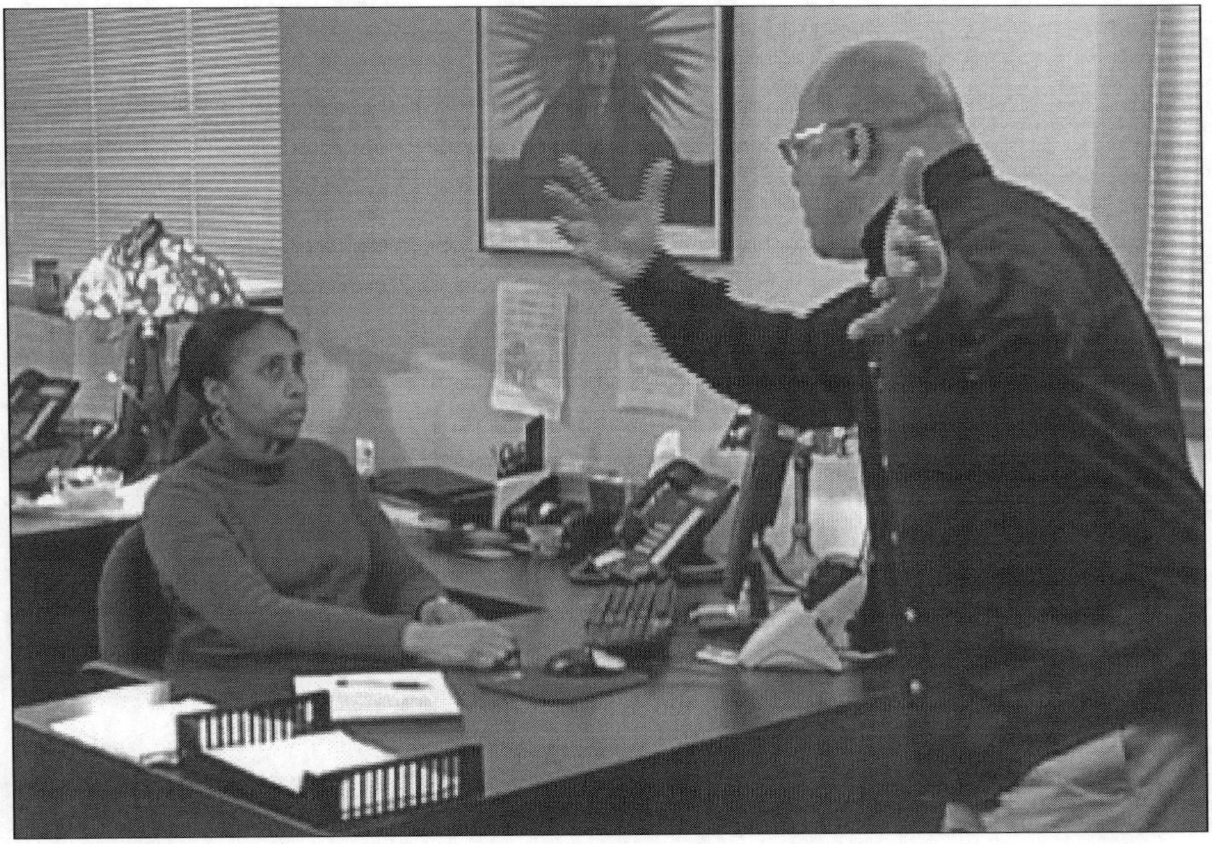

PO Box 2308, Woburn, MA 01888-0508, **p:** 781-729-3736, **www.EmbracingCulture.com**
PO Box 6401, Manchester, NH 03108, **p:** 1-888-678-CCCS

Get to know how you operate your memory in your daily activities.
Now that we have talked about things that block us, let's talk about things that help us.

Q: When you go food shopping, what do you do in order to buy everything you need?

____

____

____

Some individuals are visual learners, others are verbal or kinesthetic. Most people have a mixture of styles.

Q: For interpreters, if you know you are a visual learner, what technique(s) can you use to recall and retrieve information from your memory?

____

____

____

Q: If you know you are a verbal learner, what technique(s) can you use to recall and retrieve information from your memory?

____

____

____

Q: If you know you are a kinesthetic learner, what technique(s) can you use to recall and retrieve information from your memory?

____

____

____

If you are a visual learner you might use note-taking;
If you are a verbal learner you might repeat things to yourself (echoing);
If you are a kinesthetic learner you might use finger counting.

Memory Aids:

Visualization and Mind Mapping, Note-Taking, Finger-counting, Echoing, Anchoring

1. **Visualization**:
   This is one of the most important techniques for accurate consecutive interpretation. In visualization, the interpreter sees images that will remind him or her of the spoken words. At first it might feel awkward for the inexperienced interpreter to convert words into images instead of worrying about the words themselves.

EXERCISE

Draw a picture for ureter (s) and urethra

Mind Mapping:

With this memory aid technique, the interpreter should find a key idea and connect the idea, through association, to other pre-existing ideas. This helps the interpreter to understand and remember new information. For example, if the main idea for the interpretation is gallbladder stones, you might want to imagine a fragile bag full of heavy stones, a bag which doesn't seem to want to open. You then see a person curled up in pain, unable to carry the bag. The real story is that this patient has terrible pain due to gallbladder stones. In this mind mapping, visualization is used. Interpreters can also use written words and literally write one idea in the center of a page and then branch out with all kinds of words or ideas. Later on begin to develop relationships and connections with this journey of letting your ideas or images go loose!

Mind maps (or similar concepts) have been used for centuries in learning, brainstorming, memory, visual thinking, and problem solving. A mind map is often created around a single word or text, placed in the center, to which associated ideas, words and concepts are added.

Research mind mapping or go to http://www.mapyourmind.com/howto.htm and review the 8 steps one should take while practicing mind mapping.

EXERCISE

Read to your colleague the following information. Ask for repetition of the information by using mind mapping.

The provider is explaining to the patient's mother about the tetanus shot:
This shot is also called lockjaw. It kills about one out of every three people who get the disease. It is caused by germs that make a toxin (poison) after entering the body, usually by a cut or a scrape. The tetanus vaccine is usually combined with the diphtheria vaccine and given as one shot called td. People vaccinated as children need booster shots every ten years.

2. Note-taking:

Any notes should always be taken in the target language. If you take notes or shorthand however, avoid getting hung up on word searches. This can create undue anxiety, derail the thought process, and limit your ability to retain an entire message. The interpreter needs to take notes by using her/his own symbols such as arrows, boxes circles, etc. Some interpreters use abbreviations, although it is not highly recommended. At times, interpreters have difficulty distinguishing between words with similar roots and get into trouble when relaying meaning. In note-taking, interpreters need to connect the sequence of ideas and completely understand the meaning. Interpreters might want to write down numbers. It is very important for the interpreter to pay special attention to the first and last sentences spoken.

3. Finger Counting:

An interpreter has to recall three important points. A patient states that he has the worst headache, and chest pain that travels down his shoulder. The interpreter presses three fingers: one for headache, the second for chest pain, and the third for traveling pain. As soon as the interpreter presses finger number one, the thought "worst headache" comes to mind; finger two, chest pain; and finger three, a traveling pain down the shoulder.

4. Echoing Key Words:

An interpreter understands the meaning of a key word and repeats the word. When reminded of this key word, the entire meaning of the message comes to your mind naturally. These words are like anchors of meaning stored in a concise way in the active memory. Because this word was processed and its meaning understood by the interpreter, most likely the interpreter will access it quickly and be able to relay the entire meaning of the message.

5. Anchoring:

When an interpreter is not able to convey a complete message there is a tendency for the interpreter to feel lost. In any triadic encounter, there will be times when the interpreter will not recall the complete message. It is our obligation to not only be accurate but also complete. However, when providers are asked to repeat everything again they often don't remember exactly what they said, but they remember meaning and it takes time for the provider to recall the information and retrieve it. Interpreters when unable to recall a complete thought, instead of asking for repetition, might want to repeat the last word, or concept, that they recall; therefore, helping the provider remember. This technique is equally helpful to the provider, the patient and interpreter, because it cuts off unnecessary repetitions, reduces anxiety and frustration, and saves time.

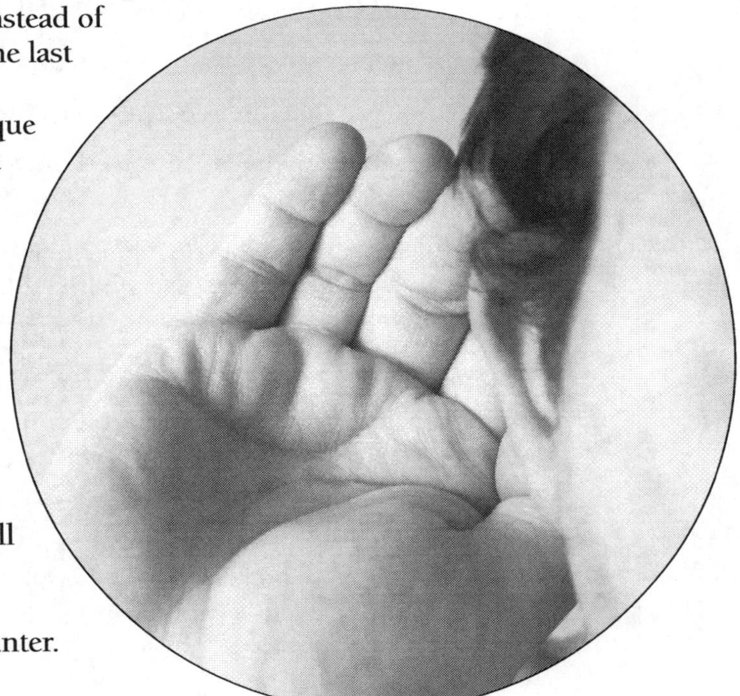

Remember that one minute of sustained speech corresponds to an average of 150 words. Thus, a skilled consecutive interpreter employs a variety of memory aids with a view to preserving accuracy. Memory is like a muscle, and it needs to be exercised. It is important that you practice all the memory aids in order for you to choose the ones that fit you best, and are most appropriate for each particular triadic encounter.

PO Box 2308, Woburn, MA 01888-0508, **p:** 781-729-3736, **www.EmbracingCulture.com**
PO Box 6401, Manchester, NH 03108, **p:** 1-888-678-CCCS

Memory Aids

PRACTICE #1

INSTRUCTIONS

I One of your colleagues is going to read an entire sentence and you are going to repeat the sentence as closely as possible.

II Please listen to the sentence carefully, apply any of the techniques you have learned to help you with your memory, such as fingercounting, echoing, visualizing, mind-mapping, note-taking, etc.

III Repeat the first sentence as soon as your colleague finishes.

IV After repeating the sentence, share your understanding of the information with your colleague .

For example, this sentence was about….. and I seem to have liked the ….. (technique).
For example, this sentence was about….. and I seem to have liked the ….. (technique).

Case A.

#1: Keep the dressing clean and dry.

#2: Wash the area gently with mild soap and warm water.

#3: For discomfort, take the medication as prescribed by your doctor.

#4: Apply a cream to the area. You need only to apply a thin coating of the ointment three times a day.

#5: If the affected area is an arm, leg, or head, you should elevate the part (above the level of your heart) for at least the first 24 hours after the burn. This will help decrease swelling and pain.

#6: Drink plenty of fluids the first 24 hours.

#7: Notify the Emergency department if you did not receive a tetanus shot and have not had one within a 5 year period. If you have had a tetanus shot within a 5 year period, you do not require another.

#8: Return to the Emergency Department if you notice any of the following: foul odor; excessive drainage; increased pain, swelling or redness; the dressing becomes wet or dirty; any lumps in the groin or under the arm of the injured side; chills or fever greater than 100 degrees Fahrenheit; red streaks going away from the affected area.

Case B.

#1: You have developed a local reaction to an insect bite.

#2: The area may become swollen, red and sometimes itchy.

#3: Insect bites may sometimes get infected. Keep the area clean.

#4: You may use cool compresses to the affected area in order to provide you with some relief.

#5: If you can tolerate aspirin, it might also help you to decrease the pain and inflammation.

#6: In case you have the following symptoms you must call your doctor immediately or return to the Emergency Room: increase in swelling, redness, and the amount of pain; red streaks going away from the reaction site; or any other signs of infection, such as drainage or yellowish pus; or, if you develop hives, shortness of breath, or light-headedness.

Case C.

#1: I am going to give you the following medications: Phenergan 25mg tablets: take one orally every 6 hours as needed for nausea. Dispense thirty. No refill. Generic substitute OK. Vicodin: 5mg: take 1 to 2 orally every 24 hours. Dispense fifteen. No refills. Generic substitute OK.

PO Box 2308, Woburn, MA 01888-0508, **p:** 781-729-3736, **www.EmbracingCulture.com**
PO Box 6401, Manchester, NH 03108, **p:** 1-888-678-CCCS

REFLECTION

What was easy? What was difficult?

____

____

____

What was case A referring to? What about case B?

____

____

____

Was there a difference when you knew what the instructions were referring to?

____

____

____

Which tools did you use for…

List of symptoms ____

Numbers ____

Names of medications ____

What did you learn about the way your brain processes and retrieves information?

____

____

____

REFLECTION *(continued)*

Overall which type/s of memory did you use to retain and recall each exercise?

Verbal? ______________________________

Visual? ______________________________

Kinesthetic? ______________________________

If you relied heavily on visual memory, how often did you mix up the order of information in the message?

____

____

____

____

Did you add or distort message meaning?

____

____

____

____

If you used primarily verbal memory, what associations and comparisons did you utilize as memory aids?

____

____

____

____

PO Box 2308, Woburn, MA 01888-0508, **p:** 781-729-3736, **www.EmbracingCulture.com**
PO Box 6401, Manchester, NH 03108, **p:** 1-888-678-CCCS

REFLECTION *(continued)*

If you used kinesthetic memory, how often did you gesture with your hands?

Was there a particular object which you held on to during the exercise?

Did you find yourself sitting in a specific position?

If you used a combination of the methods listed above, did you consciously do so or was it something that came naturally?

PRACTICE #2

In language pairs, practice converting the following instructions into your Target Language.

Case A.

Nurse to the patient: Here is the instruction sheet on how to care for your burn at home:

Keep the dressing clean and dry. Wash the area gently with mild soap and warm water.

For discomfort, take the medication as prescribed by your doctor.

Apply a cream to the area. You need only to apply a thin coating of the ointment three times a day.

If the affected area is an arm, leg, or head, you should elevate the part (above the level of your heart) for at least the first 24 hours after the burn. This will help decrease swelling and pain.

Drink plenty of fluids the first 24 hours.

Notify the Emergency department if you did not receive a tetanus shot and have not had one within a 5 year period. If you have had a tetanus shot within a 5 year period, you do not require another.

Return to the Emergency Department if you notice any of the following: foul odor; excessive drainage; increased pain, swelling or redness; the dressing becomes wet or dirty; any lumps in the groin or under the arm of the injured side; chills or fever greater than 100 degrees Fahrenheit; red streaks going away from the affected area.

Do you have any questions?

PO Box 2308, Woburn, MA 01888-0508, **p:** 781-729-3736, **www.EmbracingCulture.com**
PO Box 6401, Manchester, NH 03108, **p:** 1-888-678-CCCS

Lesson Three: Homework
Memory and Memory Aids

1. Go over your notes for today's class and read section "Additional Resources"
2. Read and practice ALL role-plays for this lesson – practice CIFE and all the memory aids
3. Continue developing your glossary
4. Translate the parts of the brain into your Target Language

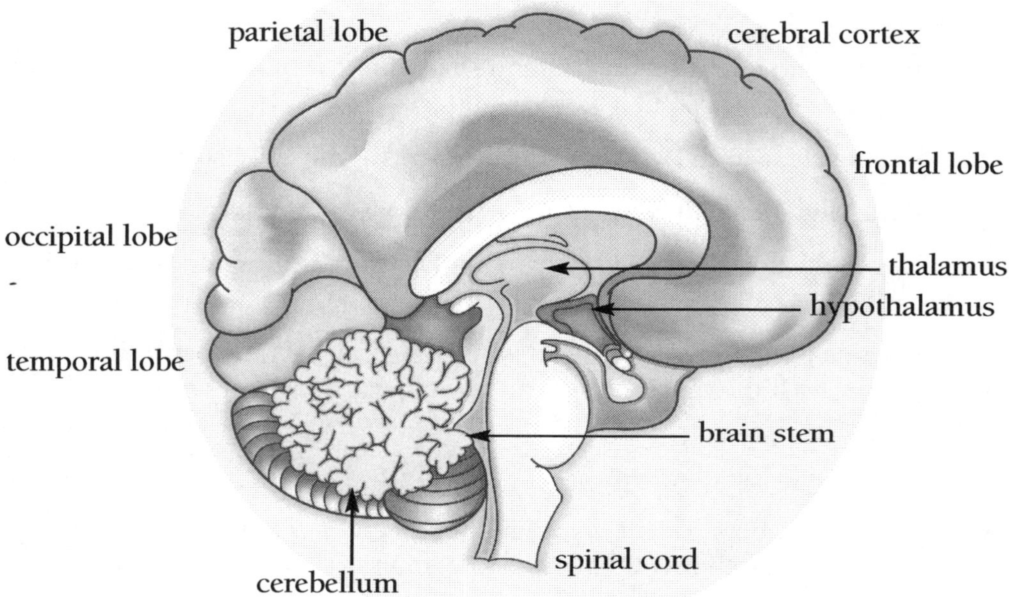

English	Target Language
a. frontal lobe	
b. parietal lobe	
c. temporal lobe	
d. occipital lobe	
e. cerebral cortex	
f. thalamus	
g. hypothalamus	
h. brain stem	
i. cerebellum	
j. spinal cord	

Matching Exercise 1:

	Associate Memory	1	Type of memory where one stores organized and clustered information for easy recall. This information can be stored for years and the quantity of information can be infinite.
	Concentration	2	To commit to memory
	Cortex	3	The process of remembering, recalling, registering and retaining information that has been learned or experienced within a time frame (from immediate to hours, days, years or decades).
	Emphasis of ideas	4	Difficulty in learning due to an impasse with
			self-confidence regarding the comprehension of a particular area. For example an interpreter may be very good as an interpreter but has a mental block about working with computers.
	Episodic memory	5	A special system of developing a technique to remember more than 7 items through associative linking
	Immediate Memory	6	A visual tool which helps the interpreter retain information and be accurate.
	Kinesthetic Memory	7	Information organized in a thoughtful way
	Linking	8	Developing unique memory tools
	Logical sequence	9	The ability to fully direct one's attention to an important objective by avoiding getting distracted by circumstantial objects
	Long- Term Memory	10	The outer or superficial layer of gray matter called cerebrum and cerebellum
	Memory	11	The importance of paying specific attention to ideas
	Memory retention	12	The type of memory where an interpreter might remember an incident, (for example, a book or business lunch).
	Mental blocking	13	Memory based on muscle skills. For example, some people use lots of hand gestures as descriptions. Others learn how to ride a bicycle but stop riding for several years. As soon as they get on a bicycle, they remember how to ride.
	Mind Mapping	14	The process of storing information in long-term memory. After a medical terminology class on the meaning of certain prefixes, roots and suffixes, an interpreter should retain information that will facilitate the prompt identification of those word parts. For example as soon as the interpreter hears the word vaginitis and s/he understands the meaning of the suffix "itis" s/he will know that vaginitis is as an inflammation of the vagina.

continued

PO Box 2308, Woburn, MA 01888-0508, **p:** 781-729-3736, **www.EmbracingCulture.com**
PO Box 6401, Manchester, NH 03108, **p:** 1-888-678-CCCS

Matching Exercise 1 *(continued)*

	Mnemonics	15	A supportive technique to help a person store information in long-term memory. It can be done by repeating the experience and using different memory approaches such as verbal, visual and/or kinesthetic.
	Note taking	16	People can only register what they absorb. One can not forget what has not been registered or selected as important. Registration happens when a person is first exposed to information, and is a first step to retention and recall.
	Order	17	Seeking out memory to help with recognition and recall.
	Originality	18	A connection where the axon or neuron terminal makes contact with the dendrite or neuron receptors. This connection generates an electrical impulse that inhibits or creates a nerve impulse.
	Perception	19	Mainly used by the left side of the brain. Interpreters implementing verbal memorization techniques may make many associations and comparisons and tend to be less sure of their accuracy.
	Recall	20	Mainly used by the right side of the brain. Some researchers believe that visualization is a more direct way of learning new information. However, visualizers tend to change the order of information and at times introduce new information. Interpreters implementing visual memorization techniques seem more sure of their accuracy, but may actually be less accurate.
	Recognition	21	The ability to grasp the meaning of information at an appropriate level. To understand is to have a clear idea, to achieve or to grasp the nature, significance or explanation of something.
	Registration	22	Also known as recent memory and is limited to less that a dozen items. This is a transitional station for holding information. As information gets stored, coded and clustered, it is deposited in long-term memory. Short term-memory can last from 25 minutes to a few days.
	Reinforcement	23	A type of memory that is based on general knowledge consisting of facts, concepts and rules. Part of the interpreter's general memory is the need to be accurate with the interpretation. Otherwise, s/he could cause irreparable damage to a patient. Literally, a patient could die as a result of a poor interpretation.

continued

Matching Exercise 1 *(continued)*

	Retention	24	Recalling information by revisiting a situation that is based in the past and is triggered as you enter the environment. For example, every time you go to a certain deli, you re-experience or recognize time spent with your mother-in-law before she passed away.
	Retrieval	25	To make the connections from one idea to another. To develop a relationship between ideas or associations
	Sematic memory	26	An order of ideas; new learning that is clustered by topics.
	Short term memory	27	Temporary memory that is limited in capacity to about 7 objects. It lasts an average of 5-7 seconds. A mental health provider may check immediate–memory by asking that a patient recalls three items (table, cover, pencil). An interpreter needs to simply convey the same words once without any further explanations so the test is valid.
	Synaptic connection	28	A memory technique, usually done in writing by circling a key idea and placing it at the center of a page. From that circle the interpreter may associate other ideas, words or concepts by developing a map. As the interpreter goes through this process, s/he is transfering information from short term memory into long term memory.
	Understanding	29	The capacity that one has to retain information within the three main types of memory: immediate, short term and long term.
	Verbal memory	30	Retrieving information from a memory entered in your consciousness voluntarily or involuntarily. The memory is stored, and even if it seems to "go away" for a short moment it will come back,(some examples are song lyrics and faces of people you know).
	Visual memory	31	People can only register what they absorb. One can not forget what has not been registered or selected as important. Registration happens when a person is first exposed to information, and is the first step in retention and recall.

continued

PO Box 2308, Woburn, MA 01888-0508, **p:** 781-729-3736, **www.EmbracingCulture.com**
PO Box 6401, Manchester, NH 03108, **p:** 1-888-678-CCCS

Matching Exercise 2:

Working with potential mechanical blockers

Pronounce words correctly in English.
Match word with best sentence.
Find appropriate word in your target language.

	WORD	SENTENCE	TARGET
	Affect	1 a device, drug or chemical agent that prevents conception.	
	Affect	2 birth control, family planning.	
	Bare	3 to shorten, ex: contract a muscle.	
	Bear	4 an explicit bilateral commitment by two parties. Ex: a psychotherapist and patient to a defined course of action to attain the goal of the psychotherapy.	
	Bear	5 to acquire by contagion or infection. Ex: contract measles, "How did your daughter contract the measles?"	
	Class	6 A downward spiral in the economic condition of a company or even a country.	
	Class	7 A temporary mental state or chronic mental disorder characterized by feelings of sadness, loneliness, despair, low self-esteem, etc.	
	Contraceptive	8 displacement of a part downward or inward. *(Sometimes a provider will press down on your arm to check for edema—swelling.)*	
	Contraception	9 A condition of one's health status; a condition of the weather; in between poor and good.	
	Contract	10 tolerate receiving or giving pressure. Ex:______ the pain, ______ down.	
	Contract	11 without clothing; nothing extra; the bare truth	
	Contract	12 Outcome. Ex.: Mrs. Smith had an exam, how did she ______?	
	Depression	13 Cause a reaction to---How does the antibiotic affect you?	
	Depression	14 How you present yourself, manner, facial expression, etc. *(What was his affect?)*	
	Depression	15 a group of students.	

continued

Matching Exercise 2 *(continued)*

	WORD	SENTENCE	TARGET
	Fair	16 An animal	
	Fair	17 A person's idea or thought.	
	Fair	18 A written decision by a judge.	
	Fare	19 A group of bacteria, strain, virus	
	Inflammation	20 To appear for examination, treatment, etc./said in reference to a patient	
	Infection	21 " the patient presents with ______"	
	Opinion	22 A fundamental pathologic process consisting of a dynamic complex of cytologic and chemical reactions that occur in the affected blood vessels and adjacent tissues in response to an injury or abnormal stimulation caused by a physical, chemical or biologic agent incuding: "Cardinal signs are: Rubor, redness; calor, heat (or warmth); tumor, swelling; and dolor, pain. Some or all of them may be present; irritated area internal or external, often red, sensitive to touch or movement/various causes	
	Opinion	23 a gift	
	Present	24 Declaration of words. Ex: He did state the following words to me.	
	Presents	25 To hit someone/something with force	
	Present	26 An illegal work stoppage.	
	Resume	27 To cross out, delete a verbal or written (*a letter or word; Judge: "______ that last statement from the record!"*) or "Please put a ______ through the incorrect word in the sentence."	
	Resume	28 A medical condition/AVC	
	Right	29 Legal directives, benefits.	
	Right	30 A method of applying one's thoughts to paper by pen, type/computer.	
	Write	31 choice cut of meat, fish, chicken	
	Sprain	32 having a part in something (*I have a personal --- ______ in this issue.)*	
	Strain	33 a large nail-type wedge (*wooden or metal*) Ex: tent ______/pen.	
	Strain	34 political union. In which ______ do you live?	

continued

PO Box 2308, Woburn, MA 01888-0508, **p:** 781-729-3736, **www.EmbracingCulture.com**
PO Box 6401, Manchester, NH 03108, **p:** 1-888-678-CCCS

Matching Exercise 2 *(continued)*

	WORD	SENTENCE	TARGET
	Steak	35 Physical, mental, emotional condition, ex: What is the patient's mental/physical status?	
	Stake	36 Gently touch, rub. Ex: "______ the cat gently."	
	Stake	37 A specific fee/amount charged to ride the bus, taxi, airplane, etc	
	State	38 *(Pronounced – reh-zoo-may)* curriculum vitae	
	State	39 Family or group of viruses, bacteria/class *(ex: a rare strain of TB)*	
	State	40 Correct, opposite of left, opposite of wrong	
	Strike	41 Invasion of the body with organisms that have the potential to cause disease. Ex: staph infection, streptococcus i. *(strep throat)*,cryptogenic i.. bacterial, viral or other i. the source of which is unknown.UTI	
	Strike	42 The cause of a reaction or symptom: asthma trigger; activating mechanism/piece of an armed weapon/gun. "Don't pull the ______"	
	Strike	43 Produce – The tomato plant will ______ 5 quarts	
	Stroke	44 Give way to. When two people disagree, each must______ a little to the other	
	Stroke	45 To injure by overuse or improper use(usually refers to a muscle tear)	
	Trigger	46 *(Pronounced-re-zoom)* continue a previously stopped action	
	Trigger	47 An injury to a ligament as a result of abnormal or excessive forces applied to a joint, but without dislocation or fracture.	
	Yield	48 A description of skin tone: sunburns easily	
	Yield	49 Equal and just treatment of a matter. *(Kids often say: That's not ______!!)*	

Lesson Three: Role-Plays
Memory and Memory Aids

Work individually at first:

- Read the entire role-play
- Get a general sense of its meaning
- Circle the most challenging medical terms
- Apply the Samurai! technique to those terms
- Read the role-play again for a deeper understanding
- Find an accurate equivalent in the target language

Work in a language-specific group of friends, fellow students or colleagues:

- Share your doubts
- Ask for other ways of expressing the same meaning
- Develop a glossary
- Check the dictionary
- Practice the role-plays – remember to do CIFE for all your role-plays
- Have your colleagues observe you and provide feedback on your accuracy and register.
- These colleagues can keep track of any omissions, additions, mistakes or distortions in your interpreting and point these out to you in a follow-up discussion.

Student Interpreter Evaluation

Student Name ____________________ Date ________

Language ____________________

Mode of Interpreting (check one): ☐ Consecutive ☐ Simultaneous

Role-Play/System ____________________

Areas Observed ____________________

Accuracy

Register ____________________

Omissions ____________________

Additions ____________________

Distortions ____________________

Pronunciation ____________________

Speaker's emotions conveyed? ____________________

Explain ____________________

Technique

General flow ____________________

Flow when requesting clarification ____________________

Speed ____________________

Eye Contact ____________________

Distracting Habits ____________________

Ethical Issues

Answered questions for patient? ____________________

Advised patient? ____________________

Vocabulary Expansion Recommendations

____

____

Other Recommendations

____

____

Language Coach Signature ____________________ Date ________

PO Box 2308, Woburn, MA 01888-0508, **p:** 781-729-3736, **www.EmbracingCulture.com**
PO Box 6401, Manchester, NH 03108, **p:** 1-888-678-CCCS

Role-Play 13: Medical History

	Pronunciation	Additions	Omissions	Mistakes
MD: Hi. I am Dr. Orr. I am sorry you had to wait a bit longer than normal, but I had to attend to an emergency.				
PT: I understand. As a doctor, you must be so busy!				
MD: Let's review your medical history. Did you have any severe illnesses during childhood?				
PT: One time, my mother had to isolate me from my siblings. One side of my throat swelled up, and then the other side. I forgot the name of the illness. But the doctor said that if I were a boy, I could have become infertile.				
MD: Humm, it sounds like you had mumps.				
PT: Yes, that's it!				
MD: Did you ever have chicken pox?				
PT: Doctor, I'm not sure, but I once had blisters all over my face and body. My mother told me not to squeeze them, or else I would be scarred. In my country, we call it varicella. Is this the same illness you're talking about?				
MD: Yes. We only have fifteen minutes so we need to go over these questions as quickly as possible. Can you limit your answers to yes or no? Have you ever had surgery or been hospitalized?				
PT: Not that I know of.				
MD: Have you ever had any blood transfusions?				
PT: Oh no! As one of Jehovah's Witnesses, my Bible-trained conscience would not allow me to have a blood transfusion.				
MD: I will write down, "patient refuses blood transfusion because of her religious beliefs." Perhaps you should carry a card in case of an emergency. Do you have a health proxy and is anyone aware of your decision in this matter?				
PT: Yes, I carry a Medical Directive in my wallet at all times, and several of my family members have copies of my health proxy. I've brought a copy for you to keep in my file.				
MD: OK. Have you ever had any history of the following: High blood pressure? Diabetes? Heart problems? Psychiatric problems or any other significant illness?				

continued

Role-Play 13 *(continued)*

	Pronunciation	Additions	Omissions	Mistakes
PT: (Shakes her head as a "no" to all these illnesses.) Once I got shingles, is that important? It was several years ago, and I just got a touch of it, not too bad!				
MD: I will write it down in your medical history. Now let's go over your medication history. Are you allergic to any medications?				
PT: No.				
MD: Are you taking any over-the-counter medications, vitamins or other remedies?				
PT: Oh no! I am pretty healthy. Once in a while I take some Tylenol for a headache.				
MD: Are you allergic to medications or food?				
PT: No.				
MD: Now I am going to ask you about your family's health history, any diabetes, asthma or cancer?				
PT: (Shakes her head indicating "no" to all these illnesses).				
MD: Any high blood pressure, thyroid or kidney disease?				
PT: My grandfather had trouble with kidney stones.				
MD: Maternal or paternal grandfather?				
PT: My mother's father. She used to tell me stories about him passing out because of the pain.				
MD: Any heart disease, tuberculosis or alcoholism?				
PT: No, once in a while my father drank a bit too much beer.				
MD: Did his drinking ever affect the family, or did he change his behavior?				
PT: A little bit. My mother would tell him he had enough. He was funny when he was a bit touched!				
MD: Let me ask you about your menstrual cycle. Date of your first period? Is your menstrual flow regular?				
PT: I get my periods every 28 days. The flow is good, heavy in the beginning, and less by the fifth day, and almost nothing by the seventh day.				
MD: I can see that you had two normal pregnancies. Are you on any type of contraceptive presently?				
PT: My husband and I use the rhythm method and it has worked well for us.				

continued

PO Box 2308, Woburn, MA 01888-0508, **p:** 781-729-3736, **www.EmbracingCulture.com**
PO Box 6401, Manchester, NH 03108, **p:** 1-888-678-CCCS

Role-Play 13 *(continued)*

	Pronunciation	Additions	Omissions	Mistakes
MD: As you know, you are taking lots of risks. Do you want to get pregnant again?				
PT: My husband and I would not mind having another cutie, but we hope that we have some more time in between pregnancies.				
MD: Was your Mother ever on DES when pregnant for you?				
PT: Is that the medication that was supposed to help with nausea but resulted in many babies being born deformed?				
MD: No, that was Thalidomide. But DES is a type of estrogen, a hormone that was used to prevent miscarriages and may cause cancer in the vagina.				
PT: No, I don't think so.				
MD: When was your last Pap smear? And your mammogram?				
PT: Two years ago. I am due for one. Should I have a mammogram?				
MD: It can never hurt to at least have a record of a mammogram as a baseline. You are still young and you do not have a family history of breast cancer, so we are not in a rush. But when you have a minute you may want to schedule it! Let me listen to your heart and lungs. Please let me know if the stethoscope is a bit cold. I am warming it up with my hands. Please take a deep breath. Good. Now breathe in and out, once again, in and out. Good. Hold your breath in, ...let go. I can hear some rales. It sounds like you have a bit of asthma. Do you smoke or are you just getting over a cold?				
PT: No, smoking is not good. I do get tired and a bit short of breath if I run, and at times I feel a bit of a wheeze.				
MD: You may need an inhaler just to help you when your chest feels tight. I will ask the nurse to show you how to use the inhaler in case you ever need it. You may inhale two puffs before exercising or when you are in the middle of a cold.				

continued

Role-Play 13 *(continued)*

		Pronunciation	Additions	Omissions	Mistakes
PT:	I once tried my husband's inhaler and I got a bit jerky.				
MD:	Yes, it almost has the affect of a stimulant, as your heart rate goes up and you may feel a bit shaky.				
PT:	I will learn how to use the inhaler, but I will avoid it by all means!				
MD:	I see that you got all you immunizations when you were a child. Do you need a PPD test for your work?				
PT:	Yes, I work with kids and I just need to remind you that in my country I took the BCG vaccine and I always show positive with my skin test.				
MD:	Perhaps we can just take an X-ray. I will order it.				
	Break It Down	☐	☐	☐	☐

☐ **CIFE with patient** ☐ **CIFE with provider** ☐ **FLOW** ☐ **REGISTER**

Role-Play 13: Glossary

PO Box 2308, Woburn, MA 01888-0508, **p:** 781-729-3736, **www.EmbracingCulture.com**
PO Box 6401, Manchester, NH 03108, **p:** 1-888-678-CCCS

1. Pathology (diseases, conditions)

2. Laboratory Tests and Diagnostic Procedures

3. Treatment Procedures

4. Idiomatic Expressions (if any)

5. Other (vocabulary in this particular role-play that you feel is important/relevant or that you anticipate problems with)

Role-Play 14: Cold

	Pronunciation	Additions	Omissions	Mistakes
Patient: I have been feeling tired and tomorrow is my daughter's birthday. Doctor, can you give me something to get me back to normal?				
MD: Hmm, you are looking for a miracle drug! Let me ask a few questions and see what I can do for you. How old is your daughter?				
Patient: She's thirteen going on twenty. She has an older boyfriend. She is a good kid, but you need to always watch out for craziness. A good kid can go bad because of the wrong friends.				
MD: You know, my kids are still young, but I understand that having a teenage girl is always hard for a father. But it is possible to successfully negotiate around friends while keeping the channels of communication open. You pick your fights and give a little, and your family will survive the teenage years!				
Patient: See, she talks with her mom. We are separated and my wife is coming after me for alimony besides the money I already pay for child support.				
MD: The best thing is to leave the money matters to the adults. I wish you all the best. Let's go over your symptoms.				
Patient: OK.				
MD: Do you have a scratchy throat, nasal or ear congestion?				
Patient: I feel that my head is going to explode. You know when you can hear the echo of your own voice in your head? That is the way I feel right now.				
MD: You told me earlier that you felt fatigue. Did I ask you about hoarseness? You sound a bit hoarse. Is it getting better or worse?				
Patient: I guess I have the flu. But then again, maybe I have a cold.				
MD: Your fever is pretty low and your symptoms are not quite as severe as flu symptoms. You know, with the flu, the symptoms can last for a few weeks. Anyway, the treatment for colds and the flu is similar.				
Patient: OK.				
MD: Drink a lot of fluids to help your body to get rid of the virus. You can buy over- the-counter decongestants like Sudafed, but do not overdo it with the medication. One inexpensive treatment is to gargle with warm salt water. Another recommendation is to stop smoking. It will help you now and in the future. We will discuss the smoking when you are ready. I have a lot of non-smoking programs in your area that you can check out when you are ready.				

continued

PO Box 2308, Woburn, MA 01888-0508, **p:** 781-729-3736, **www.EmbracingCulture.com**
PO Box 6401, Manchester, NH 03108, **p:** 1-888-678-CCCS

Role-Play 14 *(continued)*

	Pronunciation	Additions	Omissions	Mistakes
Patient: Doctor, can I ask you if you smoke?				
MD: I used to smoke until I started to treat patients with all kinds of bronchitis and lung cancer. For your body aches you can also buy over-the-counter medications such as Tylenol or Aspirin. Call me if your symptoms become a lot worse.				
MD: Symptoms to watch out for include: severe, unusual headaches; and coughing up rusty, gray, green or bloody phlegm. Also, check for fever over 101°.				
Patient: You know, I'm feeling better already. It really helped to talk about my family.				
MD: I am glad you came today. When you are ready to talk some more, I can refer you to a family therapist. By the way, if you do get real chest pain, particularly when you are spitting up phlegm, or if you get an earache with intense pain when swallowing, contact my office right away.				
Patient: OK, Doctor. Should I take one of those flu shots that old people get?				
MD: Flu shots are good for everyone. It's just that children and the elderly have more vulnerable immune systems, and we need to protect them first.				
Patient: I know. I was just joking with you. I like you, Doctor. You make me comfortable and you are not stuck-up, like those doctors who walk around with their noses in the air.				
MD: Thanks. Patients like you make a difference, but I am still going to be nagging you about your smoking! Come back in three weeks for a follow-up and then we can talk about various smoking-prevention programs. In the meantime, when you sneeze, wash your hands.				
Patient: OK, Doctor.				
Break It Down	☐	☐	☐	☐

☐ **CIFE with patient** ☐ **CIFE with provider** ☐ **FLOW** ☐ **REGISTER**

Role-Play 14: Glossary

continued

1. Pathology (diseases, conditions)

2. Laboratory Tests and Diagnostic Procedures

3. Treatment Procedures

4. Idiomatic Expressions (if any)

5. Other (vocabulary in this particular role-play that you feel is important/relevant or that you anticipate problems with)

Role-Play 15: Strep Throat

	Pronunciation	Additions	Omissions	Mistakes
MD: Hello, Carmelita! I heard that you are not feeling well today. Let me ask your mom a few questions and I will be with you in a few minutes. Meanwhile, you can play with the puzzle on that table if you like.				
MD: (to mother) So, can you tell me more about Carmelita's throat and her general health?				
Mother: I noticed that Carmelita went to bed pretty early last night. She is usually a night owl. She woke up this morning and she was a bit crabby. She complained of a headache and muscle aches all over her body. She didn't even want to eat breakfast! She seemed a bit warm to me, but I don't have a thermometer at home. Did she have a fever when the nurse checked her this morning?				
(Doctor examines the daughter)				
MD: No actually, she does not have a fever. Her temperature is 98.6°. Her neck feels fine; just a bit tender. Carmelita, I am going to ask you to stick your tongue out and open your mouth as wide as possible. I am going to touch the back of your throat with this long cotton swab. I will be so fast that you'll hardly feel it. OK, looks pretty good inside, I do not see any signs of strep.				
PT: Mom do you have a Kleenex? (She coughs.)				
MD: Your mom told me about your muscle aches. Do you have a headache also?				
PT: Yup!				
MD: The good news is that most likely Carmelita does not have strep. The bad news is that she is going to feel a bit yucky for the next three days. A virus causes this sore throat, so we do not treat it with an antibiotic. You may want to give Carmelita children's Tylenol, Panadol or Tempra. But don't give her aspirin. She should drink a lot of fluids and rest for the next three to five days. You may want to get a cool mist humidifier for her room.				

continued

Role-Play 15 *(continued)*

	Pronunciation	Additions	Omissions	Mistakes
Mother: I have a vaporizer that I would use when she used to get that terrible croup. You remember, right? I still get a bit panicky when she shows any sign of a cold or cough. But I guess she's improved a lot.				
MD: Well, with the croup you get a hyper kid, and with a cold you get a calmer but crabbier kid. If the sore throat bothers her a lot, you may give her some throat lozenges or she can try to gargle with warm water and salt. That was my mother's favorite treatment. If you notice any changes or if her fever rises to 99.8° or above, contact my office right away.				
Mother: You may think that I am overreacting by bringing her to see you so soon, but as I told you I am traumatized from all the croup episodes.				
MD: Do not worry. The signs of strep are basically a fever with all the symptoms she is having now. It is difficult for a parent to differentiate strep or an infection caused by the bacteria called streptococcus from a simple viral infection.				
PT: Doctor, can I have ice cream?				
Break It Down	☐	☐	☐	☐

☐ **CIFE with patient** ☐ **CIFE with provider** ☐ **FLOW** ☐ **REGISTER**

Role-Play 15: Glossary

continued

PO Box 2308, Woburn, MA 01888-0508, **p:** 781-729-3736, **www.EmbracingCulture.com**
PO Box 6401, Manchester, NH 03108, **p:** 1-888-678-CCCS

1. Pathology (diseases, conditions)

2. Laboratory Tests and Diagnostic Procedures

3. Treatment Procedures

4. Idiomatic Expressions (if any)

5. Other (vocabulary in this particular role-play that you feel is important/relevant or that you anticipate problems with)

Role-Play 16: Neuropraxia

Mrs. Sum just went home after having a coronary bypass. All her children, grandchildren and great grandchildren were happy to have her back home. She had many pills, but actually fewer pills than before she went to the hospital with chest pain. She did have medicine to help her sleep which she used occasionally at night. Last night she could not sleep and took her sleeping pill. She slept really well, but awoke unable to bend her wrist. She was scared and thought she might have had a stroke. She went to see her primary care doctor.

	Pronunciation	Additions	Omissions	Mistakes
PT: Hello doctor, I want to thank you for coming to see me in the hospital.				
MD: That's fine, Mrs. Sum, you did so well under the care of the cardiologist and the thoracic surgeon, I felt like a "third wheel."				
PT: Well, now I need you Dr. Can I tell you what happened?				
MD: Please do.				
PT: Well, last night I awoke and I could not bend my left wrist.				
MD: You can't flex it like this or extend it like that?				
PT: It bends down (flexes) without a problem. But I cannot bend it up (extend).				
MD: When did you first notice this?				
PT: This morning. I awoke with this problem.				
MD: Did you hit or strain your wrist?				
PT: No, not that I can remember.				
MD: Did you sleep well last night?				
PT: Oh, too well. I took the sleeping pill and did not wake up for 10 hours. When I woke up I could not move my wrist.				
MD: How is your neck? Do you have any pain when you move your neck? Do you have any pain in your arm or hand when you move your neck?				
PT: No, my neck is fine.				
MD: Well, let me examine you. First, please move your chin to your chest. Now tilt your head back so you look up at the ceiling. Look to your right, to your left. Now touch your right ear to your right shoulder, touch your left ear to your left shoulder. Good.				

continued

PO Box 2308, Woburn, MA 01888-0508, **p:** 781-729-3736, **www.EmbracingCulture.com**
PO Box 6401, Manchester, NH 03108, **p:** 1-888-678-CCCS

Role-Play 16 *(continued)*

		Pronunciation	Additions	Omissions	Mistakes
	Now grab my fingers, push me away, and pull me towards you. Shrug your shoulders. Don't let me bend your wrists. Hmm, it's weak here. Spread your fingers and don't let me close them. Hold your fingers together and don't let me pull them apart. Now I'll check the strength of your legs. Lift this knee up. Don't let me push it down. Lift the other knee up and don't let me push it down. Now straighten your leg and don't let me bend it. Now straighten your other leg and don't let me bend it. Point your toes up toward your nose and don't let me bend them back. Follow my finger with your eyes. Touch my finger with your finger, then touch my nose.				
PT:	Doctor, what is the matter?				
MD:	Well, your reflexes are fine. I think you put pressure on your nerve while asleep. This is called neuropraxia. It is very common in people who fall asleep on their arms. It will improve in 4 weeks. In the meantime, we'll check a cervical spinal film to make sure there is nothing wrong with your neck. Also, I'll ask occupational therapy to give you a splint to help keep your wrist from dropping.				
PT:	You don't think I had a stroke.				
MD:	It's not likely. You have distal wrist dysfunction, no other signs of neurological dysfunction. I'll call you when I have the neck film. I expect some arthritis but nothing serious. Do you need a pain pill?				
PT:	No, actually I do not have any pain.				
	Break It Down	☐	☐	☐	☐

☐ **CIFE with patient** ☐ **CIFE with provider** ☐ **FLOW** ☐ **REGISTER**

Role-Play 16: Glossary

______________ ______________ ______________

______________ ______________ ______________

______________ ______________ ______________

______________ ______________ ______________

continued

1. Pathology (diseases, conditions)

2. Laboratory Tests and Diagnostic Procedures

3. Treatment Procedures

4. Idiomatic Expressions (if any)

5. Other (vocabulary in this particular role-play that you feel is important/relevant or that you anticipate problems with)

PO Box 2308, Woburn, MA 01888-0508, **p:** 781-729-3736, **www.EmbracingCulture.com**
PO Box 6401, Manchester, NH 03108, **p:** 1-888-678-CCCS

Lesson Three: Additional Resources
Memory and Memory Aids

The Brain
Evolution of the Brain throughout History

One theory states that the human brain developed through time from a simple reptilian brain, which was used to look for food and defend themselves. As reptiles were exposed to different challenges, this simple brain turned into the limbic system where animals developed new features such as love and the ability to experience smell, fear, pain and pleasure. *(Minninger)* With the continuation of new challenges, the brain again developed, this time into a more sophisticated system called the neocortex. *(Minninger)*

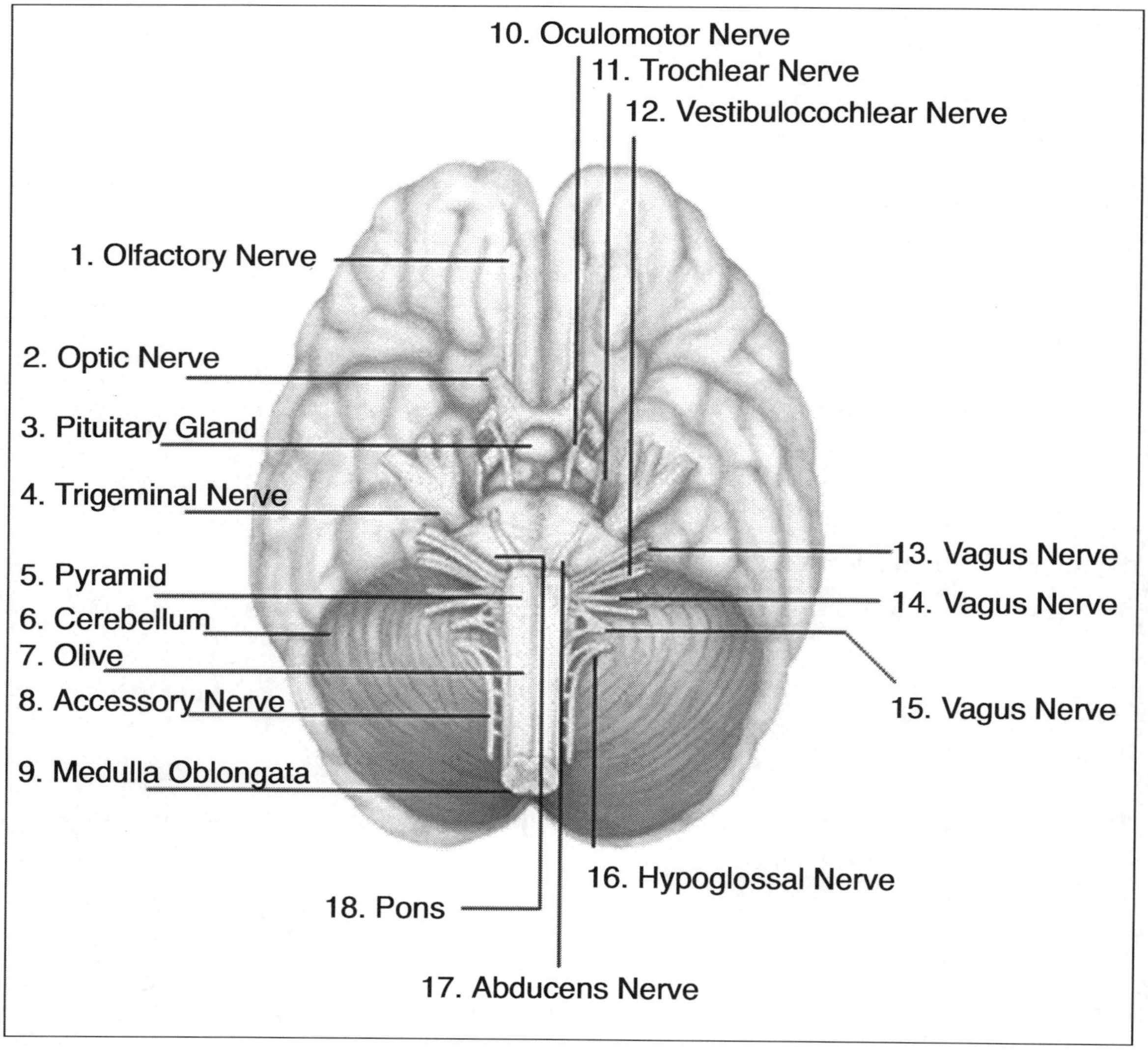

The Incredible Brain

This incredibly organized gray matter is 150 million years old and weighs an average of 2.97 pounds. Scientists understand only about 1% of how it functions. *(Buzan)(Minninger)*

The brain is divided into four parts: the cerebrum, the cerebellum, the brain stem and the diencephalon. The cerebrum is the most important and largest part of the brain. Much of the mental process happens in the cerebrum. In fact, it controls all of the body's voluntary activities and most of its involuntary activity. The cerebellum controls balance and coordination. (Buzan) The brain stem consists of the pons and the medulla oblongata. This section is responsible for vital functions (heart rate, breathing, emotions, temperature, alertness, sleep). The diencephalon is situated between the brain stem and the cerebrum. It influences, among other things, mood, body movements associated with strong emotions, emotional and visual responses to odors, and the endocrine system.

The Neocortex

The neocortex is what makes humans so special. It bestows upon us the ability "to consciously change behavior." It lets us "store logic, language, mathematics and speculation about the future." (Minninger)

Through PET scans, scientists have divided the brain into the following functional areas: sensory (sense of touch, awareness of spatial relations, academic skills), auditory, motor (motor integration, voluntary movement), visual (visual perception, visual input, reading-recognition and perception of printed words), language (memory, receptive language, language comprehension, musical awareness, sequencing skills), pre-motor (orientation, control of head and eye movements) and frontal (higher mental functions-controlling attention, motivation, emotion control, social behavior, judgment, problem-solving, decision-making, expressive language). *(Buzan)(Minninger)*

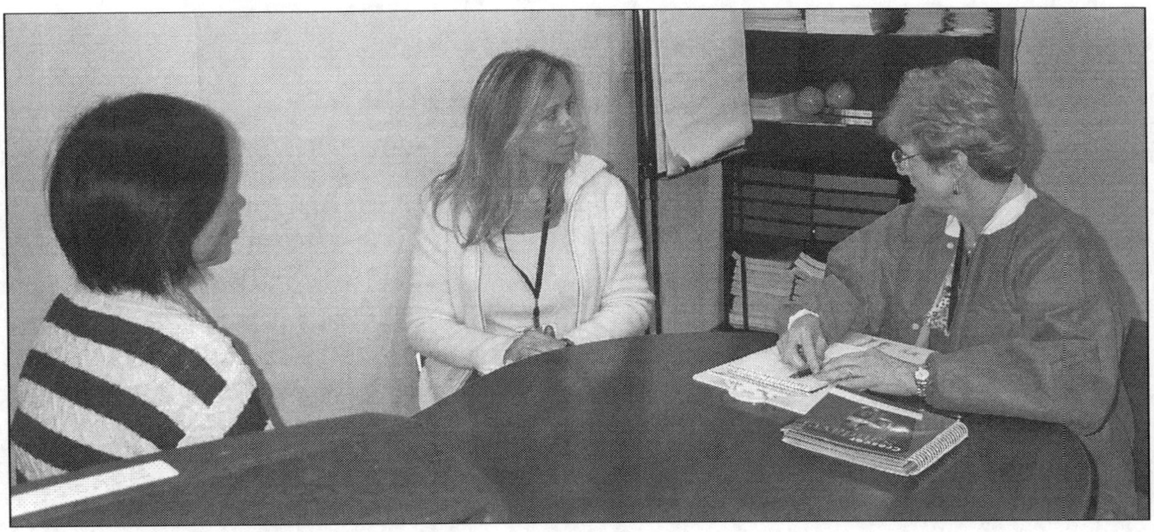

PO Box 2308, Woburn, MA 01888-0508, **p:** 781-729-3736, **www.EmbracingCulture.com**
PO Box 6401, Manchester, NH 03108, **p:** 1-888-678-CCCS

The Two Brains

Recently, scientists discovered that people have two upper brains; the left and right cortices. Each cortex deals with different types of mental activity. Both sides are connected through the Corpus Callosum, a network of complex nerve fibers. (Minninger)

The Left Cortex

The left cortex is understood as the "activity side" of the brain (words, logic, numbers, sequence, linearity, analysis, lists).

The Right Cortex

On the other hand, the right cortex is the side of the brain where an individual is more in the "alpha wave or the resting stage." (This refers to rhythm, special awareness, gestalt-whole picture, imagination, day-dreaming, color and dimension). The close interaction of the two brains is an asset for consecutive interpretation. Not everyone has fully developed both sides of the brain, but with exercise, one can begin to strengthen the different sides and the aspects they represent. The brain is like a muscle; if exercised, it will bring a vast array of abilities to the individual. (1)

LEFT	RIGHT
"activity side"	"alpha wave"
words	"resting"
logic	rhythm
numbers	gestalt
sequence	imagination
linearity	daydreaming
analysis	color
lists	dimension

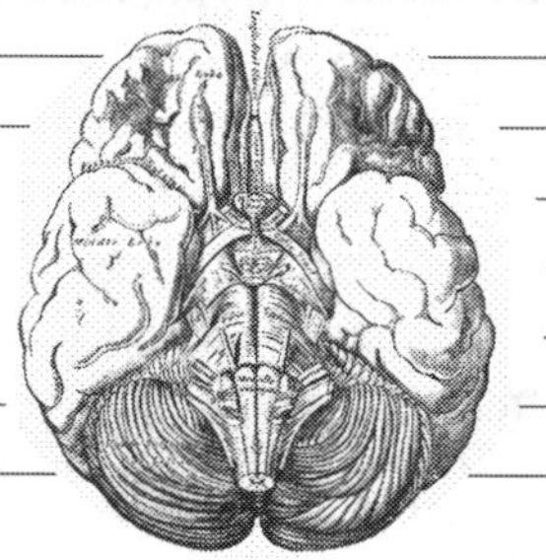

The Neuron

The basic unit of the nervous system and brain is called a neuron. It is a single cell. Each cell has a cell body with a nucleous and multiple projections. These projections are called neurites. One neurite carries electrical impulses toward the cell body and is called a dendrite. The neurite that carries impluses away from the cell body is called an axon.

The neurons communicate with each other by having the axon of one cell body in contact with the dendrite of another. The electrical impulses from one neuron stimulate impulses in the next. The point of contact for the axon of one neuron stimulating the dendrite of the next is called a synapse. The axon terminal fibers ends in a synaptic knob. Within each knob are multiple small vesicles, or small storage apparatus, that contain chemicals. These chemicals are called neurotransmitter molecules. They are released by the synaptic vesicles into the space between the synaptic knob and the membrane of the next dendrite called the synaptic cleft. The neurotransmitters excite channels in the target membrane to allow positive ions to pass through and begin an electrical stimulus of the next cell.

Different neurons will have different neurotransmitters in the vesicles. The major neurotransmitters are serotin, norepinephrine and dopamine. These neurotransmitters are released by the vesicles and cross the synaptic cleft to stimulate an impulse in the dendrite's end. After the release and the stimulus occurs, the neurotransmitter is reabsorbed into the multiple vesicles in the synaptic knob. The neurotransmitters not only allow stimulus to develop in the following dendrite, but can support mood. There are new drugs to support mood and fight depression which do their tasks by preventing the re-uptake of the neurotransmitter into the vesicle and out of the cleft. Drugs like Prozac, inhibit the re-uptake of serotonin in the cleft. Then, with more serotin floating in the cleft allowing continued stimulation of the following dendrites, patients' mood is enhanced.

Receiving and Processing Information

Information from the senses or from thoughts are processed in many different parts of the brain. One part of the brain will process information from the sensory organs, one part will process thoughts and initiate or coordinate voluntary movements. All the information processing, and interaction of events in the brain are facilitated by the multiple neurons locked in an array of cells in the brain.

Memory

The brain remembers information through the interaction of neurons which code, transmit, and store the information as electrical signals.

Memory is held by the brain's ability to generate new cells as well as derive new protein molecules and new interconnections. The hippocampus, whose name reflects its resemblance to a seahorse, is the part of the brain that helps select where important and relevant aspects of memories are held. There are three levels of memory: sensory, short-term and long-term. First is the brief sensory memory (from sensory organs consisting of seeing, listening, smelling. These are stored only for milliseconds. If retained and interpreted, the memory becomes short-term memory for a few moments. If the memory is transferred to long-term memory is said to be consolidated.

Memory is affected by how we react and understand what we see, hear and feel. Individuals have a tendency to create their own realities when they hear a message.

PO Box 2308, Woburn, MA 01888-0508, **p:** 781-729-3736, **www.EmbracingCulture.com**
PO Box 6401, Manchester, NH 03108, **p:** 1-888-678-CCCS

Interpreters Need to Be Aware....

of the human tendency to eliminate, add or misconstrue a message. This happens because the meaning of a message is first filtered by the many variables affecting the interpreter. For example, an interpreter may interpret for a patient with HIV. Perhaps the patient states that he noticed small lumps on his neck. The interpreter might be upset by hearing this message, especially if s/he has had the experience of past interpretation for patients with HIV who have complained of large lumps on different parts of their bodies. The interpreter, without even being aware, could change the message from "small" to "large" lumps. This happens because the interpreter was impressed by the emotional component of the HIV situation of the patient, and in fact s/he was not hearing the patient but was hearing his/her voice based on his/her experience.

Interpreters throughout their training will acquire quite a bit of medical knowledge intentionally designed to help interpreters quickly navigate through meaning and vocabulary; there is always a danger that interpreters may not be paying attention to all the words used in the medical encounter, because they are familiar with a certain amount of information regarding the topic being discussed. Interpreters must be good listeners so that they can be accurate with a complete message. Playing provider is dangerous and may kill a patient.

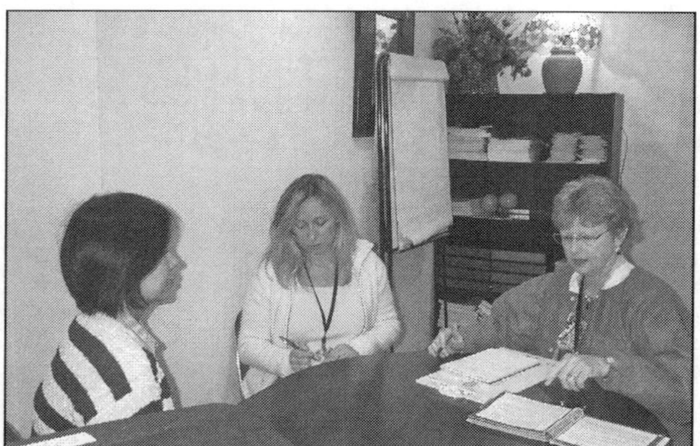

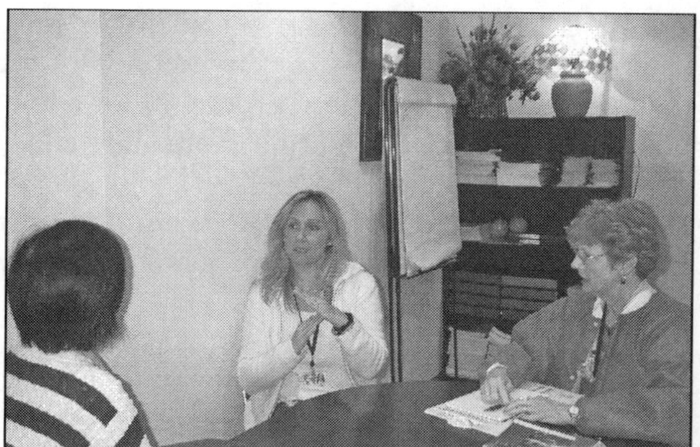

Interpreter Evaluation Tool based on the IMIA standards.

Name:____________________________Target Language:____________Date: ___/___/___

OBSERVATION

1 PRE SESSION

Client/patient	Yes	No
1. Introduction?		
2. Interpreter helped client with registration?		
3. Interpreter explained the usage of the first person?		
4. Interpreter informed client of confidentiality policy?		
5. Interpreter informed client that everything said during the session will be interpreted?		
6. Did the interpreter handle the waiting period appropriately?		
7. Did the interpreter appropriately acknowledge similarities and differences?		

Provider	Yes	No
8. Introduction?		
9. Interpreter explained the usage of the first person?		
10. Interpreter informed the provider that everything said during the session will be interpreted?		

2 THE TRIADIC RELATIONSHIP

Interpreter/provider and client	Yes	No
1. Did the interpreter appropriately arrange seating?		
2 Did the interpreter show appropriate eye contact?		
3 Did the interpreter appropriately handle the comments from client or provider?		
4 Did the interpreter stay in the room alone with client?		
5 Did the interpreter help with medical procedures?		

6 Who makes the decision of when to stay behind the curtain?
○ Interpreter ○ Client ○ Provider

PO Box 2308, Woburn, MA 01888-0508, **p:** 781-729-3736, **www.EmbracingCulture.com**
PO Box 6401, Manchester, NH 03108, **p:** 1-888-678-CCCS

3 INTERPRETATION TECHNIQUE

Interpreter	Yes	No
1. Usage of First Person?		
2. Omissions?		
3. Additions?		
4. Meaning/Accuracy?		
5. Meaning /Completeness?		
6. Keeps appropriate flow?		
7. Asks for clarification?		
8. Checks with client if he/she understood everything?		
9. Mode of interpretation: consecutive, simultaneous, sight and summary?		
10. Memorization techniques: note-taking, echoing key words and finger counting?		

4 KNOWLEDGE OF MEDICAL TERMINOLOGY

Strengths: ______________________________

Weaknesses: ______________________________

Areas for growth: ______________________________

5 FOLLOW-UP

FOLLOW-UP	Yes	No
1. Interpreter helps client with follow-up visits?		
2. Interpreter helps client getting home?		
3. Interpreter does not provide advice when asked for his or her opinion?		
4. Interpreter handled a distraught client appropriately?		

6 CULTURAL KNOWLEDGE/CLARIFICATION

CULTURAL KNOWLEDGE/CLARIFICATION	Yes	No
1. Interpreter clarified cultural meaning by checking with appropriate party?		
2. Interpreter understood vocabulary used by both, provider and client?		
3. Interpreter understands client's immigration history?		
4. Interpreter shows how to best address client by showing respect?		
5. Interpreter asks permission to become a cultural coach when appropriate?		
6. Interpreter showed respect for client's own individuality?		
7. Interpreter understands provider and client's communication styles?		
8. Interpreter understands USA medical system and that of client's native country?		

SELF- OBSERVATION:

7 ETHICS

ETHICS	Yes	No
1. Do you accept gifts?		
2. Do you share your opinion regarding controversial beliefs?		
3. Do you ask questions to clients/personal/clinical?		
4. Do you provide your telephone number?		
5. Do you give your opinion when asked by the clients?		
6. Do you deliberately delete information for political/ religious /personal beliefs?		
7. Do you call clients at home when not asked by provider to do so?		
8. Do you drive clients to places?		
9. Do you give money to clients?		
10. Do you make remarks that are pejorative against anyone?		
11. Do you use power of knowledge for personal gains?		
12. Do you discuss prior sessions with different providers?		
13. Do you tell clients what to say in the session?		
14. Do you discuss the sessions and identify clients/providers?		

PO Box 2308, Woburn, MA 01888-0508, **p:** 781-729-3736, **www.EmbracingCulture.com**
PO Box 6401, Manchester, NH 03108, **p:** 1-888-678-CCCS

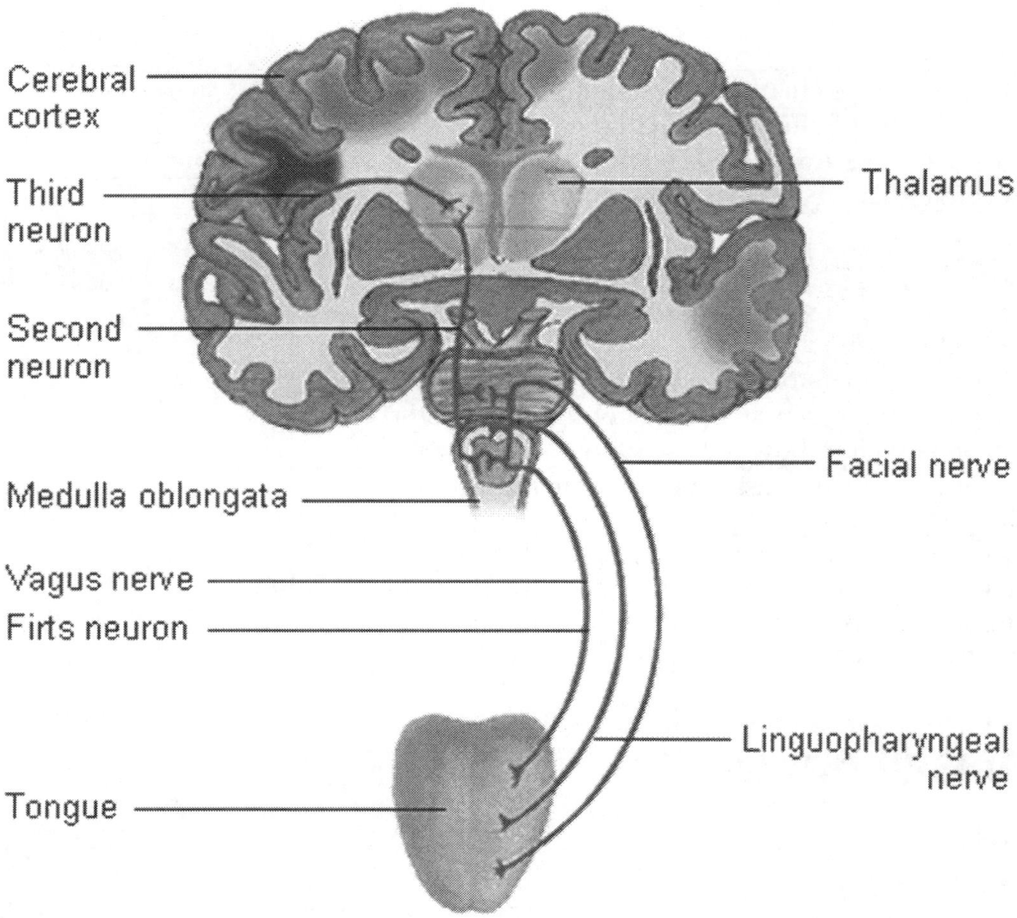
Cerebral cortex
Third neuron
Thalamus
Second neuron
Facial nerve
Medulla oblongata
Vagus nerve
Firts neuron
Linguopharyngeal nerve
Tongue

Notes

Lesson Four:
How Providers Communicate with Each Other About a Patient

Understanding Goals

Students will be able to:

- practice note-taking
- understand the provider's clinical thinking through SOAP
- learn common symbols and abbreviations
- learn different types of pain
- familiarize themselves with interpreting jargon

Key Concepts

- SOAP
- Note-taking
- Sight Interpretation

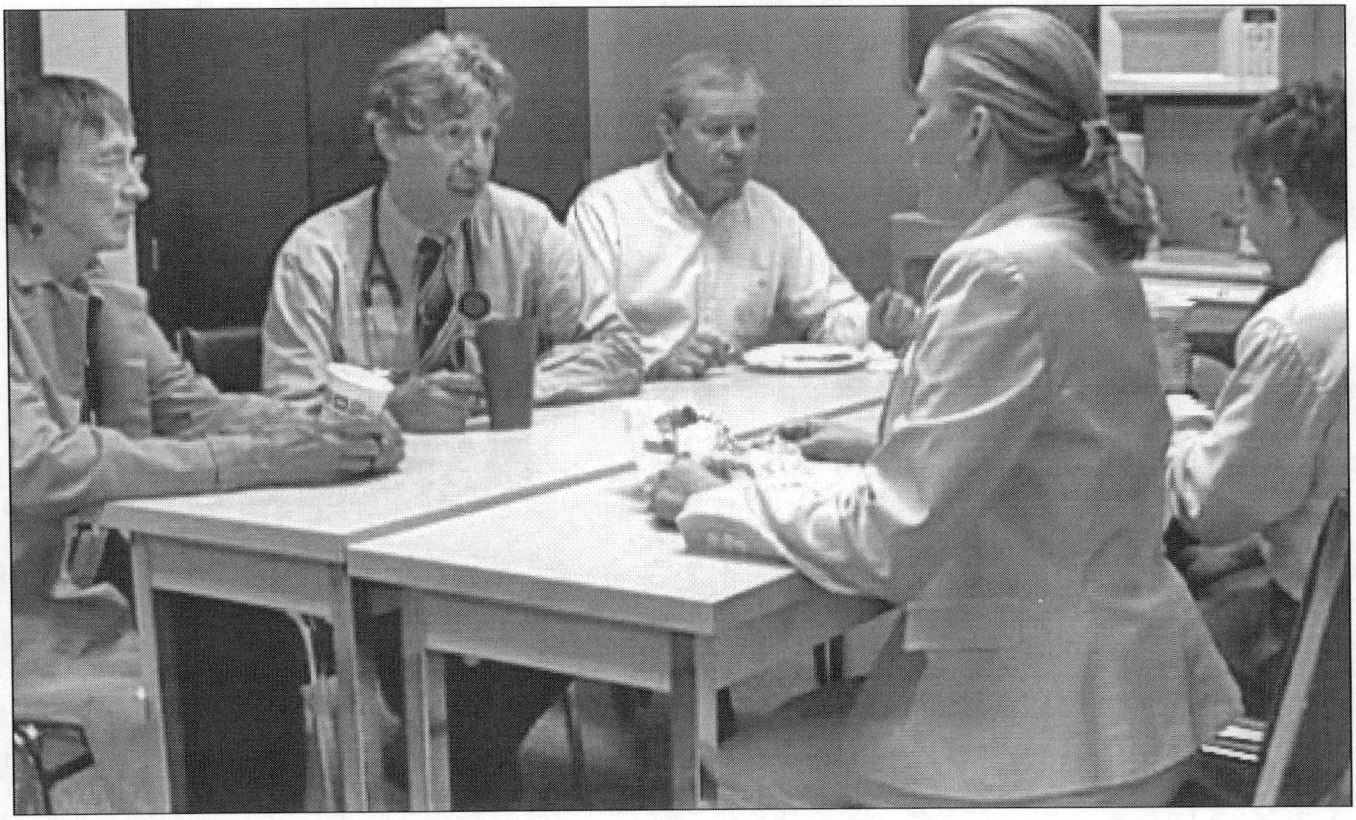

PO Box 2308, Woburn, MA 01888-0508, **p:** 781-729-3736, **www.EmbracingCulture.com**
PO Box 6401, Manchester, NH 03108, **p:** 1-888-678-CCCS

Quiz

THE ART OF MEDICAL INTERPRETATION®

Lesson Four: Quiz
How Providers Communicate with Each Other About a Patient

Mark each item "True" or False."

1. Notes should be a supplement or aid to memory, not a replacement of memory.
   ○ True ○ False
2. When using abbreviations, vowels are better memory aids than consonants.
   ○ True ○ False
3. The four parts of SOAP are: Subjective, Objective, Assessment, and Payment.
   ○ True ○ False
4. The part of SOAP when patients are able to relate their complaints that brought them to visit a doctor is called "objective."
   ○ True ○ False
5. Whenever interpreters use notes to aid their memories, they must inform both the patient and the provider that the notes are just an aid that will help achieve completeness and accuracy, and that the paper will be destroyed and discarded before leaving the room.
   ○ True ○ False
6. In note-taking, interpreters can use many different symbols borrowed from other sciences, such as lines of negation and emphasis, directional arrows representing movement or causation, slashes indicating relationships; and common punctuation marks.
   ○ True ○ False
7. BP stands for blood pressure.
   ○ True ○ False
8. A throbbing pain is the one that gives you a sensation as if you had a lesion caused by contact with heat or fire.
   ○ True ○ False
9. Providers rule out the most serious conditions through "differential diagnosis."
   ○ True ○ False
10. When a general practitioner comes up with a differential diagnosis and a clinical opinion such as, "I believe you have kidney stones and not appendicitis," he is in the "Plan" part of SOAP.
    ○ True ○ False
11. Providers during SOAP, repetitively ask different questions with the objective of prying into patient's lives. Therefore, interpreters do not need to interpret repeated questions.
    ○ True ○ False
12. Interpreters should remember that all clinicians are trained to apply the principles of SOAP and in doing so; they may ask the same questions over and over.
    ○ True ○ False
13. D&C stands for dilation and curettage.
    ○ True ○ False
14. STD stands for sexually transmitted dilemma.
    ○ True ○ False

Lesson Four: Class Activities
How Providers Communicate with Each Other About a Patient

1. You have already learned about memory aids that can help you be complete and accurate with your interpretation: visualization, finger counting, echoing, and anchoring. Let's now take a deeper look at note-taking, which requires a specific set of skills.

ACTIVITIES

Watch the video "*ACEBO*" and mark the statements that follow as True (T) or False (F). Correct the false statements..

1. There is only one way of taking notes.
   ○ True ○ False

   ____

2. You should not take notes on every word.
   ○ True ○ False

   ____

3. Note-taking is visual.
   ○ True ○ False

   ____

4. Note-taking is oriented to words, not concepts.
   ○ True ○ False

   ____

5. Notes tend to be horizontal.
   ○ True ○ False

   ____

6. When using words, words should be written down in the target language.
   ○ True ○ False

   ____

PO Box 2308, Woburn, MA 01888-0508, **p:** 781-729-3736, **www.EmbracingCulture.com**
PO Box 6401, Manchester, NH 03108, **p:** 1-888-678-CCCS

What is your first impression about the note-taking strategies that were mentioned in the video?

What looked easy? What looked challenging?

Take a couple of minutes to jot down symbols or abbreviations you use or have used when taking notes.

Points to Remember:

Note-taking in the context of consecutive interpreting, both in the legal and medical settings, is highly personalized and depends largely on the interpreter's background and training. Whatever your note-taking style, here are some points to remember:

- While some interpreters are familiar with shorthand, it is wise to exercise caution when using that skill. Shorthand is word-oriented, and we have learned that interpreters, both legal and medical, must focus more heavily on the meaning and content of a message than on the individual words used.
- Notes are merely memory supplements, or aids. To facilitate rapid recall, make sure your notes are both legible and logical.
- Notes tend to be vertical lists symbolizing concepts. In note-taking, interpreters may use many different symbols, such as lines of negation and emphasis, directional arrows representing movement or causation, slashes indicating relationships, boxes as substitutes for places or objects; and common punctuation marks.

- Abbreviation is a common form of note-taking. But beware: When abbreviating a word or concept, avoid using common prefixes, such as "pre-" and "post-." Rather, use a series of letters that will help you easily recall the desired word or concept. Remember, consonants are better memory aids than vowels!

Above all things, keep your notes brief and to the point.

Ethical Considerations When Using Note-Taking

Interpreters need to be aware that many patients have come from a politically oppressed environment or that they themselves have experienced some sort of personal abuse or trauma. In these situations note-taking may be a reminder of past abuse by a person with authority, such as a police interrogator. In these cases, interpreters need to exercise their best judgment. Interpreters should never leave the triadic encounter with any information of the patient, as it is protected by HIPAA. CCCS advises that you follow your institution's policy. You may inform both the patient and the provider that your notes are just an aid that will help you be complete and accurate with the message, and that you destroy the paper and discard it in the room.

SOAP

2. Have you ever thought why every time you go see a doctor they all seem to ask you the same questions over and over again? Well, that is not random. There is a pre-set structure to every medical triadic encounter.

ACTIVITIES

Watch the video *"The Healthcare Interpreter's Tools for Successful Communication in the Triadic Encounter, Volume 3: Clinical Insight in Medical interpretation"* and answer the questions that follow:

1. What does SOAP stand for? What is SOAP?

Subjective, Objective, Assessment, Plan

2. What is included in the "SUBJECTIVE?"

Presenting Problem presented by patient

3. Differential Diagnosis is one of the elements of the "subjective." What does Differential Diagnosis mean?

Elimination process most serious → less serious

4. What was Mr. Maciel complaining of?

pain chest – walk

Problem
Chronology
Progress
Location
Quality
Intensity
Quantity
Aggravating
Associated sy
Past History – Treatment
Current Medication / Diagnosis

PO Box 2308, Woburn, MA 01888-0508, p: 781-729-3736, www.EmbracingCulture.com
PO Box 6401, Manchester, NH 03108, p: 1-888-678-CCCS

5. What might that be a sign of?

6. How does the provider rule out the most serious condition?

7. What is included in the "OBJECTIVE?"

8. How does the interpreter remain respectful to the patient's privacy? What else could the interpreter have done?

9. What is the "ASSESSMENT?"

10. How may the "PLAN" be divided?

11. In Mr. Romero's vignette:

What is the Subjective?

What is the Objective?

What is the Assessment?

What is the Plan?

Subjective

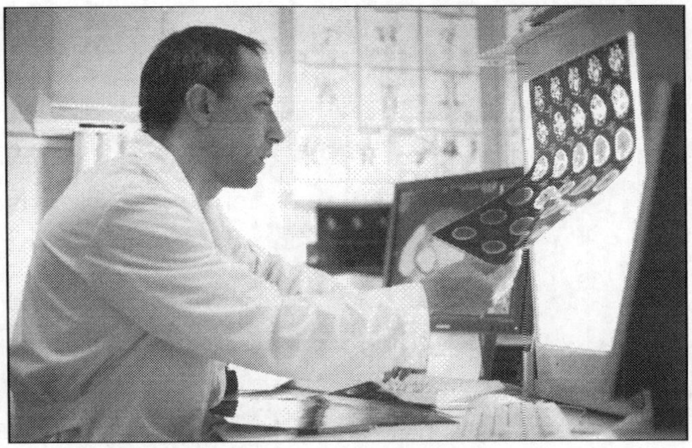

The term "subjective" refers to the patient's presenting problem. A presenting problem is defined as that which the patient brings to the session, or the patient's complaint. Examples of the subjective or presenting problem are statements such as "I have a terrible headache" or "It feels like I have an elephant sitting on my chest."

Objective

The "objective" represents the questions and actions of a provider needed for differential diagnosis. To a medical provider, the "objective" is something tangible to be measured and reported. Examples of the objective in a medical session are the measurement of vital signs or lab test results. Medical providers will try to evaluate the medical seriousness of a symptom, perhaps by checking a patient's temperature or listening to a patient's heartbeat.

Mental health providers will look for what is behind the presenting problem. This is often termed the "real" problem. In a mental health session, a patient may present chest pain, but if a medical condition is ruled out, then the patient will likely tell the clinician that life at home or at work is very stressful. In this case "stress" in the home or at work is the objective.

Assessment

"Assessment" is when the clinician comes up with a differential diagnosis and a clinical opinion. For example, a general practitioner may say, "I believe you have kidney stones and not appendicitis."
At times, a provider may not find evidence of a physical ailment or may perceive a "hidden agenda" on the part of the patient. Subsequently, the provider will begin to check-in with the patient regarding the possibility of a different diagnosis.

Plan

The term "plan" refers to a set of actions to further diagnose or treat an existing condition. For example, the provider may say to the patient, "I have ruled out a myocardium infarction but I still want you to take this nitroglycerine pill whenever you have chest pain. When I see you in a few weeks, you can let me know if the pill has helped you at all."

PO Box 2308, Woburn, MA 01888-0508, **p:** 781-729-3736, **www.EmbracingCulture.com**
PO Box 6401, Manchester, NH 03108, **p:** 1-888-678-CCCS

3. SOAP Notes: Case Study

1) Describe which parts of the case best translate into which four components of the SOAP Notes (Subjective, Objective, Assessment and Plan).
2) We are going to act out this case as a role play with two goals in mind:
   A. Use of medical terminology English to Target language. In this case the interpreter uses consecutive interpreting and is only a conduit of the message.
   B. Practice of the role of Medical Interpreting (Pre-session and during session, listening carefully for omissions, deletions, completeness and accuracy of interpreting).

MD: What brings you here today?

Patient: It hurts, it hurts.

Mother: You know, she gets these ear infections all the time.

MD: hmm… has this happened before?

Mother: Yes, after swimming, or when she has a cold, but what scared me is that this morning when I went to pick her up from bed, there was blood on her pillow case.

I checked her nose and it looked fine, but when I looked inside her ear I could see some dry blood in it. Do you think that the airplane ride made the infection worse?

MD: I have seen kids with bleeding ears after a trip. Let me take a look and I will let you know what I think is going on.

Patient: It hurts, I want my mommy!

MD: I am sorry you are feeling this much pain. I can see quite a bit of fluid in her ears. When I touch your earlobe, does it hurt?

Patient: Yes, it hurts a lot!

MD: You have otitis. You also seem to have a bit of fever. The good news is that your neck is not stiff, so we don't have to worry about meningitis. Let me give you some Tylenol right now. I'm also going to ask your mom if you have any allergies I should know about.

Mother: When she was a baby she had a bit of diarrhea, and later on she developed a slight rash when she took amoxicillin.

MD: Let's try 250mg of Ceftin twice a day. Please call our hotline if she gets a reaction. I also would like to know if the fluid continues to build up after the treatment.

Mother: OK.

MD: Sometimes the fluid in the ears does not completely clear. This could be a result of a possible bacterial resistance to this particular antibiotic. Or it could mean that the fluid is a result of a viral infection and not bacterial.

Mother: Should we have the fluid removed? I have heard that the fluid can cause some hearing loss. Is that true?

MD: Let's wait and see if this antibiotic does a good job clearing the infection. If the ears are still full of fluid and your daughter is still in pain or shows a loss of hearing, then we can consider a simple procedure that is called Myringotomy or Tympanotomy.

Mother: Is this the same as having the "tubes" in your ears cleared?

MD: Exactly, this procedure would involve a small hole in the ear drum and the suction of fluid. There are some areas where we cannot immediately access the drainage with this procedure so we insert a very small pressure equalizing tube or "PE tube" made of a material such as steel, Teflon or silicone. This tube is left in the ear through the opening.

This is a very simple procedure, but kids like to move around during it so we are now administering general anesthesia. No hospitalization is required, just a day surgery. The Eustachian tube would be left in place for about one year.

Mother: I hope she will do well with the medications.

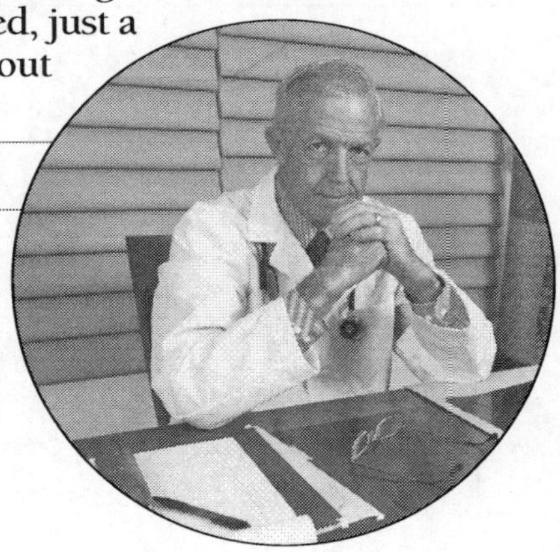

PO Box 2308, Woburn, MA 01888-0508, **p:** 781-729-3736, **www.EmbracingCulture.com**
PO Box 6401, Manchester, NH 03108, **p:** 1-888-678-CCCS

4. SOAP is not just a pre-set structure to the medical triadic encounter, but it is also a written document as a way for providers to communicate with each other. Take a look at the following medical chart:

> Patient Name: Fatma Nazur DOB: 8/1/1958
> Record No. MMOO250033
> Date: 4/27/2008

> **S** – Pt. here for nausea and RLQ acute pain; unable to walk; pt. in great distress. NKDA, NKA.
>
> **O** – BP 190/90; Wt. 155 lb ; CT ABD W/ CONT; U/A
>
> **A** – 2-mm right UVJ stone with mild hydronephrosis. 3-mm right intrarenal kidney stone
>
> **P** – Rest; drink plenty of fluids; Phenergan, 25 mg po t.i.d.; Vicodin 5 mg b.i.d. po

What is the story? What are the patient's complaints?

____

____

What tests did they do to determine if there is something to the patient's story?

____

____

What kind of plan does the doctor offer?

____

____

What do the following abbreviations stand for?

ABBREVIATION	MEANING
DOB	
pt	
RLQ	
NKDA	
NKA	
BP	
WT	
CT	
ABD	
CONT	
U/A	
UVJ	
po	
t.i.d.	
b.i.d.	

PO Box 2308, Woburn, MA 01888-0508, **p:** 781-729-3736, **www.EmbracingCulture.com**
PO Box 6401, Manchester, NH 03108, **p:** 1-888-678-CCCS

SYMBOLS and ABBREVIATIONS

Complete the following sentences using medical abbreviations:

Sentences and Abbreviations

1. Ms. Jones has the __________ of sick sinus syndrome. That is why she has the pacemaker. She presented to the __________ with a fall and they found out she had fainted.
2. Patient is an __________ who fell and has a __________ of her wrist. They have to take her to the __________ to reduce the fracture under anesthesia.

   She was on coumadin, so her__________ is elevated. She has a fever and her blood test shows her __________is also elevated. She has also fractured her nose, so we will have to page the __________ resident on call.
3. The patient has a discharge from his urethra. We will send him to the __________ clinic.
4. How long have you had __________? Do you also get chest pain when you climb stairs?
5. Have you ever had a skin test for __________. It is very common on the Island you visited last year on vacation.
6. She is having uterine contractions. Let's page the __________ doctor to come and examine her.
7. Please take one baby __________ daily to help prevent heart attacks.
8. The patient's __________ is too high if we don't get it down soon, she could have a __________ and suffer a severe neurological deficit. When that happens we will need to get a __________ to image her brain and determine what kind of stroke she might have. We cannot use an __________ to image her because she has a pacemaker.
9. Do you know if Mrs. Jones wants us to do __________ if her heart were to stop?
10. It is time to stop the patient's __________ antibiotics. I will __________ them in the morning and I will start an oral medicine for her to take__________.
11. When was Mrs. Jones born? On the chart it says her __________ is 12/4/60, but she appears to be at least 70 years old.
12. There is a pulmonary nodule on Mrs. Flores' __________. We have to check the old one to see if this nodule is old or new.

Lesson Four: Homework
How Providers Communicate with Each Other About a Patient

1. Go over your notes for today's class and read section "Additional Resources"
2. Review medical symbols and abbreviations in the manual
3. Read and practice ALL role-plays for this lesson and add words to your glossary
4. Review and translate the Types of Pain table into your Target Language

Types of Pain

TYPES	MEANING	TARGET
Ache	Suffer a continuous pain	
Band Like	A pain that encircles an area and feels tight; a squeezing type of pain	
Burning	A pain that feels like you have a lesion caused by contact with heat or fire	
Cramping	A spasmodic muscular contraction	
Dull	A pain lacking force or intensity but present	
Grabbing	A sudden snatch, a grasp	
Lancinating	A piercing or stabbing pain, a sharp pain	
Needle Like	A sharp pain as if being punctured with a needle	
Pressure	The feeling that there is some type of weight or the application of some type of force against a part of the body	
Searing	A burning pain, the feeling of sudden intense heat	
Sharp	A cutting or penetrating pain by a sharp or pointing instrument	
Shooting	A piercing or sharp pain	
Splitting	A pain that makes one feel ripped apart	

PO Box 2308, Woburn, MA 01888-0508, **p:** 781-729-3736, **www.EmbracingCulture.com**
PO Box 6401, Manchester, NH 03108, **p:** 1-888-678-CCCS

5. Explain the following terms in your own words.

TERM	
Accuracy	
Additions	
Advocate	
CIFE	
Clarifier	
Conduit	
Confidentiality	
Consecutive	
Culture broker	
Culture coach	
Distortions	
Impartiality	
Interpreting modes	
Omissions	
Sight translation	
Simultaneous	
Source language	
Target language	
Transparency	
Use of the first person	

Lesson Four: Role-Plays
How Providers Communicate with Each Other About a Patient

Work individually at first:
- Read the entire role-play
- Get a general sense of its meaning
- Circle the most challenging medical terms
- Apply the Samurai! technique to those terms
- Read the role-play again for a deeper understanding
- Find an accurate equivalent in the target language

Work in a language-specific group of friends, fellow students or colleagues:
- Share your doubts
- Ask for other ways of expressing the same meaning
- Develop a glossary
- Check the dictionary
- Practice the role-plays remember to do CIFE for all your role-plays
- Have your colleagues observe you and provide feedback on your accuracy and register.
- These colleagues can keep track of any omissions, additions, mistakes or distortions in your interpreting and point these out to you in a follow-up discussion.

Student Interpreter Evaluation

Student Name ______ Date ______

Language ______

Mode of Interpreting (check one): ☐ Consecutive ☐ Simultaneous

Role-Play/System ______

Areas Observed ______

Accuracy

Register ______

Omissions ______

Additions ______

Distortions ______

Pronunciation ______

Speaker's emotions conveyed? ______

Explain ______

Technique

General flow ______

Flow when requesting clarification ______

Speed ______

Eye Contact ______

Distracting Habits ______

Ethical Issues

Answered questions for patient? ______

Advised patient? ______

Vocabulary Expansion Recommendations

______

______

Other Recommendations

______

______

Language Coach Signature ______ Date ______

PO Box 2308, Woburn, MA 01888-0508, **p:** 781-729-3736, **www.EmbracingCulture.com**
PO Box 6401, Manchester, NH 03108, **p:** 1-888-678-CCCS

Role-Play 17: High Blood Pressure

	Pronunciation	Additions	Omissions	Mistakes
MD: Hello Mr. Gonzalez. I have the results of the last four blood pressure tests that you did with our nurse practitioner.				
Mr. G.: What do you think?				
MD: Well, your weight continues to rise and so does your blood pressure. You know, if you could lose just five pounds, it would impact well on your blood pressure.				
Mr. G.: I do try, Doctor, but when I come home from work, it is so late and I am so hungry. Marta cooks for me and I love to eat her food.				
MD: Well, Mr. Gonzalez, you can eat her food but if you don't eat anything all day and come home starving, you will end up eating huge portions. And if you eat a large portion late at night, the fat will stay on. The trick is to eat several small meals a day and make the last one early in the evening.				
Mr. G.: That is tough to do. If I eat two meals a day, I'll just come home and eat again at dinner. I'll eat twice as much and gain more weight.				
MD: Why don't you try it my way for two weeks and see if there is a difference? Anyway, now I am going to have to start you on a medicine to help bring your blood pressure down. If you can lose the weight, we might be able to stop the medicine later. But now, after four months, it's time to begin a medication.				
Mr. G.: Oh no! Listen, I'll try the diet for two weeks. Let me see if I can stick with it. If not, I'll take the pill.				
MD: OK, I'll make you an appointment with Diane. If you lose a pound in two weeks or stay at the same weight, we'll put off the medicine. But if you gain a pound or more, we'll start the pill. It's called hyrodrocholorthiazide and it gets rid of excess fluid. This helps control the blood pressure.				
Mr. G.: You'll see. I'll do it right this time.				

continued

Role-Play 17 *(continued)*

	Pronunciation	Additions	Omissions	Mistakes
MD: Good. Also, it is time for you to have an EKG to make sure your heart is not enlarged from high blood pressure. And by the way, I see that in the Dominican Republic you had a TB test that was positive. It has been two years since you had a CXR and we need to take another picture to ensure that you don't have active TB. So we'll do a CXR as well as the EKG before you leave today.				
Mr. G.: OK, as long as you don't have to draw blood.				
MD: No, I have what I need for now. But if we start the medicine, I'll have to order blood tests to watch your kidney function and your potassium.				
Mr. G.: Well, there's one more reason to lose weight. I'll do it.				
Break It Down	☐	☐	☐	☐

☐ **CIFE with patient** ☐ **CIFE with provider** ☐ **FLOW** ☐ **REGISTER**

Role-Play 17: Glossary

PO Box 2308, Woburn, MA 01888-0508, **p:** 781-729-3736, **www.EmbracingCulture.com**
PO Box 6401, Manchester, NH 03108, **p:** 1-888-678-CCCS

1. Pathology (diseases, conditions)

2. Laboratory Tests and Diagnostic Procedures

3. Treatment Procedures

4. Idiomatic Expressions (if any)

5. Other (vocabulary in this particular role-play that you feel is important/relevant or that you anticipate problems with)

Role-Play 18: Stroke

		Pronunciation	Additions	Omissions	Mistakes
MD:	Mr. Sylvestre, I have reviewed your CT scan.				
S:	Yes, Doctor.				
MD:	It shows that you have had a CVA, a small stroke in the left part of your brain that controls your right side and that is why it is difficult for you to move your right arm and hand.				
S:	I understand.				
MD:	Also, it touched the area on the left side of your brain that controls your speech, which is why initially, when you had the stroke, you couldn't speak or move your right side. It immediately got better along with your strength and that bodes well for a speedy recovery.				
S:	Should I also get an MRI?				
MD:	No, luckily, I think we got all the information we need. I will need to get an EKG, and a special echocardiogram called a transesophageal echo. This stroke occurred at the same time that you had the blood clot in your leg. I want to make sure that you don't have a hole in your heart, which would allow a clot in the leg to travel to the head. We also have to check ultrasounds of your carotids to make sure there is no clot there contributing to the stroke.				
S:	So what if you find a hole in my heart?				
MD:	We'll have several choices. One is to just continue giving you coumadin to thin your blood for the rest of your life. Second, we can arrange for a mesh to be inserted via a catheter to close off the hole. Third, we can have an open-heart surgical repair of the defect.				
S:	I hate surgery.				
MD:	Well, if that's the case, you're in luck, because it is reasonable to continue the coumadin. But it means monthly blood tests and visits with the nurse practitioner.				
S:	Compared to heart surgery, that sounds good. Is the mesh placement dangerous?				

continued

PO Box 2308, Woburn, MA 01888-0508, **p:** 781-729-3736, **www.EmbracingCulture.com**
PO Box 6401, Manchester, NH 03108, **p:** 1-888-678-CCCS

Role-Play 18 *(continued)*

	Pronunciation	Additions	Omissions	Mistakes
MD: It's a new procedure, fairly well tolerated, but we don't know a lot about how long it lasts or its long-term safety. Why don't we see what the echo shows and then we'll talk some more?				
S: OK, and I will continue the coumadin. Yes, that's important.				
Break It Down	☐	☐	☐	☐

☐ CIFE with patient ☐ CIFE with provider ☐ FLOW ☐ REGISTER

Role-Play 18: Glossary

1. Pathology (diseases, conditions)

2. Laboratory Tests and Diagnostic Procedures

3. Treatment Procedures

4. Idiomatic Expressions (if any)

5. Other (vocabulary in this particular role-play that you feel is important/relevant or that you anticipate problems with)

continued

PO Box 2308, Woburn, MA 01888-0508, **p:** 781-729-3736, **www.EmbracingCulture.com**
PO Box 6401, Manchester, NH 03108, **p:** 1-888-678-CCCS

Role Play 19: Pediatrics Symptom Checklist (PSC)

Emotional and physical health go together in children. Because parents are often the first to notice a problem with their child's behavior, emotions, or learning, you may help you child get the best care possible by answering these questions.

Please mark under the heading that best describes your child:

	Never	Sometimes	Often
1. Complains of aches and pains			
2. Spends more time alone			
3. Tires easily, has little energy			
4. Fidgety, unable to sit still			
5. Less interested in school			
6. Has trouble with teacher			
7. Acts as if driven by a motor			
8. Daydreams too much			
9. Distracted easily			
10. Is afraid of new situations			
11. Feels sad, unhappy			
12. Is irritable, angry			
13. Feels hopeless			
14. Has trouble concentrating			
15. Less interested in friends			
16. Fights with other children			
17. Absent from school			
18. School grades dropping			
19. Is down on him or herself			
20. Visits the doctor and doctor finds nothing wrong			
21. Has trouble sleeping			
22. Worries a lot			
23. Wants to be with you more than before			
24. Feels he or she is bad			
25. Takes unnecessary risks			
26. Gets hurt frequently			
27. Seems to be having less fun			

continued

	Never	Sometimes	Often
28. Acts younger than children his/her age			
29. Does not listen to rules			
30. Does not show feelings			
31. Does not understand other people's feelings			
32. Teases others			
33. Blames other for his/her troubles			
34. Takes things that do not belong to him/her			
35. Refuses to share			
Total Score			

Does your child have any emotional or behavioral problems for which she or he needs help?
◯ Yes ◯ No

Are there any services that you would like your child to receive for these problems?
◯ Yes ◯ No

If yes, what services?

____

____

____

____

____

Role-Play 19: Glossary

______________ ______________ ______________

______________ ______________ ______________

______________ ______________ ______________

______________ ______________ ______________

______________ ______________ ______________

PO Box 2308, Woburn, MA 01888-0508, **p:** 781-729-3736, **www.EmbracingCulture.com**
PO Box 6401, Manchester, NH 03108, **p:** 1-888-678-CCCS

1. Pathology (diseases, conditions)

2. Laboratory Tests and Diagnostic Procedures

3. Treatment Procedures

4. Idiomatic Expressions (if any)

5. Other (vocabulary in this particular role-play that you feel is important/relevant or that you anticipate problems with)

Role-Play 20: Practice Sight Interpretation:

- Read the document
- Understand overall message
- Circle words that need clarification
- Ask provider to stay in the room for clarification
- Read the document from English to Target Language

Document #1

CONTACT LENS FOLLOW UP CARE AGREEMENT

Additional care requirements come with wearing contact lenses. This sheet summarizes our office policies and general advice regarding the lenses.

FOLLOW-UP CARE

Follow up appointments are essential to successful lens wear. You will need a follow up visit in a week and then, in a month. A valid contact lens prescription does not exist until these visits are completed. Your contact lens order may be delayed or cancelled if these visits are not kept.

POSSIBLE ADVERSE REACTIONS

Red eyes, discomfort, corneal ulcers, and partial or total loss of vision are all possible complications of wearing contact lenses. The chances of these problems occurring can be substantially reduced by following the doctor's advice on lens care, maintaining personal hygiene, and keeping your follow-up and annual appointments.

If you experience discomfort, redness, light sensitivity, or blurry vision, remove the contact lenses and call this office immediately. Do not ignore these symptoms!

FEES

Eye exams, fitting fees, and contact lens fees are not refundable for any reason. Your fitting fee covers three months of follow-up care. The office will charge a fee for an office visit if you neglect to keep your appointments and visits extend beyond three months.

EXAMS

An annual contact lens exam is necessary to ensure the health of your eyes and the accuracy of your prescription. **Contact lens prescriptions expire one year from the date of initial exam. Contact lens replacements are not allowed beyond one year without an annual contact lens exam.**

PO Box 2308, Woburn, MA 01888-0508, **p:** 781-729-3736, **www.EmbracingCulture.com**
PO Box 6401, Manchester, NH 03108, **p:** 1-888-678-CCCS

FOR NEW CONTACT LENS WEARERS...
It is impossible to determine in advance your success with contact lenses. Certain personal, physiological, and environment factors may adversely affect the success of lens wear and may necessitate a change in the recommended wearing schedule or termination of lens wear. These factors include, but are not limited to, poor lens hygiene, allergies, and certain medications.

Your doctor will outline a wearing schedule for you to become accustomed to your lenses. You must follow the schedule and recommended cleaning system, and notify the doctor of any problems with the lenses as soon as possible.

YOUR WEARING SCHEDULE: *(new wearers only)*
Wear your contact lenses 3 or 4 hours only the first day. Increase 1 or 2 hours per day for the next six days, up to 8 hours maximum. At your follow-up visit, your doctor will instruct you on your future schedule of contact lens wear.

FOR CONTINUING WEARERS...
Your doctor will again stress the necessity of an annual contact lens exam in order to reassess the contacts you are wearing, your cleaning system, and any changes in the health of your eyes. Sometimes it may be necessary to change your lens type, lens size/shape, wearing schedule or cleaning system to maintain good ocular health.

We reserve the right to terminate a patient from a lens program due to poor compliance or abuse. Fees are not refundable.

I understand and agree with all of the above. I agree to follow the doctor's advice for continued safe contact lens wear.

Signature ______________________________ Tech initials ____________

Print Name ______________________________ Date ________________

Document # 2

PEDIATRIC IMMUNIZATION CONSENT FORM

I have received and have read the information contained in the Vaccine Information Statement(s) concerning the vaccine(s) checked below:

_______	Diphtheria, pertussis, and tetanus (5/17/07)*	_______	Hepatitis B (7/11/01)*
_______	Polio (1/1/00)*	_______	Hemophilus B conjugate (12/16/98)*
_______	Measles, mumps and rubella (1/15/03)*	_______	Varicella (1/10/07)*
_______	Tetanus/diphtheria (Td) (6/10/94)*	_______	Influenza (VIS updated yearly)*
_______	Hepatitis A (3/21/06)*	_______	Pneumococcal Conjugate (9/30/02)*
_______	MMRV (1/15/03, 1/10/07)*	_______	Rotavirus (4/12/06)*
_______	HPV (2/2/07)*	_______	Dtap-IPV-Hep B (5/17/07),1/1/00,7/11/01)*
_______	Meningococcal Vaccine (11/16.06)*	_______	Tdap Vaccine (7/12/06)*

I have had an opportunity to ask questions, which have been answered to my satisfaction. I understand the benefits, potential side effects, and risk of the vaccine(s) checked.

_______ My child will receive all vaccines checked above.

_______ My child will receive the following vaccines:

If you are a patient 18 years or older please check one of the following:

_______ I will receive all vaccines checked

_______ I will receive the following vaccines:

_______ I am refusing vaccines today for my child or myself.

Signature of patient/parent of guardian ______________________________ Date _______

**Dates in parentheses correspond with the dates on the vaccine information statements.*

PO Box 2308, Woburn, MA 01888-0508, **p:** 781-729-3736, **www.EmbracingCulture.com**
PO Box 6401, Manchester, NH 03108, **p:** 1-888-678-CCCS

Document # 3

(For confidentiality purposes this note was created based on a non-existent patient. So name of patient and identification data and name of hospital were created for the purpose of this exercise)

Note to the interpreter: The first and the last page are perhaps the only information an interpreter will be asked to sight translate right after the patient is ready to be discharged from the hospital.

AUSTIN HOSPITAL

X-RAY REPORT

Cindy Collins	4-28-08	4-27-08
PATIENT NAME	DATE	DATE OF SERVICE

The results of your x-rays performed in the Emergency Department are now complete.

- ○ Enclosed is a copy of your x-ray report.
- ○ Please follow-up with your private physician.
- ○ Please call us for additional treatment instructions.

You may contact the QA nurse at 781-729-2600, Monday-Friday from 8:00am to 3:00pm if you have any questions or concerns.

REPRINT

DEPARTMENT OF RADIOLOGY

AUSTIN HOSPITAL

4000 Boston Ave, Austin, Mass. 01890

ACCT NO: 36925000913 EXAMS TYPED 13:07:55 ON 4-27-08 FILE NO: 369250009

Collins, Cindy	Female 049 YR (S)	
MDR NO: 000210031	Dr. Drew, Anthony	ROOM: E.R.
EXAM: 221444002 CT ABD W/ WO CON		EXAM DONE: 4-27-08

CT ABDOMEN W/WO CONT 04/27/08 245. EC7355-08 70100

Abdominal Pain:

computerited tomography

Technique: 5mm thick spiral CT slices are obtained from the axial plane through the urinary tract. 100 cc of IV contrast was then given and repeat imaging was performed through the abdomen and pelvis.

Finding: Fatty infiltration of the liver is seen. The liver is enlarged, measuring 18mm in craniocaudal length. Spleen, pancreas, adrenals, and left kidney are within normal limits. The right kidney shows 3-mm right intrarenal kidney stone. There is also mild hydroureteronephrosis extending to the right UVJ where there is a 2-mm stone. Visualized osseous structures demonstrate no acute finding. No pelvic mass lesion appreciated. Visualized lung bases show dependent changes posteriorly. Vascular calcification is seen. Evaluation of the bowel is limited secondary to lack of oral contrast. Bilateral BTL clips are noted. No lymphadenopathy seen by CY size criterion.

Impression: 2-mm right UVJ stone with mild hydronephrosis. 3-mm right intrarenal kidney stone.
Hepatomegaly: Fatty liver
Vascular Calcification.
BTL.
Electronically signed by: James, Butterfly, M.D on 4/27/08 1:07pm
Dictated by: Butterfly, James
Transcribed BY/ON: ZAL 4/27/08

Report Status: Final

THIS REPORT IS VERIFIED AND FINALIZED ONLY IF SIGNED BY A RADIOLOGIST.

Collins, Cindy
CTAWW 36925000913 Page 1

THIS REPORT IS BEING TRANSMITTED WITHOUT REVIEW IMMEDIATELY FOLLOWING TRANSCRIPTION. THIS REPORT IS VERIFIEDAND FINALIZED ONLY IF SIGNED BY THE RADIOLOGIST. THE FINAL SIGNED REPORT IS ON FILE IN THE RADIOLOGY DEPARTMENT.

General Instructions
Austin Hospital
400 Boston Ave. Austin, Mass. 01890
4/27/2008 3:44

Patient: Collins, Cindy
MRN: 000210031 Acct#: 3692500913
Sex: F DOB: 08/01/58 Age 49 yr.

Thank you for visiting the Austin Hospital Emergency Department. You have been evaluated today by Butterfly, MD for the following condition(s):

- ○ Renal colic
- ○ Right ureterolithiasis.

Instructions: Rest. Drink Plenty of Fluids.

Warnings: Further evaluation is necessary in order to conduct further tests and assess the possibility of serious illness. It is very important to follow up with a physician.

GENERAL WARNINGS: Return to the Emergency Department or contact your physician immediately if your condition worsens or changes unexpectedly, if not improving as expected, or if other problems arise.

Prescription Medications: Phenergan 25mg tablets: take one orally every 6 hours as needed for nausea. Dispense thirty (30). No refill Generic substitute OK.
Vicodin: 5mg: take 1 to 2 orally every 24 hour. Dispense fifteen (15). No refills Generic substitute OK.

Follow-up: Follow-up with a neurologist- as recommended by your primary care physician. Follow up with your doctor Monday.

Understanding of the discharge instructions verbalized by patient.

You have been given the following additional information:
KIDNEY STONE (W/ COLIC)
MEICATION PHENERGAN

Patient Signature: ______________________________

Document # 4

PATIENT ROUTING SLIP

Internal Medicine

Before leaving our office today, please arrange for the next steps in your care indicated with a (check mark)

Check-out Desk

Please schedule any follow-up appointments with the following provider:

Schedule an appointment or test with a specialist:

○ <1 week ○ 1-2 weeks ○ 2-4 weeks* ○ routine

**Please talk with the check-out staff about booking specialty appointments. Please note numbers are listed on the back.*

Please call to schedule the following tests or appointments:

○ Mammography
○ Colonoscopy/Flex Sig ________
○ Bone Density

Please obtain the following materials:

○ Colorectal Screening Kit ○ Printed prescriptions ○After Visit Summary
○ Out of work/school note: ___ through___ ___ Letter for

○ Prior Authorization Form (drug name, dose & reason)

○ Health Education Handouts: ○ On Printer

Lab / Radiology

Please complete Lab and X-ray Testing:

○ Laboratory: ○ Today
○ Future ____________
○ Future Fasting ____________
○ 1-2 weeks before next visit/Fasting

○ EKG (In Lab): ○ Today
○ 3-4 days before the next visit

Fasting means nothing to eat drink (except water) 10-12 hours before the test.

○ Radiology:
○ Return to clinical area after testing
Lab hours: Monday – Friday 7:45 am–6:00pm

Pharmacy

○ Please pick up your prescriptions ___ #of scripts to be picked up

Thank you for choosing to receive your care from us. Please feel free to contact my office if you have any medical problems or concerns. Any member of our team will be happy to assist you.

FOR ADDITIONAL HEALTH INFORMATION, PLEASE VISIT OUR WEBSITE AT WWW.CCCSORG.COM

PO Box 2308, Woburn, MA 01888-0508, **p:** 781-729-3736, **www.EmbracingCulture.com**
PO Box 6401, Manchester, NH 03108, **p:** 1-888-678-CCCS

Role-Play 20: Glossary

1. Pathology (diseases, conditions)

2. Laboratory Tests and Diagnostic Procedures

3. Treatment Procedures

4. Idiomatic Expressions (if any)

5. Other (vocabulary in this particular role-play that you feel is important/relevant or that you anticipate problems with)

Lesson 4: Additional Resources
How Providers Communicate with Each Other About a Patient

SOAP NOTES: Understanding clinician-to-clinician communication

SOAP is an acronym for **subjective, objective, assessment** and **plan**. SOAP notes are a tool that helps clinicians formulate their questions by organizing a medical session into four main parts. SOAP notes have proved effective when used to gather information for diagnostic purposes and can help to build rapport between the patient and the provider.

In the process of gathering information, clinicians need to be culturally sensitive and make sure that linear questions regarding the pain scale (i.e. "Can you describe your pain on a scale of 1-10?") and end-of-life issues are asked according to the patient's personal belief system. In order to elicit accurate information from their patients, many providers have put forth a conscious effort to use open-ended questioning.

Often, interpreters comment that when there is more than one clinician involved in a session, patients can become frustrated. This frustration can increase due to the providers' tendency to ask the same questions over and over. The patient may even come to the conclusion that the providers are not communicating well with each other. However, clinicians have long understood that patients answer differently to different providers. Much of a patient's reaction is determined by momentary feelings regarding his/her health and regarding the provider. Therefore, repeated questioning is crucial to the formulation of a differential diagnosis.

As clinicians listen to the patient's presenting problem, a series of possible diagnoses arises. Clinicians first attempt to rule out the most serious diagnoses. This is called "differential diagnosis." For example, a patient presenting a headache will first be asked a series of questions that will enable the provider to rule out a diagnosis of brain cancer. After repeated questioning, the provider might finally settle for a diagnosis of stress-induced migraine headaches.

The interpreter should remember that all clinicians are trained to apply the principles of SOAP and consistently do so in each clinical interaction.

PO Box 2308, Woburn, MA 01888-0508, **p:** 781-729-3736, **www.EmbracingCulture.com**
PO Box 6401, Manchester, NH 03108, **p:** 1-888-678-CCCS

Medical Abbreviations and Symbols:

Providers use a variety of abbreviations and symbols as short cuts to describe and document procedures, names of illnesses and medical actions. Here are some examples:

Abbreviation	Meaning
AIDS	acquired immunodeficiency syndrome
aq	water (aqua)
ASA	aspirin
BID, b.i.d.	twice a day (bis in die)
BIN, b.i.n.	twice a night
BP	blood pressure
CBC	complete blood (cell) count
COLD	chronic obstructive lung disease
CONT	contrast
COPD	chronic obstructive pulmonary disease
CPR	cardiopulmonary resuscitation
C-section	caesarian section
CT	computed tomography (CAT Scan)
CVA	cerebral vascular accident
CVS	cardiovascular system
C/W	consistent with
CXR	chest x-ray
DC	discharge
D & C	dilation and curettage
DOB	date of birth
DT	delirium tremens; duration of tetany
D/T	due to
Dx	diagnosis
EKG	electrocardiogram
ENT	ear, nose and throat
ER	emergency room
Fx	fracture
FHT	fetal heart tone
GI	gastrointestinal
HIV	human immunodeficiency virus
IUD	intrauterine device
IV	intravenous
LOL	little old lady
MI	myocardial infarction
MRI	magnetic resonance imaging
NKA	no known allergies

Abbreviation	Meaning
NKDA	no known drug allergies
OB	obstetrics
OB-GYN	obstetrics and gynecology
OR	operating room
OT	occupational therapy
Pap	Pap smear, stain, or test
PID	pelvic inflammatory disease
po	by mouth
PP	after meals
PT	physical therapy
pt	patient
PE	physical examination
qd	every day (quaque die)
qid	four times a day (quater in die)
q.l.	as much as desired (quantum libet)
RLQ	right lower quadrant
Rx	prescription
SOB	shortness of breath
STD	sexually transmitted disease
TB	tuberculosis
tid	three times a day
U/A	urinalysis
URI	upper respiratory infection
UVJ	uretero vesical junction
VD	venereal disease
VO	verbal order
WBC	white blood cells
wt	weight
X Cover	cross covering or covering for another clinician
=	equal or equals
②	not equal
⑧	greater than
⑦	less than
+	increase
_	decrease
+/-	positive, negative or minus

PO Box 2308, Woburn, MA 01888-0508, **p:** 781-729-3736, **www.EmbracingCulture.com**
PO Box 6401, Manchester, NH 03108, **p:** 1-888-678-CCCS

Should one be a Clarifier or a Culture Coach when Interpreting for Different Types of Pain?

Interpreters are faced with a multitude of challenges in interpreting and describing those different types of pain. Are all of us, providers, patients and interpreters able to accurately interpret the following types of pain?

1. Dull
2. Searing
3. Sharp
4. Annoying

Are these descriptions already culture bound? The challenge is in the accuracy of meaning through the conversion from one language to another. Furthermore, English speakers often have a different understanding of the multiple types of pain. Although pain is a universal experience, the description of it is more personal.

Did you grow up in a family being told that you should not be a complainer? If yes, most likely, you will be the type of patient who will go to the emergency room with some chest pain when you are having a heart attack. Some of us describe sharp pain as if it were a needle or a knife penetrating. Others may describe a toothache as excruciating or an uncomfortable ache. Does your provider have the same meaning as your understanding for a particular type of pain? Providers are individuals and they also have their own experiences in feeling, understanding and describing pain.

According to Edward Hall on beyond the culture, 1997, "Language used to describe culture is by nature poorly adapted to this difficult task. Language is too linear, not comprehensive enough, too slow, too constrained, too unnatural, too much of a product of its' own evolution and too artificial."

There are different types and intensities and forms of pain. Pain can be physical, emotional, social and spiritual. It can be mild, uncomfortable, distressing, terrible, excruciating. Pain can be acute, recent or chronic when it continuous for more than 3 months and longer or it lasts longer than its expected healing time frame.

According to Paul Brodwinn et al in the book *Pain as Human Experience*, different cultures may describe pain as "It seems as if pepper were put into my brain" or " I have a bear headache" or as often we hear from Azorean patients 'os meus miolos vão rebentar ou explodir." One way of saying it in English is, "the inside of my brain is going to burst or explode." Or a patient coming into the emergency room suffering from a heart attack or severe angina may say , "I feel like I have an elephant or truck on top of my chest."

Whose job is it to make sure that both the speaker and the interpreter are in agreement with the description or naming of the particular pain being mentioned? Should an interpreter be a conduit, a clarifier and or culture broker and always ask for the provider's or patient's description of type of pain? How may our own personal experience of pain impact our accuracy level?

The IMIA Standards of Practice, 1995, on page 35 specifically mention that interpreters are "committed to transmitting accurately and completely the content and spirit of the original message into the other language without omitting, modifying, condensing or adding." Also, on page 32, the interpreter "is aware of and able to identify personal biases and beliefs that may interfere with the ability to be impartial, and has the moral fortitude to withdraw if unable to be impartial."

We are left with the understanding that when an interpreter cannot find an exact word for the word describing the pain, that an interpreter should ask for a description and interpret the speaker's description. The interpreter having difficulty finding the exact word should abstain from describing the pain, but involve the respective party on the description. Another way, less time consuming, but with greater potential for error, is for an interpreter to describe the pain to her/ his best judgment and let the speaker know that this is how it was interpreted.

The role of the culture coach when dealing with interpreting issues regarding the intensity of pain seems appropriate when a patient is asked by the provider, "from scale 1-10 how much doest it hurt?" The interpreter sees the patient's hesitance and possible difficulty describing it or even when a patient quickly answers but the body language is not congruent with the number. An interpreter, as per IMIA Standards, may want to inform both parties, provider and patient, of this possible misunderstanding.

Often, the medical culture is a more linear cause and effect and the patient culture is more circular, a story teller. The patient may relate to the pain by describing that the pain is as bad as when her mother went to the hospital or that is so bad that it stops her from going to work. But this same patient may not be able to illustrate the intensity of the pain by using a number. Although the scales with the different facial expressions are visual and a bit more concrete, but often they are still too abstract and not always the best technique to identify the intensity of the pain.

The feedback I get from some providers is that interpreters cannot always act as culture brokers as the session is happening. Providers appreciate the partnership with the interpreters, but perhaps the culture brokering should be at the beginning or end of a session. Here are the following tips for interpreters in the role of culture coaches: Is this about me? Can I wait? How is this intervention going to affect the provider-patient relationship?

PO Box 2308, Woburn, MA 01888-0508, **p:** 781-729-3736, **www.EmbracingCulture.com**
PO Box 6401, Manchester, NH 03108, **p:** 1-888-678-CCCS

Interpreter Evaluation Tool based on the IMIA standards.

Name:______________________________Target Language:_____________Date: ___/___/___

OBSERVATION

1 PRE-SESSION

Client/patient	Yes	No
1. Introduction?		
2. Interpreter helped client with registration?		
3. Interpreter explained the usage of the first person?		
4. Interpreter informed client of confidentiality policy?		
5. Interpreter informed client that everything said during the session will be interpreted?		
6. Did the interpreter handle the waiting period appropriately?		
7. Did the interpreter appropriately acknowledge similarities and differences?		

Provider	Yes	No
8. Introduction?		
9. Interpreter explained the usage of the first person?		
10. Interpreter informed the provider that everything said during the session will be interpreted?		

2 THE TRIADIC RELATIONSHIP

Interpreter/provider and client	Yes	No
1. Did the interpreter appropriately arrange seating?		
2 Did the interpreter show appropriate eye contact?		
3 Did the interpreter appropriately handle the comments from client or provider?		
4 Did the interpreter stay in the room alone with client?		
5 Did the interpreter help with medical procedures?		

6 Who makes the decision of when to stay behind the curtain?
○ Interpreter ○ Client ○ Provider

3 INTERPRETATION TECHNIQUE

Interpreter	Yes	No
1. Usage of First Person?		
2. Omissions?		
3. Additions?		
4. Meaning/Accuracy?		
5. Meaning/Completeness?		
6. Keeps appropriate flow?		
7. Asks for clarification?		
8. Checks with client if he/she understood everything?		
9. Mode of interpretation: consecutive, simultaneous, sight and summary?		
10. Memorization techniques: note taking, echoing key words and finger counting?		

4 KNOWLEDGE OF MEDICAL TERMINOLOGY

Strengths: ______________________________

____

____

____

____

Weaknesses: ______________________________

____

____

____

____

Areas for growth: ______________________________

____

____

____

____

____

PO Box 2308, Woburn, MA 01888-0508, **p:** 781-729-3736, **www.EmbracingCulture.com**
PO Box 6401, Manchester, NH 03108, **p:** 1-888-678-CCCS

5 FOLLOW-UP	Yes	No
1. Interpreter helps client with follow-up visits?		
2. Interpreter helps client getting home?		
3. Interpreter does not provide advice when asked for his or her opinion?		
4. Interpreter handled a distraught client appropriately?		

6 CULTURAL KNOWLEDGE/CLARIFICATION	Yes	No
1. Interpreter clarified cultural meaning by checking with appropriate party?		
2. Interpreter understood vocabulary used by both, provider and client?		
3. Interpreter understands client's immigration history?		
4. Interpreter shows how to best address client by showing respect?		
5. Interpreter asks permission to become a cultural coach when appropriate?		
6. Interpreter showed respect for client's own individuality?		
7. Interpreter understands provider and client's communication styles?		
8. Interpreter understands USA medical system and that of client's native country?		

SELF- OBSERVATION:

7 ETHICS	Yes	No
1. Do you accept gifts?		
2. Do you share your opinion regarding controversial beliefs?		
3. Do you ask questions of clients/personal/clinical?		
4. Do you provide your telephone number?		
5. Do you give your opinion when asked by the clients?		
6. Do you deliberately delete information for political/ religious /personal beliefs?		
7. Do you call clients at home when not asked by provider to do so?		
8. Do you drive client to places?		
9. Do you give money to clients?		
10. Do you make remarks that are pejorative against anyone?		
11. Do you use power of knowledge for personal gains?		
12. Do you discuss prior sessions with different providers?		
13. Do you tell clients what to say in the session?		
14. Do you discuss the sessions and identify clients/providers?		

Lesson Five:
Cross Cultural Competency for Healthcare Interpreters

Understanding Goals

Students will be able to:

- learn about culture competency
- learn about the many layers of culture
- understand how to apply culture competency tools in the triadic encounter
- review and practice the role of the culture coach or culture broker
- learn about US medical system and patient's rights

Key Concepts

- Culture
  The Onion Concept
- Intention vs. Impact
  Stereotypes vs. Generalizations
  Checking-in vs. Assumption
- Conflict Resolution
  Settling vs. Solving
- Culture Anchoring
  Explanatory Model
- Culture Competency Continuum
  Culture Competency Models
- Illness vs. Disease
  Culture of Medicine
  Patient Centered Treatment
  Literacy vs. Health Literacy
- Culture Coach
  Six WS
  ADA
  Sexual Harassment
  Patient Bill of Rights
  Consent forms

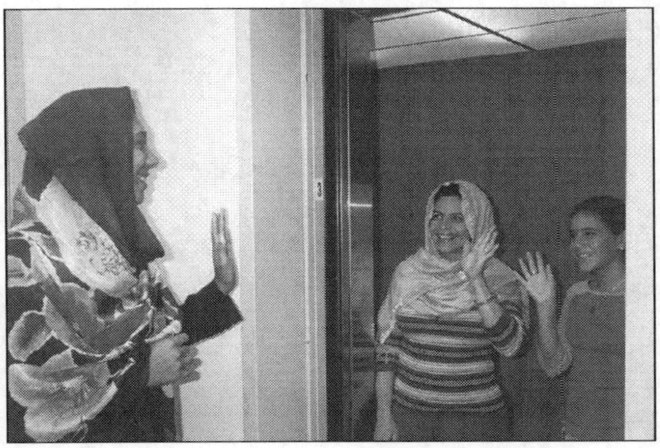

PO Box 2308, Woburn, MA 01888-0508, **p:** 781-729-3736, **www.EmbracingCulture.com**
PO Box 6401, Manchester, NH 03108, **p:** 1-888-678-CCCS

Lesson Five: Quiz
Cross Cultural Competency for Healthcare Interpreters

Mark each item "True" or False."

1. One needs to be aware of intention and impact.
   ○ True ○ False

2. When a patient takes a long time answering the medical provider, the interpreter should interrupt the patient politely and request that his/her answers be shorter.
   ○ True ○ False

3. One should always treat others the same way one would like to be treated.
   ○ True ○ False

4. Cultural competency is a stage of integration of new knowledge so the interpreter needs to tell everyone how one particular ethnic group behaves regarding authority.
   ○ True ○ False

5. It is rude not to shake hands when first meeting a person.
   ○ True ○ False

6. People who speak with strong accents are not very educated.
   ○ True ○ False

7. An interpreter should always act as a culture broker.
   ○ True ○ False

8. An interpreter who acts as a culture broker should only coach the provider.
   ○ True ○ False

9. Rituals and celebrations help build a person's roots and sense of honor.
   ○ True ○ False

10. If respect gets broken, one can still repair it by being self-righteous.
    ○ True ○ False

11. An interpreter may coach a patient in what is culturally appropriate while waiting for the provider.
    ○ True ○ False

12. If you speak a language that is shared by several countries you do not need to become familiar with linguistic differences.
    ○ True ○ False

13. The Immigration Grieving Stages are only experienced by first generation immigrants.
   ○ True ○ False

14. All immigrants experience the Honeymoon Stage when arriving to the US.
   ○ True ○ False

15. An immigrant who is experiencing the loss of homeland over-idealizes the homeland.
   ○ True ○ False

16. An interpreter should act as a culture broker when asked to interpret for advance directives (end of life issues).
   ○ True ○ False

17. We are all born with the knowledge of a culture; culture is not learned.
   ○ True ○ False

18. Culture is always related to ethnicity and race.
   ○ True ○ False

19. Culture is the defining factor in one's identity.
   ○ True ○ False

20. All patients can relate to a pain scale of 1-10.
   ○ True ○ False

21. As you develop cultural competency, you have less of a need to check your assumptions.
   ○ True ○ False

22. The most desirable mode of interpreting is "word for word."
   ○ True ○ False

23. The interpreter who asks a provider for clarification is not well trained.
   ○ True ○ False

24. Interpreters and providers who work well together do not need a pre-or post-session.
   ○ True ○ False

25. To save time, staff interpreters may start the interview process before the provider arrives.
   ○ True ○ False

PO Box 2308, Woburn, MA 01888-0508, **p:** 781-729-3736, **www.EmbracingCulture.com**
PO Box 6401, Manchester, NH 03108, **p:** 1-888-678-CCCS

26. Interpreters are hired by the clinic and they should represent the provider's interests in the triadic encounter.
   - O True
   - O False

27. Immigrants going through the honeymoon stage of the Immigration Grieving Stages often express ambivalence about immigration.
   - O True
   - O False

28. Only newly arrived immigrants experience a grieving process.
   - O True
   - O False

29. Roots are based on beliefs that are not always present at a conscious level.
   - O True
   - O False

Mark the item that best completes the sentence.

30. A culture broker is an interpreter who:
   A. tells staff how to be more sensitive to the patient's culture.
   B. tells patients all about how to deal with the "American medical system."
   C. coaches a medical provider on different ways of approaching a cultural conflict.
   D. advocates patient rights

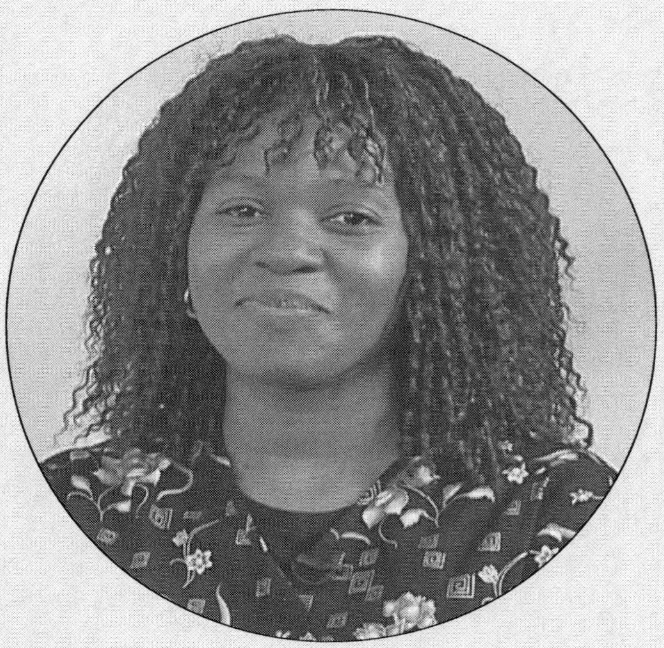

Lesson Five: Class Activities
Cross Cultural Competency for Healthcare Interpreters

EXERCISE
Review

Directions: Read the following Pain Assessment Questionnaire. Remember that, as an interpreter, you will not be asked to apply this questionnaire, however we would like you to be familiar with this terminology as well as the type of questions.

In pairs, ask your colleague to imagine the worst pain s/he has ever felt. Use the tool to assess the type, frequency, and intensity of his or her pain. Remember to take turns. Do not forget to add the new words to your glossary.

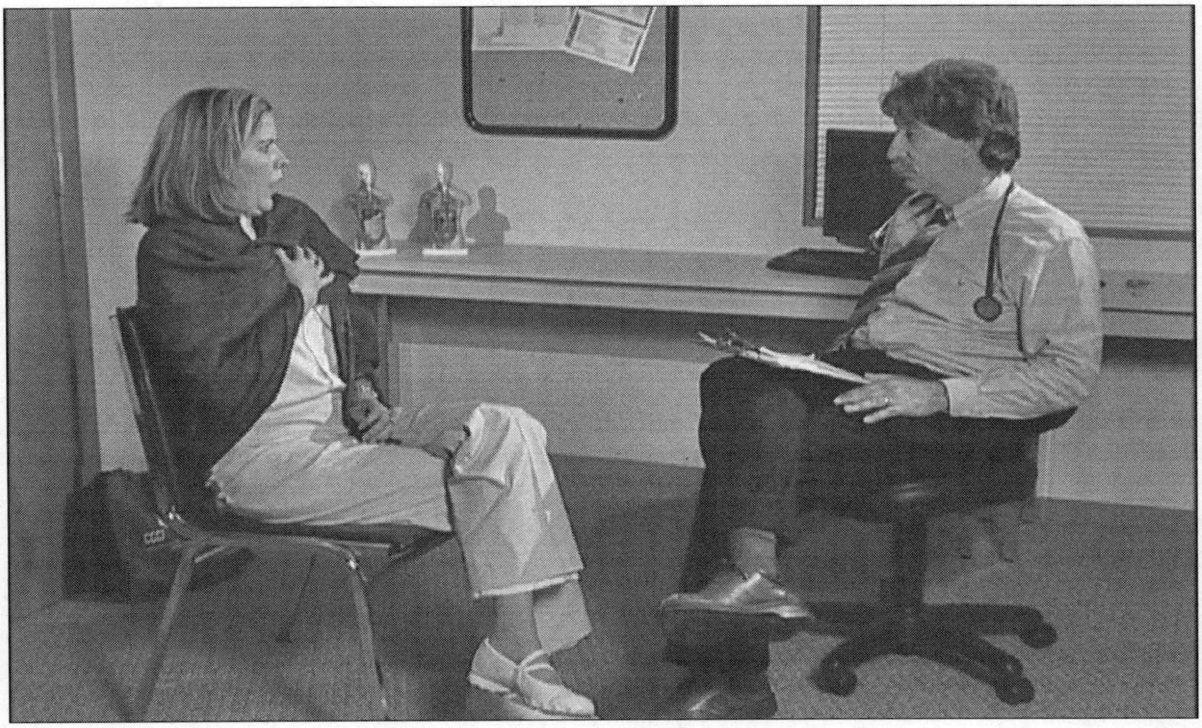

PO Box 2308, Woburn, MA 01888-0508, p: 781-729-3736, www.EmbracingCulture.com
PO Box 6401, Manchester, NH 03108, p: 1-888-678-CCCS

Pain Assessment Tool

Does the patient have any Diagnosis(es) which would give reason to believe he/she would be in pain?

○ Yes ○ No **If yes, describe cause and origin of pain:** ________________ .

Does the patient verbalize pain? ○ Yes ○ No **If yes, date of pain onset:**__/___/__

As the patient describes it, what does the pain feel like? *(check all that apply)*

○ Aching ○ Heavy ○ Tender ○ Splitting ○ Tiring ○ Exhausting ○ Throbbing
○ Shooting ○ Stabbing ○ Sharp ○ Cramping ○ Hot/Burning ○ Other ___________

Pain Location/Type/Frequency/Intensity

**If the patient is able, identify pain type(s) and locations and record below. Label sites as* A, B, C, D. Code pain type, frequency and intensity, as applicable.

Type	**Code**	**Site A**	**Site B**	**Site C**	**Site D**
	I = Internal A =Acute E = External C = Chronic				
Frequency	**Code**	**Site A**	**Site B**	**Site C**	**Site D**
	O = Occasional F = Frequent C = Constant				
Intensity	**Scale**	**Site A**	**Site B**	**Site C**	**Site D**
	|-----|-----|-----|-----|-----|-----|-----|-----|-----| 1 2 3 4 5 6 7 8 9 10 ○ No Pain = _____ ○ Moderate Pain = _____ ○ Worst Pain = _____				
		Site A	**Site B**	**Site C**	**Site D**
At Present:					
1 Hour After Medication:					
3 Hours After Medication:					
Worst It Gets:					
Best It Gets:					

Has the patient had any of the following changes in daily activities or habits?

○ Insomnia ○ Other sleep disturbances ○ Loss of appetite/weight loss ○ Constipation
○ Incontinence ○ Decreased ability to concentrate ○ Changes in mood/emotions
○ Withdrawal from activities or relationships ○ Decrease/Increase in Physical activity

This pain assessment tool was copied from the author's personal records when she visited the emergency room in 2008.

Nonverbal/Noncognitive Signs of Pain

**Check Yes or No for each of the following nonverbal/noncognitive signs which could indicate the presence of pain.*

Facial Expressions:	Vocalizations:	Body Actions/Observed Behaviors
Yes / No Grimacing/distorted face	Yes / No Moaning	Yes / No Thrashing
Yes / No Clenched jaw/teeth	Yes / No Grunting	Yes / No Pounding
Yes / No Frowning/scowling	Yes / No Gasping	Yes / No Biting
Yes / No Tightly shut lips	Yes / No Crying	Yes / No Rocking
Yes / No Glazed eyes	Yes / No Screaming	Yes / No Threatening gestures
Yes / No Wrinkled brow	Yes / No Cursing	Yes / No Altered gait/posture
Yes / No Turned down mouth		Yes / No Strenuous breathing
Yes / No Tearing		Yes / No Knees up to abdomen
		Yes / No Fidgeting
		Yes / No Pacing
		Yes / No Irritability
		Yes / No Clenched fists
		Yes / No Wringing of hands
		Yes / No Increased hand movements
		Yes / No Striking out at others

THINK

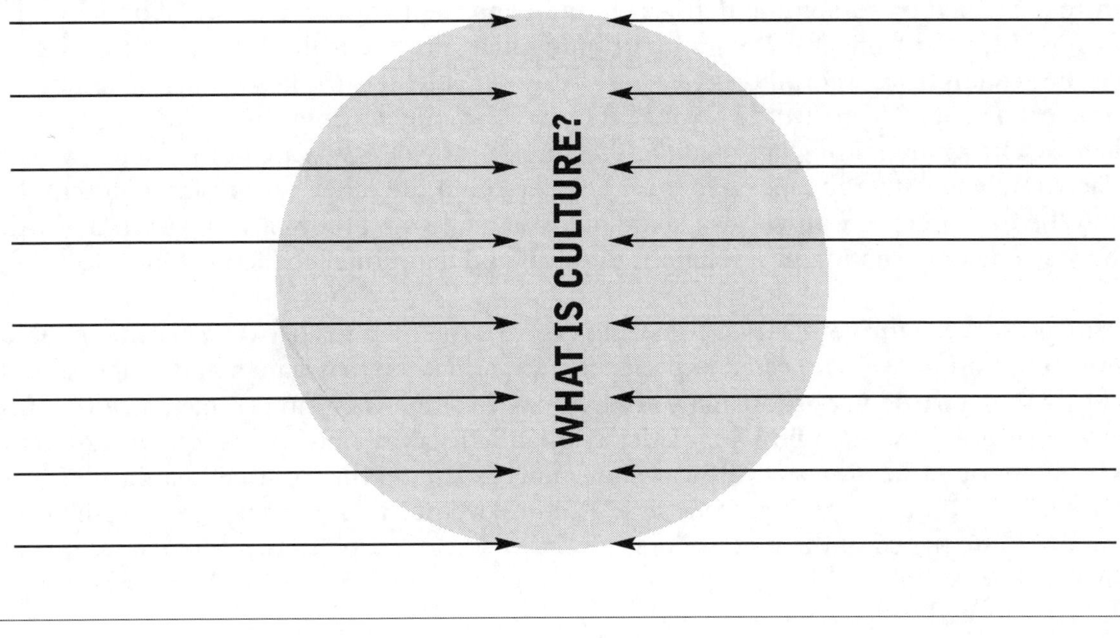

PO Box 2308, Woburn, MA 01888-0508, **p:** 781-729-3736, **www.EmbracingCulture.com**
PO Box 6401, Manchester, NH 03108, **p:** 1-888-678-CCCS

What do we have in common right now? What brought us together right this moment?
Look around the room and share what we have in common and different among us.

In Common	Different

Culture is defined by something that we **share in common** with an individual or a group that **makes us different from another** group or individual. Culture is fluid, is on-going, and it is not static. For example, as interpreters we share our own culture – *the importance of accuracy, where interpreters do not interpret word by word but convey meaning by keeping the same register without adding, distorting or omitting information*. We are not providers, we are not patients, we simply and accurately facilitate the message from one person to the other, **we are interpreters**! But within the interpreter group we also share our differences and they can consist of many different aspects: gender, age, nationality, religion, physical and emotional challenges and more.

Culture is *localized* through very unique and discrete interactions between specific people. By paying attention to these repeated experiences, an individual may gain some insight about the world view of a particular group and or individual. In some ways, interpreters need to think of their jobs as not only providing linguistically qualified services but also as ambassadors to our newly emerging profession as healthcare interpreters. Due to the fact that healthcare interpreting is still an emerging profession, it is important that interpreters follow through and become well informed of the medical culture they navigate, such as the understanding of HIPAA, Patient's Rights, the requirements for the Joint Commission and the professional standards for medical providers.

Culture is fluid, is on-going, and is adaptable. It is a liberating feeling to know that one can always repair a certain rigidity in values, assumptions, and beliefs that define a culture. So, from one formed impression of a culture (rigid), one individual or group can interrupt this journey of missed behaviors and expectations by asking for assistance and by acknowledging mistakes and growing from them by setting new paths, understandings and behaviors.

How are providers, patients and interpreters similar? How are they different?

	Providers	Patients	Interpreters
Similar			
Different			

What you just did was to create again another set of behaviors that connects and differentiates you from another group based on expectations and assumptions.

In order for us to function in a society and in the world, we all need to follow a path of guidelines, laws that in turn are influenced by beliefs and values that in turn are defined by our assumptions and expectations. The problem is that when we do not check the assumptions /beliefs with the individual and we embrace them as the truth for all group members, we are essentially expressing a form of ethnocentrism which typically leads to an unhealthy rigidity by ignoring the individuality that all people bring to a group or a dynamic.

PO Box 2308, Woburn, MA 01888-0508, **p:** 781-729-3736, **www.EmbracingCulture.com**
PO Box 6401, Manchester, NH 03108, **p:** 1-888-678-CCCS

Understanding Your World View

EXERCISE

The words below will evoke a belief or a thought from you. Individually, take a few minutes and write down what comes to your mind when you hear these words. As you have completed this exercise, pair up with a colleague in your class that you do not know well and share your notes and impressions.

1. World ____________
2. Country of origin ____________
3. Education ____________
4. Provider ____________
5. Emergency Room ____________
6. Intensive Care Unit ____________
7. Clinical Assistant ____________
8. Sexual Activity ____________
9. Police ____________
10. Family ____________
11. Religion ____________
12. Profession ____________
13. Work ____________
14. I ____________

Write down one word that you may want to work on at some point soon in your life:

____

Fortunately we, as human beings, need to relate to others and feel that we are part of a culture or cultures. We communicate with each other at different levels: emotionally, physically and spiritually. As a result, we pass on messages that often we are not even aware of at a conscious level, but that are loaded with values and beliefs.

The following exercise will give you an opportunity to move on from how you understand the world but also how the world and certain societies have defined our worlds.

Understanding Your Society

EXERCISE

Divide into small groups and take turns reading and reacting to the following statements:

1. Boys do not cry, you are not a girl!
2. He was a Jew!
3. You do not know what really happened unless you were sleeping under their bed.
4. You can not judge a book by its cover.
5. You seem to have a dark cloud over your shoulders.
6. He looks like a terrorist.
7. There is so much food in this country that being hungry is not an excuse.
8. People who receive government aid are lazy.
9. You are such an immigrant!
10. You are so ethnic!
11. Girls talk too much!

According to Huges (1976), culture is a "learned configuration of images and other symbolic elements (such as language) widely shared among members of a given society or social group which, for individuals, functions as an orientational framework for behavior."

Words are powerful tools that often represent one's world view. They can serve as a bridge for emotional support to some when the same words in fact can be divisive and offensive. Words are one part of the puzzle, the window that may define one's culture. Verbal and the written form of the usage of words is a way of expressing values, culture, register, feelings, emotions, beliefs and more, but we all know that often, words and thoughts are misinterpreted or misrepresented, even by those who share the same language.

PO Box 2308, Woburn, MA 01888-0508, **p:** 781-729-3736, **www.EmbracingCulture.com**
PO Box 6401, Manchester, NH 03108, **p:** 1-888-678-CCCS

This is why interpreters need to keep a speaker's register and when in doubt of its meaning or ability to accurately understand it, interpreters are instructed to ask for a **break down**. In the USA when a provider sees a patient holding on to his chest and stating that s/he feels pain just as if an elephant was seating in her/ his chest, the "medical world view" is that this is a patient that needs to be seen right away.

Medicine has its own culture, and the culture of medicine is different from department to department and from provider to provider. There is a certain hierarchy where certain behaviors and words are more tolerated than others and it all comes down to who has the most power in the group. Also, there are certain behaviors that are allowed among providers but never towards a patient. These behaviors can set a tone of arrogance and a certain "click" feeling to the outsiders but it can also create an emotional escape when the job stress is unbearable.

Interpreters may feel offended when they listen to a provider vent about a patient. It is not unusual for one profession to create acronyms when trying to briefly present a patient to a colleague. The provider may say: *"This LOL (Little Old Lady) is a GOMER (Get out of my emergency room), she keeps misusing the emergency room for her bladder control issues instead of going to her primary care provider."*

Interpreters, and even other colleagues of his provider, may be left with an uneasy feeling although they may smile or not correct the statement when they listen to the expression LOL.

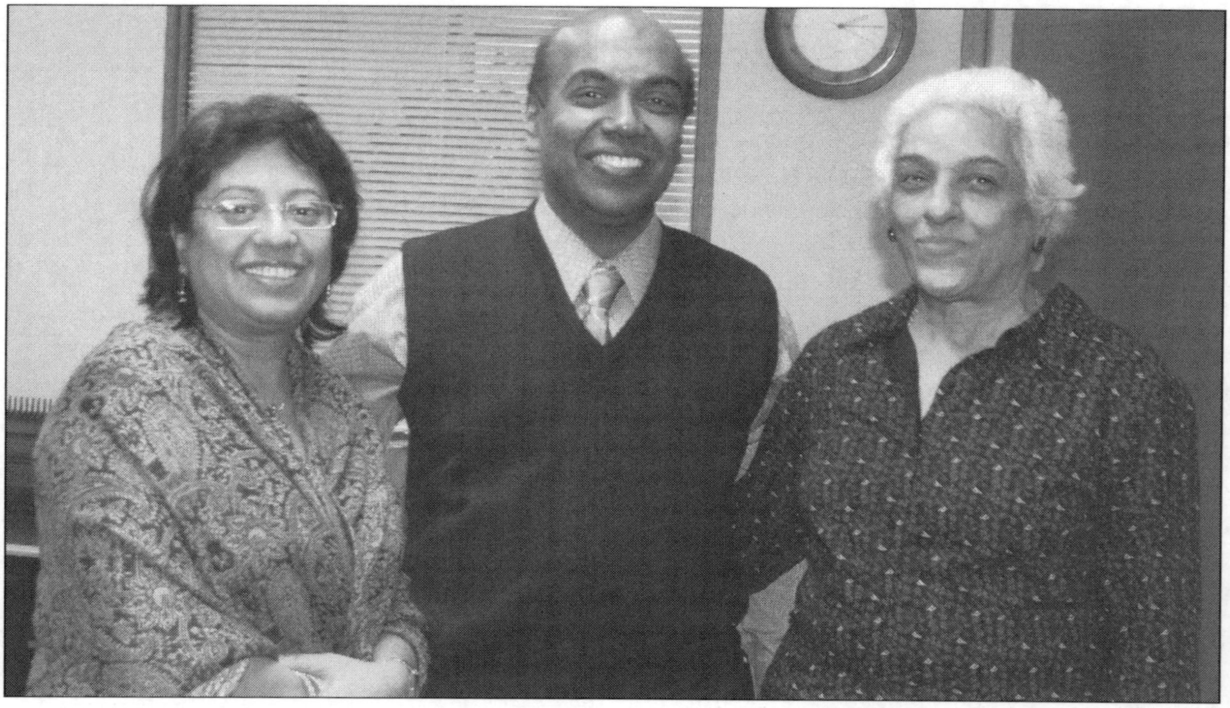

Stereotypes and Generalizations

THINK

How do you define a stereotype? to extend some

~~Inclusion of~~ characteristics ~~of~~ to a determined type of people ~~and~~ habits

Can you give an example of a stereotype you grew up with?

Girls always should help mothers at home

How do you define a generalization?

Dotar a un grupo de gente de las mismas ideas / estilo de vida

Can you give an example of a generalization?

los latinos llegan tarde

What is the difference between the two?

Generalización – nivel más abierto

Stereotype – someone putting sth on a group ("insulting")

PO Box 2308, Woburn, MA 01888-0508, **p:** 781-729-3736, **www.EmbracingCulture.com**
PO Box 6401, Manchester, NH 03108, **p:** 1-888-678-CCCS

APPLY CRITICAL THINKING

Please review the following case study and answer the questions in a small group format:

Case study #1:

Clinical Assistant: Good morning, how can I help you? (Happy and a bit loud.)

PT: I have an appointment with Dr. Peters at 12PM. (Low voice)

Clinical Assistant: And you are...Oh my God, do I need help with this name! I will just call you Ms A. Nowadays, not only do I have to do my job, but I have to adjust my tongue so that I can pronounce all these foreign names! (Louder)

PT: (Silence) Excuse me! (Low voice and a bit shy.)

Clinical Assistant: Don't worry, I have a dental assistant that speaks your language and I am sure you are going to like her. She looks just like you and speaks with all our foreign patients. (Laughing and loud)

PT: Excuse me, I am here to see Dr. Peters and I am speaking English with you. I do not need anyone to speak for me! You Americans hear an accent and get all bent out of shape! (Angry and loud)

Clinical Assistant: OK, Ms. A. Just have a seat and I will tell Dr. Peters about your situation. (Looking down and low voice.)

PT: I also would like for you to call me by my name and not by my initials. My name is Araujo and not Ms. A. (Angry and firm.)

Clinical Assistant: All right...all right... one more thing we have to do... I need to check if the information in the computer is still all correct... You are still at 46 Harvard Street? (Loud and a bit frustrated)

PT: Yes.

Clinical Assistant: And do you still have this number (781) 396-0000? (Loud)

PT: Yes.

Clinical Assistant: Wow, you're not like the others. They move around so much that I can't even reach them. (Frustrated, a bit loud)

PT: Excuse me, you are making so many assumptions that you are making me real mad! *(Loud)*

Clinical Assistant: I was just trying to tell you that you are different from your people. You seem to stay at one address just like us Americans. I was not saying anything bad, but I am sorry if I have offended you. (Frustrated, but not as loud as in the past exchanges). *(silence)*

Clinical Assistant: I was just trying to help you. Sorry if I'm too direct, but if you have a problem, you need to speak up. (apologetic)

PT: Yes, you offended me, but at least we are now both looking at each other. (low)

Questions

Take a look at the interactions that may have contributed to an unfortunate escalation of angry exchanges.

Note at least two forms of stereotypes in this interaction. Why did you consider them stereotypes?

____

____

____

____

Can you point out a generalization that turned into a stereotype?

____

____

____

____

If you were Ms. Araujo, how would you have handled this situation?

____

____

____

____

When did this intense exchange begin to calm down?

____

____

____

____

PO Box 2308, Woburn, MA 01888-0508, **p:** 781-729-3736, **www.EmbracingCulture.com**
PO Box 6401, Manchester, NH 03108, **p:** 1-888-678-CCCS

Stereotypes are gross generalizations in which the individual is never consulted. Female drivers may feel a lot of shame and self-blame when they get into a car accident. They may be reacting to the stereotype that "women are bad drivers."

Stereotypes are hurtful. They are rigid descriptions of a person's values, interactions and expectations. They put people into boxes and deny the opportunity for someone to open those boxes. Stereotypes are based on assumptions that were never checked with an individual. Stereotypes can have a positive/negative impact. In the US, it is commonly understood that Asian students are good at math and are in general great academically. So, often, Asian students when not accomplished academically may feel the double edge of "you are smart, how come you are not doing this well?" Or may feel afraid to ask for clarification or help so that they meet society's expectations. In Massachusetts, there are communities where the student suicide rate among Asian refugees is higher than other ethnic groups. Stereotypes do not connect but isolate people.

Generalizations almost seem like stereotypes, but the difference is that a generalization is inclusive of the individuality that each situation may present, whereas a stereotype (a formatted set of rigid values) is stated with certainty and finality, ignoring individuality and denying the humanity of the individual. Be careful! Interpreters are often caught in situations where in order for them to be believable they feel the need to resort to stereotypes. If you need to make a generalization, preface it with the words "it seems…," "it appears…," 'I've seen that…," or "I understand….," "I have observed…." By using "bad female drivers" as an example of a stereotype, I made a generalization that women may feel shame, and they may blame themselves for an accident. A woman reading this might never experience this at all. She could be offended by my comments and become angry at me.

Did you notice the difference when you make a statement that starts with "it may feel that women," instead of "all women feel"? It is important to allow the individual to speak for himself/herself and not assume without checking. This process of checking in has to be done in a respectfully way, by first finding common ground with that person and group and by asking permission for clarification. One needs to be a guest and create an equal balance in a dynamic of checking in an assumption. Not everyone is willing and ready to divulge or to be a coach to all at all times!

THINK

Revisit your first impression of the first time you ever met someone different from you.

What did you think of this person and group?

Would you have done anything different if you met this person or group now?

PO Box 2308, Woburn, MA 01888-0508, **p:** 781-729-3736, **www.EmbracingCulture.com**
PO Box 6401, Manchester, NH 03108, **p:** 1-888-678-CCCS

Dominant vs. Non-dominant Culture

"Every individual is born into a world already defined by existing cultural patterns. No person, no society, can ever become completely emancipated from past culture...All that we learn from history is that man does not learn from history, nevertheless, we cannot escape our history, either as individuals or societies." *Social Casework, 39 # 8, October 1958, The Concept of Culture by Dr. Teicher.*

We are all influenced by our own biases and our world view. However it is important for one to be aware of the power that one may carry! There are two types of cultures:

- dominant
- non-dominant

EXERCISE

Describe some of the aspects of a dominant and non-dominant culture in your community:

Dominant	Non Dominant

In some circumstances, a dominant culture may become non-dominant, when the social situation changes. For example, Portuguese immigrants are stereotyped as being hard workers but not very bright. In this case, the Portuguese person is not part of the dominant culture. But what if the circumstances changed?

A **dominant culture** is defined as the ethnic and racial group that runs the economic, political and social aspects of a society. All expectations and policies are based on this group's ways of relating to the world, to their God, to work ethics and values. A dominant culture is then one that, through economic or political power, is able to impose on a subordinate culture or cultures **(non-dominant)** its values, language, ways of being and behaving in the world. In the USA, the dominant culture has European Calvinist ancestry and influences.

However, there is a demographic shift in the United States. According to the USA census, the estimated Hispanic population of the United States as of July 1, 2007 was 45.5 million; the projected Hispanic population of the United States on July 1, 2050 is 132.8 million. As the population is aging in many of the developed countries, immigration will increase so that the new labor force can care for their elderly population and can become productive members of our society and pay the taxes. Clearly, there is a demographic shift in the USA and globally. The financial forces are no longer about the USA, Japan and Canada. There are other countries emerging as big economic forces such as China, India and Brazil. Although interpreters and many of the immigrant groups still function and are perceived as part of the non-dominant group, soon this will no longer be true.

Becoming an interpreter during this shift is not always easy, as those who are monolingual may feel threatened and insecure in their ability to hold on to a job. The world is getting smaller and the skills needed to survive are also changing. We just hope that the largest ethnic and racially immigrant groups in the USA will not repeat history and in fact will embrace the newer groups of immigrants.

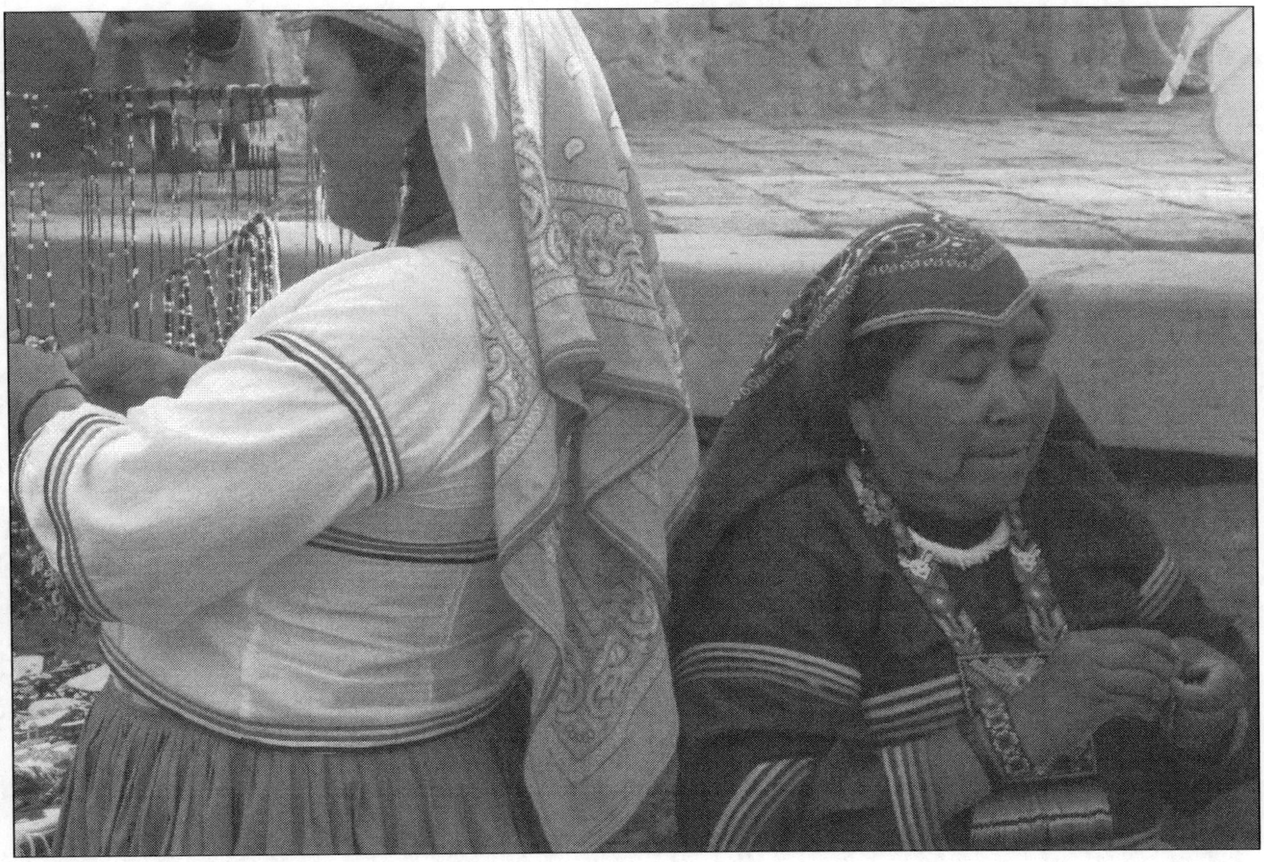

PO Box 2308, Woburn, MA 01888-0508, **p:** 781-729-3736, **www.EmbracingCulture.com**
PO Box 6401, Manchester, NH 03108, **p:** 1-888-678-CCCS

THINK

Let's say an interpreter from Lisbon, Portugal, is speaking with an Azorean client. The Azorean person also speaks Portuguese and is Portuguese, but with an accent that is clearly not from the mainland Portugal. The client may ask himself, "Can I trust this person?"

Transport this story into your own cultural reality, if not an accent it can be something else that separates you from the patient and you sense that the patients is not at ease with this difference. What would you do about it?

Which standards of practice do you think best supports your decision in this matter?

When should you let the provider know of any of your perceived patient reactions?

Historically, the Azoreans have felt misunderstood, abandoned and ridiculed for their distinct Portuguese accents. A Portuguese interpreter from the mainland all of a sudden went from the experience of non-dominant as an immigrant in the USA to dominant just because of her accent.

A series of values and historical experiences went through the Azorean person's mind. Interpreters need to be very aware of their dominant versus non-dominant roles vis a vis the particular ethnic groups that they interpret for. Fluency in a language is only one ingredient in the stew of being an interpreter! It is common for non-trained interpreters to elevate the patient's register when interpreting for the provider and lower it when speaking to the patient, in order to fit in.

What do you think of this behavior?

What do the standards of practice say about register?

Now you are asked by the provider to assist her with poor medication compliance by a patient and the provider makes a loaded statement: "This kind of uneducated people never follow-up with medications."

What should you say or do?

Is compliance with medication an issue with only uneducated people?

PO Box 2308, Woburn, MA 01888-0508, **p:** 781-729-3736, **www.EmbracingCulture.com**
PO Box 6401, Manchester, NH 03108, **p:** 1-888-678-CCCS

You can only change yourself. Try to understand what your triggers are and how you react to them, whether they evoke positive or negative feelings. We must start by understanding that we cannot change others within the course of a short interaction. Interpreters, providers and patients have feelings about each other and about what each other says, but interpreters and providers need to be impartial by not showing feelings that are inappropriate. The experience of having these feelings is a form of transparency but one cannot exhibit them throughout the triadic encounter.

Interpreters are not in the business of changing other people's belief systems but of serving as coaches and consultants to the providers so as to enhance communication and trust between patient and provider. The triadic encounter is about the patient and not about the interpreter's feelings!

Providers, interpreters and patients again may share many common personal values but when faced with each other they are automatically expected to behave a certain way.
From your observations of the triadic encounter, who do you think carries:

The most power? ____________________ The least power? ____________________.

By finding out about your values in the following exercise, we hope you will become increasingly aware of them and ensuring that they do not interfere with the patient–provider relationship.

Checking Your Values and Assumptions!

EXERCISE

Take a few minutes and complete the following evaluation alone. Choose the option that you feel best fits the situation. Join a larger subgroup and share your answers. Count how many A B and C's you have answered.

1. When addressing older persons, you call them by their:
   A. first names B. titles
   C. last names D. both A and B

   Please explain: ____________________

2. As a patient, when you feel that you have waited too long to be seen by a provider, you will probably:
   A. demand to speak to a supervisor.
   B. address the issue with a clinical assistant.
   C. wait patiently.

3. When you are sick, you feel that:
   A. you can control the illness by going to the doctor and taking the right medications.
   B. the healing process is out of your hands.
   C. you deserve to be sick because of something you have done in the past.

4. When you visit your personal healthcare provider, you:
   A. describe your pain on a pain scale of 1-10.
   B. point exactly to where it hurts.
   C. describe your pain by relating a past experience.

5. When you get a cold, you believe that:
   A. by drinking lots of fluids and resting, you will speed up your recovery.
   B. bad weather caused your cold.
   C. you didn't dress appropriately, so now you are sick.

6. You are working with a provider who tells a patient to first take care of herself and then care for her family. You personally feel that:
   A. The patient always needs to care of herself before she can care for others.
   B. There may be times when one needs to first take care of oneself in order to care for a family.
   C. The patient should take care of her children first.

7. How often do you go in for your own check-ups?
   A. Every year. It's very important to go.
   B. Only when you are sick.
   C. Never. You're too busy taking care of your family.

PO Box 2308, Woburn, MA 01888-0508, **p:** 781-729-3736, **www.EmbracingCulture.com**
PO Box 6401, Manchester, NH 03108, **p:** 1-888-678-CCCS

Please choose the option that you feel would produce the best result in the following two case studies.

8. You are interpreting for a patient's medical history, and the provider asks about the patient's sexual activity. The patient seems embarrassed and does not answer the questions. You as an interpreter should:
   A. ask the question again. *(When was the last time you had sexual intercourse?)*
   B. rephrase the question. *(Can you tell me when you last had sexual intercourse?)*
   D. use an explanatory model. *(I may need to ask you some questions that could be difficult for you to answer. These questions will help the provider to best treat you…)*

9. You are interpreting for a patient whose provider asks him to rate his pain on a scale of 1 to 10. The patient begins to tell you that the pain hurts like the time ten years ago when his aunt had a liver transplant. He then proceeds to lift up his shirt to show you the scars from an operation he had twelve years ago. You should:
   A. interrupt the patient and tell him to rate the pain from 1 to 10.
   B. tell the patient to keep his answers short.
   C. appropriately suggest the provider to use the patient's own thinking as a communication tool. *(I understand that your aunt must have been in a lot of pain when she was operated. You too must have felt pain with your operation. Now, let's go over the pain you feel today…)*

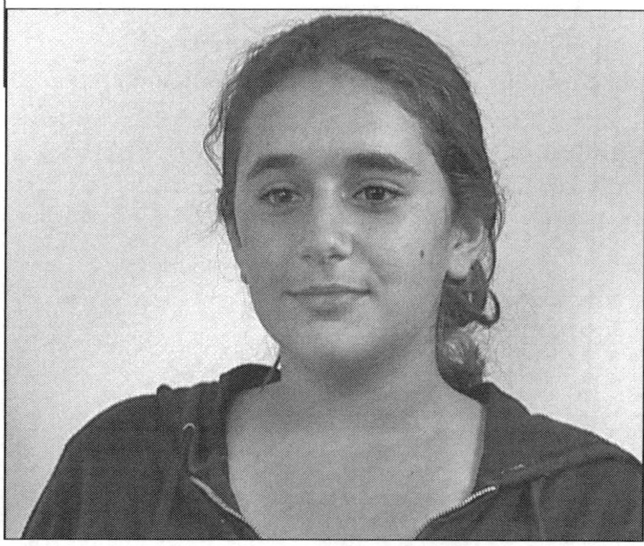

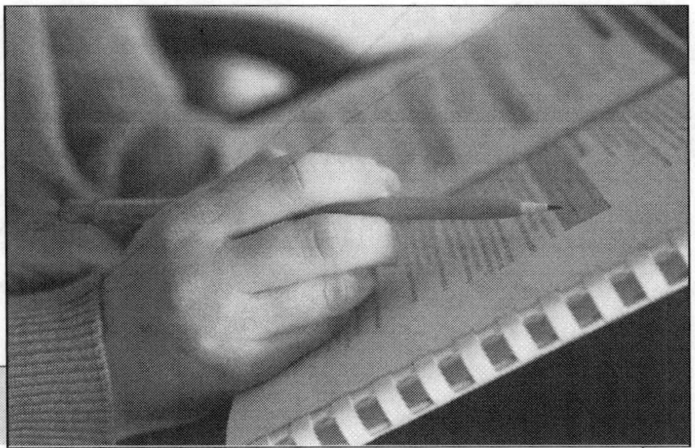

Finding out where you stand:

As you completed the above survey count how many answers you had for:

A ______________________________

B ______________________________

C ______________________________

Share with the class why you may have had a difficult time just checking one answer as requested.

Although this exercise can not determine for sure how you may orient yourself in terms of authority, time and community, it can at least give you a general idea of some of your tendencies with your thinking and behavior patterns towards some of those same variables that shape all of us, human beings.

We hope to provide you with a series of three main cultural competency models that may enable you to better understand your cultural triggers or your "fire ball" so that your professional relationship is centered and proactive instead of reactive and defensive.

PO Box 2308, Woburn, MA 01888-0508, **p:** 781-729-3736, **www.EmbracingCulture.com**
PO Box 6401, Manchester, NH 03108, **p:** 1-888-678-CCCS

The following table is demonstrative of Cultural Competency Model #1 which is called The **Three Cultural Patterns** as inspired by the readings on *Managing Diversity* by Carr-Ruffino, Norma (1996).

Model #1
Three Cultural Patterns

	Dependent	Interdependent	Independent
Authority	(Not Equal, hierarchical) May say yes to everything without meaning " Yes"	Equal	Equal May question diagnosis, wait time for appointment
Time	Circular (past and present external control) Cannot relate to pain scale 1- 10. Need to tell a story	Circular and Linear	Linear (present and future, internal control) Can respond and relate well to pain scale in an abstract way
Community	More important than the individual	Community is important as well as the Individual	Individual first, then others

Dependent Thinker

Dependent thinkers believe in the power hierarchy. They rarely express disagreement with a provider. In fact, a dependent thinker who has not developed a therapeutic relationship with the provider may say very little in a medical session. For the dependent thinker, time is important, but not as important as the ability to help and to connect with people.

When dealing with a dependent cultural pattern, a provider asking a patient to define pain on a scale of 1- 10, may get an incorrect value, simply because the patient wants to please the doctor and could never muster the courage to say that the pain scale does not make sense. Interpreters aware of this dynamic should act as culture brokers.

A dependent thinker also believes that the past is more important that the present, and the present more important than the future. It is common for patients to state that they got sick because of outside forces such as God, the weather or folk beliefs like the evil eye.

To the dependent patient, family and/or community are more important than oneself. Patients may take medications for the sake of their family members, but not because they themselves want to.

Interdependent Thinker

The interdependent pattern is a combination of independent and dependent cultural patterns. The interdependent thinker can relate to authority as both an equal and as part of a hierarchy. This person also sees the value of first taking care of others and then of oneself. This is an ideal pattern for an interpreter. Interpreters need to be flexible by avoiding being judgmental, and must understand and accept that every individual has the following four character values: **honor, respect, generosity and trust.**

Independent Thinker

Independent thinkers relate to authority as if they were at an equal level. Therefore, a patient in this case may feel very comfortable questioning a medical provider and asking him or her for a second opinion. This person also relates to time in a linear way, cause and effect. For example: You are expected to be here at 5:00PM, and you better be here on time. Time is important.

An independent thinker feels that s/he has more internal control over time and life. This is the kind of patient who will do very well with preventative type of recommendations, such as mammograms, pap-smears and other prevention oriented behaviors such as routine exercises that can enhance health (not just for pleasure).

This person is often assertive and believes that first you need to take care of yourself, so that you can take care of others. This would be the person that will not even think twice when told by the flight attendance that in case of an emergency, adults should first place the oxygen mask on themselves and then place it on the child.

Let's revisit your answers from the Exercise on checking your values and assumptions. If you answered more As, you may be the kind of person who is more of a linear thinker, more present and future oriented. If you answered more Bs, you may be more of a circular thinker where communication is story telling based and past and present are your world view. If you have answered more Cs, it may mean that you can compromise between the two worlds and you can most likely manage yourself in either world.

Read the following case individually and jot down which cultural pattern you think the provider and the patient is. Illustrate your answer by using Model # 1. Be ready to share your observations with your classmates.

APPLY CRITICAL THINKING

Case Study # 2

Ms. Nguyen is 56 years old and has a heart problem. She comes to the session late with a hospital interpreter. The doctor comes into the session worried. The visiting nurse has called him to say that Ms. Nguyen is not taking her Lasix everyday, nor is she weighing herself everyday.

Three days ago, the visiting nurse found Ms. Nguyen with extra fluid in her legs and lungs and had gained three pounds. Her oxygen saturation was low normal.

Today, the Doctor has to speak to her about her medication management. The physician asks her about her symptoms and Ms. Nguyen says that she is feeling much better now that she has started her Lasix again. She can breathe easier, her legs are not so heavy with fluid, and she is not waking up in the middle of the night to catch her breath.

The physician is happy with this report. Through the interpreter he relates to the patient that she has congestive heart failure which is from the heart's inability to squeeze the blood effectively through the body, so fluid can build up in the legs and lungs. Lasix is a diuretic, a pill to remove fluid from the body. She needs to take this pill every day to keep extra fluid from "congesting" her lungs and legs. But not only must the patient take the pill every day, she must also watch her weight every day to decide whether or not she should take extra medicine.

Ms. Nguyen nods in agreement.

Ms. Nguyen's lean weight is 125, so if she increases her weight by three pounds in 24 hours she can take two instead of one Lasix that day. If she loses three lbs in 24 hours, she should hold the Lasix and call the physician's nurse practitioner.

Ms. Nguyen nods in agreement.

The physician says this condition is something that she can live with by measuring the weight and adjusting her diuretic, Lasix, accordingly. He says that many patients are now actively involved in managing their illnesses. For instance, many people with diabetes take their blood sugars three and four times a day and give themselves fast acting insulin according to their blood sugar in order to more adequately mimic the normal pancreas' response to controlling blood sugar.

Ms. Nguyen nods in agreement.

Ms. Nguyen's case study shows the complexities of how one cannot read body language and/or words as if there was only one interpretation. An individual, in this case the provider, has to look at the entire picture – patient is gaining fluids, patient is smiling and she seems compliant, what should one do next?

Quickly review the case again and note one piece that may have been missed in the interaction patient-provider.

____

____

____

____

____

____

Perhaps the provider could have showed more empathy about Ms. Nguyen's condition, by echoing her fears, her troubles, her challenges and then explaining how the Lasix may help her. Medically, the provider was okay, but there was no teaching back request from the doctor to the patient so one will never know if the patient's nodding meant what the provider understood to be "Yes."

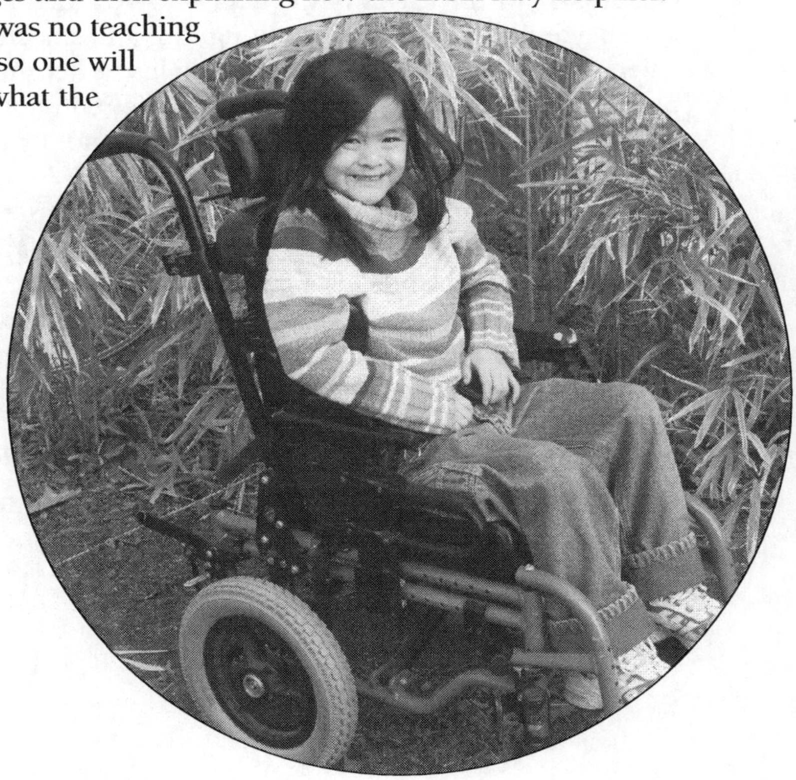

PO Box 2308, Woburn, MA 01888-0508, **p:** 781-729-3736, **www.EmbracingCulture.com**
PO Box 6401, Manchester, NH 03108, **p:** 1-888-678-CCCS

We learned that one approach (ethnocentric) to the understanding of the other's thinking and behaviors and values may not fit all! CCCS has developed two additional Culture Competency Models: **The Four Character Values** (Model #2), and Immigration as a **Grieving Process** (Model #3). These models are not only patient oriented but in fact they are presented to the interpreters because they speak for all of us, human beings, including the providers themselves. We all bring our individual, family and professional beliefs at some level into each interaction.

Imagine a beautiful tree with roots buried in the ground and a few exposed!
These roots are called **honor**. Honor keeps the tree planted firmly in the ground and feeds it. These roots are shaped by values that have passed from generation to generation.
Often, these values are difficult to explain, but most people act and behave according to unspoken expectations. If you hurt a person's honor, you must immediately stop and make amends that are in accordance with your professional guidelines.

Respect is defined be the tree's branches. It involves trying to behave in an acceptable way. Branches can be broken, and the tree will survive, but if one keeps breaking the same branch, the tree may be permanently damaged.

Generosity, or the leaves of the tree, is represented when one shows professional caring and goes beyond expectations in a thoughtful and sincere way. An example of a generous behavior is when a provider asks a patient to bring his or her medications to a medical encounter with the purposes of guiding and coaching the patient on how to best take medications. Often patients know their medication by size and color but not by name.

Trust has to be sincere and reliable and it is the essential ingredient towards a positive rapport between patient, provider, and interpreter. It is in fact a result of the interaction between honor respect and generosity. This is why we ask interpreters to interpret everything that they hear in the session, and not to expose their opinions about a medical provider or medical event. Trust can only occur if someone proves to be reliable, is qualified and does not keep digging into someone's (or is it "someone else's"?) roots.

Model #2
The Four Character Values

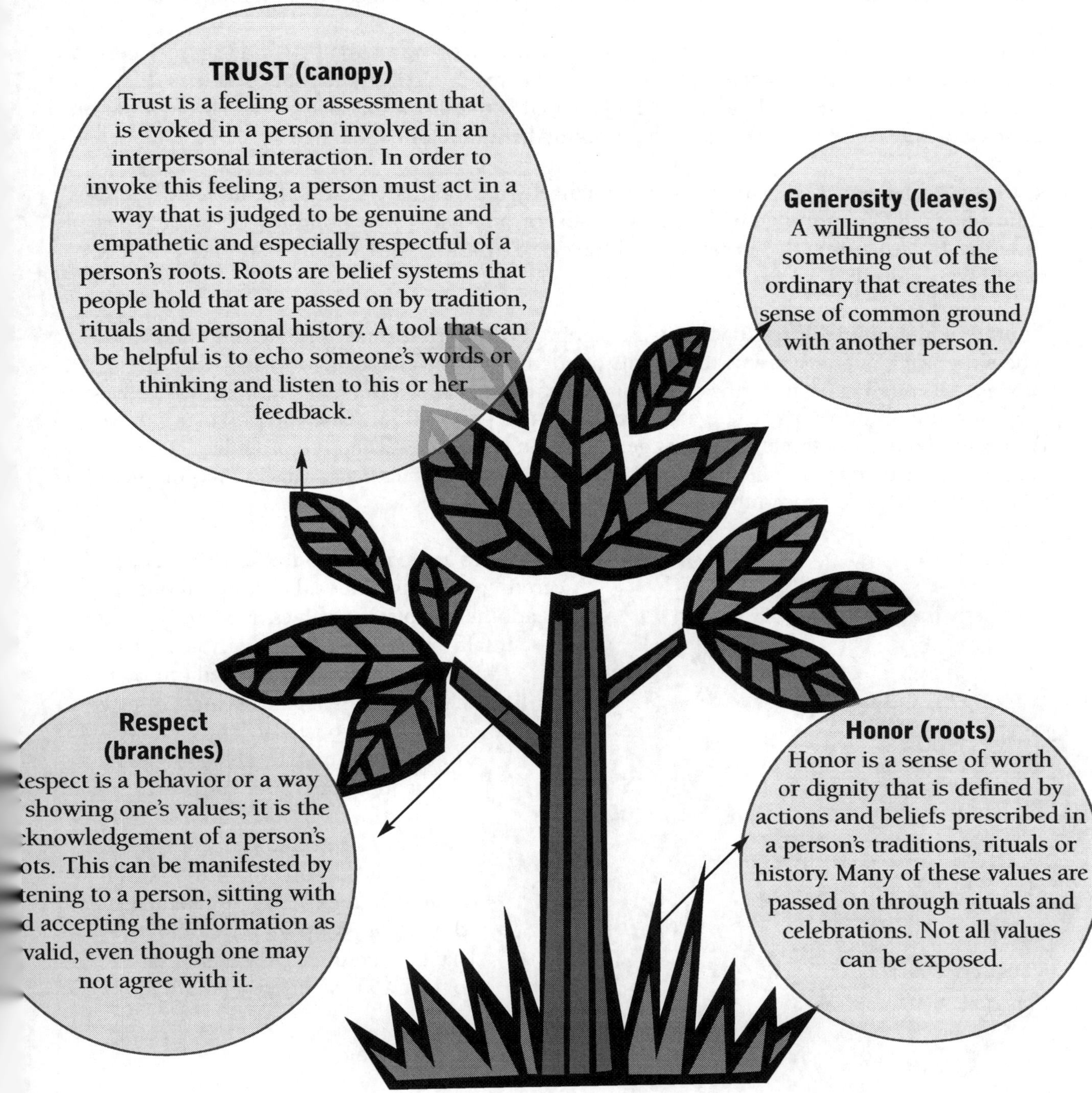

PO Box 2308, Woburn, MA 01888-0508, **p:** 781-729-3736, **www.EmbracingCulture.com**
PO Box 6401, Manchester, NH 03108, **p:** 1-888-678-CCCS

The Four Character Model establishes that all human beings share at least three common values: Honor, Respect and Generosity and that we all may break respect because we are not aware of everyone's values. One cannot break honor too many times and still build trust.

We know that broken branches or respect can grow if fixed by an apology and the tree (person) can also survive broken branches, but when one begins to dig into the roots of others, the relationship most likely will die. If a person is unable to inform that respect was broken but one senses it, a way to fix it is to explain the thinking behind it and apologize.

In the case where a female patient should medically have a pelvic exam but emotionally and/or culturally is not comfortable with having the exam, a provider may build trust if he or she is generous by explaining the importance of the exam by asking the patient if another provider would be best for her.

Another common medical situation is the signing of consent forms for procedures and tests, where the legal language seems to pay lots of attention on all that can go wrong with the surgery. Although consent forms exist in many countries, they often are short and basically state that the patient knows of the surgery, its possible risks and will not find the provider liable in the event of a bad outcome. A form of generosity in this case is when the provider acknowledges how the detailed information may be scary, and explains this is a requirement for all providers who do procedures.

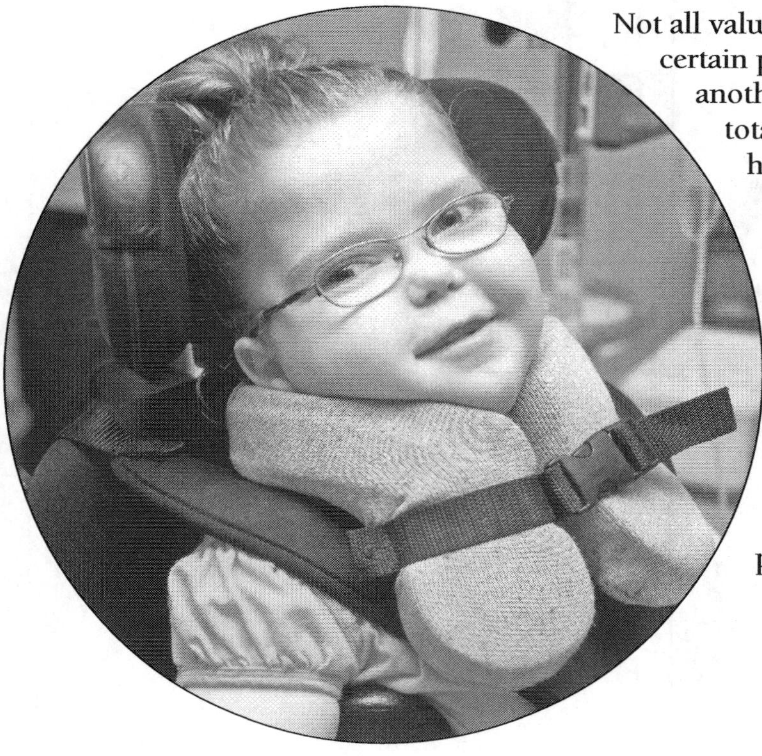

Not all values are exposed to the world and only certain people are allowed to know about another's roots and values. Not everyone is totally aware of his/her own values. As human beings, we developed our own defense mechanism to protect ourselves from being constantly emotionally injured. At some level digging into someone's roots and values may in fact be hurtful to an individual who is not ready to know about his own values and beliefs, especially if the person who is doing the digging belongs to a dominant group. In the case of the triadic encounter, they will be the provider and the interpreter.

EXERCISE

Review the following case studies and share your feedback with your classmates:

Case Study #3

After a staff meeting

After a staff meeting, a group of colleagues gathered to vent about emotions and to discuss a plan for how to handle a conflict between two other staff members.

You know, I think that Mary behaves this way because she's rough around the edges. She's from that "white trash" mentality, when you get triggered you have to fight back. But deep down, she's a really good person.

I know exactly what you are talking about!

Well, just because you're from a troubled background, it doesn't give you the right to mistreat other people.

But was she being rude, or just a bit inappropriate in the way she expressed her feelings?

I have no idea. I don't have to deal with these issues. All my colleagues are Asian. They're so quiet anyway, and they never cause trouble!

You are so lucky! Once I worked with a bunch of black people, and it was a totally different story.

I'm sorry. I'm a little confused. We started with one issue, and now we're on something quite different. Are we doing any good when we associate outcome to race or socioeconomic status?

Oh, come on! You know how these people get when they're angry.

Case Study #4

Feeling something, not sure what?

Mary came home at dinnertime to be with her partner and their new baby. She began to talk to her partner about feeling lonely at work, "Everyone seems to accept the fact that I am gay and a mother to a baby boy, but every night I am the last staff member to leave the office and everyone rushes home without saying goodbye. I feel so lonely and disconnected from everyone else!"

PO Box 2308, Woburn, MA 01888-0508, **p:** 781-729-3736, **www.EmbracingCulture.com**
PO Box 6401, Manchester, NH 03108, **p:** 1-888-678-CCCS

Case Study #5

A social time at work

A group of co-workers gather around at lunchtime on a regular basis. They all use this time to visit with each other and discuss family, life's pressures, and what they did during the weekend.

One of their animated discussions was about a wonderful weekend a coworker had with her husband. She just loves to visit Provincetown each Fourth of July! She described how much she and her husband enjoy the diversity and the feeling that everyone is welcome.

The group agreed and began to comment on the diversity in Provincetown. One of the group members added that she and her husband felt bad for all "those beautiful gay women and men." She said, "They are so gorgeous! Have you seen their bodies? My husband thinks it's such a waste."

The group laughed and some agreed with her, although another colleague commented, "But it's their choice!"

Later, an employee who overheard the group's conversation stopped by the office of a gay colleague to chat. "Did you hear what I just heard about Provincetown and what a waste it is to have all these gorgeous gay men and women?" The gay coworker was silent.

"I don't mean to offend you," the employee said, "I just miss the old times when everyone got along. Things were different when I first came to the company!"

Case Study #6

Two case managers are discussing a follow-up call with a clinician.

Mary: "You know, I was just talking to this Somali clinician about treating Somali patients. But she was so assertive that I was a bit surprised. I asked her how long she has been in the US, and she told me only 5 years. She sounded so American: so direct, and no accent at all.
Bob: "Maybe she studied English or lived abroad before coming to the States, which was not my case at all."
Mary: "Really? You were born in another country? How interesting? Tell me more about it!"
Bob: "It's a long story, but basically I worked very hard to lose my accent. I spent hours watching American movies and just repeating the words in English without even knowing their meaning. My parents speak Cantonese, but they worked very hard in making sure that we were Americans before we were Chinese!"
Mary: "So, you speak Chinese! Next time, I know who to call when I get a Chinese-speaking patient!"
Bob (smiling): "I have to go back to my desk."
Mary: "See you later."

Case Study #7

A Portuguese-speaking Cape Verdean employee

A Portuguese-speaking Cape Verdean employee who works at the front desk keeps the office cheerful with friendly "good mornings" to everyone who comes in the door. She is liked by all the staff members and has become the person that everyone confides in. She is a good listener and is very supportive of her company and colleagues.

One morning, one of her close friends and colleagues came to her and asked, "How can you be so happy all the time? I mean, we're black and the world is so unfair to black people! How can you keep it up? You know that despite the fact that everyone here is pretty nice, it's still hard for them to be around us."

PO Box 2308, Woburn, MA 01888-0508, **p:** 781-729-3736, **www.EmbracingCulture.com**
PO Box 6401, Manchester, NH 03108, **p:** 1-888-678-CCCS

Questions:

1. **How was respect broken in the above cases? Please explain.**

a. Case Study #3

____

____

____

____

b. Case Study #4

____

____

____

____

c. Case Study #5

____

____

____

____

d. Case Study #6

____

____

____

____

e. Case Study #7

____

____

____

Often we act (respect) upon our values by observing others and absorbing information that gets passed to us by generations (roots) and we are not even aware of certain beliefs as if they were implanted and show up automatically when triggered.

Can you think of a value that has registered with you? You just do it?

____

____

____

____

One value or belief that one often hears all the time is the relationship between having a foreign accent and an alright intellectual capacity. A common statement is "She is an immigrant and she is smart. Her English is so good!" or "I am sorry for writing like an immigrant!"

Being an immigrant is like being the in-laws of a country, we are loved and not so loved. If the economy goes wrong it is because of immigration, particularly first generation immigrants. They will always be the outsiders, not recognized for revitalizing economically depressed areas, for their cheap labor, and for doing the jobs rejected by the older immigrant populations.

This dichotomous feeling of love, hate, glorification of immigration and how their ancestors did better than the newly arrived group can be very much felt when patients arrive to the emergency room and are yelled about the fact that they do not speak English as if they at that moment could learn it! One needs to note that, in the future, the stress of being an immigrant will have a double edge to it due to the demographics of our newly arrived immigrants. Most countries which are giving birth at higher rates, and whose populations we need so that they can pay our taxes and take care of our aging population, are not in general from an European ancestry.

Yesterday, I heard in the National Public Radio a writer from Iran describing her and her father's experience of being Jewish in Iran. She stated that 80 years ago, her father was not allowed to go to school if it rained because Jewish people then were considered dirty and the water from the rain could contaminate the non-Jewish population. She, on the other hand, had a very different experience. Not too long ago, African countries colonized by the Portuguese were not allowed to speak their native languages, they often were ridiculed and could go to jail for it. This form of oppression was not perpetuated towards immigrants but towards native populations, but is not very different from the USA, Canada, Mexico and other countries in the Americas.

Provider's unconscious uneasiness and fears of missing the big picture when caring for LEP patients, Limited English Proficient, often becomes a barrier and clinicians may use a different thinking hat than they do when working with English speaking patients.

PO Box 2308, Woburn, MA 01888-0508, **p:** 781-729-3736, **www.EmbracingCulture.com**
PO Box 6401, Manchester, NH 03108, **p:** 1-888-678-CCCS

Review the case below and share your observations with your classmates:

Case Study #8

At a social gathering with many providers, a social worker approached an interpreter manager to share a great experience he had working with a Haitian-Creole speaking interpreter who works for a local managed care company:

"I just had a great session with an Interpreter. She was so caring, so connected. She knew exactly what to do...and she talked this Haitian family into joining the Hospice Program..."
"I first tried to explain to this family about our services and she knew right away that the family would not 'get it' so they went into another room and the interpreter talked and talked to them...I could have never done it by myself... she was so good and the family (who really needed the services) decided to join our program!"
"Hmm... and if the results were not as you expected and the interpreter had behaved the same...would you have thought so highly of the interpreter?"
"I get your point, but there is such a cultural and racial disconnect between me and the family...and poor interpreter... her boss is very cold and not nice to her...I know exactly how she feels, I do not like him myself!"
"Is this the first time that you perceived this disconnect?"
"No..."
"So, what did you do to bridge it the other times?"
"Different things.... but at least I could speak their language"
"Interesting... what about if you try those things in this case?"

Your observations:

Who knows why the interpreter decided that she could act as the provider by being alone with the patient? If an interpreter is not aware of how one feels about his or her own immigration stages, it will be very easy to fall into the trap of the provider role when requested to assist with culture misunderstanding. This is a very thin and legally dangerous line, where the interpreter may never be sued for acting as a provider, but one day when the outcome is not as expected, the interpreter may in fact get into a lot of legal trouble.

Model 3, Immigration Grieving Stages, will assist interpreters to understand how to assess dynamics between different generations of immigrants with the intent to empower interpreters to separate the interaction and the need to interpret accurately. When one feels under attack overtly or covertly, one may not be able to listen to the message completely and reacts impulsively.

The models presented in this manual are to serve as assessing tools so that you can quickly take a snapshot of the situation, take a deep breath, think of what is best for the patient, understand what the policies and laws that govern your interactions are, and later on revisit the situation so as to take a more active role in promoting change. One needs to always follow the protocol of their contracting institution.

Model #3
Immigration Grieving Stages

The immigration stages are 1-Honeymoon, 2-Anger and Loss, 3-Negotiation and Acceptance. The development of immigration as a grieving process was inspired by the reading of the book *Death and Dying* (1969) by Dr. Kübler-Ross. She developed 5 different grieving stages for patients who are dying.

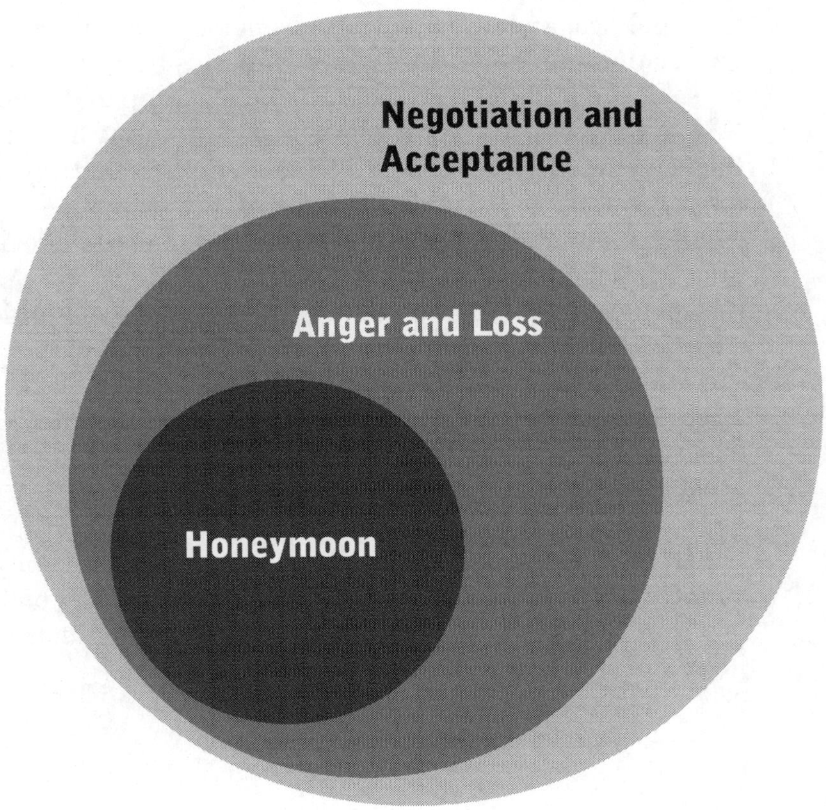

PO Box 2308, Woburn, MA 01888-0508, **p:** 781-729-3736, **www.EmbracingCulture.com**
PO Box 6401, Manchester, NH 03108, **p:** 1-888-678-CCCS

From 1985-1996, the author of this manual had a clinical practice where she treated many patients with psychosomatic and postraumatic and or depression symptoms. Patients seemed relieved from many of these symptoms when they had a chance to share their grief about leaving their homeland and were able to aknowledge the fact that immigration had changed them forever. Second generation patients seemed uneasy with the fact that they were perceived differently from the dominant group and third generation seemed totally in love with their grandparents or great grandparents' homeland.

Although this process of back and forth, falling in and out of love with the new and old country is called **Immigration Grieving Stages**, refugees also experience similar grieving. A refugee is an individual who is forced to seek safety outside his or her own country due to political, sexual orientation and or religious reasons. This person's life can not be protected by the country that he or she is escaping. In the USA refugees who do not establish themselves as permanent residents, may risk being sent back to their native country when the USA government is at peace with their country of origin.

While documented immigrants are allowed to stay in the country and can apply for citizenship after a certain amount of time living in the USA, refugees and political asylum immigrants may never be able to visit their native country. One main difference between the two is the location where the petition to stay was made. Refugee's petition to enter the country is done outside the USA and Political Asylum is done at the port of entry. If one is undocumented and living in the USA, political asylum request can be made, but immigration officers may initiate the deportation process as the asylum request is being processed. Refugees in general in the search for safety go from refugee camp to refugee camp in different countries before they get to the USA, often losing the sense of original community and culture, impacting native language fluency if one was not exposed to an academic education.

The separation from the country of birth often feels like death and a rebirth. There are three grieving stages for immigrants in general: Honeymoon, Anger-Loss and Negotiation-Acceptance. These stages can be grieved in a different order; they are not necessarily experienced as a continuum from stage one to three, they can be skipped or one may stay in one stage and never go back and forth between them. In fact, an individual may experience all the stages in one day. Refugees, documented or undocumented immigrants, may also be prone to experiencing one stage more than another if there is an organized supporting system as one arrives in the new country.

On average it takes five to ten years from the time a family or an individual considers leaving a country to be able to accomplish that. This is a costly process, and often it takes many years to pay back the expenses in addition to the on-going financial contribution one makes to their loved ones who stayed back.

Honeymoon	Anger and Loss	Negotiation and Acceptance
Falling in love with new country Falling out of love with old country	Overidealization of old country Distrust towards new country Distrust towards healthcare system and providers	Finding a balance holding on to some old behaviors and integrating new behaviors, beliefs, expectations Acknowledgement of ambivalent feelings towards immigration
Falls in love with new language	Gets irritated with false fluencies	Uses false fluencies

In the USA if one is not a Native American or a slave forced into this country one is an immigrant. Being an immigrant creates a dynamic full of mixed feelings such as hope, anger, reasoning, hardship and acceptance of a new life. Immigration happens mainly because of economic, geographic and political reasons. Some people come into this country to study or because they married someone from here, but these are not the great majority of our immigrants. There is an undertone feeling of not being good enough, of being pushed out, pushed away or rejected. This feeling may never be overtly expressed, so one may only glorify moments of success and erase out painful experiences.

It is not uncommon for one to feel this anger from immigrants who have been here longer. I believe that providers, as well as interpreter and patients, get re-traumatized from their past experiences when they themselves or their loved ones were treated differently. This could be related to an accent, inability to speak English well, different eating diets and dressing styles or other issues. The exposure to a first generation immigrant could awake past and forgotten pain leading providers at times to extremes of being too nice and not listening to a dysfunctional piece or too upset and offensive, attacking one's fabric.

The understanding of the possibility that providers may be too much in love with their country or too angry with immigrants was liberating to me as an immigrant. By finding common ground during adversity I now can connect with an individual as a human being and I can separate self from experience, from trauma, enabling me to be a better listener and a better interpreter. If the environment becomes intolerable and there is evidence of overt discrimination, an interpreter may have to resort to the policies and guidelines that legally support his/her actions.

PO Box 2308, Woburn, MA 01888-0508, **p:** 781-729-3736, **www.EmbracingCulture.com**
PO Box 6401, Manchester, NH 03108, **p:** 1-888-678-CCCS

Watch the video *Patient Diversity: Beyond The Vital Signs* by CRM Learning at www.crmlearning.com. Please identify and illustrate the behaviors that best match the concepts and words that you learned up to now:

Honor/Values	
Respect / Broken Respect	
Generosity	
Trust	
Stereotype	
Independent Thinker	
Dependent Thinker	
Other	

In Summary

An individual may not be aware of his/her ethnocentrism. These beliefs may be buried so deep in the roots of oneself that they get blocked or acted upon when triggered by an interaction or an observation. Culture is defined by Written Rules- laws, codes, standards, and Unwritten Rules- mores and the World View-a set of assumptions about a person's environment. The initial journey towards culture competency is to know one self, to be able to navigate through different cultures not always with the most comfort but with an open ear and heart. Individuals and organizations may go through different stages of a cultural continuum before reaching a level of cultural competency. This is an on-going process.

1-Denial **2- Minimization** **3-Acceptance** **4- Integration**

When challenged by new situations, we, human beings, may deny, minimize and accept our behaviors. The most difficult jump is the one from acceptance to integration. Part of integration involves understanding new information and making this information part of one's individual and organizational fabric. This is the most challenging step, because it means change and we do not always do well with change. Again, one has to let go of things and behaviors that made us feel comfortable, and feel at home.

I recall becoming very sad during my first years in the USA when I perceived people as distant and cold. I was coming from a culture of two kisses when one greeted one another and at times a hug. I walked holding hands or crossing arms with my mother until I was a young adult. It took me some grieving to adjust and understand that there were other ways of being caring and connected. Nowadays, I am able to wait for the person who will lead me to a comfortable compromise when greeting each other. In fact this loss opened me up to new opportunities and made me a better person because I got to know many different people who did not kiss or shook hands, but still were kind and warm.

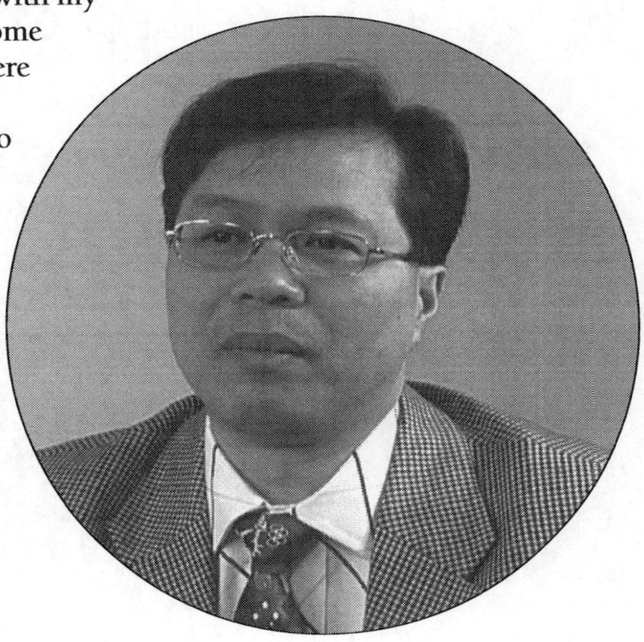

PO Box 2308, Woburn, MA 01888-0508, **p:** 781-729-3736, **www.EmbracingCulture.com**
PO Box 6401, Manchester, NH 03108, **p:** 1-888-678-CCCS

The process of integration is a stage of incorporating changes, reassessing thinking actions and doing something about it. This is the last stage of a continuum that usually starts with "denial" to "minimization" to "acceptance." For example, in my situation while interpreting that a different greeting in the USA was "cold," I used my world view (ethnocentric) by denying the possibility that there are other ways of greeting and connecting by continuing to kiss twice and shake hands. My experience, my comfort, was the base with which I judged others. Soon after being in the USA and having developed strong connections with people who lived here for many generations, I would say they are nice but there is something missing about their ability to connect and instead of greeting with two kisses I began to go for the hand shake. Then as I became more exposed to other outside cultures I realized that the handshake could also be offensive and could possibly cause more damage and tension than what was intended. Therefore I began to accept that there were other ways of greeting. This was a period of recognition of a behavior, but still I was not able to incorporate other ways of greeting besides dropping the two kisses. It took me a few "false moves" and difficult situations for me to begin to assess that my intentions were not having the results I wished so I needed to look for new ways of greeting. Now, I observe, wait for the person to lead me and I feel comfortable with using a smile, a nod with my head, bowing to a verbal acknowledgement of the presence of someone, shaking hands or two kisses when appropriate.

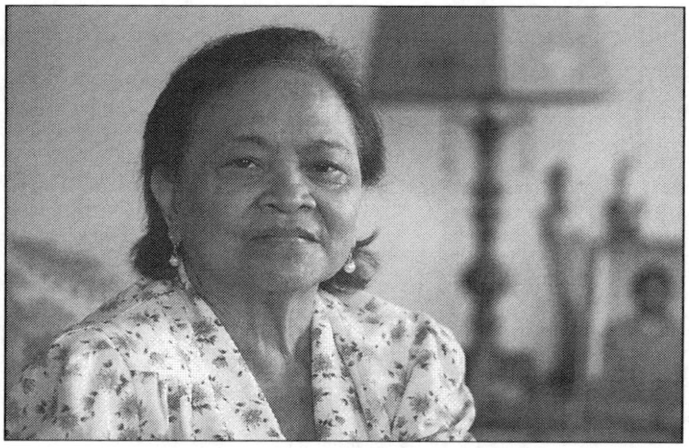

The following case study demonstrates parts of the cultural competency continuum. Read it and as a large group identify the four stages.

Case Study #9:

A hospital that was committed to developing quality interpreter services for Spanish and Portuguese speakers, all of a sudden started to also serve young women from Cambodia who were mainly using the delivery room. It had taken so many years for the hospital to get an interpreter program and according to the patient population statistics, the hospital felt very pleased with their interpreter services.

When the young Asian women started to utilize the hospital, the medical staff used their husbands to serve as interpreters in the delivery room. The hospital had very little knowledge of the Cambodian culture specifically in regards to the delivery and post-delivery process. They felt that working with the immigrant population they were presently serving was enough to help them with how to best care for the newer wave of patients.

One day, a young patient had a non-eventful delivery, went to her room and refused to drink any fluids or eat. She also refused to take a bath and wash her hair. The nurse, very kind, broke the ice in small chips and began to place them in the patient's mouth.
To her surprise this quiet, young and tired new mother, frantically and abruptly pushed the nurse's hand away.

The nurse went back to the nurse's station and complained to her colleagues that at least the Portuguese and Spanish speakers were nicer patients. When she returned to check the patient's vital signs, she had spiked a fever and she was beginning to look very lethargic. The husband was called in and meanwhile another nurse offered the patient some hot tea, which she swallowed with great thirst! She was given an IV and soon taken off it, when she volunteered to continuing drinking her tea.

PO Box 2308, Woburn, MA 01888-0508, **p:** 781-729-3736, **www.EmbracingCulture.com**
PO Box 6401, Manchester, NH 03108, **p:** 1-888-678-CCCS

In the USA, it is common to serve cold drinks and give a new mom ice chips for comfort and to make sure one gets the right amount of fluids. But in the Cambodian culture cold drinks seem to create an imbalance, when one is hot one should always drink warm drinks. The recovering mother must be protected from the yin (cold forces) for as long as thirty days postpartum. This is not only with food intake but also relates to the temperature of the rooms. Some believe that cold forces can harm a mother who is recovering from her labor. From then on, the delivery room nurses began to ask all patients if they wanted a hot or cold drink. Little did they know that in fact the Portuguese and Spanish speaking patients also preferred hot drinks over the cold ones!

In the past ten years, the Federal Government has created many guidelines and enforcement policies. The CLAS, Culture Language Assessment Standards created 14 standards that are divided into groups of three different topics: Culturally Competent Care (Standards 1-3), Language Access Services (Standards 4-7), and Organizational Supports for Cultural Competence (Standards 8-14). CLAS **mandates** are current Federal requirements for all recipients of Federal funds (Standards 4, 5, 6, and 7). See summary of standards in the attachment section of this lesson but also download complete version from http://www.omhrc.gov.

The following outline is A WALK THROUGH SEVERAL CHECKING POINTS FOR YOU as you begin this on-going journey towards culture competency. We have divided it into four phases, 1- You, 2- Your Organization, 3- The Cross Cultural Individual, 4-Integration:

PHASE I: You

Understanding your Cultural Patterns

- Interdependent
- Dependent
- Independent

Understanding in which Era You Were Born

- Who was excluded?
- Who were you afraid of?
- Who did you want to be like?

Understanding Your Immigration Stages

- Honeymoon
- Anger and Loss
- Negotiation and Acceptance

Different people evoke different feelings and stages in you. Take note of these feelings and use them as valuable tools as you team up with others different from you.

PHASE II: Your Organization

Understanding your Organization's Leadership Styles:

- Adaptive
- Authoritarian
- Defensive

Understanding your Organization's Intercultural Sensitivity Continuum:

- Denial
- Minimization
- Acceptance
- Integration

Understanding your Organization's Mission and Vision:

- Inclusive
- Exclusive
- Reactive/Proactive

Understanding How you can Contribute to your Organization:

- Knowledge Sharing
- Asks Questions, Approach Different Levels
- Formulate New Knowledge

PO Box 2308, Woburn, MA 01888-0508, **p:** 781-729-3736, **www.EmbracingCulture.com**
PO Box 6401, Manchester, NH 03108, **p:** 1-888-678-CCCS

There are simple gestures you may have towards work rituals, ceremonies, celebrations, by promoting inclusiveness and by acknowledging differences as gifts to you and the organization.

PHASE III: The Cross Cultural Individual

Understanding Individual Cultural Patterns:
- Interdependent
- Dependent
- Independent

Understanding Move to the United States:
- Immigration status
- Refugee
- Political Asylum

Understanding the Politics Between Native Country and USA:
- War
- Financial
- Jobs

Understanding Ethnic Group Values:
- Honor
- Respect
- Trust

Understanding Immigration Stages:
- Honeymoon
- Anger/Loss
- Negotiation and Acceptance

PHASE IV: Integration

It is all the information you gathered from the prior phases, you become culturally competent when you can experience discomfort and are able to travel through all these models and arrive to a stage where your knowledge has changed as a result of an adaptation and negotiation between you, your organization and your cross cultural client. This will be a continuous process of promoting new knowledge.

As we begin to understand ourselves, the culture of the organization we work for, the standards and the guidelines that shape us, and the medical profession, one needs to develop a better understanding of the role of the **culture broker**. This is a great opportunity to once again review the CHIA, IMIA and the NCHIC Health Care Interpreter Standards.

Lesson Five: Homework
Cross Cultural Competency for Healthcare Interpreters

Read the following articles:

Cross-Cultural Primary Care: A Patient-Based Approach by Dr. Emilio Carrillo et al.

Culture, Illness, and Care. Clinical Lessons from Anthropologic and Cross-Cultural Research by Dr. Arthur Kleinman et al.

1. Understanding the medical culture as not one! From the articles you have just read, explain the different concept of Illness and Disease:

ILLNESS	DISEASE

2. Write a paragraph identifying the Three Thinking Patterns and give an example of how a patient, interpreter, or provider might display characteristics of a particular pattern.

THE ART OF MEDICAL INTERPRETATION®

Homework

PO Box 2308, Woburn, MA 01888-0508, **p:** 781-729-3736, **www.EmbracingCulture.com**
PO Box 6401, Manchester, NH 03108, **p:** 1-888-678-CCCS

3. Write a paragraph differentiating stereotypes from generalizations.

4. Translate the following tables from English to Target Language:

BODY PARTS	MEANING	TARGET LANGUAGE
Brain	Part of the central nervous system contained within the cranium, comprising the prosencephalon, mesencephalon, and rhombencephalon.	
Endocrine glands	Organs that secrete hormones which are released into the circulatory system and which influence the metabolism. The glands include the pituitary, thyroid, parathyroid, adrenal, the pineal body, and the gonads.	
Eye	The organ of vision, composed of three coats: the sclera and cornea, the choroid, and the retina.	
Gallbladder	The pear-shaped reservoir for the bile on the posteroinferior surface of the liver, between the right and the quadrate lobe. Primary functions are to store, concentrate and secrete bile into the small intestine by a series of ducts. The gallbladder and these ducts are called the biliary system.	
Head	The upper, anterior, or proximal extremity of a structure or body. It contains the brain and the organs of special sense.	

continued

BODY PARTS	MEANING	TARGET LANGUAGE
Heart	The viscus of cardiac muscle that maintains the blood circulation. It is divided into four cavities: two atria and two ventricles.	
Intestines	The portion of the alimentary canal extending from the pyloric opening of the stomach to the anus. The small intestine consists of three sections: the duodenum, the jejunum, and the ileum. The large intestine consists of ascending, transverse, and descending sections.	
Kidneys	Either of the two organs in the lumbar region that filter the blood, excreting the end-products of body metabolism in the form of urine, and regulating the concentrations of hydrogen, sodium, potassium, phosphate, and other ions in the extracellular fluid.	
Liver	A large gland of a dark-red color situated in the upper part of the abdomen on the right side. Its functions include the storage and filtration of blood, the secretion of bile, the excretion of bilirubin and other substances, and numerous metabolic functions.	
Lung	The organs of respiration; they occupy the lateral cavities of the chest, separated from each other by the heart and mediastinal structures.	
Neck	A constricted portion, such as the part connecting the head and trunk of the body, or the constricted part of an organ.	
Pancreas	A large, elongated, racemose gland situated transversely behind the stomach, between the spleen and the duodenum.	
Skin	The outer covering of the body, consisting of the corium, or dermis, and the epidermis and resting upon the subcutaneous tissues.	

continued

PO Box 2308, Woburn, MA 01888-0508, **p:** 781-729-3736, **www.EmbracingCulture.com**
PO Box 6401, Manchester, NH 03108, **p:** 1-888-678-CCCS

BODY PARTS	MEANING	TARGET LANGUAGE
Spine	A strong but flexible support that holds the head and body upright and allows the upper body to bend and twist. It is made up of three main types of vertebrae: cervical, thoracic and lumbar.	
Spleen	Large, gland-like organ situated in the upper part of the abdominal cavity on the left side and lateral to the cardiac end of the stomach. Disintegrates red blood cells, sets hemoglobin free, and serves as a reservoir of blood.	
Stomach	The musculomembranous expansion of the alimentary canal between the esophagus and the duodenum. It consists of two chambers: an upper portion (cardiac end) called fondus, and a pyloric end called antum.	

Lesson Five: Role-Plays
Cross Cultural Competency for Healthcare Interpreters

Work individually at first:

- Read the entire role-play
- Get a general sense of its meaning
- Circle the most challenging medical terms
- Apply the Samurai! technique to those terms
- Read the role-play again for a deeper understanding
- Find an accurate equivalent in the target language

Work in a language-specific group of friends, fellow students or colleagues:

- Share your doubts
- Ask for other ways of expressing the same meaning
- Develop a glossary
- Check the dictionary
- Practice the role-plays remember to do CIFE for all your role-plays
- Have your colleagues observe you and provide feedback on your accuracy and register.
- These colleagues can keep track of any omissions, additions, mistakes or distortions in your interpreting and point these out to you in a follow-up discussion.

Student Interpreter Evaluation

Student Name ______ Date ______

Language ______

Mode of Interpreting (check one): ☐ Consecutive ☐ Simultaneous

Role-Play/System ______

Areas Observed ______

Accuracy

Register ______

Omissions ______

Additions ______

Distortions ______

Pronunciation ______

Speaker's emotions conveyed? ______

Explain ______

Technique

General flow ______

Flow when requesting clarification ______

Speed ______

Eye Contact ______

Distracting Habits ______

Ethical Issues

Answered questions for patient? ______

Advised patient? ______

Vocabulary Expansion Recommendations

______

______

Other Recommendations

______

______

Language Coach Signature ______ Date ______

PO Box 2308, Woburn, MA 01888-0508, p: 781-729-3736, www.EmbracingCulture.com
PO Box 6401, Manchester, NH 03108, p: 1-888-678-CCCS

Role-Play 21: Namibi suffers from sickle-cell anemia

Tembe is an African refugee. Her firstborn, Namibi, is six months old. The baby has been crying uncontrollably and does not nurse regularly. Her little hands and feet are swollen, and the whites of her eyes appear yellow. Tembe takes the baby to a local hospital. Blood tests indicate that Namibi suffers from sickle-cell anemia.

	Pronunciation	Additions	Omissions	Mistakes
MD: Tembe, I want to thank you for bringing Namibi to the hospital. As you know, the blood tests indicate that she has a genetic disease called sickle-cell anemia.				
Tembe: Thank you, doctor. But what do you mean by "genetic disease?" Is this disease something I passed on to my baby?				
MD: Well, sickle-cell anemia occurs mostly in people of African descent, and is directly related to a person's blood genotype. Most people have a blood genotype called AA. But some people, like you and your husband, inherit an A gene from one parent and an S gene from the other parent and have an AS blood genotype. You yourselves will not develop sickle-cell anemia, but there is a 1 in 4 chance that any child born to you will inherit the defective S gene from both of you. Namibi's test results indicate that she has SS blood.				
Tembe: Namibi is our firstborn. Family is very important in our African culture, and we always planned to have other children.				
MD: Considering your 25% percent chance of giving birth to a sickler child, you and your husband will want to weigh your family planning decisions carefully.				
Tembe: Is there any hope for Namibi? What can we do to make her better?				
MD: There is no known cure for sickle-cell anemia. But there are some simple things that you can do to minimize the frequency of Namibi's crises.				
Tembe: But what do you mean by crises? What will sickle cell do to her?				
MD: Red cells in the blood travel to the lungs to pick up a supply of oxygen. They then travel through arteries to all parts of the body. Eventually, the arteries narrow into tiny blood vessels so small that the red cells must travel in single file.				

continued

Role-Play 21 *(continued)*

	Pronunciation	Additions	Omissions	Mistakes
Your blood cells, like your husband's and mine, are round and move easily through small blood vessels. But in Namibi, the blood cells look more like sickles. Sickled blood cells can get stuck in the small veins of the body and impede the flow of other red blood cells. When the flow of blood to a part of the body diminishes, oxygen is cut off and the patient begins to feel pain.				
Tembe: Is there any way to stop the pain?				
MD: Some sickle-cell patients rarely feel pain. Others have crises on a monthly basis. In any case, the pain will generally diminish after a few hours or days. We usually admit crisis patients to the hospital and treat them with strong pain-killing drugs, oral and intravenous fluids, oxygen, and antibiotics.				
Tembe: Could a crisis seriously harm my baby?				
MD: A severe crisis can sometimes disrupt the normal function of the brain, lungs, heart, kidneys, or spleen.				
Tembe: Will my baby die?				
MD: Severe crises are sometimes fatal. Children with sickle-cell are at high risk for seizures and strokes, and are especially prone to infectious diseases. Of course, not everyone with sickle-cell anemia develops these symptoms.				
Tembe: You mentioned antibiotics. Will Namibi get lots of infections?				
MD: Every case is different, but infections among sickle-cell patients are common. We will start Namibi on oral penicillin twice a day. She may need to continue this treatment for a long time.				
Tembe: Is there anything I can do at home to keep her healthy?				
MD: Besides following the penicillin treatment, keep her well fed, clean and rested. Be sure to bring her to all of her scheduled check-ups. And don't hesitate to call our emergency hotline if you notice a sudden change in her condition.				
Tembe: I know that in my country, doctors give blood transfusions to sickle cell patients. Does this happen here in America too?				

continued

PO Box 2308, Woburn, MA 01888-0508, **p:** 781-729-3736, **www.EmbracingCulture.com**
PO Box 6401, Manchester, NH 03108, **p:** 1-888-678-CCCS

Role-Play 21 *(continued)*

	Pronunciation	Additions	Omissions	Mistakes
MD: Yes, blood transfusions are often used to correct anemia by increasing the number of normal red blood cells in circulation. Transfusions are also used to treat spleen enlargement in children if the condition is potentially life threatening. In addition, regular transfusion therapy can prevent recurring strokes in children at high risk of crippling nervous system complications. With time, we may have to consider transfusion therapy for Namibi.				
Tembe: Doctor, are there any alternatives to transfusion?				
MD: Why do you ask?				
Tembe: My husband and I value life, and we seek good medical care. That is why I brought Namibi to the hospital right away. But we are determined not to violate God's commandments regarding the use of blood, which have been consistent for thousands of years. The Bible clearly states that those who respect life as a gift from the Creator do not try to sustain it by taking in blood. What is more, blood transfusions increase the risk of AIDS, hepatitis and other illnesses. That is why I asked about other treatments. We are willing to give Namibi the finest in alternative care, but we will not accept blood transfusions.				
MD: Well, Tembe, I don't know how the legal and medical systems interact in your country, but here in the United States, when it comes to treating children, a hospital can get a court order overriding a parent's wishes and can secure the right as an institution to administer treatment to a minor. We will do everything in our power to treat Namibi without blood, but if in the future we feel that transfusion is necessary, the courts will have to decide what is best for her.				
Tembe: Well, doctor, I thank you for your help. Your explanations of the disease were very clear. We will follow your instructions for Namibi's immediate care. But my husband and I will also take her to see a specialist familiar with non-blood treatment alternatives.				
Break It Down	☐	☐	☐	☐

☐ **CIFE with patient** ☐ **CIFE with provider** ☐ **FLOW** ☐ **REGISTER**

continued

Role-Play 21: Glossary

1. Pathology (diseases, conditions)

2. Laboratory Tests and Diagnostic Procedures

3. Treatment Procedures

4. Idiomatic Expressions (if any)

5. Other (vocabulary in this particular role-play that you feel is important/relevant or that you anticipate problems with)

PO Box 2308, Woburn, MA 01888-0508, **p:** 781-729-3736, **www.EmbracingCulture.com**
PO Box 6401, Manchester, NH 03108, **p:** 1-888-678-CCCS

Role-Play 22: Augustin's Lung Carcinoma

Augustin is a 56-year-old French-speaking African male. He complains of breathlessness, hoarseness, coughing and hemoptysis (coughing up blood, from Greek, "Haima," meaning "blood" and "ptysis," meaning "spitting"). He has also lost a significant amount of weight over the last three months.

Augustin is a refugee in New England. He lives with a few other family members, but he is now unable to care for himself or to help his family. He is afraid that the doctor will give him bad news concerning his health and is planning to go back to his country so as not be a burden to his family and friends in the United States. But if he goes back, he risks being killed by his country's repressive government.

His family speaks some English and they are reluctant to have a non-native French interpreter. They would rather have a native of their country interpret in the session, but on this given day, that is not an option. The family expects that a native interpreter will filter the cultural appropriateness of the conversation between Augustin and his doctor when they meet alone.

An interpreter arrives just as a doctor who speaks some French is trying his best to communicate with Augustin.

		Pronunciation	Additions	Omissions	Mistakes
MD:	Bonjour Augustin, it's good to see you again. What brings you to the clinic today?				
A:	(Wheezing) I'm having a hard time breathing, doctor. I can't breath, I'm hoarse, I can't eat…I don't know what to do. I just want to go back home.				
MD:	Hmm, you say you can't eat…why is that?				
A:	I have no appetite, and I feel so weak.				
MD:	How long has this been going on?				
A:	For a few months now…I was going to come sooner, but I thought this would pass. I need to work so that my family can survive.				
MD:	I understand you are a good family man, but first you need to take care of yourself. Are there any other symptoms that you've experienced in conjunction with the hoarseness, like a loss of appetite or labored breathing?				
A:	I've had a persistent cough for a few weeks now. And I've been coughing up blood. But I know I am in God's hands.				
MD:	Are you still smoking, Augustin?				
A:	Yes, but I can quit at any time. You know, when your time comes, there is nothing you can do about it. Please do not tell my family if I have something bad, I just want to go back home. At this point in my life it does not matter if I get killed or not!				
MD:	I see that you are quite pale and that you're wheezing even when at rest. I also understand that you have been giving a lot of thought to your prognosis. Let's examine you and find out what your problem really is.				

continued

Role-Play 22 *(continued)*

	Pronunciation	Additions	Omissions	Mistakes
(MD examines Augustin)				
MD: You appear to have clubbing in your fingers. See how the tips are enlarged and the nails curved back?				
A: I noticed that, but thought it was because of the type of work I do. I work in a factory cleaning steel nails; you know how it is with all the acids we use.				
MD: Actually, clubbing is caused by low blood oxygen levels and can be a symptom of a variety of serious conditions. Another thing I noticed is that your chest is barrel-shaped and your movements seem diminished on the right side. When I listen to your chest, I don't hear any breath sounds over the right middle lobe. I'd like to run some tests to further investigate the matter.				
(Later, after examination)				
MD: Augustin, the tests reveal the presence of malignant squamous cells. Would you like to have your family present for the rest of this interview?				
A: No, let's leave them out of this. What are squamous cells?				
MD: Squamous cells are flat cells, usually found in epithelial tissue, where the body meets the outside environment. These cells can turn cancerous. I'd like you to go for a bronchoscopy so we can determine the nature of these cells.				
(Later, after bronchoscopy)				
MD: Augustin, the bronchoscopy revealed a grayish-tan tumor spreading out from your right middle bronchus and obstructing it. We know from the biopsy that the tumor is cancerous. Thankfully, surgical resection can be potentially curative in patients like you. Let's talk about your treatment options.				

The interpreter begins to feel very uncomfortable with the doctor's directness and asks the doctor to step outside. But Augustin understands some English and says, "I already knew I had cancer. I am ready for God to take me." Augustin leaves the room crying and the family looks at the interpreter with disdain. In their eyes, the interpreter is the cause of the bad news. The family insists they never want this interpreter (or this doctor) again!

Break It Down	☐	☐	☐	☐

☐ **CIFE with patient** ☐ **CIFE with provider** ☐ **FLOW** ☐ **REGISTER**

continued

PO Box 2308, Woburn, MA 01888-0508, **p:** 781-729-3736, **www.EmbracingCulture.com**
PO Box 6401, Manchester, NH 03108, **p:** 1-888-678-CCCS

Role-Play 22: Glossary

1. Pathology (diseases, conditions)

2. Laboratory Tests and Diagnostic Procedures

3. Treatment Procedures

4. Idiomatic Expressions (if any)

5. Other (vocabulary in this particular role-play that you feel is important/relevant or that you anticipate problems with)

Lesson Five: Additional Resources
Cross Cultural Competency for Healthcare Interpreters

Culture Broker

Conflicts can be used as an opportunity for sharing, growth and change. As human beings, we often react to our own unconscious analysis of a behavior or a dynamic. Our analysis, although real to us, is often blurred by our own belief systems and values. However, our response to this analysis may have a greater impact than we can predict. Interpreters will be faced with different expectations by providers and patients on what their roles should be. It is important that interpreters develop conflict resolution skills besides a greater understanding of who they are and how they can best consistently apply the standards and policies.

Being a culture broker means having some basic conflict resolution skills. Cultural conflicts can be felt when a provider is giving bad news to a patient. The provider might be clear and direct, while family members believe that bad news will kill the patient sooner than expected. There are some cultures that maintain that if a person mentions something bad, most likely that person will catch the badness. Families who believe in keeping clinical truth from patients may try, through elaborate storytelling, to avoid contact with the provider, dismiss information, argue or even attempt to remove a very ill patient from the hospital against medical advice. The "Ethical" provider feels that the truth needs to be said. From a provider's standpoint, the patient is the one who has the right to self-determination, not the family.

Wow! This is a loaded ethical situation! Interpreters should coach the provider; if they don't, the family may never again want interpreter services. It happens that, when there is such a conflict, it is almost impossible for family members to differentiate between the roles of the interpreter and the provider. Often, to them, they are all one and the same. Part of developing basic conflict resolution skills is to show the speaker that he/she is being heard. Listen. Empathize with the parties by repeating their words in a more summarized way. You may want to say, "It seems that this is the issue..." and then repeat the speaker's key words. Or you may want to say, "I hear your struggle around these issues." As soon as you empathize, you need to acknowledge that only the speaker can best express the points at hand, so you ask the speaker, "Is this true?" This questioning process is called checking in. As you do this several times, you are showing support and hopefully making someone come out of the box of "I am right and you are wrong." Every time you repeat the speaker's words, you may want to offer a bit of information about what the other party involved in the conflict might be thinking. You must always find common ground among them and never ally with one or the other side. Your job is to coach by respecting that there are people in the world with differing beliefs.

PO Box 2308, Woburn, MA 01888-0508, **p:** 781-729-3736, **www.EmbracingCulture.com**
PO Box 6401, Manchester, NH 03108, **p:** 1-888-678-CCCS

Sexual Harassment

Adapted from www.eeoc.gov
Sexual harassment at work occurs whenever unwelcome conduct on the basis of gender affects a person's job. It is defined by the Equal Employment Opportunity Commission (EEOC) as unwelcome sexual advances, requests for sexual favors, and other verbal or physical conduct of a sexual nature when:

- submission to the conduct is made either explicitly or implicitly a term or condition of an individual's employment, or
- submission to or rejection of the conduct by an individual is used as a basis for employment decisions affecting such individual, or
- the conduct has the purpose or effect of unreasonably interfering with an individual's work performance or creating an intimidating, hostile, or offensive working environment.

It is not uncommon for interpreters who grew up in different countries to feel restrained from expressing their care and admiration towards a colleague, patient or provider by using language that is perceived sexually suggestive in the USA as a way of initiating a greeting or a social relationship. Also, the same may happen from a person with power towards an interpreter.

Not too long ago we had a student at our institute who loves to bake cakes and she brought in a penis shaped cake decorated in pink frosting with the hope of sharing it with the classroom as students were presenting on the different body systems. Although the student was not targeting one person, this cake could lead to a sexually hostile environment in the classroom for other students. It would have been different if the student brought an anatomical chart with a penis and she was presenting on the reproductive system or any illness regarding the male genitals.

There is often a grey area for those who are accused of being sexually inappropriate with others, which is the freedom of expression. The first Amendment act in fact does not protect those who are in positions of power and use it to offend and intimidate other employees, colleagues, patients to the point that their work is affected, creating a sexually hostile environment. When asked about her intention, the student genuinely had a good intention and at first, although feeling a bit sad, she agreed that the impact of sharing this cake with the class may not match her initial intention which was to share a cake with her colleagues who were stressed out!
So not every behavior that makes us feel good is in fact appropriate in our USA society where laws were created to hopefully protect women and men from being discriminated and oppressed due to their gender. Although there are more cases of sexual harassment by men against women, the law forbids any form of unwelcome sexual advance against colleagues, employees, subordinates, customers, patients and others by either gender and for those cases where people are from the same gender.

Title VII applies to employers with 15 or more employees, including state and local governments. It also applies to employment agencies and to labor organizations, as well as to the federal and state government institutions. Some courts have held that individual employees cannot be liable under Title VII. Some state laws, however, do impose personal liability on individuals for perpetrating harassment. But the employer who has more than 15 employees is not exempt; therefore the employer if sued may be entitled to sue an employee back who was found guilty for damages and legal expenses from a supervisor who was aware of his or her unauthorized conduct.

There are two types of sexual Harassment:

There are two types of legally recognized way of committing sexual harassment: (1) Quid Pro Quo sexual harassment; and (2) Hostile environment harassment.

I. Quid Pro Quo Sexual Harassment

It is when the person who commits quid pro quo sexual harassment is a person with power to influence the victim's employment or educational situation like a supervisor, manager or provider. It does not matter if the victim agreed to follow through with the arrangement. An example will be the interpreter who offers to drive a client home in exchange of some sexual favor. Or a provider who keeps telling the interpreter that she or he will keep his job if they can continue seeing each other.

II. Hostile Environment Sexual Harassment

Hostile work environment sexual harassment happens when a co-worker, manager or supervisor in the work place makes unwelcome sexual advances, verbal or non-verbal, which interferes with work performance or creates an intimidating, hostile or offensive work environment. An example reported once by an interpreter from Brazil was that each time she would arrive to a clinic, the male staff at the desk would play the drums with their pens against the desk and they would make remarks such as let's go Samba together tonight! A common verbal harassment is when one makes a sexual comment about a person's clothing, anatomy or looks, or gives a neck massage or rubs one's shoulders without being asked.

Patient's Bill of Rights

Copied from http://www.cc.nih.gov/participate/patientinfo/legal/bill_of_rights.shtml

1. The patient has the right to considerate and respectful care.
2. The patient has the right to know, by name, the physician responsible for coordinating his or her care at the Clinical Center.
3. The patient has the right to obtain from his or her physician complete current information about diagnosis, treatment, and prognosis in easily understandable terms. If it is medically inadvisable to give such information to the patient, it will be given to a legally authorized representative.
4. The patient has the right to receive from his or her physician information necessary to give informed consent prior to the start of any procedure or treatment. Except in emergencies this will include, but not necessarily be limited to, a description of the specific procedure or treatment, any risks involved, and the probable duration of any incapacitation. When there are alternatives to therapeutically designed research protocols, the patient has the right to know about them. The patient also has the right to know the name of the person responsible for directing the procedures or treatment.
5. The patient has the right to refuse to participate in research, to refuse treatment to the extent permitted by law, and has the right to be informed of the medical consequences of these actions, including possible dismissal from the study and discharge from the institution. If discharge would jeopardize the patient's health, he or she has the right to remain under Clinical Center care until discharge or transfer is medically advisable.
6. The patient has the right to be transferred to another facility when his or her participation in the Clinical Center study is terminated, provided the transfer is medically permissible, the patient has been informed of the needs for and alternatives to such a transfer, and the facility has agreed to accept the patient.
7. The patient has the right to privacy concerning the medical care program. Case discussion, consultation, examination, and treatment are confidential and will be conducted discreetly. The patient has the right to expect that all communications and records pertaining to care will be treated as confidential to the extent permitted by law.

8. The patient has the right to routine services whenever hospitalized at the Clinical Center in connection with the active protocol for which he or she is eligible; these services will generally include diagnostic procedures and medical treatment deemed necessary and advisable by the professional staff. Complicating chronic conditions will be noted, reported to the patient, and treated as necessary without the assumption of long-term responsibility for their management. The patient may be returned for long-term or definitive care of these conditions to the referring physician or to other appropriate medical resources.
9. The patient has the right to expect that medical information about him or her discovered at the Clinical Center, as well as an account of his or her medical program, will be communicated to the referring physician.
10. The patient has the right, at any time during the medical program, to designate additional physicians or organizations to receive medical updates. The patient should inform the Outpatient Department staff of these additions.
11. The patient has the right to know in advance what appointment times and physicians are available and where to go for continuity of care provided by the Clinical Center when such care is required under the study for which the patient was admitted.

PO Box 2308, Woburn, MA 01888-0508, **p:** 781-729-3736, **www.EmbracingCulture.com**
PO Box 6401, Manchester, NH 03108, **p:** 1-888-678-CCCS

REFUSAL OF CARE AGAINST MEDICAL ADVICE (AMA) AND RELEASE AT SCENE (RAS)

Copied from:
http://egovwebprd.marinpublic.com/depts/HH/main/ems/documents/Policies/8104.pdf

I. PURPOSE

To provide guidelines for pre-hospital personnel dealing with patients refusing care Against Medical Advice (AMA) or patients requesting a Release at Scene (RAS)

II. DEFINITIONS

A. Against Medical Advice (AMA) – The refusal of treatment or transport, by an emergency patient or his/her designated decision maker, against the advice of the medical personnel on scene or of the receiving hospital.

B. Release at Scene (RAS) – A call outcome that occurs when the patient and the EMS personnel agree that the illness/injury does not require immediate treatment/transport via emergency/911 services and the patient does not require the services of the prehospital system.

C. Patient – Any person who seeks medical attention from 911/ EMS.

D. Patients who may legally give consent for medical treatment are:

1. At least 18 years of age
2. A minor (<18) who is lawfully married or divorced
3. A minor on active duty with the armed forces
4. A minor who seeks prevention or treatment of pregnancy or sexual assault
5. A minor who is 12 years of age or older, who seeks treatment for rape, contagious diseases, alcohol or drug abuse
6. A self sufficient minor, 15 years or older, caring for himself/herself
7. A legally emancipated minor

E. Designated Decision Maker (DDM) – An individual to whom a person or court has legally given the authority to make medical decisions concerning the person's healthcare (a parent or a Durable Power of Attorney for Healthcare).

F Competency – the ability to understand and to demonstrate an understanding of the nature and consequences of refusing medical care.

G. Emergency Medical Personnel:

EMT – P (Paramedics) – providing ALS or BLS service
EMT - 1 (Emergency Medical Technicians) – providing only BLS service

III. AGAINST MEDICAL ADVICE (AMA) POLICY

A. All emergency patients will be offered treatment and/or transport following a complete assessment.

B. Adults have the right to accept or refuse any and all pre-hospital care and transportation, provided that the decision to accept or refuse these treatments and transportation is made on an informed basis and provided that these adults have the mental capacity to make and understand the implications of such a decision.

To meet the standard of "meaningful understanding" the patient must be informed and must understand (best demonstrated by the patient's ability to restate) the nature and consequences of the consent or refusal at the time the care and/or treatment is being offered. The following information must be provided to the patient or DDM by the Emergency Medical Personnel:

1. The nature of the recommended treatment
2. The risks involved including any possible complications
3. The benefits of the treatment
4. The consequences of not seeking care and treatment - these must be reasonable for the presenting condition.

C. High-Risk Patient Complaints: Some patient complaints may represent more concerning and potentially higher risk (for the patient and medical provider) clinical conditions. These patients may warrant (but not require) receiving hospital and/or physician contact before completing an AMA with a patient of DDM. Every effort should be made to transport patients with the following complaints:

1. Patients >65 years of age who are requesting AMA
2. Chest Pain
3. SOB/Dyspnea
4. Syncope
5. Headache (new onset)
6. Seizure (new onset)
7. TIA/Resolving Stroke Symptoms
8. Traumatic Injuries
9. Pediatric Complaints
10. Pregnancy-related Issues

PO Box 2308, Woburn, MA 01888-0508, **p:** 781-729-3736, **www.EmbracingCulture.com**
PO Box 6401, Manchester, NH 03108, **p:** 1-888-678-CCCS

D. If the patient refuses transport to the recommended destination and the patient's refusal of transport would create a life-threatening or high-risk situation, obtain a Receiving Hospital Physician Consult, document the AMA, and transport the patient to the requested facility within Marin County. If this patient requests an out of county transport, a Physician Consult from the recommended destination hospital in Marin County is required.

E. If the patient cannot legally refuse care or is mentally incapable of refusing care:

1. Document on the PCR that the patient required immediate treatment and/or transport, and lacked the mental capacity to understand the risks/consequences of the refusal (implied consent), and transport accordingly.
2. Do not request a 5150 hold unless the patient requires a psychiatric evaluation
3. Treat as necessary to prevent death or serious disability and transport.
4. Consider involvement of law enforcement early if there is a threat to self, to others, or grave disability.

IV. RELEASE AT SCENE (RAS) POLICY

A. After evaluation by the EMS personnel, and the patient/DDM is deemed a competent adult, EMS personnel may release the patient at the secene as long as both the EMS personnel and the patient/DDM concur that the illness/injury does not require immediate treatment/transport via emergency/911 services and the patient does not require the services of the prehospital system.

B. EMS personnel shall advise patients of alternative care and transport options, which may include, but not be limited to:

1. Private transport to a clinic, a physician's office, or an ER.
2. Telephone consultation with a physician.

C. EMS personnel are encouraged to obtain a Receiving Hospital Physician Consult if there are any questions or concerns regarding the patient's disposition.

D. The patient or DDM shall sign the AMA/RAS Form.

E. Patients who do not have a DDM physically present may be released at the scene after telephone consent is obtained. This would most often occur with a minor when the parent is not at the scene.

V. PATIENTS TRANSPORTED AGAINST WILL:

A. Implied Consent – If the patient is not a danger to him/herself or others, yet not competent to refuse evaluation or transport, the patient should be transported to the appropriate facility under implied consent. In this case, a 5150 hold is not necessary. However, if the providers believe the patient will resist (and that it is medically necessary to transport the patient against his/her will), the providers should request police assistance in transporting the patient. The police may consider the placement of a 5150 hold on the patient, but this is not required for transport.

B. 5150 - When a patient exhibits signs of being a danger to him/herself or others, or is gravely disabled and cannot simply be treated and/or transported, the provider should notify the proper authorities to obtain a 5150, and remain with the patient until authorities have made such a determination. Patients on a 5150 hold cannot be released at the scene.

C. At no time are field personnel to put themselves in danger by attempting to transport or treat a patient who refuses. At all times, good judgment should be used, appropriate assistance obtained, and supporting documentation completed.

VI. DOCUMENTATION REQUIREMENTS (PCR):

The following items shall be included for adherence to protocol:

1. Who activated 911 and the reason for the call
2. All medical care provided including the chief complaint and level of distress of the patient, level of consciousness, and a Glasgow Coma Scale.
3. The apparent competency of the patient to sign out AMA or RAS
4. The ability of the patient/DDM to verbalize an understanding of his/her illness or injury
5. The patient/DDM has had the risks and potential outcome of nontreatment and/or non-transport explained fully to him/her by the provider, such that the patient/DDM can verbalize understanding of this information
6. The presence or absence of any impairment of the patient/DDM such as by alcohol or drugs
7. Reasons given by the patient/DDM for refusing offered care and transport. Include patient's/DDM's alternate plan if one has been stated.
8. That the patient/DDM has been informed that they may re-access 911 if necessary
9. Signature of the patient/DDM on the AMA/RAS Form, or reason why signature was not obtained

PO Box 2308, Woburn, MA 01888-0508, **p:** 781-729-3736, **www.EmbracingCulture.com**

PO Box 6401, Manchester, NH 03108, **p:** 1-888-678-CCCS

MARIN COUNTY EMS AGAINST MEDICAL ADVICE (AMA)–RELEASE AT SCENE (RAS) FORM CRITERIA FOR REFUSING CARE

The patient meets all of the following:

1. Is an adult (18 or over), or if < 18 meets the criteria stated in the AMA/RAS policy
2. Exhibits no evidence of:
   - Altered level of consciousness
   - Alcohol or drug ingestion that impairs judgment
3. Understands the nature of the medical condition, as well as the risks and consequences of refusing care

1. ACKNOWLEDGMENT OF INFORMATION:

A. __ AMA: I have been advised that medical assistance on my behalf is necessary, and that refusal of said assistance could be hazardous to my health, and under certain circumstances, including disability and/or death. I have been advised to discuss my medical complaints with my regular healthcare provider as soon as possible. Nevertheless, I refuse to accept treatment or transport to a medical facility and assume all risks and consequences of any decision.

or

B. __ RAS: I acknowledge that I may have a medical problem, which may require additional medical attention, and that an ambulance is available to transport me to the hospital. Instead, I elect to seek alternative medical care and refuse further treatment and/or transport.

2. RELEASE OF LIABILITY:

By signing this form, I am releasing the County of Marin, the responding Provider Agency(ies), and the Receiving Hospital (if contacted) of any liability or medical claims resulting from my decision to refuse the medical care/transport offered.

I have read and understand the "Acknowledgment of Information" and "Release of Liability." I also acknowledge that I have received a Notice of Privacy Practices.

Signature

Refused to sign, Reason:

Relationship *(if not the patient)*: Lawful: ☐ parent ☐ guardian ☐ conservator *(pertains to a child/dependent only)*

☐ Physician Consulted

☐ Telephone consent/refusal obtained. Witnessed by:

☐ Interpreter used

Di

Completed by *(Print)* Signature Unit #/Agency #

Patient Name AO#

DDM Date

entregado.

DISPOSITION: ☐ Released in care or custody of self.
☐ Released in custody of law enforcement

Agency Badge #

Released in care or custody of: ☐ Parent ☐ Guardian ☐ Other:__________

Instructions

1. If you change your mind or your condition changes, call 9-1-1 (in an emergency), go to an emergency department in your area, or call your private doctor (if appropriate).
2. __________
3. __________

Witness Information

Signature Name Printed

Address City State Zip

Phone: ( ) Driver's License #

An immigrant that falls in love with the new country__________ ____ the new country.

PO Box 2308, Woburn, MA 01888-0508, **p:** 781-729-3736, **www.EmbracingCulture.com**
PO Box 6401, Manchester, NH 03108, **p:** 1-888-678-CCCS

CLAS Standards for providers

Although CLAS standards were created for providers, It is important that Interpreters become familiar with them. For more information check http://www.omhrc.gov.

The Following outline was copied from the Office of Minority Health at the Department of Health and Human Services.

The CLAS standards are primarily directed at healthcare organizations; however, individual providers are also encouraged to use the standards to make their practices more culturally and linguistically accessible. The principles and activities of culturally and linguistically appropriate services should be integrated throughout an organization and undertaken in partnership with the communities being served.

The 14 standards are organized by themes: Culturally Competent Care (Standards 1-3), Language Access Services (Standards 4-7), and Organizational Supports for Cultural Competence (Standards 8-14). Within this framework, there are three types of standards of varying stringency: mandates, guidelines, and recommendations, as follows:

CLAS mandates are current Federal requirements for all recipients of Federal funds (Standards 4, 5, 6, and 7).

Standard 1: Healthcare organizations should ensure that patients/consumers receive from all staff members effective, understandable, and respectful care that is provided in a manner compatible with their cultural health beliefs and practices and preferred language.

Standard 2: Healthcare organizations should implement strategies to recruit, retain, and promote at all levels of the organization a diverse staff and leadership that are representative of the demographic characteristics of the service area.

Standard 3: Healthcare organizations should ensure that staff at all levels and across all disciplines receive ongoing education and training in culturally and linguistically appropriate service delivery.

Standard 4: Healthcare organizations must offer and provide language assistance services, including bilingual staff and interpreter services, at no cost to each patient/consumer with limited English proficiency at all points of contact, in a timely manner during all hours of operation.

Standard 5: Healthcare organizations must provide to patients/consumers in their preferred language both verbal offers and written notices informing them of their right to receive language assistance services.

Standard 6: Healthcare organizations must assure the competence of language assistance provided to limited English proficient patients/consumers by interpreters and bilingual staff. Family and friends should not be used to provide interpretation services (except on request by the patient/consumer).

Standard 7: Healthcare organizations must make available easily understood patient-related materials and post signage in the languages of the commonly encountered groups and/or groups represented in the service area.

Standard 8: Healthcare organizations should develop, implement, and promote a written strategic plan that outlines clear goals, policies, operational plans, and management accountability/oversight mechanisms to provide culturally and linguistically appropriate services.

Standard 9: Healthcare organizations should conduct initial and ongoing organizational self-assessments of CLAS-related activities and are encouraged to integrate cultural and linguistic competence-related measures into their internal audits, performance improvement programs, patient satisfaction assessments, and outcomes-based evaluations.

Standard 10: Healthcare organizations should ensure that data on the individual patient's/consumer's race, ethnicity, and spoken and written language are collected in health records, integrated into the organization's management information systems, and periodically updated.

Standard 11: Healthcare organizations should maintain a current demographic, cultural, and epidemiological profile of the community as well as a needs assessment to accurately plan for and implement services that respond to the cultural and linguistic characteristics of the service area.

Standard 12: Healthcare organizations should develop participatory, collaborative partnerships with communities and utilize a variety of formal and informal mechanisms to facilitate community and patient/consumer involvement in designing and implementing CLAS-related activities.

Standard 13: Healthcare organizations should ensure that conflict and grievance resolution processes are culturally and linguistically sensitive and capable of identifying, preventing, and resolving cross-cultural conflicts or complaints by patients/consumers.

Standard 14: Healthcare organizations are encouraged to regularly make available to the public information about their progress and successful innovations in implementing the CLAS standards and to provide public notice in their communities about the availability of this information.

PO Box 2308, Woburn, MA 01888-0508, **p:** 781-729-3736, **www.EmbracingCulture.com**
PO Box 6401, Manchester, NH 03108, **p:** 1-888-678-CCCS

Forms When Committing a Patient Into a Mental Health Hospital

Different states have different laws and the forms are also written differently. Practice your Sight translations skills at the same time you become familiar with the following forms usually given to a mental health patient who is at risk of hurting himself, herself or others. Interpreters should request the presence of a clinician when interpreting for such legal documents.

There is a difference between Informed Consent and Consent Form. Research the difference and place it in this lesson's glossary?

Commonwealth of Massachusetts
Department of Mental Health
Application for and Authorization of Temporarily Involuntary Hospitalization
M.G.L Chapter 123, Sections 12 (a) and 12 (b)
Application Pursuant to 12 (a)

1. **Application to (facility name):** ______________________
2. **I herby apply for admission of (name of patient):** ______________________

____
Address City/Town State

____
Social Security Number Date of Birth Sex: M F

To the facility named above pursuit to M.G.L. c. 123, s. 12(a). This person, in my opinion, requires hospitalization at the above named facility so as to avoid the likelihood of serious harm by reason of mental illness. Evidence supporting my opinion includes:

A. Mental Illness: For purposes of admission to an inpatient facility under section 12, "Mental Illness" means a substantial disorder of thought, mood, perception, orientation, or memory which grossly impairs judgment, behavior, and capacity to recognize reality or ability to meet the ordinary demands of life. Symptoms caused solely by alcohol or drug intake, organic damage or mental retardation do not constitute a serious mental illness. Specify evidence including behavioral and symptoms.

B. Likelihood of Serious Harm: *(check all categories that apply)*:

_____ 1. Substantial risk of physical harm to the person himself/herself as manifested by evidence of threats of, or attempts at suicide or serious bodily harm; and/or

_____ 2. Substantial risk of physical harm to other persons as manifested by evidence of homicidal or other violent behavior or evidence that other are placed in reasonable fear of violent behavior and serious physical harm to them; and/or

_____ 3. Very Substantial risk of physical impairment or injury to the person himself/herself as protect himself/herself in the community and the reasonable provision of his/her protection is not available in the community.

Specific evidence including behavior and symptoms:

____

____

____

3. **Applicant Certification** (*check all applicable boxes*):
   a. I am a: ☐ Licensed Physician ☐ Qualified (i.e Licensed) Psychologist
   ☐ Qualified(i.e.Licensed and Certified) Psychiatric Nurse Mental Health Clinical Specialist
   ☐ Police Officer
   b. I have ☐ I have not ☐ personally examined this person If not, why?

   ____

   c. ☐ I have consulted with either the receiving facility or emergency screening program.
   ☐ I have not so consulted because

Applicant's name (not patient):

(print)	Phone	
Address	City/Town	State
Applicants Signature	Date	Time

NOTE: parts 1. through 3. above, must be completed to apply for involuntary hospitalization. Authorization Pursuant to Section 12 (b)

Designated Physician* Authorization:

A. ___ I am a designated physician* of the aforementioned facility with authority to authorize admissions under section 12 (b)

B. ___ I have personally examined this person

___ within 2 hours of his/her arrival at the facility

___ more than 2 hours after his/her arrival at the facility due to the fact that I was engaged in an emergency situation.** The emergency situation was:

____

____

______________ and I examined he patient at ______________ am/pm

PO Box 2308, Woburn, MA 01888-0508, **p:** 781-729-3736, **www.EmbracingCulture.com**
PO Box 6401, Manchester, NH 03108, **p:** 1-888-678-CCCS

C. ___ This person does not require emergency for inpatient medical or surgical care.

D. ___ I have offered this person an application for Care and Treatment on a Conditional Voluntary Basis and this person:

(one of the two boxes below must be checked to proceed with section 12 (b) authorization)

☐ refused to sign or

☐ the application was rejected (if the reasons why the application was rejected must be stated on the application and the rejected application shall become part of this persons medical record at the facility.)

NOTE: 104 CMR 27.07 (1) requires that the patient be offered an opportunity to change to conditional voluntary status again within three days of admission.

E. ___ I concur with the applicant's recommendation and have completed a psychiatric examination to support this conclusion. Alternatively, I am the applicant, I have personally examined this person, and have completed sections 1, 2, 2A, and 2B on the opposite side of this form.

F. ___ In my opinion, at the present time there is no less restrictive placement that is appropriate for this person to which he or she is willing to go.

G. ___ I authorize this person's admission

H. ___ I reject this application for admission for the following reasons:

____

____

____

Designated Physicians Name (print) Phone

Address

Designated Physicians Signature

Date Time

** A Physician who meets the criteria in 104 CMR 33.03*
*** See 104 CMR 27.07 (2)*

Commonwealth of Massachusetts
Department of Mental Health
Notice of Rights

To be given to all patients admitted under M.G.L. c. 123, s. 12 (b)
Temporary Involuntary Hospitalization

You have been admitted to this facility under M.G.L c. 123, s. 12 (b) for a period of up to three (3) business days. By the end of the third (3rd) business day, if the Superintendent or other head of the facility decides that your release would create a likelihood of serious harm to you or others by reason of your mental illness, he or she may file a petition for your civil commitment to the facility for a period of up to six months. If a petition is filed, The District Court will begin the hearing within five (5) business days, not including Saturday, Sunday, or holidays, during which time you will have to remain in the facility.

At your request, we will notify the Committee for Public Counsel Services (CPCS) of your name and location. CPCS will then appoint an attorney to meet with you. Would you like CPCS contacted at this time?

☐ Yes ☐ No

If you say No and change your mind later, CPCS will be contacted at that time.

If you have been admitted to this facility under M.G.L c. 123, s. 12 (b) and have reason to believe that such admission is the result of an abuse or misuse of the admission process, you may request, on your own or through counsel, an emergency hearing in the District court in whose jurisdiction this facility is located. If you wish to file such a request, the facility will provide you with the appropriate form.

I have received and read this Notice:

Name ____________________ Date ____________

Staff witness signature ____________________ Date ____________

Should one be a Clarifier or a Culture Coach when Interpreting for Different Types of Pain?

Interpreters are faced with a multitude of challenges in interpreting and describing those different types of pain. Are all of us, providers, patients and interpreters able to accurately interpret the following types of pain?

1. Dull
2. Searing
3. Sharp
4. Annoying

Are these descriptions already culture bound? The challenge is in the accuracy of meaning through the conversion from one language to another. Furthermore, English speakers often have a different understanding of the multiple types of pain. Although pain is a universal experience, the description of it is more personal.

Did you grow up in a family being told that you should not be a complainer? If yes, most likely, you will be the type of patient who will go to the emergency room with some chest pain when you are having a heart attack. Some of us describe sharp pain as if it were a needle or a knife penetrating. Others may describe a toothache as excruciating or an uncomfortable ache. Does your provider have the same meaning as your understanding for a particular type of pain? Providers are individuals and they also have their own experiences in feeling, understanding and describing pain.

According to Edward Hall on beyond the culture, 1997, "Language used to describe culture is by nature poorly adapted to this difficult task. Language is too linear, not comprehensive enough, too slow, too constrained, too unnatural, too much of a product of its' own evolution and too artificial."

There are different types and intensities and forms of pain. Pain can be physical, emotional, social and spiritual. It can be mild, uncomfortable, distressing, terrible, excruciating. Pain can be acute, recent or chronic when it continuous for more than 3 months and longer or it lasts longer than its expected healing time frame.

According to Paul Brodwinn et al in the book *Pain as Human Experience*, different cultures may describe pain as "It seems as if pepper were put into my brain" or " I have a bear headache" or as often we hear from Azorean patients "os meus miolos vão rebentar ou explodir." One way of saying it in English is, "the inside of my brain is going to burst or explode." Or a patient coming into the emergency room suffering from a heart attack or severe angina may say , "I feel like I have an elephant or truck on top of my chest."

Whose job is it to make sure that both the speaker and the interpreter are in agreement with the description or naming of the particular pain being mentioned? Should an interpreter be a conduit, a clarifier and or culture broker and always ask for the provider's or patient's description of type of pain? How may our own personal experience of pain impact our accuracy level?

The IMIA Standards of Practice, 1995, on page 35 specifically mention that interpreters are "committed to transmitting accurately and completely the content and spirit of the original message into the other language without omitting, modifying, condensing or adding." Also, on page 32, the interpreter "is aware of and able to identify personal biases and beliefs that may interfere with the ability to be impartial, and has the moral fortitude to withdraw if unable to be impartial."

We are left with the understanding that when an interpreter cannot find an exact word for the word describing the pain, that an interpreter should ask for a description and interpret the speaker's description. The interpreter having difficulty finding the exact word should abstain form describing the pain, but involve the respective party on the description. Another way, less time consuming, but with greater potential for error, is for an interpreter to describe the pain to her/ his best judgment and let the speaker know that this is how it was interpreted.

The role of the culture coach when dealing with interpreting issues regarding the intensity of pain seems appropriate when a patient is asked by the provider, "from scale 1-10 how much doest it hurt?" The interpreter sees the patient's hesitance and possible difficulty describing it or even when a patient quickly answers but the body language is not congruent with the number. An interpreter, as per IMIA Standards, may want to inform both parties, provider and patient, of this possible misunderstanding.

Often, the medical culture is a more linear cause and effect and the patient culture is more circular, a story teller. The patient may relate to the pain by describing that the pain is as bad as when her mother went to the hospital or that is so bad that it stops her from going to work. But this same patient may not be able to illustrate the intensity of the pain by using a number. Although the scales with the different facial expressions are visual and a bit more concrete, but often they are still too abstract and not always the best technique to identify the intensity of the pain.

The feedback I get from some providers is that interpreters cannot always act as culture brokers as the session is happening. Providers appreciate the partnership with the interpreters, but perhaps the culture brokering should be at the beginning or end of a session. Here are the following tips for interpreters in the role of culture coaches: Is this about me? Can I wait? How is this intervention going to affect the provider – patient relationship?

PO Box 2308, Woburn, MA 01888-0508, **p:** 781-729-3736, **www.EmbracingCulture.com**
PO Box 6401, Manchester, NH 03108, **p:** 1-888-678-CCCS

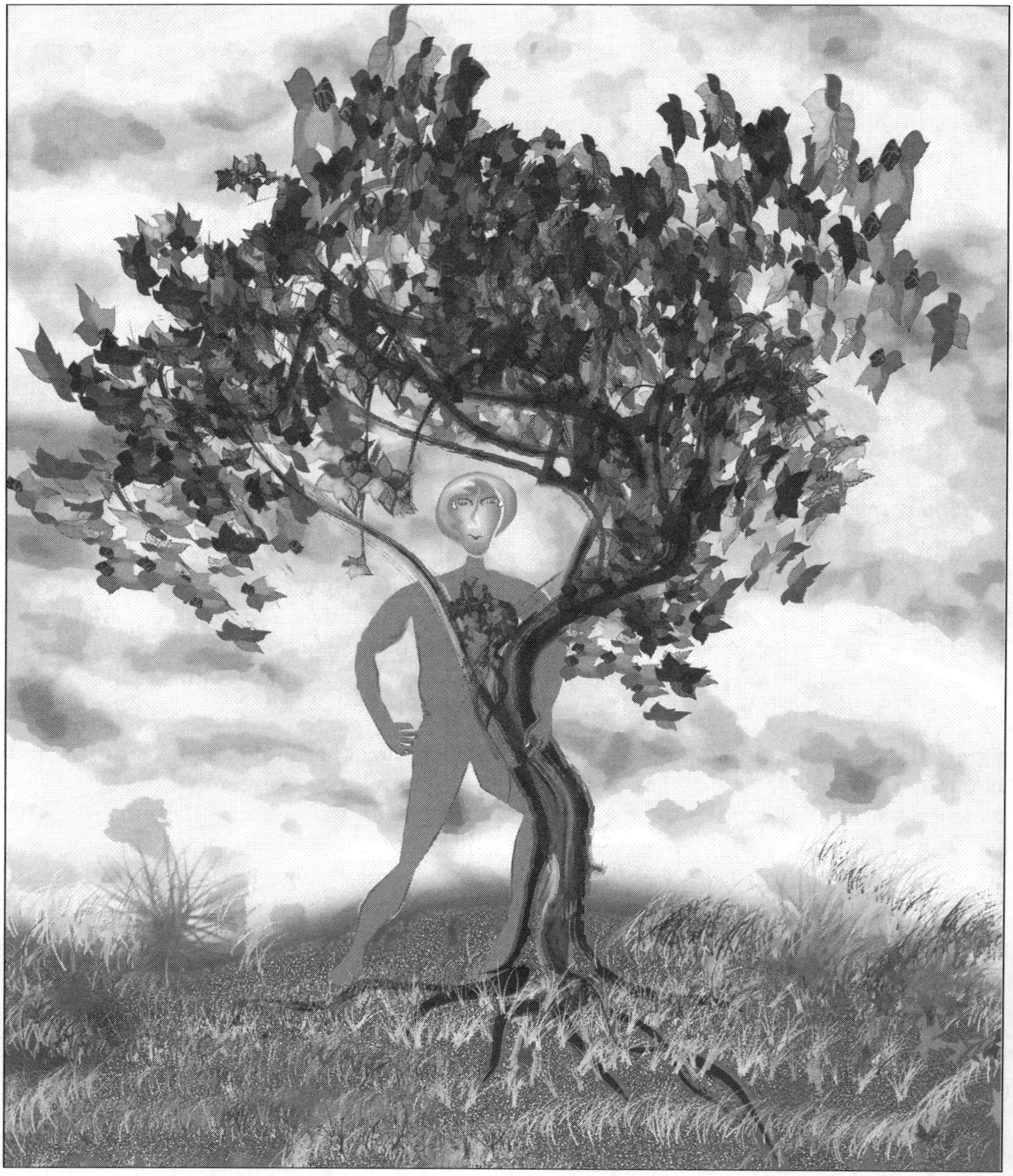

Lesson Six:
The Samurai! Technique and the Cardiovascular System

Understanding Goals

Students will be able to:

- review learned concepts
- learn about different Medical Specialties
- learn about the Samurai! Technique
- understand major organs, organ systems and their respective functions (Cardiovascular System)
- sharpen their consecutive interpreting skills through role play-practice

Key Concepts

- Medical Specialties
- Samurai! Technique
- Word Formation – Prefix, Root, Suffix
- Cardiovascular System

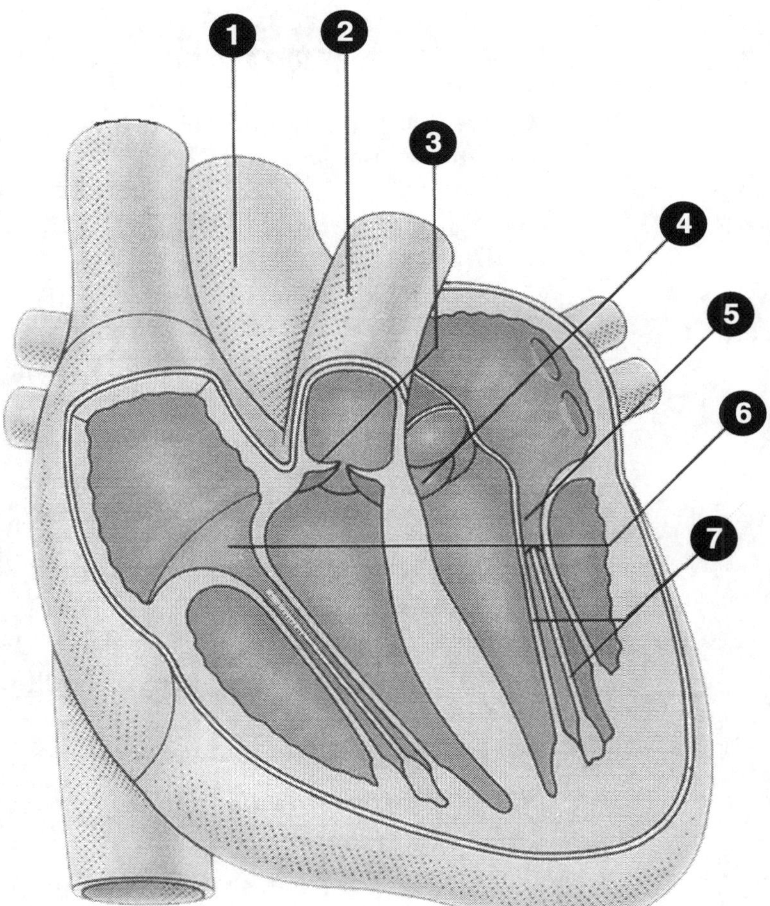

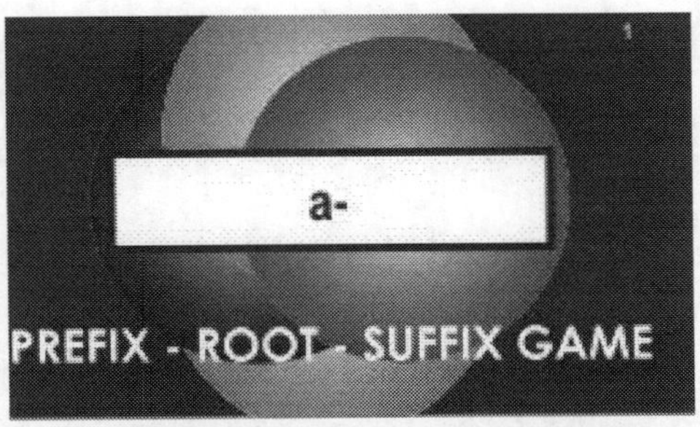

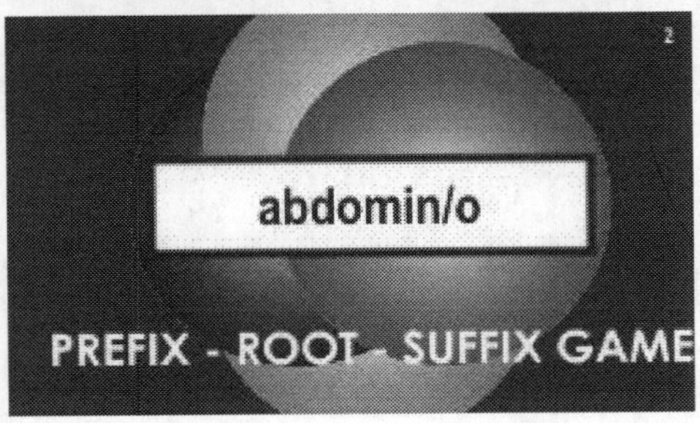

PO Box 2308, Woburn, MA 01888-0508, **p:** 781-729-3736, **www.EmbracingCulture.com**
PO Box 6401, Manchester, NH 03108, **p:** 1-888-678-CCCS

Lesson Six: Quiz
The Samurai! Technique and the Cardiovascular System

Mark each item "True" or "False."

1. Most medical words have originated from Latin and Greek.
   ○ True ○ False
2. "-ist" is a suffix that means "to remove."
   ○ True ○ False
3. Urology is a specialty that treats both men and women.
   ○ True ○ False
4. An internist is a physician in training.
   ○ True ○ False
5. A word root is usually accompanied by a prefix or a suffix, or sometimes by both.
   ○ True ○ False
6. The root often gives information regarding the body part or function in question.
   ○ True ○ False
7. The root "psych/o" refers to the heart.
   ○ True ○ False
8. A prefix is placed after a word or word root to modify its meaning.
   ○ True ○ False
9. A suffix is usually preceded by a dash when the suffix is written alone.
   ○ True ○ False
10. "O" is the most frequently used combining vowel which is inserted to make a word easier to pronounce.
    ○ True ○ False
11. Hyperglycemia means "low sugar."
    ○ True ○ False
12. Necrosis: "Necro-" in this word is a suffix that means "death."
    ○ True ○ False
13. The thick muscular tubes that carry oxygenated blood are called veins.
    ○ True ○ False
14. The thin, more distensible tubes carrying deoxygenated blood are called arteries.
    ○ True ○ False
15. Arteries are depicted as red (carrying oxygenated blood) and veins are depicted as blue (carrying deoxygenated blood).
    ○ True ○ False
16. A stimulant is a type of medicine that thins the blood.
    ○ True ○ False
17. A heart murmur is the sound of blood flowing through the heart.
    ○ True ○ False
18. When blood backs up into the lungs, we call it congestive heart failure.
    ○ True ○ False
19. A Gerontologist specializes in dental problems of the elderly.
    ○ True ○ False
20. When we hear the word "Leukemia" we think about white blood cells.
    ○ True ○ False

Lesson Six: Class Activities
The Samurai! Technique and the Cardiovascular System

REVIEW

Read and role-play the following case:

1. Describe which parts of the case pertain to which four components of the SOAP Notes (Subjective, Objective, Assessment, and Plan)
2. Practice the use of medical terminology, English to Target Language, and abbreviations
3. Practice interpreting in the consecutive mode, pre-session and session. Avoid omissions and deletions, while concentrating on completeness and accuracy of interpreting.

CASE:

Fatuma's Leg Pain

Fatuma comes to the ER complaining of a sudden onset of severe pain and weakness in her left leg. She is 51 years old.

MD:	What brings you here today?
F:	I've had terrible pain in my left leg! I can't move it; if I do, the pain gets worse. I can't even move my toes.
MD:	How long have you had this pain?
F:	Well, I've always had leg pain. But it's been much worse during the past few days.
MD:	I can see from your chart that you smoke. How long have you been a smoker?
F:	Oh, I had my first cigarette when I was 16. I've been smoking ever since.
MD:	Do you follow a diet or an exercise regimen?
F:	Well, like I said before, I've had leg pain for years, so exercise is almost impossible. I don't do much of it. But that can't be what's causing this terrible pain!
MD:	Well, I can't say for sure until I send you for some lab work and exams. One of the exams is called a Doppler Ultrasound. You or someone you know may have had one in the past.
F:	I don't think so.

PO Box 2308, Woburn, MA 01888-0508, **p:** 781-729-3736, **www.EmbracingCulture.com**
PO Box 6401, Manchester, NH 03108, **p:** 1-888-678-CCCS

MD:	Well, the Doppler is a diagnostic instrument that emits an ultrasonic beam into the body and the ultrasound reflected from moving structures changes its frequency. This is called the Doppler effect. It will help us determine whether there is either peripheral vascular or cardiac disease.
F:	Heart disease? But I have leg pain, not chest pain!
MD:	I know. It is common for patients with vascular and cardiac disease to show symptoms of pain or swelling in their extremities.
	(Later, after testing)
MD:	Well, your labs came back showing leukocytosis, which means you have an abnormally high number of white blood cells. But the Doppler showed obstruction of your left femoral artery. It seems you have a large blood clot. We need to try to dissolve or remove that clot.
F:	How do you remove the clot?
MD:	Well, the treatment depends on the size and severity of the embolus, or clot. Current treatments include anticoagulants, commonly know as "blood thinner" medications and oxygen therapy, thrombolysis, or a vena cava filter. In more severe cases, surgery may be required. Surgical procedures include removing the clot through traditional or catheter-directed pulmonary embolectomy. Because your illness is in such an advanced state, I'd like us to consider surgery.
F:	But I'm in a lot of pain; won't surgery make it worse?
MD:	Actually, surgery may be the best solution for your pain. Really, the earlier the intervention, the higher the likelihood that your limb may be salvaged. In other words, if we do not follow through with treatment, you may lose your leg.
F:	Lose my leg? You're going to amputate?
MD:	Amputation is something we avoid at all costs. That's why we'd like you to consider having an embolectomy. Let me explain how it's done. Catheter-directed pulmonary embolectomy involves inserting a catheter via the femoral or internal jugular vein and using fluoroscopic guidance to navigate into the pulmonary artery. The clot is then extracted from the pulmonary bed using a cup device and syringe suction. Considering the alternative, surgery is not so bad.
F:	I just never imagined I'd have to be operated on. I thought you could just give me something for the pain. This is terrible…I can't miss work.

1. The Samurai! Technique

So, who are the medical professionals, you are most likely to meet as you get your start as a healthcare interpreter? Use the space below to brainstorm the medical professionals you are familiar with:

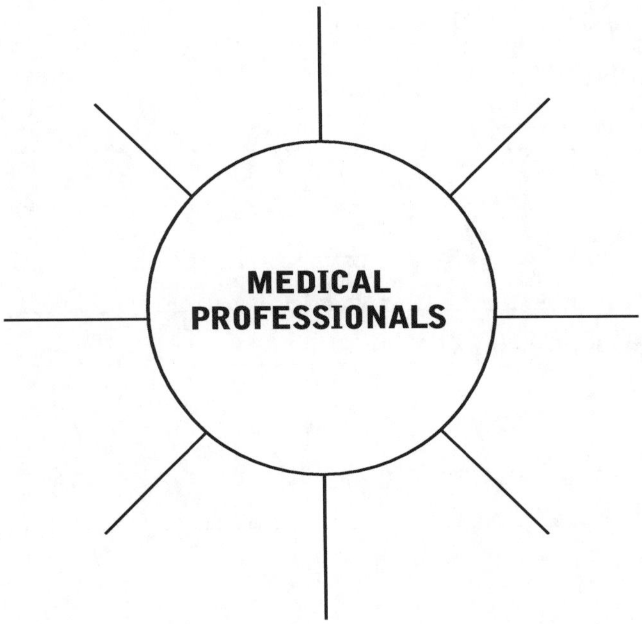

PO Box 2308, Woburn, MA 01888-0508, **p:** 781-729-3736, **www.EmbracingCulture.com**
PO Box 6401, Manchester, NH 03108, **p:** 1-888-678-CCCS

There are countless medical professions and specialties, but we have come up with a list of medical professionals you absolutely will meet and should definitely know. Examine each word carefully. **What is each specialty about?** Jot down your thoughts below.

Word	Meaning
Anesthesiologist	
Cardiologist	
Certified Nursing Assistant (CNA)	
Clinical Social Worker	
Counselor	
Dental Hygienist	
Dentist, DDS and DMD	
Dermatologist	
Emergency Medical Technician (EMT)	
Endocrinologist	
Family Practitioner	
Gastroenterologist	
Gynecologist	
Internist	
Hospitalist	
Licensed Practical Nurse, Licensed	
Vocational Nurse, LPN/LVN	
Neurologist	
Nurse Midwife	
Nurse Practitioner	
Obstetrician	
Oncologist	

continued

Word	Meaning
Occupational Therapist, OT	
Ophthalmologist	
Optometrist	
Orthopedic (Orthopaedic) Surgeon	
Pediatrician	
Pharmacist	
Physical Therapist, PT	
Physician Assistant, PA	
Psychiatrist	
Psychologist	
Radiologist	
Registered Nurse, RN	
Respiratory Therapist	
Social Worker, BA, MSW,	
LCSW, LICSW	
Surgeon	
Urologist	

PO Box 2308, Woburn, MA 01888-0508, **p:** 781-729-3736, **www.EmbracingCulture.com**
PO Box 6401, Manchester, NH 03108, **p:** 1-888-678-CCCS

EXERCISE

Mark the following statements "TRUE" or "FALSE." Correct the false ones:

1. A Physician Assistant is a doctor with just one year of experience.
   ○ True ○ False

   ____

2. A social worker only provides financial assistance to a patient or patient's family.
   ○ True ○ False

   ____

3. Urology is the specialty treating the male reproductive system.
   ○ True ○ False

   ____

4. A neurologist treats infants during the first six weeks after birth.
   ○ True ○ False

   ____

5. An oncologist treats infectious diseases of the immune system. ○ True ○ False

   ____

6. An internist is a physician in training. ○ True ○ False

   ____

7. Dermatologists administer skin allergy tests. ○ True ○ False

   ____

8. Dentists use fluoroscopy to examine the upper respiratory tract.
   ○ True ○ False

   ____

Did you notice that many of the specialties have the same ending "-ist"? Why do you think that is? What meaning does that suffix carry?

____

____

WHAT ARE PREFIXES, ROOTS AND SUFFIXES?

Most medical words have originated from Latin and Greek. We strongly recommend that medical interpreters master the chopping of medical words by looking for **Prefixes, Roots and Suffixes**. Interpreters need to learn relatively few word parts and recognize them when they see them in a word. Many word parts are used to form medical terms that pertain to various body systems.

The root is the main body of a word. All words have at least one root. A word root is usually accompanied by a prefix or a suffix, or sometimes by both. The root often gives information regarding the body part or function in question.

The ROOT gives the essential meaning of the term. What is the meaning of the following roots?

ROOT	MEANING	ROOT	MEANING
aden/o		ophtalm/o	
cardi/o		opt/o, optic/o	
col/o		orth/o	
dermat/o		ot/o	
enter/o		path/o	
gastr/o		ped/o	
gynec/o		psych/o	
hemat/o		pulmon/o	
hepat/o		rect/o	
laryng/o		rheumat/o	
nephr/o		rhin/o	
neur/o		thorac/o	
obstetr/o		ur/o	
onc/o		vascul/o	

A prefix is placed before a word or word root to modify its meaning. When written alone, a prefix is usually followed by a hyphen, indicating that another word part follows the prefix. For example, the prefix "dys-" in *dysmenorrhea* means painful or difficult.

PO Box 2308, Woburn, MA 01888-0508, **p:** 781-729-3736, **www.EmbracingCulture.com**
PO Box 6401, Manchester, NH 03108, **p:** 1-888-678-CCCS

What prefixes do you know?

____

____

A suffix is attached to the end of a word or word root to modify its meaning. A suffix is usually preceded by a hyphen when the suffix is written alone, indicating that another word part needs to precede it before a complete word can be formed. For example, the suffix "- asis" in *cholelithiasis* means the presence of a condition. Suffixes are joined to combining forms to write nouns, adjectives, or verbs. A combining vowel is inserted to make the word easier to pronounce, as in *somat/o/*, where *O* is the combining vowel). *O* is the most frequently used combining vowel.

What suffixes do you know?

____

____

Directions: Can you find the prefixes, roots and/or suffixes in the following words? Practice the Samurai! Technique by "chopping" each word into its respective word parts. Some interpreters find it easier to first look for the ending, or suffix of the word, and then work backwards to the root and prefix. Remember – not all medical terms contain both a prefix and a suffix.

MEDICAL WORD	SUFFIX	ROOT	PREFIX	MEANING
Arthralgia				
Cephalgia				
Cholecystolithiasis				
Colonoscopy				
Gastroenterologist	ist			
Hepatitis	itis			
Hyperglycemia	mia			
Hypogastric				
Mammography	graphy			
Necrosis	sis			
Neuralagia				
Osteoporosis				
Prostatectomy				
Stomatitis				
Thrombosis				
Vasectomy				

Look at the following words. What do they have in common?

Bradycardia   Cardiology   Tachycardia   Electrocardiogram

____

____

2. THE CARDIOVASCULAR SYSTEM

The Cardiovascular System assures that "good " blood (red=oxygenated) gets pumped into the different organs and parts of the body. As the "good" blood gets delivered, the "bad" blood (blue=deoxygenated) gets collected and brought back into the heart to get recycled and cleaned by the lungs. This exchange is called circulation. Blood goes around the body in a circular way. One full cycle takes about one minute in an adult at rest.

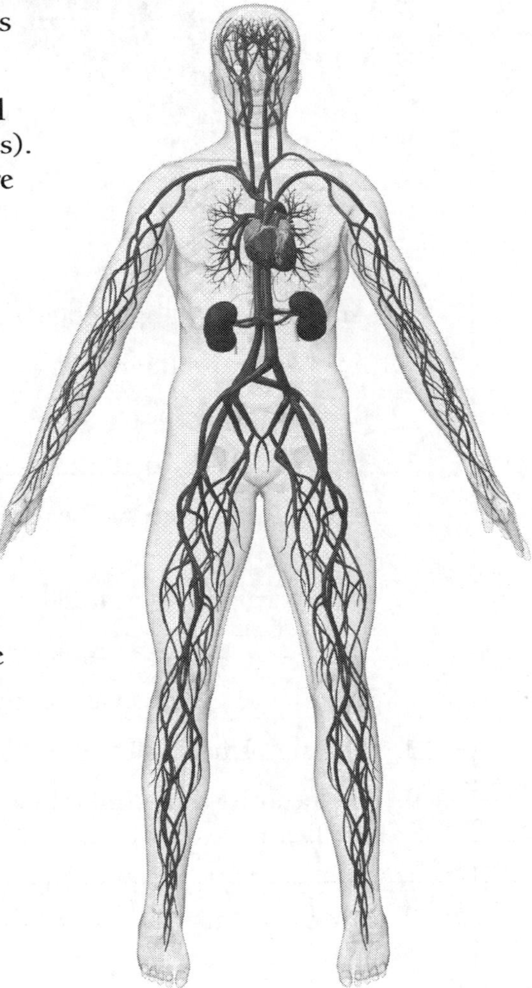

Imagine the circulatory system as a sophisticated internal system of tubes or conduits (arteries, veins and capillaries). The thick muscular tubes that carry oxygenated blood are called arteries. The thin, more distensible tubes carrying deoxygenated blood are called veins. Arteries are depicted as red (carrying oxygenated blood) and veins are depicted as blue (carrying deoxygenated blood). For blood to move through this tubular system, there needs to be a pump. The pump in our body is a four-chambered device, about the size of a fist, called the heart. The two top chambers are called the left and right atria (singular "atrium"). The lower chambers are called the left and right ventricles.

The used or deoxygenated blood enters from the upper (superior vena cava) and lower (inferior vena cava) large veins into the right side of the heart (right atrium). It goes through the tricuspid valve into the right ventricle and gets pumped out through the pulmonary artery to the lungs for oxygenation, completing one half of the circle. Once the blood has oxygen, it flows through the pulmonary vein to the left side of the heart into the left atrium. There it proceeds through the mitral valve into the muscular left ventricle. This is the real pump of the body. The muscular left ventricle pumps the blood out of the

PO Box 2308, Woburn, MA 01888-0508, **p:** 781-729-3736, **www.EmbracingCulture.com**
PO Box 6401, Manchester, NH 03108, **p:** 1-888-678-CCCS

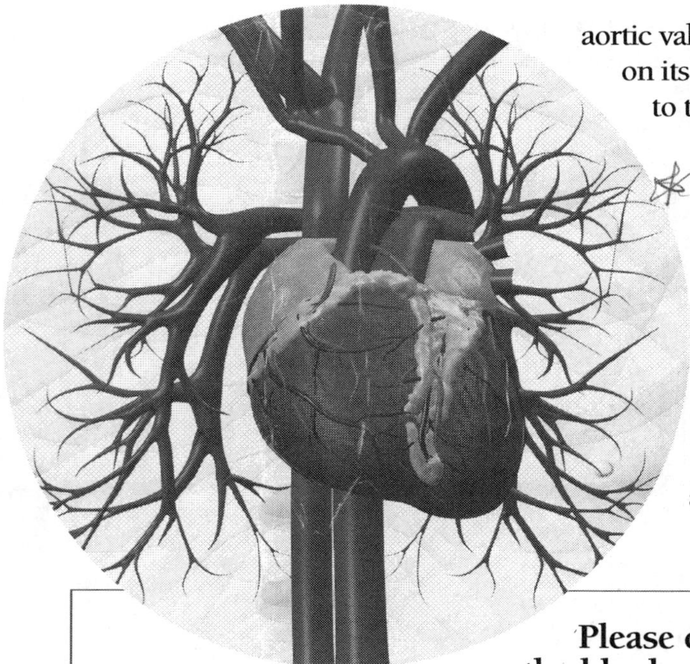

aortic valve into the aorta, which, in turn, sends blood on its circulatory voyage to the head and arms, or on to the rest of the body.

Generally, arteries carry oxygenated blood away from the heart, while veins carry deoxygenated blood to the heart. But looking closely at the pulmonary artery, we find it to be just the opposite! It carries used and deoxygenated blood from the heart. Now, looking closer at the pulmonary vein, we see it carry the oxygenated blood to the heart. Life is always filled with exceptions to the rule!

Please circle the correct answers or fill in the blanks:

1. The heart acts as the ____________ for the cardiovascular system.
2. Arteries are thick, large tubes carrying blood:
   A. away from the heart
   B. toward the heart
3. The heart is divided into ____4____ chambers.
4. Blood going from the heart into the aorta is red because the blood has just been ____________ .
5. A lay term for myocardial infarction is ____________ .
6. ____________ is a medicine that thins the blood.
7. ____________ is a weakening of an arterial wall so that it balloons out.
8. The abnormal collection of fat in both legs is called ____________ .
9. Endocarditis is an inflammation of the ____________, the smooth interior lining of the heart.
10. The painless condition that slowly adds to the harmful effects of hardening of the arteries is called ____________ or ____________ .

DIAGRAM

1. Label the atria, the ventricles, and the main artery(ies) and vein(s) shown in the diagram
2. Trace the flow of blood through the heart

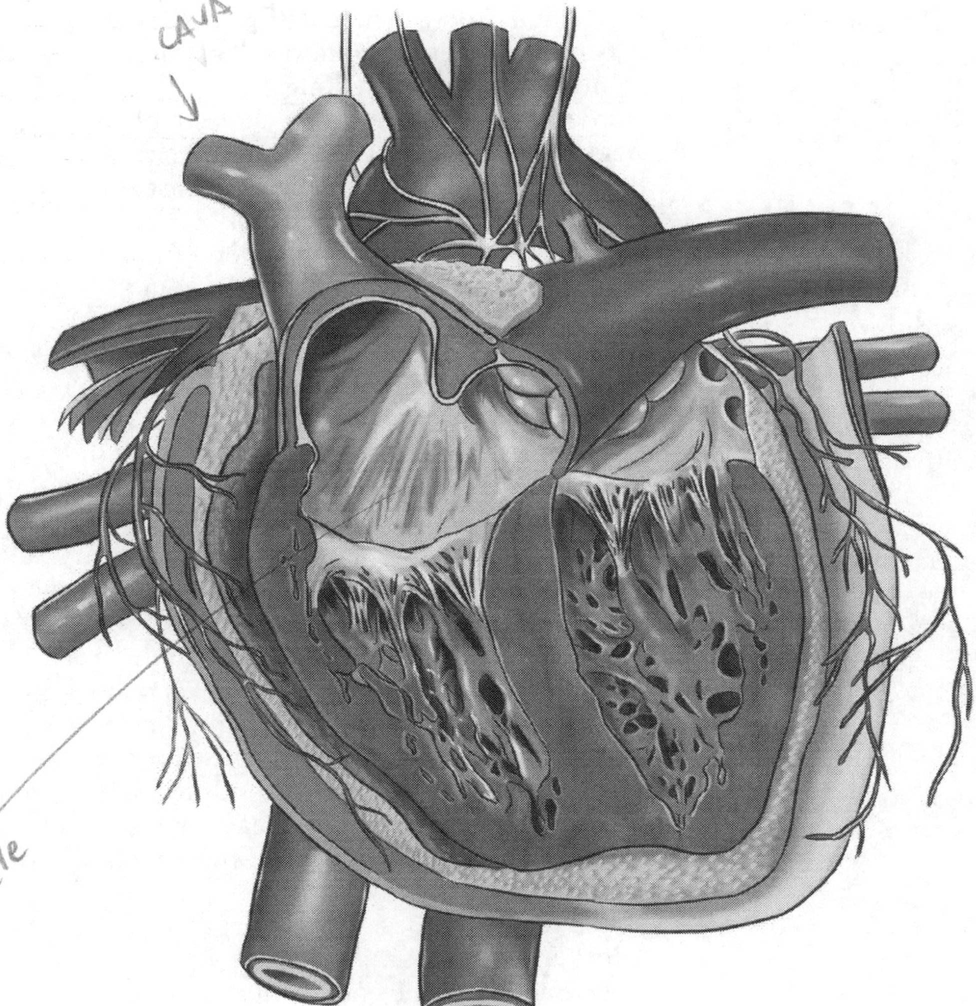

PO Box 2308, Woburn, MA 01888-0508, **p:** 781-729-3736, **www.EmbracingCulture.com**
PO Box 6401, Manchester, NH 03108, **p:** 1-888-678-CCCS

The following exercises will help you learn terminology related to the cardiovascular system.

A. Match the **illness or condition** in Column I with its meaning in Column II.

Column I	Column II
1. Artherosclerosis	A. Dilation and weakening of the ventricles preventing the heart from pumping adequate amounts of blood.
2. Myocardial Infarction	B. A swelling of one or both legs due to a possible disruption of the drainage of lymph back into the blood. It can be acquired or congenital. There is no cure for this disease.
3. Heart Murmur	C. A painful dangerous condition in which the blood clots and moves from the heart into the lungs.
4. Arrhythmia	D. Hardening of the arteries by cholesterol and inflammatory plaque.
5. Pericarditis	E. Also called heart attack. A heart attack is brought on by a hardening of the arteries and the subsequent choking off of oxygen to the heart muscle. A small clot blocks off the already small coronary artery and prevents blood from supplying the heart muscle. The pain from lack of blood to the heart is called angina.
6. Endocarditis	F. A weakening of an arterial wall so it balloons out. Sometimes these weakened states can lead to blood cutting into the thick wall of an artery and dissecting the layers of that wall. This is very painful and dangerous.
7. Cardiomyopathy	G. This is an abnormal collection of fat in both legs, mainly in the lower part of the legs or in between the calf and the ankle area. (A provider, when pressing down, leaves no pressure marks).
8. Hypertension or High Blood Pressure	H. Inflammation of the serous cover of the heart called the pericardium. The pericardium is a two layered envelop that surrounds the heart.
9. Pulmonary Embolism	I. The sound of blood flowing through the heart.
10. Aneurysm	J. A painless condition that slowly adds to the harmful effects of hardening of the arteries and eventually leads to disease in large organs supplied with blood like the kidneys, heart or brain.
11. Coronary Artery Disease	K. A person suffering from this condition suffers from tremendous pain and constriction of the heart caused by a lack of blood to the heart. This pain or sensation of pressure is also due to a lack of oxygen in the heart.
12. Lipedema	L. When the heart goes into an irregular rhythm of beating, it is called an arrhythmia.
13. Lymphedema	M. Inflammation of the endocardium, the smooth interior lining of the heart, usually caused by an infection.

1. ____ 2. ____ 3. ____ 4. ____ 5. ____ 6. ____ 7. ____ 8. ____ 9. ____ 10. ____ 11. ____ 12. ____ 13. ____

B. Match the **Laboratory Tests and Clinical Procedures** in Column I with its meaning in Column II.

Column I	Column II
1. Lipid Tests	A. Uses sound waves to make a picture of the heart.
2. Cardiac Enzymes and Troponin	B. A dye is injected into an artery of the body or of the heart. Pictures of the dye can suggest when there is hardening of the arteries or narrowing.
3. Electrocardiogram	C. A test given to determine the reason(s) for the poor functioning of the heart. Some tests simply make the patient walk quickly or run while recording the heart activity with an EKG. Other tests include EKG tracings and/or taking images of the heart made with an infusion of radioisotopes to measure the heart's ability to function.
4. Echocardiography	D. A blood test which measures the level of different types of fat in the blood – HDL, "good cholesterol," or LDL, "bad cholesterol."
5. Angiography (Catheterization)	E. A collection of enzymes that can increase in the blood stream when the heart muscle dies and allows their contents into the blood.
6. Angioplasty and Stenting	F. A 24-hour recording of the heart rhythm. The patient wears a box a little bigger than a walk-man for 24 hours. The monitor is then removed and sent to the lab.
7. Stress Testing	G. A recorder which the patient wears around his waist for 30 days.
8. Holter Monitor	H. A drawing of the electrical impulses generated by the heart.
9. Event Monitor	I. The cardiologist will put a small balloon via a catheter into an artery. The balloon is expanded and often opens the narrowing caused by arteriosclerosis. To prevent a reblockage, a wire mesh called a stent is placed into the artery.

1. ____ 2. ____ 3. ____ 4. ____ 5. ____ 6. ____ 7. ____ 8. ____ 9. ____

PO Box 2308, Woburn, MA 01888-0508, **p:** 781-729-3736, **www.EmbracingCulture.com**
PO Box 6401, Manchester, NH 03108, **p:** 1-888-678-CCCS

Watch "The Beast Within" from the *Body Story* DVD, and take a look at how delicate the human heart is as an emergency team works to save a heart-attack victim. Use the space below to take notes on what you see or what you find interesting.

Fun Facts

How well do you know your heart? *Consider this....*

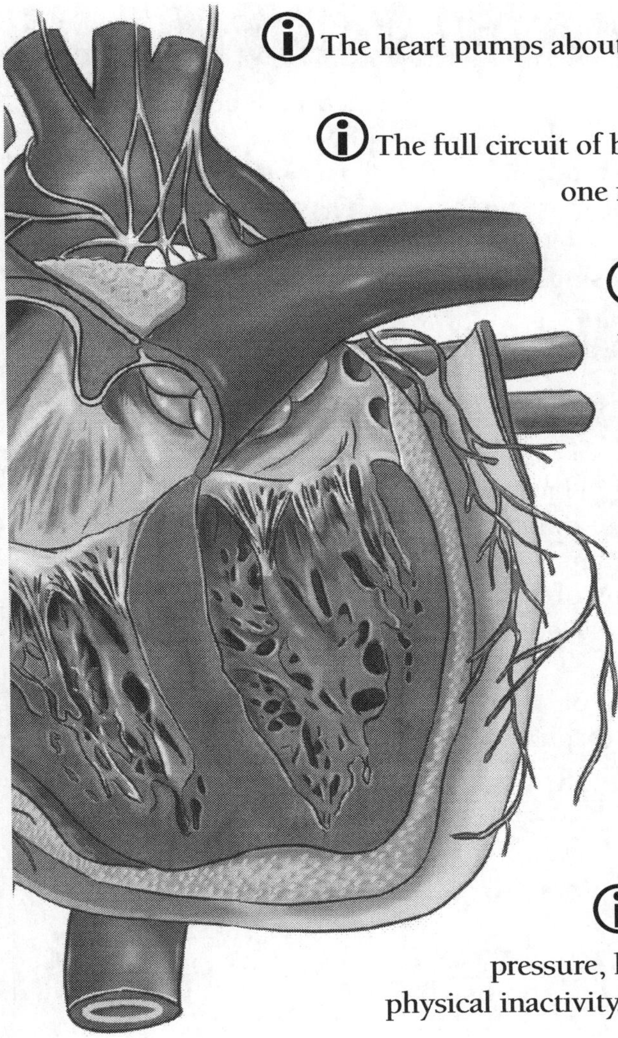

ⓘ The heart pumps about 5 to 7 quarts of blood a day.

ⓘ The full circuit of blood around the lungs and body takes about one minute when the body is at rest.

ⓘ Without control by nerves, the heart would beat about 100 beats per minute. However, parasympathetic nerves set a resting rate of 60 to 70 beats.

ⓘ One in ten American women ages 45 to 64 has some form of heart disease.

ⓘ In the United States , coronary heart disease (CHD) is the number one killer of both men and women. Each year , more than 50,000 Americans die of heart attacks caused by CHD.

ⓘ Risk factors for CHD include high blood pressure, high blood cholesterol, smoking, obesity and physical inactivity.

ⓘ Changing one's habits is the single most effective way to stop coronary heart disease from progressing. Changing your diet to low fat one, exercising regularly, and if you are a smoker, quit smoking and you will reduce your risk of heart disease.

Adapted from www.nhlbi.nih.gov/health

PO Box 2308, Woburn, MA 01888-0508, **p:** 781-729-3736, **www.EmbracingCulture.com**
PO Box 6401, Manchester, NH 03108, **p:** 1-888-678-CCCS

Lesson Six: Homework
The Samurai! Technique and the Cardiovascular System

1. **Let's test your knowledge about Medical Professionals. Without consulting the list of professions, try to match the following descriptions to the appropriate profession.**

Definition	Profession
1. A professional who fills or makes prescriptions.	A. Licensed Practical Nurse (LPN)
2. Physician who specializes in the prevention, diagnosis, and treatment of mental illness and can prescribe medication.	B. Pharmacist
3. A professional specializing in diagnosing and treating diseases of the brain, emotional disturbance, and behavior problems, and can only use talk therapy.	C. Psychiatrist
4. Professional nurse who provides direct care and makes decisions regarding plans of care for individuals and groups. They often have bachelor degree or associate degree in nursing.	D. Psychologist
5. Licensed nurses with two years of training that usually operate under the supervision of professional registered nurses or physicians.	E. Radiologist
6. A physician specialized in the branch of medicine that uses radiation for the diagnosis and treatment of disease.	F. Registered Nurse (RN)

2. **Cardiovascular System and Word Formation – Match the combining form in Column I with its meaning in Column II.**

Column I	Column II
_______ 1. arteriol/o	A. Small vein
_______ 2. phleb/o	B. Artery
_______ 3. arteri/o	C. Heart
_______ 4. angi/o	D. Small artery
_______ 5. venul/o	E. Vein
_______ 6. coron/o	F. Vessel

3. **Translate the 62 *Specialists* (found in the Additional Resources section) and their respective Departments into your TL**

Word	Target Language
1. Anesthesiologist	
2. Cardiologist	
3. Certified Nursing Assistant (CNA)	
4. Clinical Social Worker	
5. Counselor	
6. Dental Hygienist	
7. Dentist, DDS and DMD	
8. Dermatologist	
9. Embryologist	
10. Emergency Medical Technician (EMT)	
11. Endocrinologist	
12. Endodontist	
13. Epidemiologist	
14. Family Practitioner	
15. Gastroenterologist	
16. Gerondontist	
17. Gerontologist or Geriatrician	
18. Gynecologist	
19. Hematologist	
20. Hospitalist	
21. Internist	
22. Licensed Practical Nurse, LPN/LVN	
23. Medical Examiner	
24. Medical Transcriptionist	
25. Mental Health Worker	
26. Neonatologist	
27. Neurologist	
28. Nuclear medicine	
29. Nurse Midwife	

continued

PO Box 2308, Woburn, MA 01888-0508, **p:** 781-729-3736, **www.EmbracingCulture.com**
PO Box 6401, Manchester, NH 03108, **p:** 1-888-678-CCCS

	Word	Target Language
30.	Nurse Practitioner	
31.	Obstetrician	
32.	Oncologist	
33.	Occupational Therapist, OT	
34.	Ophthalmologist	
35.	Optometrist	
36.	Oral Surgeon	
37.	Orthodontist	
38.	Orthopedic Surgeon	
39.	Otologist	
40.	Otorhinolaryngologist	
41.	Paramedic	
42.	Pathologist	
43.	Pediatrician	
44.	Periodontist	
45.	Pharmacist	
46.	Physical Therapist, PT	
47.	Physician Assistant, PA	
48.	Proctologist	
49.	Psychiatrist	
50.	Psychologist	
51.	Public Health Nurse, PHN	
52.	Radiologic Technologist, RT	
53.	Radiologist	
54.	Records Technician, MRT	
55.	Registered Physical Therapist, RPT	
56.	Registered Nurse, RN	
57.	Respiratory Therapist or Pulmonary Therapist, ARRT	
58.	School Psychologist	
59.	Social Worker, BA, MSW, LCSW, LICSW	
60.	Surgeon	
61.	Traumatologist	
62.	Urologist	

4. **Translate the 14 *Illnesses or Conditions* found on page 18**

Word	Target Language
1. Artherosclerosis	
2. Myocardial Infarction	
3. Heart Murmur	
4. Arrhythmia	
5. Pericarditis	
6. Endocarditis	
7. Cardiomyopathy	
8. Hypertension or High Blood Pressure	
9. Pulmonary Embolism	
10. Aneurysm	
12. Coronary Artery Disease	
13. Lipedema	
14. Lymphedema	

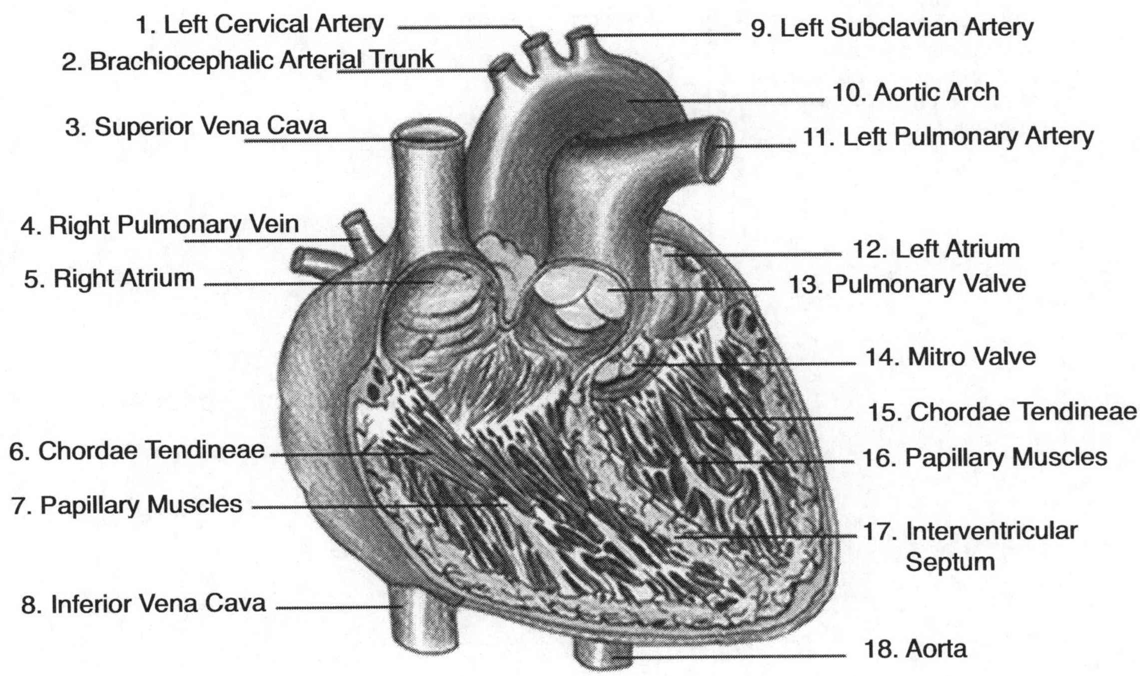

PO Box 2308, Woburn, MA 01888-0508, **p:** 781-729-3736, **www.EmbracingCulture.com**
PO Box 6401, Manchester, NH 03108, **p:** 1-888-678-CCCS

Lesson Six: Role-Plays
The Samurai! Technique and the Cardiovascular System

Work individually at first:

- Read the entire role-play
- Get a general sense of its meaning
- Circle the most challenging medical terms
- Apply the Samurai! technique to those terms
- Read the role-play again for a deeper understanding
- Find an accurate equivalent in the target language

Work in a language-specific group of friends, fellow students or colleagues:

- Share your doubts
- Ask for other ways of expressing the same meaning
- Develop a glossary
- Check the dictionary
- Practice the role-plays remember to do CIFE for all your role-plays
- Have your colleagues observe you and provide feedback on your accuracy and register.
- These colleagues can keep track of any omissions, additions, mistakes or distortions in your interpreting and point these out to you in a follow-up discussion.

Student Interpreter Evaluation

Student Name ____________________ Date

Language ____________________

Mode of Interpreting (check one): ☐ Consecutive ☐ Simultaneous

Role-Play/System ____________________

Areas Observed ____________________

Accuracy

Register ____________________

Omissions ____________________

Additions ____________________

Distortions ____________________

Pronunciation ____________________

Speaker's emotions conveyed? ____________________

Explain ____________________

Technique

General flow ____________________

Flow when requesting clarification ____________________

Speed ____________________

Eye Contact ____________________

Distracting Habits ____________________

Ethical Issues

Answered questions for patient? ____________________

Advised patient? ____________________

Vocabulary Expansion Recommendations

____

____

Other Recommendations

____

____

Language Coach Signature ____________________ Date

Role-Play 23: Shortness of Breath

	Pronunciation	Additions	Omissions	Mistakes
Myra: Oh doctor, I could not breathe, and then they told me I was an SOB!				
MD: Myra, I think in the ER they meant that you had "SOB" which means "shortness of breath."				
Myra: Oh, that's true.				
MD: Did you have chest pain?				
Myra: No, only shortness of breath.				
MD: Yes, they took a CXR and saw no pneumonia. They did a CT scan and saw no blood clot. The EKG showed lots of changes and then they did an echo, which showed that your heart was not pumping fully.				
Myra: Did I have a heart attack?				
MD: No, it looks like this came along with your cold symptoms from last week. You have an inflammation of the heart called a myocarditis. I checked a repeat EKG and echo today and I have good news. The changes are all back to normal. Are you feeling better?				
Myra: I haven't had shortness of breath in a week. When can I go back to work?				
MD: Well, let's have you rest for three more weeks. I'll check you then and if things are going well, I'll assume you've dodged a bullet, and send you back to work in a month's time.				
Myra: I don't have much sick time, Doctor.				
MD: I'll call the social worker, she'll check and see if there is disability insurance available to you while you recuperate. She'll check with your company.				
Myra: Thank you, Doctor.				
Break It Down	☐	☐	☐	☐

☐ **CIFE with patient** ☐ **CIFE with provider** ☐ **FLOW** ☐ **REGISTER**

Role-Play 23: Glossary

_______________ _______________ _______________

_______________ _______________ _______________

_______________ _______________ _______________

continued

PO Box 2308, Woburn, MA 01888-0508, **p:** 781-729-3736, **www.EmbracingCulture.com**
PO Box 6401, Manchester, NH 03108, **p:** 1-888-678-CCCS

1. Pathology (diseases, conditions)

2. Laboratory Tests and Diagnostic Procedures

3. Treatment Procedures

4. Idiomatic Expressions (if any)

5. Other (vocabulary in this particular role-play that you feel is important/relevant or that you anticipate problems with)

Role-Play 24: Fatima's Leg Pain

Fatima comes to the ER complaining of sudden onset of severe pain and weakness in her left leg. She is 61 years old.

	Pronunciation	Additions	Omissions	Mistakes
MD: What brings you here today?				
F: I've had terrible pain in my left leg! I can't move it. If I do, the pain gets worse. I can't even move my toes.				
MD: How long have you had this pain?				
F: Well, I've always had leg pain. But it's much worse in the past few days.				
MD: I see from your chart that you smoke. How long have you been a smoker?				
F: I had my first cigarette when I was 16. I've been smoking ever since.				
MD: I also see that your cholesterol and blood pressure have been high. Have you been taking your blood pressure and cholesterol medicine?				
F: I have to be honest with you doctor. I never renewed the prescriptions as they ran out. Anyway I did not feel any difference on or out of the medications... Also it does not help that my husband just got laid off and I have been very busy!				
MD: I understand. Let me examine you now.				
Examines patient				
MD: Well your left leg is weak, but what concerns me the most is that your leg is very cold and the pulses are hard to feel, especially compared to your right leg.				
F: What does that mean?				
MD: I think that you have a blockage of your femoral artery. I am going to call the vascular surgeon on call to examine you. I believe you will need a test called angiography to visualize where and how big the blockage is. Then the vascular surgeon can decide whether you need a procedure called an angioplasty which is a balloon that can open up the blockage.				
F: Let's do that.				
MD: Well, we'll see what he says. Often these large blockages can require a surgical procedure.				
Procedure called an embolectomy.				
F: Surgery. But with all this pain won't surgery make it worse?				
MD: It depends on the size and location of the blockage.				
F: I just thought you'd have to give me some pain medicine and I would be OK.				
MD: You will be feeling a lot better when that blockage is removed.				
Follow Up Visit Ten Days Later				

continued

PO Box 2308, Woburn, MA 01888-0508, **p:** 781-729-3736, **www.EmbracingCulture.com**
PO Box 6401, Manchester, NH 03108, **p:** 1-888-678-CCCS

Role-Play 24 *(continued)*

		Pronunciation	Additions	Omissions	Mistakes
MD:	Welcome back. How are you feeling?				
F:	You were right. Dr Brown, the vascular surgeon took one look at my leg and rushed me to radiology for a picture of my leg blockage.				
MD:	I heard.				
F:	He said it was very obstructed. He took the embolus out but then found other blockages that did not let my leg get better. So he did a bypass surgery.				
MD:	I know how much you disliked the idea of surgery.				
F:	I was not a happy person. But I tell you you were right in another way.				
MD:	How's that?				
F:	You said the pain would be gone and it's been gone for three to five days.				
MD:	I'm glad.				
F:	This is the best it's been in two to three years. And you know what, I can even walk up to 50 ft. without my calf giving me cramps walking. I was about to tell you about that but never got around to it.				
MD:	I hope you'll tell me what ever is going on or what is bothering you. If I had known about the leg cramps we might have sent you to Dr. Brown sooner. I also want to put you back on the meds you need for your blockage: I want you to be back on your beta blocker and your statin drug to help not only the cholesterol but fight the inflammation in your artery.				
F:	OK, but that's enough. You forget I'm on aspirin and my leg is really weak.				
MD:	Well I actually think you need another special blood pressure medication called an Ace Inhibitor. It is now felt that all patients with hardening of the arteries have better outcomes if they have one of those medicines on board.				
F:	Are you sure you're not giving me too many different medications?				
MD:	Well, I think you will need all of them but in the meantime we'll just restart the Beta Blocker and the statin and have you come back in four weeks and we'll see if you you can tolerate the Ace Inhibitor.				
F:	Don't forget I'm also on plavix and aspirin.				
MD:	I see that on your record. You should stay on the plavix for six months to a year and on the aspirin for the foreseeable future. They can cause bleeding so let me know if you have bleeding gums or blood in your urine.				
F:	I am feeling better, but I have to watch out for the medicines. It's always something.				
	Break It Down	☐	☐	☐	☐

☐ **CIFE with patient** ☐ **CIFE with provider** ☐ **FLOW** ☐ **REGISTER**

continued

Role-Play 24: Glossary

1. Pathology (diseases, conditions)

2. Laboratory Tests and Diagnostic Procedures

3. Treatment Procedures

4. Idiomatic Expressions (if any)

5. Other (vocabulary in this particular role-play that you feel is important/relevant or that you anticipate problems with)

PO Box 2308, Woburn, MA 01888-0508, **p:** 781-729-3736, **www.EmbracingCulture.com**
PO Box 6401, Manchester, NH 03108, **p:** 1-888-678-CCCS

Role-Play 25: High Blood Pressure

	Pronunciation	Additions	Omissions	Mistakes
MD: Hello Mr. Gonzalez. I have the results of the last four blood pressure tests that you did with our nurse practitioner.				
Mr. G.: What do you think?				
MD: Well, your weight continues to rise and so does your blood pressure. You know, if you could lose just five pounds, it would impact well on your blood pressure.				
Mr. G.: I do try, Doctor, but when I come home from work, it is so late and I am so hungry. Marta cooks for me and I love to eat her food.				
MD: Well, Mr. Gonzalez, you can eat her food but if you don't eat anything all day and come home starving, you will end up eating huge portions. And if you eat a large portion late at night, the fat will stay on. The trick is to eat several small meals a day and make the last one early in the evening.				
Mr. G.: That is tough to do. If I eat two meals a day, I'll just come home and eat again at dinner. I'll eat twice as much and gain more weight.				
MD: Why don't you try it my way for two weeks and see if there is a difference? Anyway, now I am going to have to start you on a medicine to help bring your blood pressure down. If you can lose the weight, we might be able to stop the medicine later. But now, after four months, it's time to begin a medication.				
Mr. G.: Oh no! Listen, I'll try the diet for two weeks. Let me see if I can stick with it. If not, I'll take the pill.				
MD: OK, I'll make you an appointment with Diane. If you lose a pound in two weeks or stay at the same weight, we'll put off the medicine. But if you gain a lb or more, we'll start the pill. It's called Hyrodrocholorthiazide and it gets rid of excess fluid. This helps control the blood pressure.				
Mr. G.: You'll see. I'll do it right this time.				

continued

Role-Play 25 *(continued)*

	Pronunciation	Additions	Omissions	Mistakes
MD: Good. Also, it is time for you to have an EKG to make sure your heart is not enlarged from high blood pressure. And by the way, I see that in the Dominican Republic you had a TB test that was positive. It has been two years since you had a CXR and we need to take another picture to ensure that you don't have active TB. So we'll do a CXR as well as the EKG before you leave today.				
Mr. G.: OK, as long as you don't have to draw blood.				
MD: No, I have what I need for now. But if we start the medicine, I'll have to order blood tests to watch your kidney function and your potassium.				
Mr. G.: Well, there's one more reason to lose weight. I'll do it.				
Break It Down	☐	☐	☐	☐

☐ **CIFE with patient** ☐ **CIFE with provider** ☐ **FLOW** ☐ **REGISTER**

Role-Play 25: Glossary

continued

PO Box 2308, Woburn, MA 01888-0508, **p:** 781-729-3736, **www.EmbracingCulture.com**
PO Box 6401, Manchester, NH 03108, **p:** 1-888-678-CCCS

1. Pathology (diseases, conditions)

2. Laboratory Tests and Diagnostic Procedures

3. Treatment Procedures

4. Idiomatic Expressions (if any)

5. Other (vocabulary in this particular role-play that you feel is important/relevant or that you anticipate problems with)

Role-Play 26: Blood Pressure Visit

	Pronunciation	Additions	Omissions	Mistakes
MD: Mrs. Silva, I am glad to see you. It has been a long time.				
SH: I've come to have you check my blood pressure.				
MD: Well, I'm happy to do that. But for all the years I've known you, I have never found you to have high blood pressure.				
SH: I know that, but I went to the drug store two months ago and just to be careful, I checked my blood pressure on the machine there and it was 150/90. Here are my notes. I have been going every week since and each time my blood pressure has been high.				
MD: Hmm, let me see. Well, let's check it now.				
(Checks blood pressure. Hortensia coughs.)				
MD: Well that's some cough. How long has that been going on?				
SH: About two months. Actually, I went to the drugstore that first day to buy a bottle of cough syrup.				
MD: Well, first let me tell you that your blood pressure today is fine. How is your weight?				
SH: I've lost 5 pounds, but I've been on that Oprah diet.				
MD: Are you smoking now?				
SH: Yes, I started again two months ago. I guess I was worried about the cough.				
MD: Are you making sputum when you cough?				
SH: Yes.				
MD: Have you seen blood in your sputum?				
SH: Yes, Doctor, that is why I am so worried. It won't stop.				
MD: OK, let me examine you now.				
(MD examines lungs, heart, abdomen, and feels for lymph nodes.)				
MD: SH, I hear some crackles in your left upper lung field. It could be pneumonia. I'd like to get a chest x-ray and some blood tests. Go on down to the lab, then come back with the x-ray.				

continued

PO Box 2308, Woburn, MA 01888-0508, **p:** 781-729-3736, **www.EmbracingCulture.com**
PO Box 6401, Manchester, NH 03108, **p:** 1-888-678-CCCS

Role-Play 26 *(continued)*

	Pronunciation	Additions	Omissions	Mistakes
(Patient goes to the lab, brings back the x-rays. MD reads them and comes back to the room.)				
MD: Well, Señora Hortensia, we have some things we need to talk about.				
Break It Down	☐	☐	☐	☐

☐ **CIFE with patient** ☐ **CIFE with provider** ☐ **FLOW** ☐ **REGISTER**

Role-Play 26: Glossary

continued

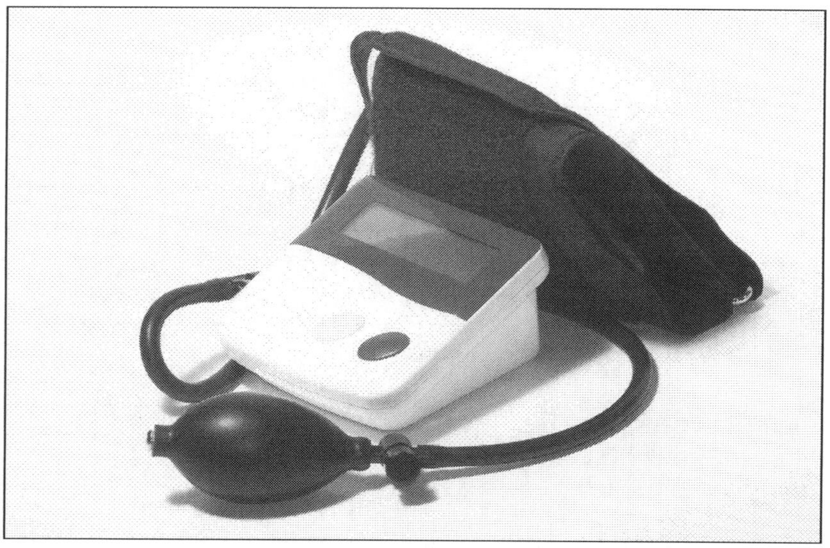

1. Pathology (diseases, conditions)

2. Laboratory Tests and Diagnostic Procedures

3. Treatment Procedures

4. Idiomatic Expressions (if any)

5. Other (vocabulary in this particular role-play that you feel is important/relevant or that you anticipate problems with)

PO Box 2308, Woburn, MA 01888-0508, **p:** 781-729-3736, **www.EmbracingCulture.com**
PO Box 6401, Manchester, NH 03108, **p:** 1-888-678-CCCS

Role-Play 27: Atrial Fibrillation

	Pronunciation	Additions	Omissions	Mistakes
MD: Hello, Mr. Sorrento. What brings you here today?				
PT: I've noticed that my heart is beating funny.				
MD: What do you mean?				
PT: It feels like it's beating in an odd way, sometimes fast, sometimes slow. It's just not regular like it used to be.				
MD: When does it do this?				
PT: All the time.				
MD: How long has this been going on?				
PT: Seven days.				
MD: Have you been feeling sweaty, getting chest pain or having shortness of breath during these last seven days?				
PT: No, not at all. Actually, I can still work out without any problems.				
MD: Has this ever happened to you before?				
PT: Sometimes, but it would always go away. This time it's not going away.				
Break It Down	☐	☐	☐	☐

☐ **CIFE with patient** ☐ **CIFE with provider** ☐ **FLOW** ☐ **REGISTER**

Role-Play 27: Glossary

continued

1. Pathology (diseases, conditions)

2. Laboratory Tests and Diagnostic Procedures

3. Treatment Procedures

4. Idiomatic Expressions (if any)

5. Other (vocabulary in this particular role-play that you feel is important/relevant or that you anticipate problems with)

PO Box 2308, Woburn, MA 01888-0508, **p:** 781-729-3736, **www.EmbracingCulture.com**
PO Box 6401, Manchester, NH 03108, **p:** 1-888-678-CCCS

Role-Play 28: Chest Pain

carro de carga

Mr. Lopes tried to work, carrying the curtain rolls; he tried to push the dollies, but he found he could not function due to his chest pain and shortness of breath. He knew it was serious and decided to go to the emergency room.

	Pronunciation	Additions	Omissions	Mistakes
MD: Mr. Lopes, what brings you to the emergency room?				
Mr. L: I have pain when I walk or work. A few days ago I felt a crushing pain in my chest and had difficulty catching my breath. I turned white, really pale, according to my friend. I sat down on a park bench and when I felt better I started to walk again but when I got up that hill to my house I felt shortness of breath again. I literally began to sweat, and felt shortness of breath and pressure, as if a large animal were sitting on my chest.				
MD: How long has it been bothering you?				
Mr. L: Since yesterday. It happens whenever I walk up a hill. You've got to fix me, because if I don't work, we can't eat! I got the pain again at work!				
MD: Do you sweat with this pain?				
Mr. L: Yes.				
MD: Do you get it when you exercise or when you are sitting still?				
Mr. L: I do not exercise. I work. I carry curtain rolls and push dollies.				
MD: Yes, I see. But the pain comes when you carry or push, not when you are at rest, right?				
Mr. L: That's right.				
MD: Do you smoke?				
Mr. L: Not really, only a pack a day.				
MD: Do you have anyone in your family with heart disease?				
Mr. L: My father had an attack when he was 45.				
MD: Any diabetes?				
Mr. L: Yes, I'm told I have a little of it. My doctor says all I have to do is take a pill. I haven't tried it yet.				
MD: OK, let me examine you and then we'll get an EKG.				

continued

Role-Play 28 *(continued)*

	Pronunciation	Additions	Omissions	Mistakes
MD: I'd like to take a look at an x ray as well and do some blood work.				
Mr. L: OK.				
(after results have arrived)				
MD: Mr. Lopes, I have some of your blood work back and the first cardiac enzyme is called troponin. It is elevated which suggests that there is damage going into the heart muscle. I also looked at your EKG and I've compared it with one you had at your physical with your primary care physician. There are changes in the electrocardiogram that suggest that the anterior wall of your heart is losing oxygen. The left side of the heart has a chamber called the left ventricle. This is the part that pumps the blood and the anterior portion of the ventricle provides most of the muscle that sends the blood all through the body. Because the heart cannot pump, the blood backs up in the lungs and you get short of breath. When blood backs up into the lungs, we call it congestive heart failure. Your chest X-ray shows signs of fluid in your lungs. I think you are having a myocardial infarction or a heart attack and it is causing your left ventricle not to work and you are in mild congestive heart failure. I have called the cardiologist, Dr. Trip. Mr. Lopes, I think he is going to want to give you some medicine that will help open your arteries. If that doesn't work, he may want to put dye in your heart's arteries in what we call a catheterization, so he can see if there's a blockage. If you have some blockage of the arteries, Dr. Trip will decide if he can do an angioplasty. That's when he puts a balloon in the artery and blows it up so that the obstructing clot and plaque get pushed to the sides of the artery and opens the flow. If you have too many blockages he can then suggest coronary artery bypass surgery, what we call a CABG. At any rate, we will see what he wants to do next. Do you have any pain now?				
Mr. L: No pain. I just got sick yesterday. (He starts to sweat.) You know, I think I feel that pressure again.				
MD: How bad on a ten scale?				

continued

PO Box 2308, Woburn, MA 01888-0508, **p:** 781-729-3736, **www.EmbracingCulture.com**
PO Box 6401, Manchester, NH 03108, **p:** 1-888-678-CCCS

Role-Play 28 *(continued)*

	Pronunciation	Additions	Omissions	Mistakes
Mr. L: What is a ten scale?				
MD: Well, you grade the pain with 0 being no pain and 10 being the worst pain you ever had.				
Mr. L: I don't know, I can't grade a pain.				
MD: Well, is it a little, slightly more than a little or a lot?				
Mr. L: It is a little. Not as bad as yesterday.				
MD: OK, we are going to give you some aspirin right now to fight the clot that we believe you have in your heart arteries and I am going to give you some IV morphine for pain. I am also going to start an IV drip of nitroglycerin that will help open your arteries so more blood can get through. I'm going to admit you to the hospital and the cardiologist will be down in a minute to help us decide what to do next. I think you will have to have the catheterization. Do you have any questions?				
Mr. L: I need to be home by tomorrow so I can go to work. Can you do all this by tomorrow?				
MD: We will do everything so that you can return to work healthy, but now your heart needs attention. Would you like me to write a note so to release you from your work?				
Mr. L: Yes, please. My wife can bring it tomorrow to my boss.				
MD: I am going to ask the nurse to begin the IV for you and she will be getting you ready upstairs.				
Break It Down	☐	☐	☐	☐

☐ CIFE with patient ☐ CIFE with provider ☐ FLOW ☐ REGISTER

Role-Play 28: Glossary

continued

1. Pathology (diseases, conditions)

2. Laboratory Tests and Diagnostic Procedures

3. Treatment Procedures

4. Idiomatic Expressions (if any)

5. Other (vocabulary in this particular role-play that you feel is important/relevant or that you anticipate problems with)

PO Box 2308, Woburn, MA 01888-0508, **p:** 781-729-3736, **www.EmbracingCulture.com**
PO Box 6401, Manchester, NH 03108, **p:** 1-888-678-CCCS

Additional Resources: The Samurai! Technique and the Cardiovascular System

WORD	TARGET	MEANING
Medical Professionals		
1. Anesthesiologist	Administers anesthesia during surgery	
2. Cardiologist	Treats diseases of the heart and blood vessels	
3. Certified Nursing Assistant (CNA)	Assistant who helps nursing staff perform uncomplicated, routine tasks.	
4. Clinical Social Worker	Social worker qualified to assess and treat patients for psychological problems, but cannot perform psychological testing or prescribe medication.	
5. Counselor	Professional who helps patients understand and solve adjustment problems.	
6. Dental Hygienist	Does prophylactic care: cleaning, teaching patients proper prophylactic care, takes X-rays.	
7. Dentist, DDS and DMD	Legally qualified practitioner of prevention, diagnosis and treatment of oral/dental deformities and disease	
8. Dermatologist	Qualified to practice prevention, diagnosis and treatment of skin disease and irregularities.	
9. Embryologist	Monitors prenatal development between the stages of ovum and fetus.	
10. Emergency Medical Technician (EMT)	Emergency paramedic	
11. Endocrinologist	Treats disorders of the endocrine glands.	
12. Endodontist	Treats diseases of pulp, does root canal work	
13. Epidemiologist	Studies factors regarding how to prevent, control, and contain communicable diseases	
14. Family Practitioner	Similar to general practice, but qualified as a specialty; also similar to internal medicine; an internist	
15. Gastroenterologist	Deals with diseases of the digestive system	
16. Gerondontist	Specializes in dental problems of the elderly	
17. Gerontologist or Geriatrician	Deals with all aspects of aging and disorders thereof	
18. Gynecologist	Concerned with female reproductive tract disorders and prenatal, delivery, and postpartum care	
19. Hematologist	Physician skilled in the diagnosis and treatment of blood and bone marrow diseases	
20. Hospitalist	Physicians, physician assistants, and nurse practitioners whose primary professional focus is hospital medicine	

continued

WORD	TARGET	MEANING
21. Internist	Focuses on medical conditions, but does not perform surgery or obstetrics	
22. Licensed Practical Nurse, LPN/LVN	Graduate of a one-year program, may perform some duties similar to a RN's in limited hospital settings	
23. Medical Examiner	Performs investigative examinations of bodies to determine the cause of death in suspicious or questionable circumstances	
24. Medical Transcriptionist	Technician who transcribes medical data	
25. Mental Health Worker	This description covers a wide variety of careers in mental health	
26. Neonatologist	Treats infants in first 6 weeks of life	
27. Neurologist	Deals with diseases and injuries to the brain, spinal cord, and nerves	
28. Nuclear medicine	Makes diagnostic and therapeutic use of radionuclides	
29. Nurse Midwife	RN with additional training; delivers in uncomplicated births	
30. Nurse Practitioner	A registered nurse with special training for providing primary health care, including many tasks customarily performed by a physician	
31. Obstetrician	Concerned with prenatal, delivery and postpartum care and disorders of the female reproductive system relating to such	
32. Oncologist	Uses radiation, surgery and chemotherapy in the treatment of tumors and cancers	
33. Occupational Therapist, OT	Trained therapist; uses self-care, work and physical recreation to increase patient mobility and coordination	
34. Ophthalmologist	Deals with eye disease and eye surgery, prescribes glasses and does eye exams	
35. Optometrist	Treats refractive errors; fits eyeglasses	
36. Oral Surgeon	Performs complicated dental extractions and treats maxillofacial trauma cases and congenital defects such as cleft palate	
37. Orthodontist	Treats malocclusion with braces and retainers	
38. Orthopedic Surgeon	Treats disorders of musculoskeletal system and joint diseases	
39. Otologist	Deals with ear surgery, hearing problems, hearing aids	
40. Otorhinolaryngologist	Treats ear, nose, and throat (ENT) disorders and performs surgery	
41. Paramedic	Ambulance attendant	
42. Pathologist	Diagnoses morbid changes in tissues from biopsy or postmortem	
43. Pediatrician	Deals with disease prevention, diagnosis and treatment of children, usually to age 16	

continued

PO Box 2308, Woburn, MA 01888-0508, **p:** 781-729-3736, **www.EmbracingCulture.com**
PO Box 6401, Manchester, NH 03108, **p:** 1-888-678-CCCS

WORD	TARGET	MEANING
44. Periodontist	Treats gum disease such as gingivitis; performs surgery, deep cleaning and gingivectomy	
45. Pharmacist	Licensed to prepare and dispense drugs	
46. Physical Therapist, PT	Performs treatment by physical means such as heat, cold, and exercise	
47. Physician Assistant, PA	Performs examinations, simple suturing, etc.	
48. Proctologist	Treats diseases of the rectum and sigmoid colon	
49. Psychiatrist	Diagnoses and treats mental disorders; may prescribe medications	
50. Psychologist	Treats emotional disorders, but in most cases cannot prescribe medications	
51. Public Health Nurse, PHN	RN with at least a BS degree; works for health departments, schools or health agencies	
52. Radiologic Technologist, RT	Takes X-ray films, prepares patients for X-ray films	
53. Radiologist	Uses radiant energy, X-rays, radium and cobalt in diagnosis and treatment	
54. Records Technician, MRT	Collects, files, organizes and retrieves medical data	
55. Registered Physical Therapist, RPT	Performs treatment by physical means such as heat, cold and exercise	
56. Registered Nurse, RN	Nurse; may work in hospitals, clinics or medical offices	
57. Respiratory Therapist or Pulmonary Therapist, ARRT	Treats patients with breathing difficulties	
58. School Psychologist	Psychologist working in a school or educational institution; treats emotional disorders but cannot prescribe medication	
59. Social Worker, BA, MSW, LCSW, LICSW	A professional trained to assist individuals and communities with emotional, financial and social well-being. There are several levels of social work, and some social workers are called 'clinicians'	
60. Surgeon	Performs general surgery	
61. Traumatologist	Deals with injury, both accidental and physiological	
62. Urologist	Treats urinary tract diseases and disorders of the male reproductive organs	

Demystifying Medical Terminology Through the Samurai! Technique

Medical terminology is traditionally intimidating. To the inexperienced interpreter, providers may seem to be speaking a foreign tongue. Medical vocabulary consists of complex terms of Greek and Latin origin, as well as slang, jargon, and abbreviations. An interpreter without this knowledge can inadvertently become an "outsider." So as medical interpreters, we have found Dr. Richard Lane's Samurai! technique to understanding medical terminology very helpful.

The Samurai! technique draws a parallel from the samurai warriors of ancient Japan to modern-day medical interpreters. The samurai were members of the warrior elite, and their distinctive trademark was the katana, or sword. As interpreters, we too are equipped with a katana, the knowledge that enables us to chop complex medical terms into smaller, easily understandable parts.

Many medical terms consist of a combination of a prefix, word root, and suffix. We have provided you with a concise list of commonly used word parts. It is imperative that you practice and learn all of the prefixes, roots and suffixes on the list. By training you, the interpreter-samurai, to recognize key word parts and abbreviations, we are giving you the tools needed to unveil the mysteries of medical terminology.

We know that mastery of medical terminology is not the sole indicator of professionalism in interpreting. However, medical terms can be intimidating if not immediately recognized, and

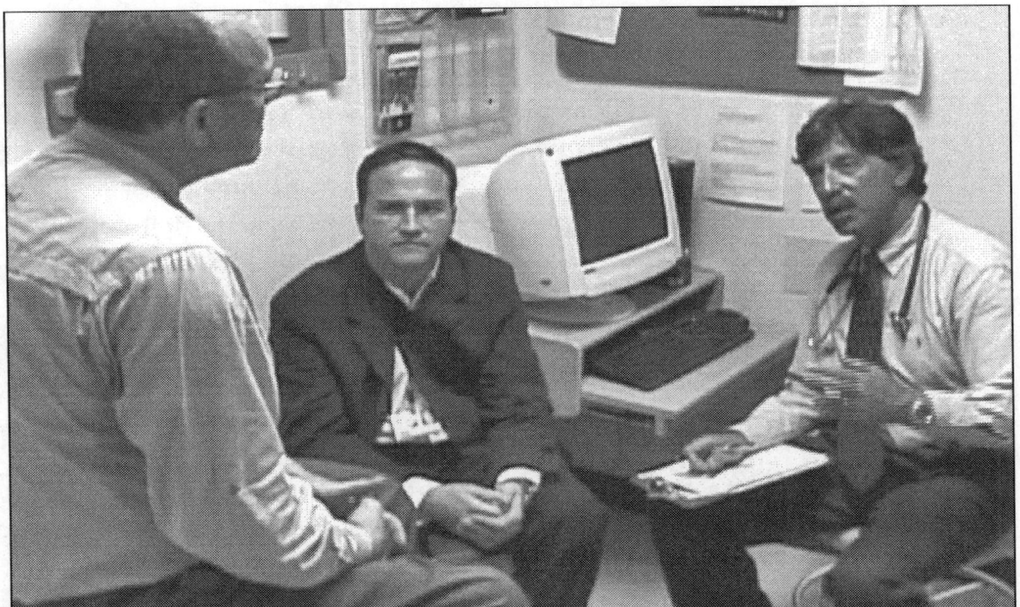

PO Box 2308, Woburn, MA 01888-0508, **p:** 781-729-3736, **www.EmbracingCulture.com**
PO Box 6401, Manchester, NH 03108, **p:** 1-888-678-CCCS

feelings of intimidation can negatively impact an interpreter's accuracy. When an interpreter is lost in a message, key words will invariably be lost in its translation. We don't expect you to become a health care provider. We simply want you to successfully manage the triadic encounter.

An interpreter familiar with medical terms and their meanings will likely interpret more quickly and with greater accuracy than an interpreter who has no clue what the provider is talking about. Also, providers generally value knowledge of medical terminology and are often more likely to trust an interpreter proficient in "medicalese." Note, however, that an interpreter should never use the power of medical language as a means of intimidating, scaring or confusing patients.

An interpreter has the ethical obligation to inform the provider when a patient seems to not understand the interpretation from English to the target language. Rather than embarrassing the patient by saying to the provider, "The patient does not understand you," the professional interpreter might solicit a simplified explanation of a term or concept by asking the provider to "break it down."

It has been suggested that the best way to make sure the patient is keeping up with the provider's register is to encourage the provider to ask the patient to recap the information out loud and to express any doubts. This technique of asking a patient to teach back has become an integral component of patient centered care approach to the patient provider dyad.

With bilingual workers, especially those who grew up in the United States, there is a tendency to perform well with medical terminology in English while repeatedly missing the target language equivalents. And because many of our non English-speaking and LEP patients will not question authority (in this case, the interpreter), providers and institutions may never become aware of this discrepancy in linguistic equivalency.

If unsupervised, the interpreter will be the only one who knows about the "misses" in the interpretation, and it takes a mature professional to acknowledge mistakes and to correct them on the spot. For example, an interpreter may understand that the English word "constipation" refers to a difficulty releasing, a normal bowel movement. However, in Portugal, the word "constipação" (a false cognate) can refer to a cold.

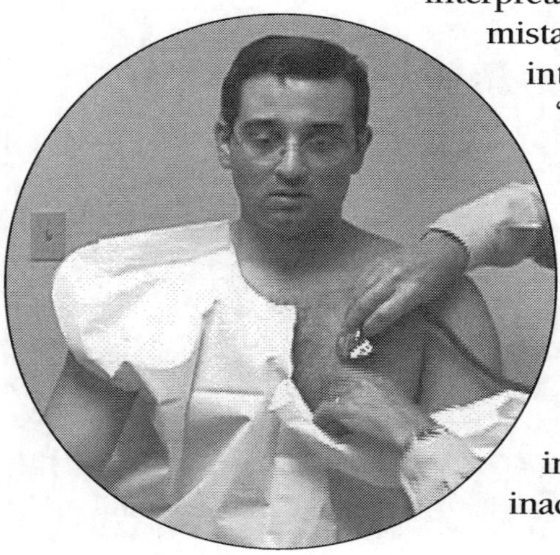

Another Portuguese term, "angina do peito" is the target language equivalent of the English word "angina," a condition where a patient suffers from chest pain. However, the Portuguese word "angina" can also refer to tonsillitis, an inflammation of the tonsils. If the interpreter does not check in with the patient to clarify meaning, the result may well be an inaccurate interpretation.

Prefix - Root - Suffix

WORD	MEANING	TARGET
a-	no, not, without	
abdomin/o	abdomen	
able, -ible	capable of, able to	
-ac, -al, -an, -ar, -ary	pertaining to	
acr/o	extremities (arms and legs)	
actin/o	light	
acu/o	sharp, severe, sudden	
ad-	toward	
aden/o	gland	
adenoid/o	adenoids	
adip/o	fat	
-al	pertaining to	
albumin/o	protein	
-algia	pain	
an-	no, not, without	
andr/o	male	
aneurysm/o	aneurysm	
angi/o	vessel	
ankyl/o	crooked, bent, stiff	
ante-	before	
anter/o	anterior, toward the front	
anti-	against, opposite	
anxi/o	uneasy, anxious	
aort/o	aorta	
-apheresis	removal	
appendic/o	appendix	
aque/o	water	
-ar	pertaining to	
-arche	beginning	
arter/o, arteri/o	artery	
arteri/o	artery	
arteriol/o	arteriole	
arthr/o	joint	
-arthria	articulate (speak distinctly)	
asthenia	weakness, debility	
-ation	process	
audi/o	hearing	
auruicul/o	ear	
aut/o	self, own	
azot/o	urea, nitrogen	

a

continued

PO Box 2308, Woburn, MA 01888-0508, **p:** 781-729-3736, **www.EmbracingCulture.com**
PO Box 6401, Manchester, NH 03108, **p:** 1-888-678-CCCS

	WORD	MEANING	TARGET
b	bacteri/o	bacteria	
	balan/o	glans penis	
	bi-	two	
	bil/i	bile, gall	
	blephar/o	eyelid	
	brachi/o	arm	
	brachy-	short	
	brady-	slow	
	bronch/o, bronchi/o	bronchi	
	bucc/o	cheek	
	burs/o	bursa (sac of fluid near joints)	
c	calc/i	calcium	
	calcane/o	calcaneus (heel bone)	
	cancer/o, carcin/o	cancer, cancerous	
	cardi/o	heart	
	carp/o	carpus (wrist bone)	
	cata-	down	
	caus/o	burn, burning	
	cauter/o	heat, burn	
	-cele	hernia	
	-centesis	puncture to remove fluid	
	cephal/o	head, toward the head	
	cerebr/o	brain, cerebrum	
	cervic/o	neck, cervix (neck of uterus)	
	-chalasis	relaxation	
	chem./o	drug, chemical	
	cholecyst/o	gallbladder	
	cholesterol/o	cholesterol (a lipid substance)	
	chrom/o	color	
	chondr/o	cartilage	
	chron/o	time	
	-cidal	pertaining to killing	
	cis/o	to cut, used primarily in words like incision (to cut into) & excision (to cut out/remove)	
	clavicul/o	clavicle (collar bone)	
	-clysis	irrigation, washing	

continued

WORD	MEANING	TARGET
coagul/o	coagulation (clotting)	
col/o	colon (large intestine)	
colp/o	vagina	
comat/o	deep sleep	
con-	together, with	
conjuctiv/o	conjunctiva	
cor/o	of or pertaining to the eye's pupil	
coron/o	heart	
corpo/o	body	
cortic/o	cortex	
crypt/o	hidden	
-cusis	hearing	
cutane/o	skin	
cyan/o	blue	
cyst/o	urinary bladder	
-cytosis	condition of cells, slight increase in numbers	
derm/o, dermat/o	skin	
-derma	skin	
desicc/o	to dry	
-desis	to bind, tie together	
di-	two	
dia-	through	
diaphor/o	sweat	
dilat/o	enlarge, expand	
-dilation	widening	
dips/o	thirst	
dist/o	far or from the point of origin or attachment	
dolich/o	long	
dors/o	back	
dorsi-	back	
duct/o	to lead	
duoden/o	duodenum	
dynam/o	power, strength	
-dynia	pain	
dys-	bad, difficult, painful	
-eal	pertaining to	
ech/o, son/o	sound	
-ectasia, -ectasis	dilatation, stretching	

c

d

e

PO Box 2308, Woburn, MA 01888-0508, **p:** 781-729-3736, **www.EmbracingCulture.com**
PO Box 6401, Manchester, NH 03108, **p:** 1-888-678-CCCS

	WORD	MEANING	TARGET
e	ecto-	out, outside	
	-ectomy	excision	
	electr/o	electricity	
	-ema	blood condition	
	-emesis	vomiting	
	-emia, hem/a, hem/o	blood, blood condition	
	-emic	pertaining to blood condition	
	en-	in	
	encephal/o	brain (en = in, cephal/o = head)	
	endo-	within	
	enter/o	intestines (usually small intestines)	
	epi	above, around	
	episi/o	vulva	
	erythr/o	red	
	-esis	condition	
	eso-	inward	
	esthesi/o	feeling	
	estr/o	female	
	ex-, exo-	out, without, away from	
	exanthamat/o	rash	
	excision	to cut out, remove	
	extra-	outside	
f			
	femor/o	femur (thigh bone)	
	fibros/o	fibrous connective tissue	
	fibul/o	fibula	
	-fida	split	
	furc/o	forking, branching	
	-fusion	to pour	
g			
	galact/o	milk	
	gastr/o	stomach	
	gen/o	producing, beginning	
	-genesis	producing, forming	
	gester/o	pregnancy	
	gingiv/o	gum	
	glauc/o	gray	
	-globin	protein	
	glomerul/o	glomerulus	
	glyc/o, glycos/o	sugar	
	gon/o	seed	

continued

WORD	MEANING	TARGET
gonad/o	sex glands	
-gram	a record	
gram/o	to record	
-graph	recording instrument	
-graphy	process of recording	
gravid/o	pregnancy	
gynec/o	women, female	
hem/a, hem/o, hemat/o	blood	
hemi-	half, partly	
hemi, semi	half	
hepat/o	liver	
hidr/o	perspiration	
holo	entire, complete	
home/o	like, resembling	
hydr/o	water	
hyper	above, excessive, more than normal	
hypn/o	sleep	
hypo	deficient, below, under	
hyster/o	uterus, womb	
-ia	condition	
-iasis	abnormal condition	
-iac, -ic, -ical	pertaining to	
ichthy/o	dry, scaly	
idi/o	unknown, individual, distinct	
ili/o	ilium, expansive portion of the hip bone	
-in, -ine	a substance	
infra-	below, inferior to, beneath	
inter-	between	
intra-	within, in	
-ion	process	
-ior	pertaining to	
isch/o	to hold back	
-ism	condition, theory	
-ist	one who	
-itis	inflammation	
-ium	membrane	
-ive	pertaining to	

g

h

i

continued

PO Box 2308, Woburn, MA 01888-0508, **p:** 781-729-3736, **www.EmbracingCulture.com**
PO Box 6401, Manchester, NH 03108, **p:** 1-888-678-CCCS

	WORD	MEANING	TARGET
k	kal/i	potassium	
	ket/o, keton/o	ketones, ketone bodies, acetones	
	-kinesis	movement	
	klept/o	to steal	
l	labi/o	lip, labia	
	lacrim/o	tear, tear duct, lacrimal duct	
	lact/o	milk	
	lapar/o	abdominal wall, abdomen	
	laryng/o	larynx (voice box)	
	-lepsy	seizure	
	-leptic	to seize, take hold of	
	leuc/o, leuk/o	white	
	-lexia	word	
	lip/o	fat, lipid	
	lithotomy	incision (for removal of a stone)	
	lith/o	stone, calculus	
	lob/o	lobe	
	-logist	one who studies, specialist	
	-logy	study or science of	
	lumph/o	lymph, lymphatics	
	lymphat/o	lymphatics	
	-lysis	loosening, dissolution, separating, dissolving	
m	mal-	bad	
	-malacia	softening	
	meat/o	meatus	
	medull/o	medulla	
	mega-	large	
	megal/o	enlargement	
	men/o	menses, menstruation	
	-meter	instrument used to measure	
	-metry	process of measuring	
	-micro	small	
	mono-	one, single	
	morph/o	shape, form	
	multi-	many	
	muscul/o	muscle	
	my/o	muscle	
	mydr/o	wide	
	myocardi/o	myocardium (heart muscle)	
	myx/o	mucus	

continued

n

WORD	MEANING	TARGET
narc/o	numbness, stupor, sleep	
nas/o	nose	
nat/i	birth	
necr/o	dead, death	
neo-	new	
nephr/o	kidney	
neur/o	nerve	
noct/i	night	
nucle/o	nucleous	
nulli-	none	

o

WORD	MEANING	TARGET
ocul/o	eye	
odont/o	tooth	
-oid	resembling	
-ole	little, small	
olig/o	scanty	
-oma	tumor (occasionally, swelling)	
onc/o	mass, tumor	
-one	hormone	
onych/o	nail	
-opia	vision	
-opsia	vision	
opt/o	eye, vision	
orchi/o	testis	
-orexia	appetite	
-orrhaphy	suturing, repairing	
-ose	sugar	
-osis	condition	
oste/o	bone	
-otia	ear condition	
-ous	pertaining to, characterized by	
ox/o	oxygen	
oxy-	swift, rapid, acid	
oxys/o	sudden	

p

WORD	MEANING	TARGET
palpebr/o	eyelid	
pancreat/o	pancreas	
para-	near, beside, abdominal, apart from, along the side of	
-pareunia	sexual intercourse	
-partum	birth, labor	
patell/a	patella	

continued

PO Box 2308, Woburn, MA 01888-0508, **p:** 781-729-3736, **www.EmbracingCulture.com**
PO Box 6401, Manchester, NH 03108, **p:** 1-888-678-CCCS

p

WORD	MEANING	TARGET
path/o	disease	
-pathy	disease	
ped/o	child, foot	
-penia	deficiency	
-pepsia	digestion	
per-	through	
-pexy	fixation	
-phagia	eating, swallowing	
phak/o	lens of eye	
pharmacy/o	drugs, medicine	
pharyng/o	throat, pharynx	
phas/o, -phasia	speech	
phleb/o	vein	
phon/o	voice, sound	
-phoresis	carrying, transmission	
phot/o	light	
phren/o	mind, diaphragm	
-phylaxis	protection	
plas/o	development	
-plasia	development, formation, growth	
-plasty	repair	
pleg/o	paralysis	
-plegia	paralysis, palsy	
pleur/o	pleura	
-pnea	breathing	
pneum/o, pneumon/o	lung, air	
pod/o	foot	
-poiesis	formation	
polio-	gray matter of brain or spinal cord	
poly-	many, much	
post-	after, behind	
poster/o	posterior, toward the back	
pre-	before	
primi-	first	
pro-	before	
proct/o	anus and rectum	
prote/o, protein/o	protein	
prostat/o	prostrate gland	
proxim/o	near	
psych/o	mind	
-ptosis	sagging, prolapse	
pulmon/o	lung	
pyret/o	fever	

continued

WORD	MEANING	TARGET	
quadri-	four		q
radi/o	rays (usually x-ray), radiant energy (this combining form is also used for radius, a bone of the forearm)		
rect/o	rectum		r
ren/o	kidney		
resection-	to cut back, or out		
retin/o	retina		
retro-	behind, back		
-rrhage	excessive bleeding		
-rrhagia	hemorrhage		
-rrhaphy	suture		
rrhytm/o	rhythm		
sacchar/o	sugar		
salping/o	uterine (fallopian) tube, oviduct, auditory (eustachian) tube		s
-schisis	to split		
sclera/o, -sclerosis	hard, hardening		
-scopy	visual examination		
sect/o	to cut		
secti/o	to cut, section, cutting into		
-sis	state of, condition		
-sol	solution		
somat/o	body		
somn/o	sleep		
-somnia	sleep		
son/o	sound		
-spasm	twitching, cramp		
sperm/o	spermatozoa, sperm cells		
-sphyxia	pulse		
spin/o	spine (backbone), spinal cord		
spleen/o, splen/o	spleen		
-stasis	stopping, controlling		
-static	pertaining to stopping, controlling		
-stenosis	tightening, stricture		
stern/o	sternum (breastbone)		
stomat/o	mouth		
-stomy	new opening		
sub-	under		
super-, supra-	above, beyond, upper		
syncop/o	to cut off, cut short		

continued

PO Box 2308, Woburn, MA 01888-0508, **p:** 781-729-3736, **www.EmbracingCulture.com**
PO Box 6401, Manchester, NH 03108, **p:** 1-888-678-CCCS

	WORD	MEANING	TARGET
t	tachy-	fast	
	tetra-	four	
	test/o	testis,testicle	
	therm/o	heat	
	thorac/o	chest	
	-thorax	pleural cavity, chest	
	thromb/o	thrombus, blood clot	
	-thymia	mind	
	-thymic	pertaining to mind	
	tom/o	cut, section	
	-tome	instrument used for cutting	
	-tomy	incision, cutting, operation, to section, make an incision	
	tone/o	to stretch	
	tonsill/o	tonsil	
	top/o	place, position	
	tox/o	poison	
	trache/o	windpipe	
	trachel/o	neck, neckline	
	trans-	across	
	tri-	three	
	trigon/o	trigone	
	-tripsy	surgical crushing	
	-trophy	nourishment, development	
u	-ule	little	
	umbilic/o	navel, umbilical cord	
	-ur/o, -urin/o, -uria	urine, urea, urinary tract, urination	
	ureter/o	ureter	
	urethr/o	urethra	
	urin/o	urine	
	uter/o	uterus, womb	
v	vag/o	vagus nerve	
	vagin/o	vagina	
	valvul/o	valve	
	vas/o, vascul/o	blood vessel	
	ven/o	vein	
	ventr/o	belly, side of body	
	ventricul/o	ventricle (of brain or heart), lower heart chamber	
	vesic/o	urinary bladder	
	viscer/o	internal organs	

continued

WORD	MEANING	TARGET
vitr/o	vitreous body (of the eye)	
vitre/o	glassy	
vol/o	volume	
voyeur/o	to see	
vulv/o	vulva	
xanth/o	yellow	

V

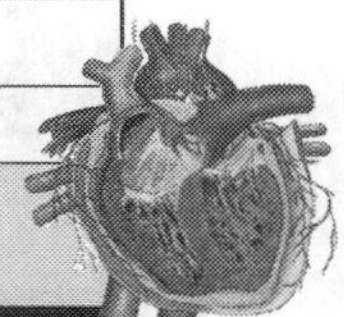

Cardiovascular System / Vocabulary

Main Organs and Body Structures	Target
Aneurysm	
Aorta	
Arteries	
Arteriole	
Atrioventricular valves	
Atrium (plural: atria)	
Bicuspid valve	
Blood vessels	
Bundle of his	
Capillaries	
Chordae tendineae	
Cusps	
Deoxigenated blood	
Diastole	
Endocardium	
Epicardium	
Fibrous connective tissue	
Heart	
Mitral valve	
Myocardium	
Oxygen	
Parietal layer	
Pericardial cavity	
Pericardium	
Pulmonary artery	
Pulmonary valve	
Pulmonary vein	
Semilunar valve	
Septum (plural:septa)	
Sinoatrail node	
Superior vena cava	
Systole	

continued

PO Box 2308, Woburn, MA 01888-0508, **p:** 781-729-3736, **www.EmbracingCulture.com**
PO Box 6401, Manchester, NH 03108, **p:** 1-888-678-CCCS

Main Organs and Body Structures	Target
Tricuspid valve	
Veins	
Ventricles	
Venule	
Visceral layer	

Main Tests and Procedures	Target
Anastomosis	
Aneurysmectomy	
Angiography	
Angioplasty	
Aortography	
Arteriography	
Atherectomy	
Automatic implanted	
Cardioverter defibrillator	
Cardiac catheterization	
Cardiac enzyme studies	
Cardiac MRI	
Cardiopulmonary resuscitation (CPR)	
Coagulation tests	
Coronary bypass surgery	
Defibrillation, cardioversion	
Digital subtraction	
Angiography	
Doppler ultrasonography	
Duplex scanning	
Echocardiography	
Electrocardiography	
Endarterectomy	
Holter monitoring	
Intraluminal coronary artery	
Stent placement	
Lipid profile	
Lipoprotein electrophoresis	
Pacemaker	
Pericardicentesis	
Sclerotherapy	
Serum enzyme tests	
Stress test	
Thrombolytic therapy	
Troponini	
Valve replacement	
Valvuloplasty	
Vena cava filter	

Blood and The Immune and Lymphatic Systems

Main Organs and Body Structures	Target
Anisocytosis	
Erythrocyte	
Erythropoiesis	
Erythropoietin	
Hematopoiesis	
Hemocytoblast	
Hemolysis	
Immunoglobulins	
Kuper cells	
Leukocyte	
Leukocytosis	
Lymphoblast	
Lysosomes	
Macrophage	
Monoblast	
Myelogenous	
Myeloid	
Natural killer (nk) cell	
Normochromia	
Osteoclast	
Pathogen	
Phagocyte	
Poikilocytosis	
Reticulocyte	

Main Illnesses	Target
Adenoiditis	
Aids	
Anaphylaxis	
Anemia	
Asplenia	
Cytomegalovirus	
Elephantiasis	
Epstein-Barr virus	
Erythremia	
Hematoma	
HIV-positive	
Hyperchromia	
Hypersensitivity	
Hypersplenism	

continued

PO Box 2308, Woburn, MA 01888-0508, **p:** 781-729-3736, **www.EmbracingCulture.com**
PO Box 6401, Manchester, NH 03108, **p:** 1-888-678-CCCS

Main Illnesses	Target
Hypocrhomia	
Hypogammaglobulinemia	
Immunodeficiency	
Karposi sarcoma	
Leukemia	
Lymphadenitis	
Lymphadenopathy	
Lymphangioma	
Lymphatic carcinoma	
Lymphedema	
Lymphoid aplasia	
Lymphoma	
Mononucleosis	
Phlebitis	
Pneumonia	
Sarcoidosis	
Systemic lupus	
Erythematosus	
Thrombosis	
Tonsillitis	

Main Tests and Procedures	Target
Antiglobulin test	
Antinuclear antibody titer	
Bone marrow aspiration	
Biopsy	
Bone marrow	
Transplantation	
Cd4 cell count	
Chemotherapy	
Electrophoresis	
Hematocrit (hct)	
Hemostasis	
Immunization	
Immunosuppression	
Lymphangiography	
Splenomegaly	
Splenorrhaphy	
Thymectomy	
Tissue typing	
Transplantation	
Western blot	

Lesson Seven:
The Digestive System

Understanding Goals

Students will:

- review learned concepts
- practice the Samurai! Technique
- understand major organs, organ systems and their respective functions (Digestive System)
- sharpen their consecutive interpreting skills through role-play practice

Key Concepts

- Digestive System

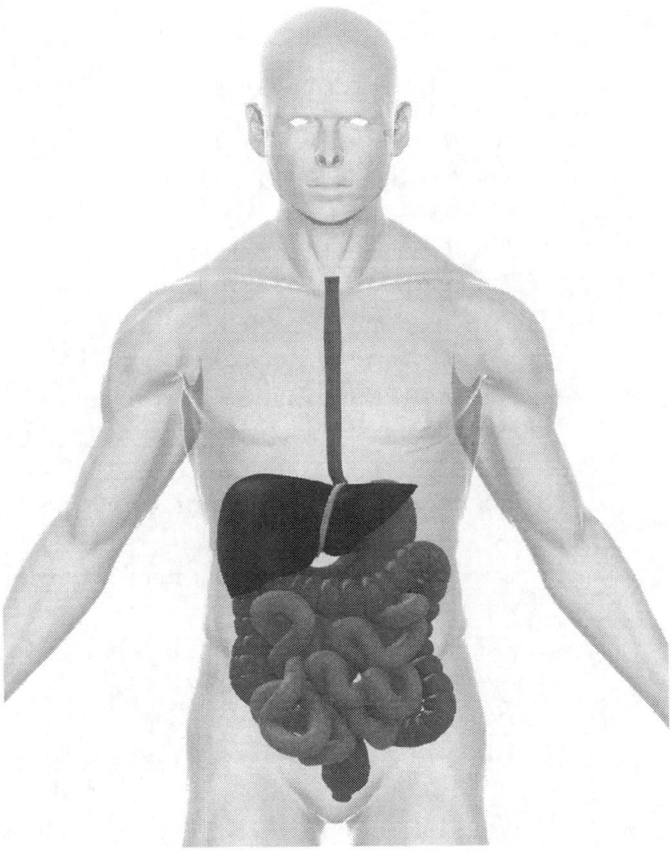

PO Box 2308, Woburn, MA 01888-0508, **p:** 781-729-3736, **www.EmbracingCulture.com**
PO Box 6401, Manchester, NH 03108, **p:** 1-888-678-CCCS

Quiz

THE ART OF MEDICAL INTERPRETATION®

Lesson Seven: Quiz
The Digestive System

Mark each item "True" or "False."

1. Heartburn is a symptom of acid reflux. It can be caused by eating chocolate or drinking alcohol or caffeine.
   ○ True ○ False
2. Most peptic ulcers can be treated with medicine, thus avoiding surgery.
   ○ True ○ False
3. Hepatitis C is passed by sexual contact so patients with this disease should stop all sexual contact with their partners.
   ○ True ○ False
4. Gastroenteritis is caused by gallstones.
   ○ True ○ False
5. An outpouching of the colon is a diverticulum. If it gets inflamed, we say the patient has diverticulitis.
   ○ True ○ False
6. The breaking down of starch into component sugars is an example of how the digestive system breaks down nutrients mechanically.
   ○ True ○ False
7. All chest pain is caused by problems of the heart.
   ○ True ○ False
8. The liver, gallbladder and pancreas all connect to the small intestine at the duodenum.
   ○ True ○ False
9. The small intestine only functions as a transport tube. It provides no other functions.
   ○ True ○ False
10. The appendix has no known contribution to digestion.
    ○ True ○ False
11. The liver and the pancreas are both vulnerable to the effects of excessive alcohol use.
    ○ True ○ False
12. The gastrointestinal tract is 90 feet long and it has six sections: oral cavity, esophagus, stomach, small intestine, tongue, and teeth.
    ○ True ○ False
13. The food being digested in the stomach is now called bolus.
    ○ True ○ False
14. The duodenum is the last part of the small intestine.
    ○ True ○ False
15. The last part of the colon, just before the anus has an s-shape and it's called the sigmoid colon.
    ○ True ○ False
16. The gallbladder is an organ on the underside of the liver that produces urine.
    ○ True ○ False
17. In addition to producing enzymes that breakdowns proteins, fats and carbohydrates, the pancreas also produces insulin.
    ○ True ○ False

Lesson Seven: Class Activities
The Digestive System

gallbladder removed

ENT, otorrinolaringologo

REVIEW

A. Match the combining form (root word) in column I with its meaning in column II:

	Column I	Column II
I	1. cholecyst/o	A. Mouth
C	2. col/o	B. Endocrine and exocrine gland near the stomach
J	3. duoden/o	C. Large intestine
G	4. gastr/o	D. Liver
D	5. hepat/o	E. Anus and rectum
F	6. ile/o	F. Third part of the small intestine
A	7. or/o	G. Stomach
B	8. pancreat/o	H. Throat
H	9. pharyng/o	I. Gallbladder
E	10. proct/o	J. First section of the small intestine

B. Using the root words above, write down as many words as you remember:

~~Cholesterol~~

Colitis

Oral cavity

Gastroenteritis Gastric Gastritis

Hepatitis

Pancreatitis

Pharyngitis Pharynge

PO Box 2308, Woburn, MA 01888-0508, p: 781-729-3736, www.EmbracingCulture.com
PO Box 6401, Manchester, NH 03108, p: 1-888-678-CCCS

Introduction to the Digestive System

How much do you know?

1. Label the main organs of the digestive system in the diagram below in English and in your TL
2. Briefly explain the function of each organ
3. Write one paragraph summarizing the path of food through the digestive system

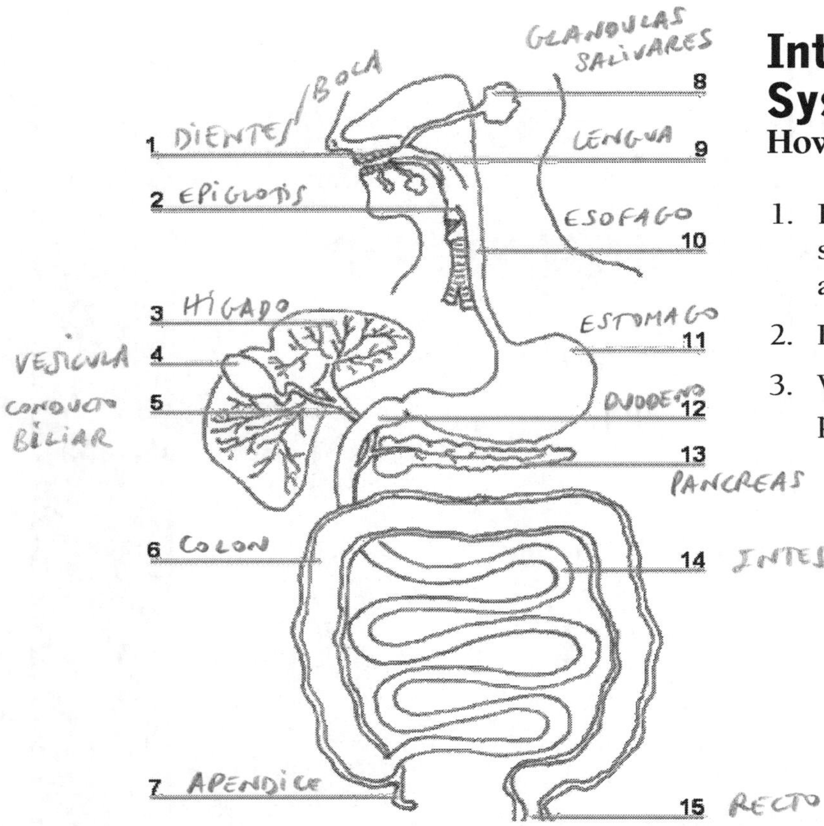

	ORGAN	FUNCTION
1	Mouth/teeth	CHEW THE FOOD
2	EPIGLOTIS VALV.	CLOSES THE TRAQUEA WHEN FOOD COMES IN.
3	LIVER	BREAKS FAT DOWN, MAKES PROTEIN.
4	GALLBLADER	STORES AND CONCENTRATE THE BILE FROM THE LIVER
5	GALLBLADER DUCT (BILE DUCT)	WHERE THE BILE GOES THROUGH TO THE SMALL
6	COLON	WATER AND SALT ABSORVED AND THE REST INTO FECES
7	APPENDIX	GETS INFLAMED IF FOOD GETS CAUGHT IN IT
8	SALIVARY GLANDS	PRODUCES SALIVA THAT CONTAINS AMYLASE
9	TONGUE	AIDS IN SHAPING FOOD INTO A BOLUS
10	ESOPHAGUS	PROPELS THE BOLUS INTO THE STOMACH
11	STOMACH	ENZYME CALLED PEPSIN - BREAKS DOWN FOOD
12	DUODENUM	
13	PANCREAS	PRODUCES INSULINE
14	SMALL INTESTINE	SECRETION OF ENZYMES FOR DIGESTION
15	ANUS	

The Digestive System

The digestive system is the system responsible for taking energy and nutrients from the environment, allowing the body to use them, and depositing waste products back into the environment. The digestive system takes food and breaks it down both physically and chemically so the body can extract energy and nutrients from it. This system breaks down food, stores it, digests it and eliminates waste. The digestive system consists of (1) the gastrointestinal tract and (2) the accessory organs.

1. The Gastrointestinal Tract

The gastrointestinal tract runs from the mouth to the anus. It is 30 feet long and has six sections: oral cavity, esophagus, stomach, small intestine, large intestine, and anus. There are also six accessory digestive organs: the salivary glands, tongue, teeth, gall bladder, pancreas, and liver.

The Oral Cavity

The first section of this 30-foot long gastrointestinal tract is the oral cavity, consisting of the mouth and pharynx. In the mouth are the teeth, tongue and salivary glands. The teeth break food down into smaller chunks that can be swallowed. These smaller chunks are then broken down further by chemical processes. The tongue is a mucous covered muscle that shapes the chewed food. The salivary glands moisten the chewed food and begin the chemical breakdown with amylase, converting complex carbohydrates into their component sugars.

Try this: Put a piece of unbuttered bread in your mouth and just chew it. At some point you will notice that the bread begins to taste sweet. It is at this moment that amylase is breaking down the carbohydrate called starch into sweeter sugars you can taste. This is chemistry at work.

The chewed food, which is called a bolus, moves from the mouth into the throat or pharynx. Because the pharynx leads into the larynx (or voice box) as well as the esophagus, it can transport both air and bolus. In this case, muscles will then propel the bolus from the pharynx into the esophagus. During swallowing, the larynx rises up and presses against a piece of cartilage called the epiglottis. It closes off the opening to the trachea and allows the bolus to move into the esophagus without "going down the wrong pipe."

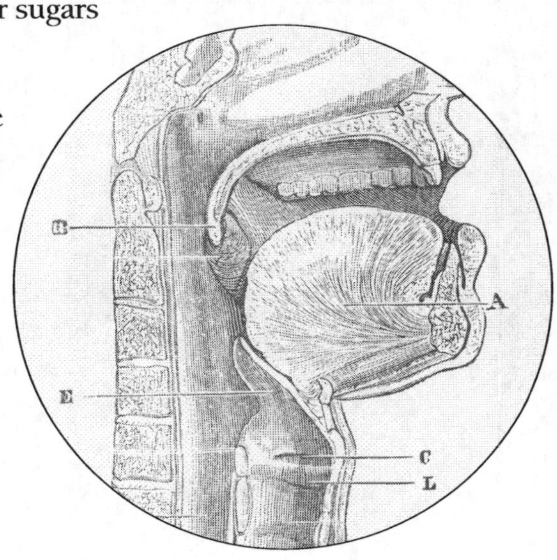

PO Box 2308, Woburn, MA 01888-0508, p: 781-729-3736, www.EmbracingCulture.com
PO Box 6401, Manchester, NH 03108, p: 1-888-678-CCCS

The Esophagus

The esophagus is a 10-inch long muscular tube that sequentially propels the bolus into the stomach.

Did you know you can swallow upside down? Why is this? It is because of the orderly contraction of the muscles of the esophagus that propels food to the stomach. It doesn't matter if you're upside down or right side up. The orderly progression of muscle contraction in the digestive tract is called peristalsis. Sometimes the muscles in the esophagus do not contract in order. When that happens, people can get chest pain that feels like a heart attack. Therefore, keep in mind that all chest pain is not from the heart. Peristalsis occurs throughout the GI tract. When the bolus gets to the bottom of the esophagus, the lower esophageal sphincter opens and allows the bolus into the stomach. If this sphincter is weakened by structural abnormalities or by chemicals like alcohol, chocolate or caffeine, acid can climb up the esophagus causing a burning pain. This is called acid reflux. When the bolus gets into the stomach, the action begins.

Stomach

Where is the stomach exactly? When a lot of people point to where they think their stomach is, they're actually pointing at the location of their large and small intestines. In other cultures, a person might point to other regions such as the chest. The truth is that the stomach is the j-shaped organ in the left upper quadrant of the abdomen.

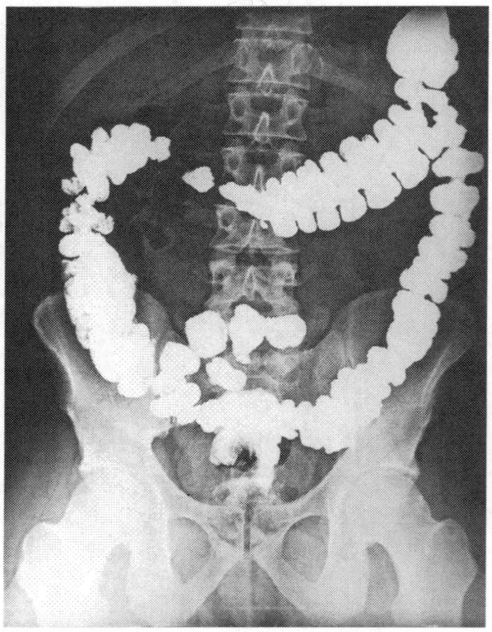

The stomach makes an enzyme called pepsin, which works with gastric acid to break proteins into smaller units called peptides. An enzyme from the pancreas, called lipase, breaks down fat into glycerol and fatty acids. Amylase, this time from the pancreas, continues to work on starch. The stomach makes hydrochloric acid, which helps to activate pepsin. The acid can also kill bacteria. Food passes from the mouth in about one minute. It takes two to three seconds to be swallowed by the esophagus. Then it stays two to four hours in the stomach being digested.

The food being digested in the stomach is now called chyme. The stomach squirts the chyme into the small intestine through its distal opening called the pyloric sphincter.

Small Intestine – Duodenum, Jejunum, and Ileum

The small intestine consists of the duodenum, jejunum and ileum. It is the major site of digestion and absorption of nutrients.

The **duodenum**, the first part of the small intestine, is approximately 10 inches long (25cm) and was measured in the old days as "twelve fingerbreadths" long. The word duodenum comes from the Latin, duodeni, which means "twelve each." The duodenum is the place where the liver, gallbladder, and pancreas inject their respective enzymes and digestive juices. The common bile duct and pancreatic duct meet there in the ampulla of Vater. Here the pancreas puts in lipase and amylase. It also contributes trypsin and chymotrypsin that split proteins into smaller units as well.

The next section of the small intestine is the **jejunum**, approximately 8 feet long. It comes from the Latin word, jejunus, which means "devoid of nutritive value." Perhaps this was because there was no obvious function of the jejunum other than as a transport tube. We'll discuss why this was found not to be true in a moment.

The **ileum**, being 12 feet long, is the third and final section of the small intestine. The word ileum comes from the Latin word for groin or viscera. Cells in the stomach secrete a protein called intrinsic factor. This combines with vitamin B12 to allow B12 to be absorbed into the blood stream. This absorption occurs in the ileum. People who have inflammation of the ileum or ileitis lose the ability to absorb the B12-intrinsic factor complex and thus become Vitamin B12 deficient. This is sometimes called pernicious anemia.

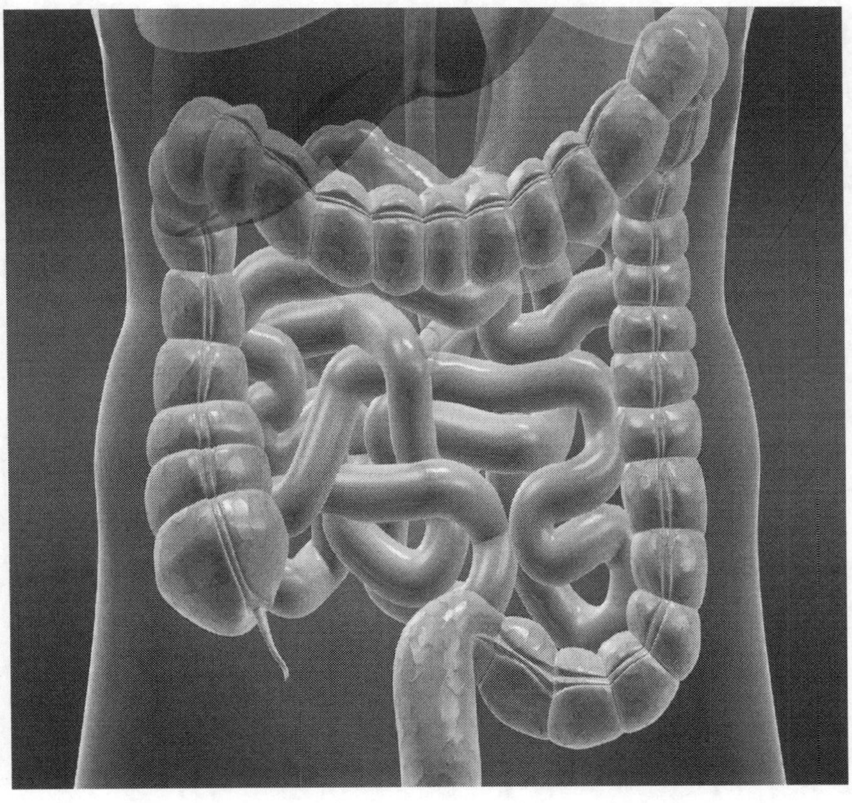

PO Box 2308, Woburn, MA 01888-0508, **p:** 781-729-3736, **www.EmbracingCulture.com**
PO Box 6401, Manchester, NH 03108, **p:** 1-888-678-CCCS

The small intestine is more than just a transporting tube. In the walls of the small intestine are cells that secrete enzymes that continue the digestive process. Enzymes like maltase, sucrase and lactase are secreted here. They convert disaccharide sugars into monosaccharide sugars that are more easily absorbed into the blood stream. Peptidase, also found in the intestinal wall, breaks down large peptides (protein building blocks) into smaller peptides and amino acids. Why is this important? If there is an infection or inflammation of the small intestine, the cells that make these enzymes are sloughed off and the enzymes temporarily are not produced. So the big disaccharide sugars like lactose are not broken down. They stay in the lumen (central opening) of the intestine. Large molecules attract water so that the inside of the lumen has more water. The more water, the looser the stool and hence you get diarrhea. It is also here that those with lactose intolerance have their deficit: no cells making lactase. Without lactase, more lactose remains in the small intestine causing more diarrhea and pain.

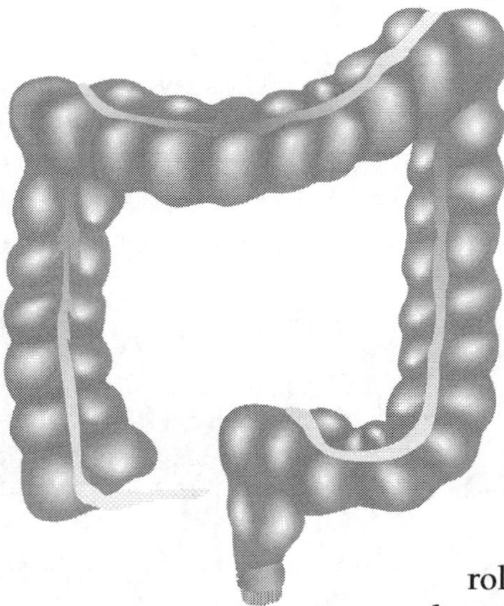

Large Intestine or Colon

From the small intestine, the further digested chyme goes into the large intestine. The large intestine is also called the colon and is 5 feet long. Here, water and salt are further absorbed into the body by cells in the lining of the lumen. The remaining material is pressed into feces and stored for excretion. The first part of the large intestine is the cecum. The cecum has a small ribbon-like appendage called the appendix. If foodstuffs get caught here, the appendix can become inflamed. This is called appendicitis. At present, the appendix has no known positive role in digestion. The last part of the colon before the anus is an s-shaped section called the sigmoid colon.

The Anus

The anus consists of a series of smooth muscles that open upon relaxing, allowing the feces to be moved out by peristalsis in the large intestine.

Chyme may travel through the small intestine in 1 to 4 hours. It may go through the colon anywhere from 10 hours to several days. Thus the total transit time of food digestion and absorption is 14 hours to several days. The longer the transit time, it is thought, the more exposure the digestive tract has to carcinogens and toxins. It is felt that high fiber diets improve transit time. Those who subsist on high fiber diets tend to have a lesser incidence of colon cancer.

2. The Accessory Organs

There are six accessory digestive organs: the salivary glands, tongue, teeth, liver, gall bladder, and pancreas.

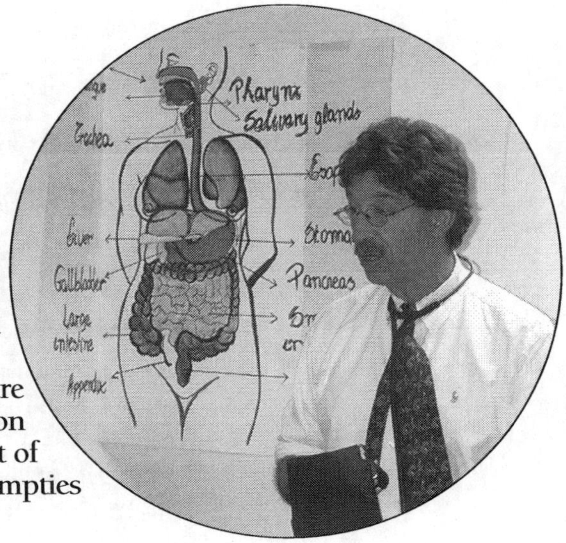

The Salivary Glands

The salivary glands are three sets of glands in the area surrounding the mouth. They produce saliva, which moistens food and makes it easier to form a bolus. Saliva also contains amylase, which breaks down carbohydrates. The parotid gland is a large pancake-shaped gland located in front of each ear. It gets inflamed with certain viral infections like mumps. There are two submandibular glands located back at the lower jawbone on either side. There are two sublingual glands located at the front of the mouth under the tongue. Each gland has a tiny duct that empties saliva into the mouth.

The Tongue

The tongue, as described earlier, is a smooth mucous covered muscle. It aids in speech and in shaping food material into a bolus to be swallowed.

The Teeth

The teeth crush and tear food so it can be easily swallowed.

The Liver

The liver is a large rust-colored organ in the right upper quadrant of the body. Its many functions include producing cholesterol and making bile from the breakdown of fat and old red blood cells. It also makes protein and stores iron, glycogen and vitamins. The liver cells make bile, which is passed on through tiny ducts that merge to form the common hepatic duct. The bile moves down the common hepatic duct through the cystic duct to the gall bladder where it is stored and concentrated. When the body eats a fatty meal the gall bladder contracts and squeezes, forcing bile back up the cystic duct to the common bile duct and into the duodenum through the ampulla of Vater.

The Gallbladder

The gallbladder is an organ on the underside of the liver on the right side of the abdomen. The function of the gallbladder is to store and concentrate the bile that is produced in the liver before the bile is secreted into the intestines.

The Pancreas

The pancreas is a long thin gland that sits under the liver and over the duodenum. It produces enzymes, as we have discussed, that break down proteins, fats and carbohydrates. It also produces sodium bicarbonate that neutralizes stomach acid. The enzymes are secreted into ductules, which converge to form the pancreatic duct. This duct goes into the ampulla of Vater along with the common bile duct. Both bile and pancreatic enzymes flow into the duodenum here. The pancreas is also the gland that makes insulin. This hormone is crucial in helping the body obtain energy. It allows glucose to be absorbed into the cells where it is used to produce energy.

PO Box 2308, Woburn, MA 01888-0508, p: 781-729-3736, www.EmbracingCulture.com
PO Box 6401, Manchester, NH 03108, p: 1-888-678-CCCS

EXERCISE

TEST YOUR UNDERSTANDING!

Match each description with its respective organ or disease:

______	1. A smooth mucous covered muscle.	A.	Chyme
______	2. A long thin gland that sits under the liver and over the duodenum. It produces enzymes.	B.	Ulcer
______	3. The third and final section of the small intestine.	C.	Gallbladder
______	4. Food being digested in the stomach.	D.	Appendix
______	5. Frequent or lasting indigestion is often a warning sign of this condition.	E.	Tongue
______	6. The stomach squirts the chyme into the small intestine through this opening.	F.	Pyloric sphincter
______	7. Sac that stores bile.	G.	Sigmoid colon
______	8. S-shaped lower portion of the large intestine.	H.	Ileum
______	9. Organ that makes bile, stores sugar, and produces proteins to clot blood.	I.	Pancreas
______	10. Small sac that hangs from the beginning of the large intestine.	J.	Liver

EXERCISE

Fill in the blanks:

1. The gastrointestinal tract is __________ feet long and food can take __________ hours to __________ days to pass from mouth to anus in the digestive system.

2. Saliva moistens the food and also contains __________, an enzyme that breaks starches down into their component sugars.

3. The liver has many functions and one of them is to create __________, a digestive juice made from degraded blood pigments, which helps to digest fats.

4. The __________ is a gland that makes amylase, as do the salivary glands. It also makes other enzymes that break down fats and proteins, and manufactures __________, which is important for absorbing glucose into cells.

Illnesses and Conditions of the Digestive System

Now that we talked about how the digestive system operates, let's learn about diseases. Below you will find summaries of some common illnesses of the digestive system.

EXERCISE

Divide into groups. Divide the illnesses accordingly. Study them well and prepare to give a short presentation to the class about them.

ILLNESS	MEANING	TARGET
1. Acid Reflux	A backflow of stomach contents upward into the esophagus. Symptoms will occur if the lower esophageal sphincter is weak or if it is stimulated to open inappropriately. Chocolate, alcohol, caffeine and the hormonal changes of pregnancy can cause the sphincter to open. The chief symptom is heartburn.	
2. Acute Pancreatitis	Acute or sudden inflammation of the pancreas heralded by pain, nausea and vomiting. The most common causes are gallstones and alcohol damage to the pancreas.	
3. Alcoholic Hepatitis	A range of inflammations of the hepatocytes caused directly by the effect of alcohol on the liver as well as by acetaldehyde, which is a metabolite of alcohol digestion.	
4. Anal Fissure	A tear or ulcer in the lining of the anus.	
5. Cirrhosis	Consists of bands of scar tissue which destroy not only the hepatocytes themselves but also the ductules which bring bile and other products out of the liver in well organized canals or ducts. This destruction leads to increased backpressure when blood from the portal vein goes into the liver to bring deoxygenated blood to the liver. The back flow is called portal hypertension and ultimately this leads to lower extremity edema, hemorrhoids in both the esophagus (varices) as well as in the rectum.	
6. Constipation	Condition of uncomfortable or infrequent bowel movements.	
7. Diarrhea	Increase in the volume, wateriness or frequency of bowel movements.	
8. Diverticular Disease	Fifty percent of Americans over the age of 50 get sac-like, out- pouching of any portion of the gastrointestinal tract, though this is most often found in the large intestine. The presence of a diverticulum is called diverticulosis. An inflammation or infection inside an out-pouching is called diverticulitis.	

continued

PO Box 2308, Woburn, MA 01888-0508, **p:** 781-729-3736, **www.EmbracingCulture.com**
PO Box 6401, Manchester, NH 03108, **p:** 1-888-678-CCCS

ILLNESS	MEANING	TARGET
9. Food Poisoning	A subset of gastroenteritis. It can be caused by ingesting food with bacteria that has toxins, or by chemical toxins in seafood or in plants such as mushrooms. Lactose intolerance may cause symptoms strong enough to be called gastroenteritis. Some heavy metals such as arsenic lead, mercury or cadmium in food can cause nausea, vomiting and diarrhea, while many antibiotics can cause abdominal cramps and diarrhea.	
10. Gallstones	Stones made of bile pigment and cholesterol can form in the gall bladder or common bile duct. If the stone is blocking the cystic or common bile duct when a fatty meal causes the gallbladder to contract, pain can occur because there is no egress of the bile and pressure builds acutely in the biliary system. Secondly, any blockage of the bladder or of a duct allows bacteria to fester and grow. This is called cholecystitis when the bladder is blocked, and cholangitis when the duct is blocked. If the stones block lower in the duct and obstruct the pancreatic duct, acute pancreatitis can occur.	
11. Gastroenteritis	A syndrome of nausea, vomiting and diarrhea that can be produced by bacteria, such as salmonella, campylobacter, or E. coli. Some viruses, intestinal parasites and chemical toxins can all cause this syndrome. The chief downside here is the inflammation of the small intestine, which causes diarrhea, and the loss of protein and water through the small and large intestine. Vomiting can also lead to dehydration and abnormalities of the electrolytes. Electrolytes are minerals that become ions in solution. An ion carries an electrical charge thus these minerals are "electro" lytes. One electrolyte that is heavily involved is potassium. When someone has gastroenteritis, much potassium is excreted out of the system through diarrhea and vomitus. Low potassium can cause heart problems. Little children are at great risk from gastroenteritis. They can become quite dehydrated in a short time with this illness.	

continued

ILLNESS	MEANING	TARGET
12. Hemorrhoids	Swollen veins in the walls of the rectum and anus. They are equivalent to varicose veins in the lower extremities.	
13. Hepatitis	Inflammation of the liver is usually caused by viruses, especially Hepatitis A, B, C and D. Hepatitis can be acute or chronic. There are non-viral causes as well, which include herbal supplements, toxic chemicals and alcohol.	
14. Hepatomegaly	Enlargement of the liver caused by acute hepatitis, fatty infiltration, congestion with blood (i.e. CHF) or a tumor.	
15. Inflammatory Bowel Diseases	Inflammatory disorders in which the intestine becomes inflamed, often causing recurring cramps and diarrhea. Two forms of this condition are Crohn's Disease and Ulcerative Colitis.	
16. Irritable Bowel Syndrome	Disorder of motility of gastrointestinal tract that produces abdominal pain, constipation or diarrhea. It is a diagnosis of exclusion. That means that all other infectious or structural causes need to be ruled out in most patients before the diagnosis of irritable bowel syndrome can be given.	
17. Jaundice	Yellow discoloration of the skin and the whites of the eyes caused by abnormally high levels of the blood pigment, bilirubin, in the blood. This can be caused by a loss of functional hepatocytes in acute hepatitis or by the obstruction of the biliary tree by gallstones or a tumor.	
18. Liver Encephalopathy	Decreased brain function or coma due to increased build-up of toxic substances usually removed by the liver.	
19. Pancreatic Carcinoma	Originates in pancreatic ducts and is associated with tobacco smokers and those with chronic pancreatitis. Prognosis is poor, with around 2% surviving five years after the diagnosis. The actual cause is unknown. Symptoms include a dull abdominal pain radiating to the back with nausea and weight loss.	

PO Box 2308, Woburn, MA 01888-0508, **p:** 781-729-3736, **www.EmbracingCulture.com**
PO Box 6401, Manchester, NH 03108, **p:** 1-888-678-CCCS

EXERCISE

TEST YOUR UNDERSTANDING!

Using your knowledge from last class and what you are learning today, Match the illnesses/conditions in Column I with its meaning in Column II. Use the Samurai! technique:

	Column I	Column II
_______	1. Jaundice	A. Pain of the stomach
_______	2. Hepatitis	B. Stones made of bile pigment and cholesterol that can form in the gallbladder or common bile duct.
_______	3. Hepatomegaly	C. Yellow discoloration of the skin and other tissues
_______	4. Cirrhosis	D. Chronic disease of the liver with degeneration of liver cells.
_______	5. Gallstones	E. Inflammatory disorders in which the intestines become inflamed.
_______	6. Inflammatory bowel disease	F. Enlargement of the liver.
_______	7. Stomatitis	G. Inflammation of the mouth
_______	8. Gastralgia	H. Inflammation of the liver

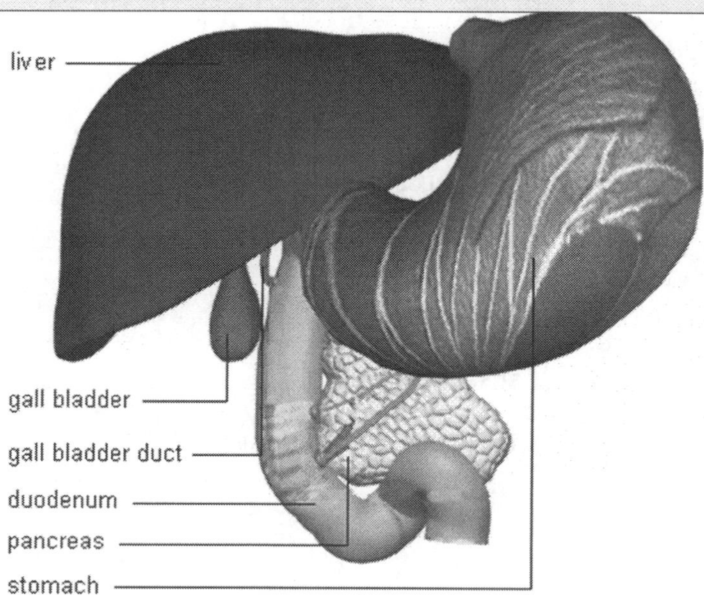

Food Poisoning is one of the diseases of the Digestive System. Watch the video "Spreading Menace" from the *Body Story* DVD to learn more about this common disease. Use the space below to take notes on what you see or what you find interesting.

What is the treatment for Food Poisoning?

PO Box 2308, Woburn, MA 01888-0508, **p:** 781-729-3736, **www.EmbracingCulture.com**
PO Box 6401, Manchester, NH 03108, **p:** 1-888-678-CCCS

EXERCISE

In the Additional Resources section of this lesson you will find a list of MAIN TESTS AND PROCEDURES related to the Digestive System. Using your "Samurai" skills, match the test or procedure in Column I with its description in Column II.

	Column I	Column II
______	1. Cholecystectomy	A. Direct visual inspection of the rectum and lower intestine
______	2. Colonoscopy	B. Surgery that removes all or part of the stomach
______	3. Gastrectomy	C. A passage done via surgery that allows fecal material to be excreted from the ileum to an opening in the abdominal wall
______	4. Gastrostomy	D. Removal of the gallbladder via open surgery or laparascopy
______	5. Sigmoidoscopy	E. Direct visual examination of the colon
______	6. Ileostomy	F. Surgical creation of a passage through the abdominal wall into the stomach for putting feeding preparations directly into the stomach

Lesson Seven: Homework
The Digestive System

1. Go over your notes for today's class and read section "Additional Resources"
2. Read and practice ALL role-plays for this lesson
3. Continue developing your glossary
4. Translate the gastrointestinal tract and the accessory organs into your TL.

Word	Target Language	Word	Target Language
1. oral cavity		9. anus	
2. esophagus		10. salivary glands	
3. stomach		11. tongue	
4. small intestine		12. teeth	
5. duodenum		13. liver	
6. jejunum		14. gallbladder	
7. ileum		15. pancreas	
8. large intestine		16. appendix	

5. Translate the 19 common illnesses of the Digestive System:

Word	Target Language	Word	Target Language
1. acid reflux		11. gastroenteritis	
2. acute pancreatitis		12. hemorrhoids	
		13. hepatitis	
3. alcoholic hepatitis		14. hepatomegaly	
4. anal fissure		15. inflammatory bowel disease	
5. cirrhosis		16. irritable bowel syndrome	
6. constipation			
7. diarrhea		17. jaundice	
8. diverticular disease		18. liver encephalopathy	
9. food poisoning		19. pancreatic carcinoma	
10. gallstones			

THE ART OF MEDICAL INTERPRETATION®

Homework

PO Box 2308, Woburn, MA 01888-0508, **p:** 781-729-3736, **www.EmbracingCulture.com**
PO Box 6401, Manchester, NH 03108, **p:** 1-888-678-CCCS

6. Translate the main tests and procedures of the Digestive System

Word	Target Language
1. abdominal CT scan	
2. abdominal MRI	
3. abdominal ultrasound	
4. barium tests	
5. cholangiography	
6. cholecystectomy	
7. colonoscopy	
8. colostomy	
9. endoscopy	
10. gastrectomy	
11. gastrointestinal endoscopy	
12. gastrostomy	
13. hemorrhoidectomy	
14. ileostomy	
15. LFTs	
16. laparoscopy	
17. occult blood test	
18. sigmoidoscopy	
19. stool culture	
20. UGI series	

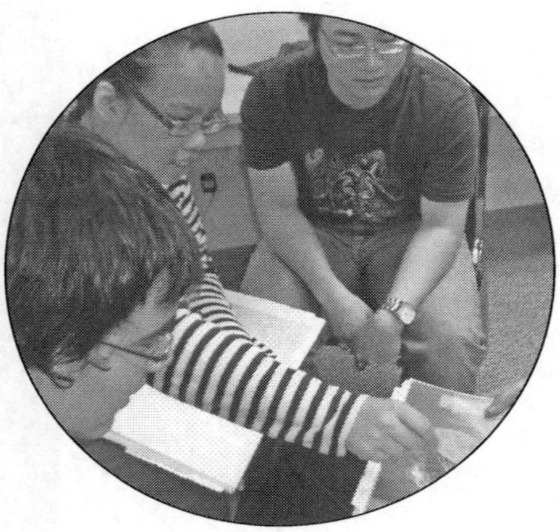

Lesson Seven: Role-Plays
The Digestive System

Work individually at first:

- Read the entire role-play
- Get a general sense of its meaning
- Circle the most challenging medical terms
- Apply the Samurai! technique to those terms
- Read the role-play again for a deeper understanding
- Find an accurate equivalent in the target language

Work in a language-specific group of friends, fellow students or colleagues:

- Share your doubts
- Ask for other ways of expressing the same meaning
- Develop a glossary
- Check the dictionary
- Practice the role-plays remember to do CIFE for all your role-plays
- Have your colleagues observe you and provide feedback on your accuracy and register.
- These colleagues can keep track of any omissions, additions, mistakes or distortions in your interpreting and point these out to you in a follow-up discussion.

Student Interpreter Evaluation

Student Name ______ Date ______

Language ______

Mode of Interpreting (check one): ☐ Consecutive ☐ Simultaneous

Role-Play/System ______

Areas Observed ______

Accuracy

Register ______

Omissions ______

Additions ______

Distortions ______

Pronunciation ______

Speaker's emotions conveyed? ______

Explain ______

Technique

General flow ______

Flow when requesting clarification ______

Speed ______

Eye Contact ______

Distracting Habits ______

Ethical Issues

Answered questions for patient? ______

Advised patient? ______

Vocabulary Expansion Recommendations

______

______

Other Recommendations

______

______

Language Coach Signature ______ Date ______

PO Box 2308, Woburn, MA 01888-0508, **p:** 781-729-3736, **www.EmbracingCulture.com**
PO Box 6401, Manchester, NH 03108, **p:** 1-888-678-CCCS

Role-Play 29: Appendicitis

		Pronunciation	Additions	Omissions	Mistakes
MD:	So, Fatima, can you tell me more about your pain? You sounded pretty miserable on the phone!				
PT:	I guess I have a pretty bad case of the flu. I have been feeling chills and running a low fever. I feel nauseated, and now I cannot stand the pain in my stomach! (points to the lower right side of the abdomen) I've been going to the bathroom more than usual, and I have some diarrhea. I feel so bloated!				
MD:	Can you tell me more about the type of pain and describe in more detail where it started?				
PT:	This is a pretty sharp pain. It started first around my navel and now it seems to be going down to the right side of my abdomen. I am having some difficulty walking because the pain is so bad!				
MD:	Hmm, let me examine you. I am going to press with my two fingers and I will let go of them quickly. Does it hurt? Does it hurt when I press and when I let go?				
PT:	I feel so nauseated! I guess that it hurts all over my tummy. I do not know.				
MD:	Is there a chance that you could be pregnant?				
PT:	Doctor, I am too busy for this type of monkey business!				
MD:	I am sorry that sometimes I have to ask difficult questions. Hmm, let me examine you again! Now I am going to press with my two fingers. Does it hurt?				
PT:	Yes.				
MD:	It looks like appendicitis and you may need an appendectomy done today. Do you want to call anyone in your family?				
PT:	I will call my godmother and my friend from work since my parents are not feeling well. Wow! I am having difficulty walking, I guess I will just walk all bent over.				
MD:	Why don't you lie down? And I will check the area of the appendix again. Is it tender here? And here? Is it worse? Yes, you are having a rebound type of pain with your symptoms worsening. I am going to call the IV nurse to give you some extra fluids and medication. You will be in the operating room very soon. I will give you the telephone to make your call and you just stay lying down.				
PT:	This is a pretty sharp pain. Can I die from this?				

continued

Role-Play 29 *(continued)*

	Pronunciation	Additions	Omissions	Mistakes
MD: We are going to remove an organ, the appendix, that has no known function in the human body, but when it gets infected and it bursts into your abdomen, you get peritonitis and it can become pretty critical. This is why we are not waiting too long to remove it!				
PT: I feel so nauseated! It hurts all over my tummy.				
MD: We are going to take care of you right away. I am not even sending you for a CT scan (computed tomography) since the lab is busy and I am pretty certain that you have peritonitis as a result of this appendicitis. When was the last time you ate any solids?				
PT: I have not eaten anything. I guess I just lost my appetite.				
MD: No problem. You are sure you have had protected intercourse? I will run a few blood and urine tests anyway. Your symptoms and your fever seem to have gotten worse in the past 24 hours. Here is the cup, we need a clean urine sample and I will ask the nurse to help you with the preparation.				
PT: I feel a very sharp pain all over my tummy; it also feels like someone is grabbing my groin.				
MD: When you cough, does it hurt?				
PT: Yes, it does hurt; I feel that my whole tummy is one big ache.				
MD: Your white blood cells count came back pretty elevated and you do not have a urinary tract infection. Also, you were right, your pregnancy test is negative.				
PT: I feel so nauseated!				
MD: The nurse will stay with you and get you ready for the operating room. Meanwhile, I am going to get the consent forms ready and make sure that the operating room is all set for you.				
PT: Could I have done something about this to prevent all this trouble?				
MD: Not really. Some people believe that diets high in greens and tomatoes help, but you did the right thing by coming in now and not waiting any longer. We want this appendix out before any major rupture.				
Break It Down	☐	☐	☐	☐

☐ CIFE with patient ☐ CIFE with provider ☐ FLOW ☐ REGISTER

PO Box 2308, Woburn, MA 01888-0508, **p:** 781-729-3736, **www.EmbracingCulture.com**
PO Box 6401, Manchester, NH 03108, **p:** 1-888-678-CCCS

Role-Play 29: Glossary

1. Pathology (diseases, conditions)

2. Laboratory Tests and Diagnostic Procedures

3. Treatment Procedures

4. Idiomatic Expressions (if any)

5. Other (vocabulary in this particular role-play that you feel is important/relevant or that you anticipate problems with)

Role-Play 30: Gallbladder

Antonio Machado smokes too much. He also likes thick black coffee. Somehow, between his cigarettes and his coffee, he finds the strength to work three jobs. He is sending money to his family in Minas Gerais, Brazil. If he didn't have to sleep, Antonio says with a laugh, he'd get another job. Over the last three months, the already wire-thin Antonio has lost seven pounds. He can't eat as much as before. Whenever he has feijoada (Brazilian bean stew), or when he eats Kentucky Fried Chicken and french fries, he gets a pain in his right side just below his rib cage.

	Pronunciation	Additions	Omissions	Mistakes
MD: Good morning, Mr. Machado. What brings you to the clinic?				
Antonio: Well, I have this pain in my stomach when I eat.				
MD: How long has this been going on?				
Antonio: About three months.				
MD: Does it happen with all your meals or only certain ones?				
Antonio: Usually at dinner and sometimes at lunch. Oh, yes, we had brunch at Denny's last week and it happened then too.				
MD: What foods give you this pain?				
Antonio: Well, french fries and feijoada.				
MD: I'm sorry, what is feijoada?				
Antonio: It's beans and pork in a kind of stew, a real Brazilian delicacy.				
MD: So, if you eat foods that have fat or oil you get this?				
Antonio: Yes. I know that if I just avoided them I'd be ok, except I like to eat them. I get tired of eating just rice and salad. Anyway, the other night, I had this pain for three hours. I couldn't even stay at work. For a while, I had a fever. But it passed.				
MD: Where does it hurt?				
Antonio: Right here under my right rib cage. It's like a big cramp.				
MD: Have you had any nausea or vomiting? Any diarrhea?				
Antonio: No.				
MD: Have you noticed that your stools are black and tarry, or is there any red blood in your stools?				
Antonio: My stools are sometimes black. But I haven't seen any blood!				
MD: Have you taken any medicine?				

continued

PO Box 2308, Woburn, MA 01888-0508, **p:** 781-729-3736, **www.EmbracingCulture.com**
PO Box 6401, Manchester, NH 03108, **p:** 1-888-678-CCCS

Role-Play 30 *(continued)*

	Pronunciation	Additions	Omissions	Mistakes
Antonio: Yes, Pepto Bismol. It does not help at all.				
MD: Do you have a family history of gallstones?				
Antonio: Yes. My mother and grandmother both had them.				
MD: OK, let's examine you.				
(Examines Patient)				
MD: You have pain in your right upper quadrant. That suggests to me that you may have gallstones. I will send you to the lab for some blood tests and arrange for you to have an ultrasound of your abdomen so we can see how your biliary tract looks. In the meantime, I will give you a medicine called Zantac. Although I think you have gallstones, the black stools and the abdominal pain could also be from an ulcer. Also, Pepto Bismol can cause black stools. But in your exam today, I found no blood in your stool, so I am thinking more and more that this is gall bladder trouble. If your tests confirm this, I'll send you to the surgeon, Dr. Spievack.				
Antonio: Surgeon! You mean I might need surgery? But I need to work.				
MD: Well, let's see what the tests show. There is a new type of gall bladder surgery that will allow you to go back to work within 10 days. It is done with a laparascope. But, don't worry. I'll call you and let you know if you need to see the surgeon.				

(Later)

Antonio to the interpreter: I feel so lonely in this country. I do not speak English well. In my country I was a respected man, but here I am nothing. Do you mind that I call you directly at home whenever I need an interpreter? I am comfortable with you. I will only call you for an emergency.

Break It Down	☐	☐	☐	☐

☐ CIFE with patient ☐ CIFE with provider ☐ FLOW ☐ REGISTER

Role-Play 30: Glossary

_______________ _______________ _______________

_______________ _______________ _______________

continued

1. Pathology (diseases, conditions)

2. Laboratory Tests and Diagnostic Procedures

3. Treatment Procedures

4. Idiomatic Expressions (if any)

5. Other (vocabulary in this particular role-play that you feel is important/relevant or that you anticipate problems with)

PO Box 2308, Woburn, MA 01888-0508, **p:** 781-729-3736, **www.EmbracingCulture.com**
PO Box 6401, Manchester, NH 03108, **p:** 1-888-678-CCCS

Role-Play 31: Hepatitis

Prueba de evaluación

		Pronunciation	Additions	Omissions	Mistakes
MD:	Well, Mr. Garza, the insurance screening test came up with abnormalities on your blood test.				
PT:	Yes, doctor, over the phone you said something about my liver.				
MD:	Yes, one of the tests that measures the health of the cells of the liver was elevated.				
PT:	Well, I came in for the repeat test last week, how was that?				
MD:	It was pretty good. The test from before was still elevated and another test like it, both called transaminases, was also elevated but nothing else was abnormal.				
PT:	What is going on?				
MD:	Your liver is slightly inflamed. The two transaminases are elevated in a way that suggests that either you have taken a toxin that may have hurt the liver, or you might have an infection called viral hepatitis.				
PT:	How can we find out?				
MD:	Have you ever had liver inflammation before?				
PT:	Not that I know of.				
MD:	Do you use alcohol?				
PT:	Yes, I drink whenever I go out.				
MD:	How often is that?				
PT:	About two or three times a week, and I have one or two drinks.				
MD:	What do you like to drink?				
PT:	Oh, I like beer and a whiskey chaser. *(Note: a whiskey chaser is when a person consumes a lager or beer immediately after the whiskey.)*				
MD:	Well, it's possible that this elevation may be caused by your use of alcohol. Do you think you could completely stop drinking alcohol for three weeks and then come back for a repeat blood test?				
PT:	Sure, no problem. But what if it's caused by a virus? Shouldn't we check and see if I have one of those diseases?				
MD:	Of course. We can check the tests for viral hepatitis today. Then, you should come back in three weeks after not drinking alcohol to see if the tests improve.				
PT:	OK.				
	Break It Down	☐	☐	☐	☐

☐ **CIFE with patient** ☐ **CIFE with provider** ☐ **FLOW** ☐ **REGISTER**

continued

Role-Play 31: Glossary

1. Pathology (diseases, conditions)

2. Laboratory Tests and Diagnostic Procedures

3. Treatment Procedures

4. Idiomatic Expressions (if any)

5. Other (vocabulary in this particular role-play that you feel is important/relevant or that you anticipate problems with)

PO Box 2308, Woburn, MA 01888-0508, **p:** 781-729-3736, **www.EmbracingCulture.com**
PO Box 6401, Manchester, NH 03108, **p:** 1-888-678-CCCS

Role-Play 32: Bowel Movements

Mrs. Bettencourt goes to the clinic quite often. She is well over fifty, but you'd never guess it. She has a hypothyroid condition and frequent difficulty moving her bowels. Sometimes, she'll go a week without having a bowel movement. Her mother died of colon cancer last year.

	Pronunciation	Additions	Omissions	Mistakes
Mrs. B: I can't move my bowels again. I think you should re-check my Thyroid. Last time this happened, I got better on more thyroid medication.				
MD: OK. Do you feel cold when others feel warm?				
Mrs. B: In this weather, I always feel cold. I'm from a tropical climate. In my country, we are not used to this weather.				
MD: Have you seen blood in your stool?				
Mrs. B: No. (Answers abruptly.)				
MD: (Noticing patient's concern) You seem concerned…what's wrong?				
Mrs. B: My mother had blood in her stool and at first they thought she had hemorrhoids. Then they did a test and found out she had colon cancer. She died last summer.				
MD: I'm sorry. You know, you are fifty now, and as a precautionary measure, it's reasonable for you to have a screening sigmoidoscopy. Actually, though, since your mother had colon cancer, it would be a good idea for the GI specialist to look at your whole colon through a procedure called colonoscopy.				
(pause)				
But I do think this is your usual constipation. We'll treat it by checking your TSH and adjusting the thyroid medicine if need be. I also want you to take two packets of Metamucil per day and drink lots of fluids. In the meantime, I'll send you to see Dr. Wyman. He'll discuss doing the colonoscopy. Before you see him, you'll need to do these stool hemoccults. Is there anything else?				
Mrs. B: Well, I have had a runny nose and I'm feeling a little stuffy, but my chief concern is my constipation.				
Break It Down	☐	☐	☐	☐

☐ CIFE with patient ☐ CIFE with provider ☐ FLOW ☐ REGISTER

Role-Play 32: Glossary

_______________ _______________ _______________

_______________ _______________ _______________

continued

1. Pathology (diseases, conditions)

2. Laboratory Tests and Diagnostic Procedures

3. Treatment Procedures

4. Idiomatic Expressions (if any)

5. Other (vocabulary in this particular role-play that you feel is important/relevant or that you anticipate problems with)

Role-Play 33: Kidney Stones

Salvador has always been very healthy. Occasionally, he would notice some blood in his urine after he'd get a twinge of pain in his right flank (lower back). It would always go away and he'd have no problems. He did not have health insurance for many years. Now, he and his wife own a cleaning business with five employees doing houses and offices. He is busier than ever, especially since his wife is pregnant and no longer able to help with the business like she used to. Today, he comes in to the clinic. He complains of horrible pain in his flank. He is urinating bright red. Something is wrong and Salvador is worried.

	Pronunciation	Additions	Omissions	Mistakes
NP: So, you're urinating blood?				
Salvador: *(Standing up, pacing in the room)* Yes, but can you help me with this pain? It is horrible.				
NP: How long have you had it?				
Salvador: For about a day. It started yesterday morning. It starts here and goes down into my groin. I can't sleep or think. Can you fix this?				
NP: Well, we certainly can try. Have you had any nausea or vomiting?				
Salvador: No, but I feel like it when the pain gets worse. I am a little dizzy. I haven't felt like eating or drinking anything since yesterday.				
NP: OK, we'll examine you and check your urine.				
Salvador: Can you give me something for my pain?				
NP: Let me examine you quickly.				
(Examines patient and runs tests.)				
NP: Well, your blood pressure is a little low. You have pain in your right flank and blood in your urine. I think you have kidney stones.				
(pause)				
I am going to give you some fluids in an IV and a shot for pain. We're going to send you to the Mount Auburn emergency room so they can run a spiral CAT scan of your abdomen to verify that you do have stones. If so, you'll probably go home with medication for pain.				
Salvador: Will I have to stay in the hospital?				

continued

Role-Play 33 *(continued)*

	Pronunciation	Additions	Omissions	Mistakes
NP: Only if you can't keep any food or fluids down after you are treated, or if the urologist finds that the stones are in a position that requires something more than watchful waiting.				
Salvador: Is this serious?				
NP: The pain can be very bad, but if it is what I think it is, it will pass soon and you will be fine.				
Salvador: Thank you. Ai! The pain is bad. Anytime you're ready for a shot, I'm ready.				
Salvador to the interpreter: You know, I'm not sure what to tell my wife. I'm a good man, not like some of my employees. They go downtown for the women...you know what I mean. I forgot to ask the doctor when I can be with my wife again. What do you think?				
Break It Down	☐	☐	☐	☐

☐ **CIFE with patient** ☐ **CIFE with provider** ☐ **FLOW** ☐ **REGISTER**

Role-Play 33: Glossary

PO Box 2308, Woburn, MA 01888-0508, **p:** 781-729-3736, **www.EmbracingCulture.com**
PO Box 6401, Manchester, NH 03108, **p:** 1-888-678-CCCS

1. Pathology (diseases, conditions)

2. Laboratory Tests and Diagnostic Procedures

3. Treatment Procedures

4. Idiomatic Expressions (if any)

5. Other (vocabulary in this particular role-play that you feel is important/relevant or that you anticipate problems with)

Role-Play 34: Heartburn

Filomena was worried. For the past six weeks, when she would go to bed after dinner, she would wake up with burning chest pain. She tried antacids, but to no avail. Five years ago, her mother died in the night of a heart attack. Filomena's symptoms seem so similar to her mother's that she felt the need to go to the doctor.

	Pronunciation	Additions	Omissions	Mistakes
MD: What can I do for you?				
Filomena: I have chest pain.				
MD: When do you get it?				
Filomena: At night. It wakes me from sleep.				
MD: Do you get this when you exert yourself?				
Filomena: No.				
MD: Do you get sweats, palpitations or shortness of breath with it?				
Filomena: No. Do you think it's my heart?				
MD: I don't know yet, but let me ask you some more questions. What time do you eat dinner?				
Filomena: I work second shift. I get home at midnight, eat and go to bed.				
MD: Do you ever get heartburn?				
Filomena: What is heartburn?				
MD: It is a burning pain that climbs from your stomach up into your chest after eating fatty or greasy foods.				
Filomena: That is exactly how my pain feels.				
MD: So it is not a pressure pain?				
Filomena: No, it is a burning pain.				
MD: Let's do an EKG and I'll examine you.				
Examines patient				

continued

PO Box 2308, Woburn, MA 01888-0508, **p:** 781-729-3736, **www.EmbracingCulture.com**
PO Box 6401, Manchester, NH 03108, **p:** 1-888-678-CCCS

Role-Play 34 *(continued)*

	Pronunciation	Additions	Omissions	Mistakes
MD: Well, I think you have heartburn from what is called esophageal reflux. Sometimes after a big meal, if you go right to bed, the acid your stomach produces to digest the food goes up the esophagus and causes a burning pain that is heartburn. It's worse if you drink coffee, or eat chocolate or fatty foods. After you eat dinner, you should wait at least two hours before going to bed. I will also give you a pill to take twice a day that will help. I'll see you in six weeks and you can let me know how the symptoms are. I'd like you to do three of the hemocult cards to make sure you're not putting out any blood in your gastrointestinal tract.				
Filomena: You mean the EKG says my heart is OK?				
MD: Your EKG, your complaint, and your exam all suggest that your heart is fine. But to make this go away you're going to have to follow the dietary suggestions I just made.				
Filomena: I'm very relieved.				
Filomena to the Interpreter: Do you have a moment? The doctor seemed very nice. What do you think? Sometimes doctors are in a rush and they do not have time for patients like me. I'll see you next week when I come to the hospital to take care of my bills. It is so cold out there. Please don't forget that I'll be back next week.				
Break It Down	☐	☐	☐	☐

☐ **CIFE with patient** ☐ **CIFE with provider** ☐ **FLOW** ☐ **REGISTER**

Role-Play 34: Glossary

continued

1. Pathology (diseases, conditions)

2. Laboratory Tests and Diagnostic Procedures

3. Treatment Procedures

4. Idiomatic Expressions (if any)

5. Other (vocabulary in this particular role-play that you feel is important/relevant or that you anticipate problems with)

PO Box 2308, Woburn, MA 01888-0508, **p:** 781-729-3736, **www.EmbracingCulture.com**
PO Box 6401, Manchester, NH 03108, **p:** 1-888-678-CCCS

Lesson 7: Additional Resources
The Digestive System

MAIN TESTS AND PROCEDURES

WORD	MEANING	TARGET
1. Abdominal computed tomography (CT scan)	Computer-enhanced two-dimensional x-ray images of the abdominal organs	
2. Abdominal magnetic resonance imaging (MRI)	Magnetic imaging test that creates images of abdominal organs and tissues in all three planes of the body	
3. Abdominal ultrasound	Uses sound waves to produce images of internal organs and other structures of the abdomen	
4. Barium x-ray studies (Barium Swallow, Upper GI with small bowel follow through, Barium Enema).	The use of barium that is put into the gastrointestinal tract via swallowing or enemas to outline the esophagus, stomach, duodenum or intestines on x-ray of the particular part	
5. Cholangiograpghy	X-ray examination of the bile ducts	
6. Cholecystectomy	Removal of the gallbladder via open surgery or laparascopy	
7. Colonoscopy	Direct visual examination of the colon for a tumor or other abnormality	
8. Colostomy	Surgically created passage from the colon to the abdominal wall for excretion of fecal waste when the colon is blocked and feces can not get to the anus	
9. Endoscopy	Direct visual examination of internal structures of the digestive system using a fiber-optic tube	
10. Gastrectomy	Surgery that removes all or part of the stomach	
11. Gastrointestinal endoscopy	Visual examination of the gastrointestinal tract using an endoscope	
12. Gastrostomy	Surgical creation of a passage through the abdominal wall into the stomach for putting feeding preparations directly into the stomach	
13. Hemorrhoidectomy	Excision of hemorrhoids by surgery or use of rubber bands	
14. Ileostomy	A passage done via surgery that allows fecal material to be excreted from the ileum to an opening in the abdominal wall	

continued

WORD	MEANING	TARGET
15. Liver Function Tests (LFTs)	Measurement of liver enzymes and other substances in the blood	
16. Laparoscopy	Direct visual examination for diagnosis and treatment of abnormalities in the abdomen	
17. Occult blood test (OB)	Test for microscopic blood in the stool	
18. Sigmoidoscopy	Direct visual inspection of the rectum and lower intestine to detect polyps or cancer	
19. Stool culture	Test to find organisms in the stool (feces) that can cause gastrointestinal symptoms and disease	
20. Upper Gastrointestinal Series (UGI series)	X-ray series using barium swallowed into the esophagus and stomach to outline the lining of the esophagus, stomach, duodenum and sometimes the small bowel	

DIGESTIVE SYSTEM VOCABULARY

Main Organs And Body Structures:

Vocabulary Word	Target Language
Anus	
Appendix	
Bile	
Colon	
Cystic duct	
Duodenum	
Esophagus	
Gallbladder	
Hepatic duct	
Ileum	
Jejunum	
Large intestine	
Liver	
Oral cavity	
Pancreas	
Pancreatic duct	
Peritoneum	
Rectum	
Salivary glands	

continued

PO Box 2308, Woburn, MA 01888-0508, **p:** 781-729-3736, **www.EmbracingCulture.com**
PO Box 6401, Manchester, NH 03108, **p:** 1-888-678-CCCS

Vocabulary Word	Target Language
Small intestine	
Stomach	
Tongue	
Teeth	
Gums	
Lip	
Abdomen	
Mandible	
Palate	
Throat	
Pyloric sphincter	
Sigmoid colon	
Bile	
Bilirubin	
Sugar	
Lipid	
Saliva	
Enzyme	

Main Illnesses:

Vocabulary Word	Target Language
Acid reflux	
Appendicitis	
Acute pancreatitis	
Alcoholic hepatitis	
Anal fissure	
Cholecystitis	
Cholelithiasis	
Cholestasis	
Cirrhosis	
Constipation	
Diarrhea	

continued

Vocabulary Word	Target Language
Diverticular disease	
Food poisoning	
Gallstones	
Gastroenteritis	
Hemorrhoids	
Hepatitis	
Hepatomegaly	
Inflammatory bowel disease	
Irritable bowel syndrome	
Jaundice	
Liver encephalopathy	
Pancreatic carcinoma	

Main Tests and Procedures:

Vocabulary Word	Target Language
Abdominal computed tomography (CT scan)	
Abdominal magnetic resonance imaging (MRI)	
Abdominal ultrasonography	
Appendectomy	
Barium tests	
Cholangiography	
Cholecystograph	
Cholecystectomy	
Cholecystojejunostomy	
Colonoscopy	
Colostomy	
Enterocolostomy	
Endoscopic retrograde	
Gastrectomy	
Gastrointestinal Endoscopy	
Gastrointestinal series (GI)	

PO Box 2308, Woburn, MA 01888-0508, **p:** 781-729-3736, **www.EmbracingCulture.com**
PO Box 6401, Manchester, NH 03108, **p:** 1-888-678-CCCS

Vocabulary Word	Target Language
Gastrojejunostomy	
Gastroscopy	
Gastrostomy	
Hemorrhoidectomy	
Ileostomy	
Laparoscopy	
Liver biopsy	
Liver Function Tests (LFTs)	
Nasogastric intubation	
Sigmoidoscopy	
Stool culture	
Vagotomy	

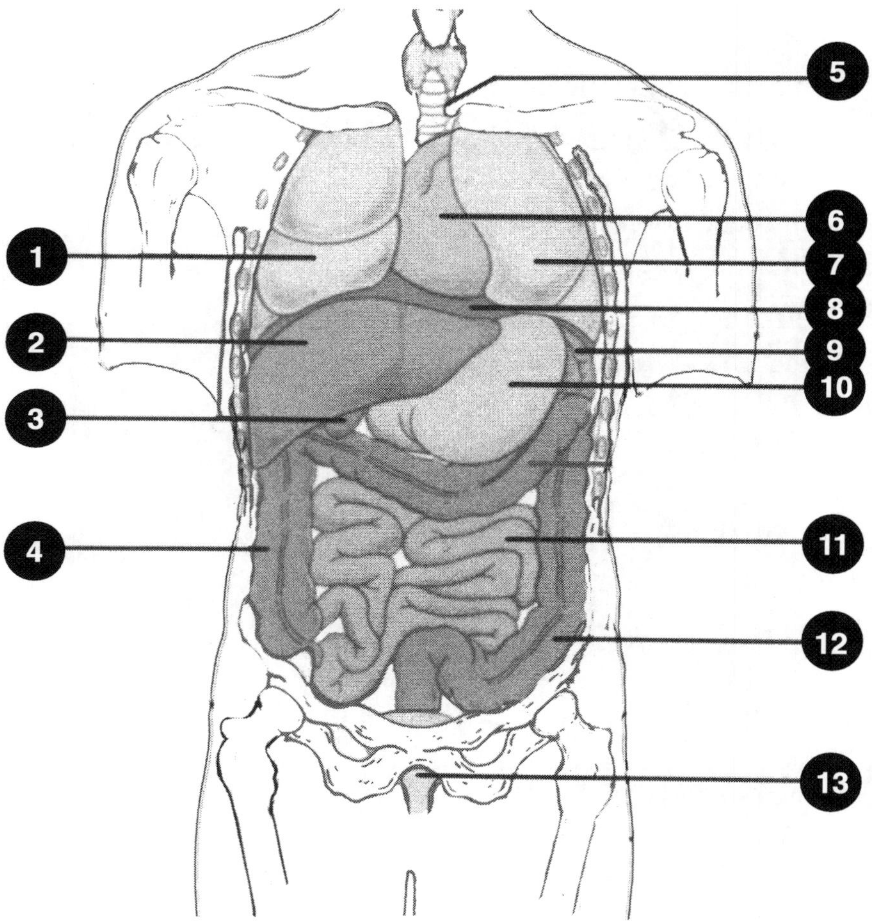

Lesson Eight: Skeletal System

Understanding Goals

Students will:

- review learned concepts
- practice the Samurai! Technique
- identify the major bones of the skeletal system
- learn about bone fractures
- sharpen their consecutive interpreting skills through role-play practice

Key Concepts

- Skeletal system
- Fractures
- Sprains
- Register

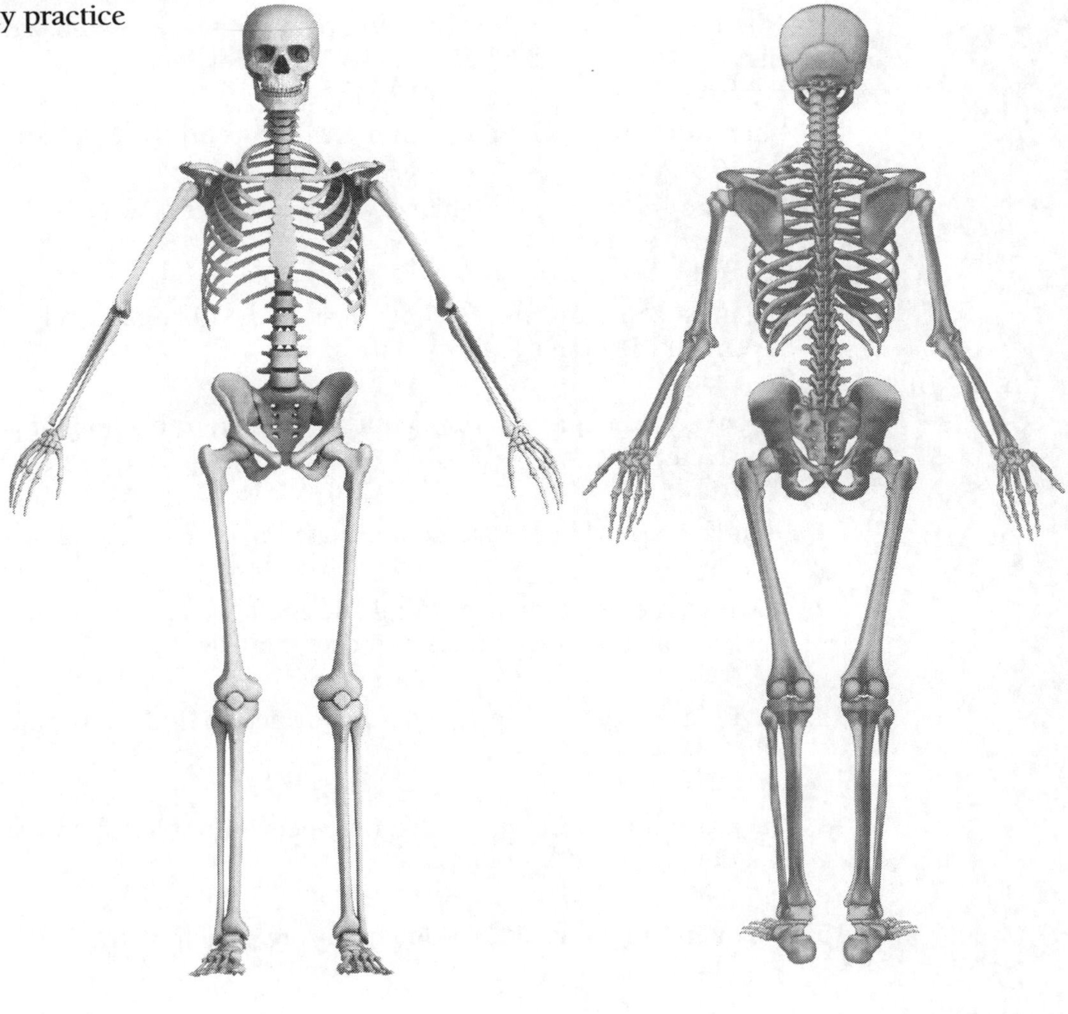

PO Box 2308, Woburn, MA 01888-0508, **p:** 781-729-3736, **www.EmbracingCulture.com**
PO Box 6401, Manchester, NH 03108, **p:** 1-888-678-CCCS

Lesson Eight: Quiz
Skeletal System

Read the following statements and determine if they are true or false, then circle the appropriate answer next to the statement.

1. Bones are amazingly strong due to the vast amount of mass they contain.
   - ○ True ○ False
2. Ossification is a process by which the cartilage slowly hardens as mineral salts are deposited.
   - ○ True ○ False
3. Bone growth continues until ages 27 to 35.
   - ○ True ○ False
4. A fracture happens when the joints are stretched beyond capacity.
   - ○ True ○ False
5. Displaced or dislocated bones are set back in their proper positions through a procedure called REDUCTION.
   - ○ True ○ False
6. When there is no need to have an operation to set a bone back to its proper position, this is known as a CLOSED REDUCTION.
   - ○ True ○ False
7. A sprain happens when there is a break, rupture, or crack in a bone or cartilage.
   - ○ True ○ False
8. A compound fracture is when several bones break at the same time without breaking the skin.
   - ○ True ○ False
9. The most common sites for fractures are the tibia, the neck of the femur, the elbow, the end of the radius and tip of the ulna.
   - ○ True ○ False
10. When a cancer spreads from a different organ into a bone it is called "Secondary bone cancer."
    - ○ True ○ False
11. Gout is a type of bone cancer stimulated by excess of uric acid.
    - ○ True ○ False
12. When women stop menstruating and their levels of estrogen decrease, they become more prone to bone fractures and osteoporosis.
    - ○ True ○ False
13. The nuclear scanning test that is performed to find abnormalities in the bone is called "Bone scan."
    - ○ True ○ False
14. The procedure through which a limb gets immobilized with a splint during a first-aid situation is called "splinting."
    - ○ True ○ False
15. The main functions of the bone tissue are to help with bone movement.
    - ○ True ○ False

Lesson Eight: Class Activities
The Skeletal System

REVIEW

A. Do you still remember what the following root words mean?

1. oste/o ______________________________
2. chondr/o ______________________________
3. arthr/o ______________________________
4. ten/o ______________________________
5. tendin/o ______________________________
6. my/o ______________________________
7. myos/o ______________________________
8. cost/o ______________________________
9. vertebr/o ______________________________
10. cervical refers to the ______________________________
11. thoracic refers to the ______________________________
12. lumbar refers to the ______________________________

B. Using the roots words above, write down as many words as you remember:

______________	______________	______________
______________	______________	______________
______________	______________	______________
______________	______________	______________
______________	______________	______________
______________	______________	______________

PO Box 2308, Woburn, MA 01888-0508, **p:** 781-729-3736, **www.EmbracingCulture.com**
PO Box 6401, Manchester, NH 03108, **p:** 1-888-678-CCCS

Introduction to the Skeletal System

How much do you know?

How many bones do you know from the top of your head? In this lesson, we will focus on the 20 most common broken bones.

1. Label the main bones in the diagram below.
2. Label the bones in your target language. You may use a bilingual medical dictionary, encyclopedia or glossary, or a target language atlas of anatomy to find an equivalent name for each bone.

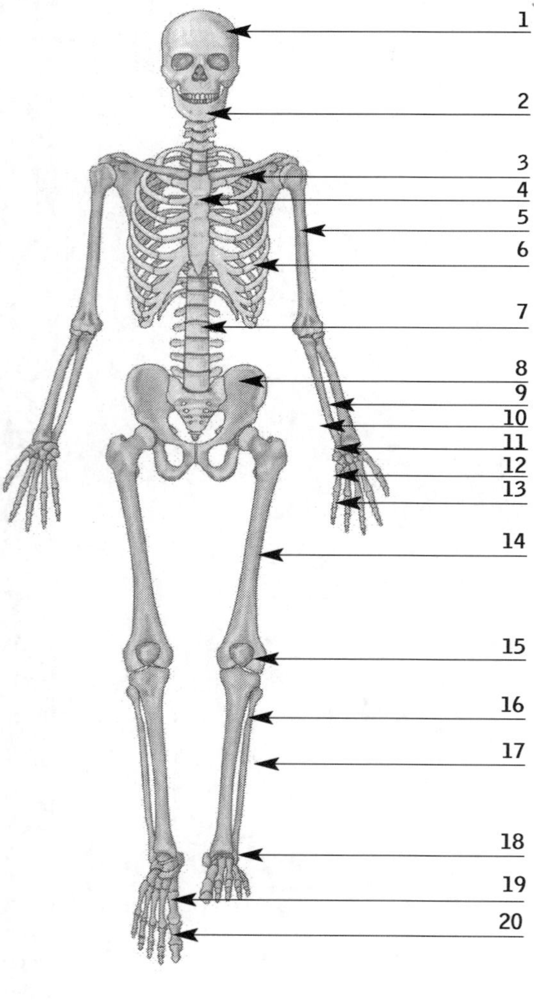

	ENGLISH	TARGET
1	Cranium	Craneo
2	mandible	Mandibula
3	clavicle	Clavicula
4	sternum	Esternon
5	Humerus	Humero
6	Ribs	Costillas
7	~~Lumbar~~ vertebrae	Columna Vertebral
8	Pelvis	Pelvis
9	Radius	Radio
10	Ulna	~~Ulna~~ cúbito
11	Carpals	Carpo
12	Metacarpals	Metacarpo
13	Phalanges	Falanges
14	Femur	Femur
15	Patella	Rótula (paleta)
16	Tibia	Tibia
17	Fibula	~~Fibula~~ Perone
18	Tarsals	Tarso
19	metatarsals	metatarso
20	Phalanges	Falanges

You probably noticed that some bones are usually known by a different name from the one your instructor used. Do you still remember the term we used to refer to the level of language one uses? If you remembered **REGISTER**, you are right.

Fill in the table:

High Register	Low Register
mandible	jaw bone
sternum	breast bone
	foot
clavicle	collar bone
carpals	
	hand bones
vertebra	
	hips
	ankle bones
phalanges	
metatarsals	
scapula	

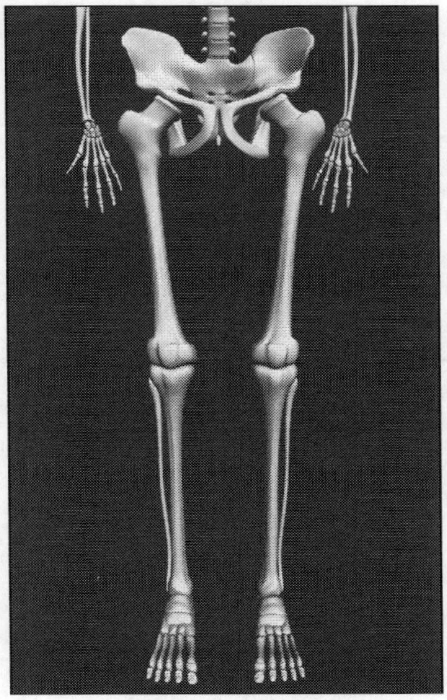

1. THE SKELETAL SYSTEM

Bones are considered connective tissue. They are amazingly strong for the amount of mass they contain. The cells of the bones and protein fibers are interspersed in a gel consisting of water, minerals, and carbohydrates; which is continually breaking down and rebuilding. The building block of cortical bone is the osteon. It is rod-shaped and consists of a central canal surrounded by concentric layers called lamellae. In each layer or lamella, fibers of a protein called collagen are woven in such a way that gives added strength to the bone. Within the bone gel or matrix are osteocytes, which lay down new bone. Osteoclasts tear down the bone system.

The main functions of bone are to support soft tissue, to protect the body, to assist with body movement, to serve as a reservoir for mineral storage, to assist with the formation of red blood cells and to store energy via the adipose tissue created by the yellow bone marrow.

PO Box 2308, Woburn, MA 01888-0508, **p:** 781-729-3736, **www.EmbracingCulture.com**
PO Box 6401, Manchester, NH 03108, **p:** 1-888-678-CCCS

Bones are described in four different ways according to their shapes: 1- long (arms and legs), 2 - short (wrists and ankles), 3 - flat (ribs, skull), 4 - irregular (vertebrae along the spine).

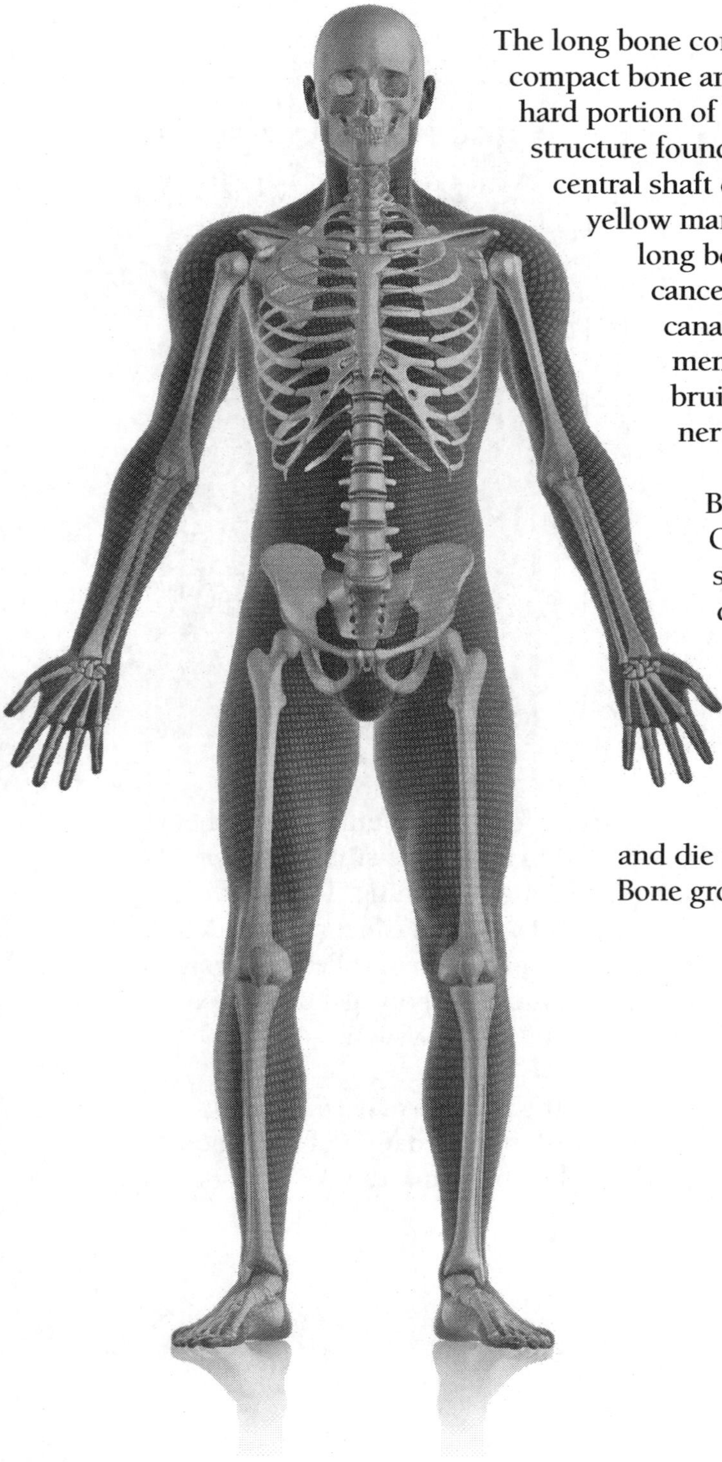

The long bone consists of three major portions: the spongy bone, compact bone and the medullary bone. The cortical bone is the long hard portion of long bones. Cancellous refers to the porous, spongy structure found within the central part of a long bone. Within the central shaft of a long bone is the medullary canal,which contains yellow marrow, fatty tissue, and blood vessels. The ends of long bones have marrow, which produces blood cells. The cancellous tissue surrounds the marrow. The medullary canal is connected to the periosteum which is the thin membrane that covers the bone surface. When a bone is bruised or broken, it is the periosteum with its plentiful nerves that makes bone pain so difficult to bear.

Bones are descended from ancestor cartilage. Ossification is a process by which the cartilage slowly hardens as mineral salts like calcium are deposited. At the end of long bones, there is cartilage covering the bone instead of periosteum. Also at the end of long bones is an area called the epiphyseal plate. This plate is the source of bone growth. Cartilage cells proliferate and form columns pushing older cells toward the middle of the bone shaft. As chondrocytes enlarge and die the space they occupied is filled by new bone cells. Bone growth continues until ages 17 to 21.

Test Your Understanding.

Mark each item "True" or "False"

1. The tissues of the bones are layered in a gel consisting of proteins, blood cells, and amylase.
   - O True O False
2. Cortical bone is the spongy structure found within the central part of a long bone.
   - O True O False
3. Ossification is a process by which the cartilage slowly hardens as mineral salts are deposited.
   - O True O False
4. Osteoclasts are builders.
   - O True O False

Watch the video "Breaking Down" from the *Body Story* DVD to learn about how bones break and heal. Use the space below to take notes on what you see or what you find interesting. Then, answer the questions that follow.

____

____

1. Why is it that we all walk differently?
2. *Bones are alive*. Why do we say that?
3. What is the difference between osteoclasts and osteoblasts?
4. Why does our body release endorphins?
5. What are stem cells?
6. What is a hematoma?
7. What bone did Lisa break?
8. What kind of fracture did she suffer?

PO Box 2308, Woburn, MA 01888-0508, **p:** 781-729-3736, **www.EmbracingCulture.com**
PO Box 6401, Manchester, NH 03108, **p:** 1-888-678-CCCS

2. Bone Fractures

A fracture is a break, rupture, or crack in a bone or cartilage. There are many types of fractures. There are **simple (closed)** fractures and **compound (open)** fractures. In a simple fracture, the broken bone is not visible through the skin, and does not cause the skin to break. In a compound fracture, the skin may break and the bone may separate from its other half. A compound fracture should be considered a medical emergency and reparative surgery considered before five hours.

Within these two main categories are many subdivisions. When bones are broken totally apart into two or more pieces, fractures can be described as **complete**. If the bone is merely cracked or partially broken, the fracture is described as **incomplete**.

If bones are not aligned they are called **displaced**. A fracture that causes a break straight across the bone is a **transverse fracture**. A fracture that causes the bone to shatter into fragments is called a **comminuted fracture**. A break that twists the bone diagonally, often with jagged ends is called a **spiral fracture**. A **greenstick fracture** is when the long bone bends and cracks obliquely on only one side. The tibia, the neck of the femur, the elbow, the end of the radius and tip of the ulna (the wrist) are common sites of fractures.

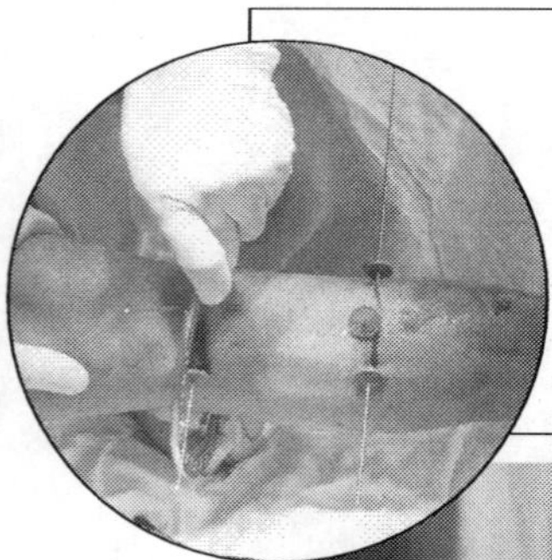

Please draw corresponding types of fracture:
Greenstick Spiral Comminuted Transverse

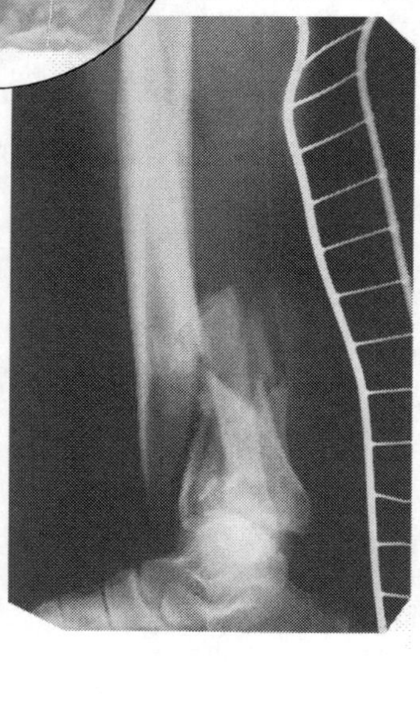
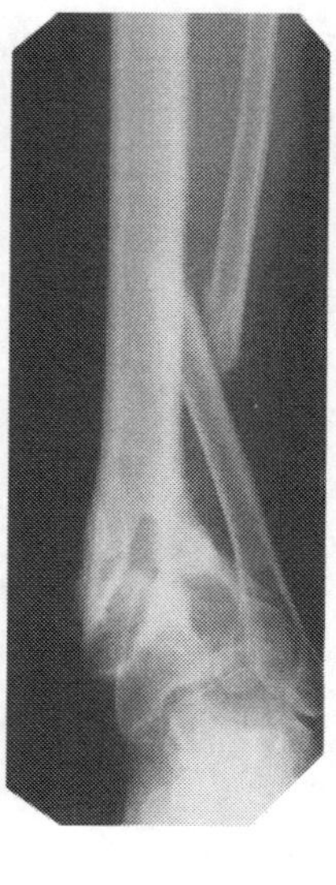
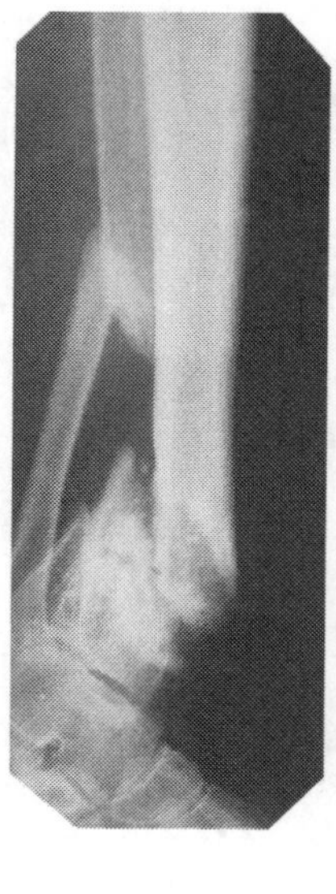
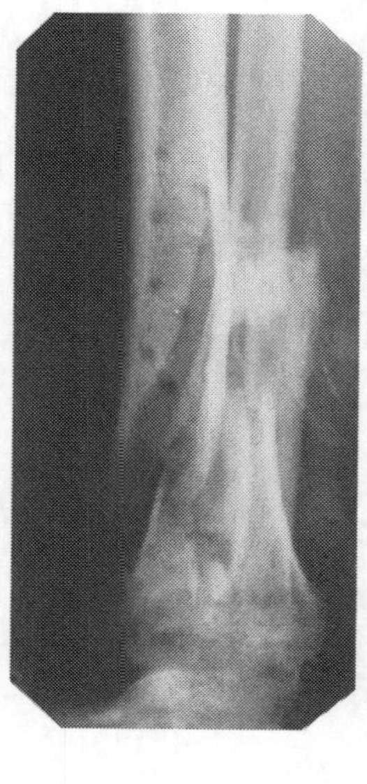

EXERCISE

Organize the information above in the following table. The first one has been done for you:

Pertaining to:

Skin

simple = closed	≠	compound = open

Pertaining to:

Degree of broken bone

	≠	

Pertaining to:

Direction

	≠	

Pertaining to:

Number

	≠	

PO Box 2308, Woburn, MA 01888-0508, **p:** 781-729-3736, **www.EmbracingCulture.com**
PO Box 6401, Manchester, NH 03108, **p:** 1-888-678-CCCS

The PROCEDURE of setting displaced or dislocated bones back in their proper positions is called **reduction**. Setting a bone without an operation is **closed reduction**. If an operation is performed, the procedure is called **open reduction**.

For a list of *main tests and procedures*, consult the Additional Resources section for this lesson.

3. Sprains

Patients often come to the emergency room because of sprained ligaments. A sprain happens when the joints are stretched beyond capacity. There are two types of sprains: partial or complete tears. When ligament fibers are torn, causing pain, swelling or bruising, a patient may have a partial sprain. But if the ligaments are completely severed and, in addition to pain and swelling, there is a loss of movement in the joint, it is probable that the patient has a complete tear.

COMMON BONE DISORDERS

(For list and definitions, consult the table in the Additional Resources section for this lesson)

Practice the Samurai! Technique to match the complaints with their definition:

______	1. arthralgia	a. a fast-growing malignant tumor of skeletal tissue
______	2. osteosarcoma	b. forward curvature of the lumbar spine
______	3. bursitis	c. inflammation of a bursa
______	4. chondralgia	d. bone pain
______	5. chondritis	e. pain in a joint
______	6. lordosis	f. pain originating in the cartilage
______	7. ostealgia	g. inflammation of a bone
______	8. osteitis	h. inflammation of the cartilage
______	9. osteomyelitis	i. inflammation of the bone, bone marrow, and surrounding soft tissue.

Lesson Eight: Homework
The Skeletal System

1. Go over your notes for today's class and read section "Additional Resources"
2. Read and practice ALL role-plays for this lesson
3. Continue developing your glossary
4. Translate the types of fractures:

Type	Translation	Type	Translation
1. simple		8. single	
2. closed		9. multiple	
3. compound		10. comminuted	
4. open		11. linear	
5. complete		12. transverse	
6. incomplete		13. spiral	
7. greenstick			

5. Translate the 19 common illnesses of the Skeletal System:

Type	Translation	Type	Translation
1. arthritis		6. osteoporosis	
2. bone cancer		7. paget's disease	
3. gout		8. rheumatoid arthritis	
4. osteoarthritis			
5. osteomalacia			

6. Translate the main tests and procedures:

Type	Translation	Type	Translation
1. amputation		8. casting	
2. arthrocentesis		9. splinting	
3. arthrography		10. traction	
4. arthroscopy		11. laminectomy	
5. bone scan		12. myelography	
6. casting		13. open reduction	
7. closed reduction		14. sequestrectomy	

PO Box 2308, Woburn, MA 01888-0508, **p:** 781-729-3736, **www.EmbracingCulture.com**
PO Box 6401, Manchester, NH 03108, **p:** 1-888-678-CCCS

Lesson Eight: Role-Plays
The Skeletal System

Work individually at first:
- Read the entire role-play
- Get a general sense of its meaning
- Circle the most challenging medical terms
- Apply the Samurai! technique to those terms
- Read the role-play again for a deeper understanding
- Find an accurate equivalent in the target language

Work in a language-specific group of friends, fellow students or colleagues:
- Share your doubts
- Ask for other ways of expressing the same meaning
- Develop a glossary
- Check the dictionary
- Practice the role-plays remember to do CIFE for all your role-plays
- Have your colleagues observe you and provide feedback on your accuracy and register.
- These colleagues can keep track of any omissions, additions, mistakes or distortions in your interpreting and point these out to you in a follow-up discussion.

Student Interpreter Evaluation

Student Name ____________________ Date ________

Language ____________________

Mode of Interpreting (check one): ☐ Consecutive ☐ Simultaneous

Role-Play/System ____________________

Areas Observed ____________________

Accuracy

Register ____________________

Omissions ____________________

Additions ____________________

Distortions ____________________

Pronunciation ____________________

Speaker's emotions conveyed? ____________________

Explain ____________________

Technique

General flow ____________________

Flow when requesting clarification ____________________

Speed ____________________

Eye Contact ____________________

Distracting Habits ____________________

Ethical Issues

Answered questions for patient? ____________________

Advised patient? ____________________

Vocabulary Expansion Recommendations

____

____

Other Recommendations

____

____

Language Coach Signature ____________________ Date ________

Role-Play 35: Bones

Mr. N is a 60 year old man who played soccer all his life. He loved to run, play soccer with his grandkids and take long walks with his wife. He plays league soccer and despite his age, is able to play almost all of each game. Six weeks ago, he fell while playing and twisted his knee. His knee became swollen; the next day he realized that he had knee pain every time he'd take a step.

Mr. N called his primary care doctor who sent him to the orthopedic physician's assistant in the health center. The PA examined the knee and sent Mr. N for an MRI and made a follow up with the orthopedic doctor. He is now at the orthopedic doctor's office for his first visit with her.

	Pronunciation	Additions	Omissions	Mistakes
MD: Hello, Mr. N, I am Dr. Severs, and I have spoken to Kevin about your case. How is your knee pain?				
Mr. N: Well, every time I take a step, it feels like there is a nail in my knee. I twisted the knee and it is very painful.				
MD: Can you bend the knee?				
Mr. N: Only so far. Maybe 30 degrees.				
MD: Does your knee ever buckle? (give way).				
Mr. N: No, not so far. But I am concerned because usually when I twist or hurt something, it is better in four or five days. I am still hurting after six weeks.				
MD: Well, Mr. N, let me examine your knee and we'll talk about that and what the MRI showed.				
Mr. N: OK.				
(MD examines patient)				
MD: Well, Mr. N, the exam shows tenderness along your medial joint line. You have an effusion (water on the knee). However your ligaments are strong and are not damaged. The MRI shows that you have torn your medial meniscus. It is flapping in the breeze, so to speak, and I think you will need surgery to fix this.				
Mr. N: I will need surgery at this age?				
MD: Yes, but the good news is that it is arthroscopic surgery.				
Mr. N: Why is that good news?				
MD: Well, instead of opening up the knee and fixing the meniscus, we are able to insert a fiber optic tube into the joint without opening it up, and clip the meniscus with micro tools and vacuum the unneeded clipped portion of the cartilage right out of the joint.				

continued

PO Box 2308, Woburn, MA 01888-0508, **p:** 781-729-3736, **www.EmbracingCulture.com**
PO Box 6401, Manchester, NH 03108, **p:** 1-888-678-CCCS

Role-Play 35 *(continued)*

	Pronunciation	Additions	Omissions	Mistakes
Mr. N: How long do I have to be in the hospital?				
MD: Well, you are pretty healthy without other illnesses, I don't think you'll need to go to the hospital. We can do it at our surgicenter downtown. Usually it's just a half a day, and you spend the night at home. Some people go back to work in one to three days. I will ask your PCP to do a preoperative evaluation and if he agrees, we can do this at the surgicenter.				
Mr. N: What happens after the surgery?				
MD: Well, first you go to the recovery room where your temperature, blood pressure and other vital signs are monitored. It's there that you'll get your first oral pain killer to take effect as the anesthesia wears off.				
Mr. N: Dr., I come from the old school regarding any pain killers, just live with the pain and it will get better as long as the surgery did the trick!				
MD: I understand, but sometimes the pain killer in the beginning is a way to help temporarily so when you arrive home you'll be in good shape. After you get home, you will need to ice your knee. In fact, I will order a special icing and pressure system for you to use for the month. Also, when you get home you should take it easy but you can bear weight as tolerated. You'll be given crutches to help you walk. I will give you a narcotic pain medicine to use every four hours. If your kidneys and stomach are in good shape, I can give you a non-steroidal anti-inflammatory medicine to use as well , and that should decrease the amount of narcotic you'll need for pain control. Around a week or ten days after the surgery, you can begin physical therapy.				
Break It Down	☐	☐	☐	☐

☐ CIFE with patient ☐ CIFE with provider ☐ FLOW ☐ REGISTER

Role-Play 35: Glossary

______ ______ ______

______ ______ ______

______ ______ ______

continued

1. Pathology (diseases, conditions)

2. Laboratory Tests and Diagnostic Procedures

3. Treatment Procedures

4. Idiomatic Expressions (if any)

5. Other (vocabulary in this particular role-play that you feel is important/relevant or that you anticipate problems with)

PO Box 2308, Woburn, MA 01888-0508, **p:** 781-729-3736, **www.EmbracingCulture.com**
PO Box 6401, Manchester, NH 03108, **p:** 1-888-678-CCCS

Role-Play 36: Wrist

Ms. W is a marvel. She is 70 years old and she still works at the curtain factory. She takes care of her grandson, who is a senior in high school and doing very well. She volunteers at the church several nights a week. As she walked to work early one January morning, she slipped on a patch of ice and tried to break her fall with her right hand. She landed hard and hurt her wrist and her hip. She did not lose consciousness; but when she tried to get up she had pain in her hip and she could not move her wrist. Someone called 911 and she was brought to the emergency room.

At the emergency room, she had a set of x-rays taken. The emergency room MD comes in to speak with her:

	Pronunciation	Additions	Omissions	Mistakes
MD: Hello Ms W. So how are you doing?				
Ms. W: OK. But I am having pain when I walk and I cannot move my wrist. This is not good. I have to work and I have to walk to the bus; and then at work, I use my hands and arms to wrap the rolls of curtains.				
MD: Well, the wrist is clearly broken. Both the distal radial bone and the distal ulna are fractured. The fracture is not displaced, so we can put you in a splint, wait a week for the swelling to go down and then put you in a cast.				
Ms. W: How long does the cast stay on?				
MD: Usually it stays on for 6-8 weeks, with another splint to give support after that.				
Ms. W: How long before I can return to work?				
MD: Well, as regards to your wrist, it takes six to 12 weeks after such a fracture before you can use the wrist for strenuous activities such as wrapping curtain rolls.				
But I am also concerned about your hip. Are you having pain when you walk?				
Ms. W: Yes, every time I get up or sit down, or walk down the corridor it hurts.				
MD: Hmm. Well the X-ray shows no fracture in the pelvis or hip. Here, let me examine your hip again. (**MD:**examines patient's hip)				
MD: Well, I can see you have pain with movement, but your range of motion is excellent. I think I will send you back to have an MRI of your pelvis and hips to make sure you did not fracture something that was not seen on the plain films.				

continued

Role-Play 36 *(continued)*

	Pronunciation	Additions	Omissions	Mistakes
Patient goes to MRI and returns.				
MD: Well, you did fracture your inferior pubic ramus. It's a pelvic bone. The good news is that you don't need surgery. The pelvic rami fracture heals without surgery. It is painful but at least you'll avoid general anesthesia.				
Ms. W: You said it was painful?				
MD: Yes, because every time you get up or sit down, you put some pressure on the bone that is fractured; but it heals on its own. I will give you some oxycodone, which is a form of narcotic. You take it every four hours and you can take one or two at a time depending on whether you grade your pain as moderate or severe.				
Ms. W: I cannot hold anything in my right hand, and I cannot walk well. My grandson goes to high school and is not around enough to help me. What can I do?				
MD: Well, I'll call the hospital's case manager. Your insurance, which is Medicare, will pay for a stay in a sub acute rehabilitation center. There, the physical therapists will help you learn to walk with a walker that will only require one hand to manage. You can bear weight as you tolerate it, because a little weight bearing helps speed up your healing.				
Ms. W: Well, why do I need a cast on my wrist? Couldn't using and moving the wrist speed the healing for the wrist in the same way?				
MD: No, it's a different part of the body and more unstable because of the constant movement of the wrist. Once the cast is removed, you can wear a brace for a few weeks afterwards.				
Break It Down	☐	☐	☐	☐

☐ CIFE with patient ☐ CIFE with provider ☐ FLOW ☐ REGISTER

Role-Play 36: Glossary

_______________ _______________ _______________

_______________ _______________ _______________

_______________ _______________ _______________

continued

PO Box 2308, Woburn, MA 01888-0508, **p:** 781-729-3736, **www.EmbracingCulture.com**
PO Box 6401, Manchester, NH 03108, **p:** 1-888-678-CCCS

1. Pathology (diseases, conditions)

2. Laboratory Tests and Diagnostic Procedures

3. Treatment Procedures

4. Idiomatic Expressions (if any)

5. Other (vocabulary in this particular role-play that you feel is important/relevant or that you anticipate problems with)

Role-Play 37: Broken Ankle

Mr. Borges is from Argentina. He works with a cousin who builds houses. His specialty is placing rocks in intricate patterns to make wonderful patios and rock walls. He has an eye for beauty and he is a perfectionist. He is known to have taken down an entire wall when rocks too big at the base altered the pattern. Five days ago, a large rock fell off a wall he was building at a home in Lynnfield. It hit Mr. Borges on the foot. He has been limping since then. Last night, he could not sleep. He finally agreed to go to the Emergency Room.

	Pronunciation	Additions	Omissions	Mistakes
MD: Mr. Borges, the nurse has told me that you hurt your foot and we have already gotten X-rays. I want to tell you that you have broken the lateral malleolus. It is the distal end of the fibula, which is the smaller bone going from your knee down to the outside of your ankle.				
Mr. B.: I want to work. Can you fix it so I can go back to work?				
MD: Tell me when this occurred and how it happened.				
Mr. B.: Well, it happened at the beginning of the week, about five days ago. A rock we were using on a rock wall fell on my foot. I kept working. It was not so bad, but it has been quite painful lately. I could not sleep at all last night.				
MD: Well, you broke your ankle. Luckily the skin did not break at all so this is not a compound fracture. There still is a significant amount of swelling. I can put a splint on your foot and for the next five days you need to keep your leg elevated. Then you can come back here to our Ortho Clinic and we'll put on a walking cast.				
Mr. B.: Can I go back to work?				
MD: My advice is that you don't work for the first five days with the splint on. We want the swelling to go down. You'll need to keep your leg up. You'll also need to put ice on the ankle for 30 minutes four times a day.				
Mr. B.: Can I work when you give me the cast?				
MD: Yes, I think you can, especially if you don't drop any more rocks on your foot. By the way, I'll give you some anti-inflammatory pills to help with the swelling and the pain.				
Mr. B.: Thank you Doctor, but I am not worried about the pain. I am worried about not working.				

continued

PO Box 2308, Woburn, MA 01888-0508, **p:** 781-729-3736, **www.EmbracingCulture.com**
PO Box 6401, Manchester, NH 03108, **p:** 1-888-678-CCCS

Role-Play 37 *(continued)*

	Pronunciation	Additions	Omissions	Mistakes
MD: If there is anything good about this visit it's that from reviewing your chart, I see that the skin rash on your arms and face is getting better. Are you using the cream for the itching?				
Mr. B.: Yes, but I'd much rather have the itching than this pain! I could work with the itching.				
MD: I understand, and I am sorry about all the troubles, but the good thing is that nowadays you do not have to stay in the cast as long as in the past. Within just 4-5 weeks we may be able to stabilize your ankle with a special boot, giving you a bit more freedom and mobility.				
Mr. B.: I think I'm still in shock. I have worked with these rocks for so many years, and this had to happen to me now?				
MD: I'll complete the forms so that you can receive workman's compensation or would you like to speak to one of our wonderful social workers?				
Mr. B.: My situation is complicated, and I would rather you not report anything. I will talk to my boss.				
MD: You let me know. Here is a letter stating that you have to stay off your feet for the next week until I see you again. Please contact us immediately if you find your leg hot or swollen or if you have a fever or you see a red line. Keep your leg up, keep moving or wiggling your toes, and rest. No work!				
Break It Down	☐	☐	☐	☐

☐ **CIFE with patient** ☐ **CIFE with provider** ☐ **FLOW** ☐ **REGISTER**

Role-Play 37: Glossary

______________ ______________ ______________

______________ ______________ ______________

______________ ______________ ______________

______________ ______________ ______________

______________ ______________ ______________

______________ ______________ ______________

continued

1. Pathology (diseases, conditions)

2. Laboratory Tests and Diagnostic Procedures

3. Treatment Procedures

4. Idiomatic Expressions (if any)

5. Other (vocabulary in this particular role-play that you feel is important/relevant or that you anticipate problems with)

PO Box 2308, Woburn, MA 01888-0508, **p:** 781-729-3736, **www.EmbracingCulture.com**
PO Box 6401, Manchester, NH 03108, **p:** 1-888-678-CCCS

Role-Play 38: Arthritis

	Pronunciation	Additions	Omissions	Mistakes
PT: Doctor, I have noticed a few changes since I turned 50, but I am a bit concerned about the most recent one. A few months ago, I began to notice that my rings do not slide on and off of my fingers as easily as they did in past. I blamed my weight, but soon after I began to feel pain in my knuckles. See how red and swollen they are?				
MD: Do they hurt when I touch them?				
PT: Yes, but it's mostly like the pain is coming from the inside.				
MD: Any family history of arthritis?				
PT: Yes! My mother's half brother. I remember that when I was a child, his hands were deformed. The fingers were bent. He was a court stenographer, and he had to give up his job because he couldn't type any more.				
MD: Anyone else in your family with a history of arthritis?				
PT: Yes, my mother suffered from a bone condition. I guess that my genes aren't so good after all.				
MD: What kind of work do you do?				
PT: I use my hands a lot. I write for a community newspaper. I used to crochet quite a lot, but I've been so busy lately.				
MD: Is there anything you do to ease the pain?				
PT: I love to run hot water over my hands.				
MD: I will order a few blood tests. I can send you for an X-ray, but from just looking at you joints, it seems that you already have some bony spurs. It looks like you have osteoarthritis.				
PT: What can I do about it?				
MD: Massage therapy will help you with managing the pain. Even the usage of your fingers such as going back to your crochet little by little can help manage the pain. You can useTylenol as needed. I would stay away from nonsteroidals like Motrin because they can cause gastritis or kidney failure.				
PT: Doctor, can you tell me more about this illness? Is it an autoimmune disorder?				

continued

Role-Play 38 *(continued)*

	Pronunciation	Additions	Omissions	Mistakes
MD: I do not think that this is rheumatoid arthritis. You are not complaining of any fatigue, or of losing significant weight. I do not see or feel any subcutaneous nodules. But we'll order some blood tests to check the anti-nuclear antibody and the rheumatoid factor just to make sure there is no autoimmune activity.				
Break It Down	☐	☐	☐	☐

☐ **CIFE with patient** ☐ **CIFE with provider** ☐ **FLOW** ☐ **REGISTER**

Role-Play 38: Glossary

continued

PO Box 2308, Woburn, MA 01888-0508, **p:** 781-729-3736, **www.EmbracingCulture.com**
PO Box 6401, Manchester, NH 03108, **p:** 1-888-678-CCCS

1. Pathology (diseases, conditions)

2. Laboratory Tests and Diagnostic Procedures

3. Treatment Procedures

4. Idiomatic Expressions (if any)

5. Other (vocabulary in this particular role-play that you feel is important/relevant or that you anticipate problems with)

Role-Play 39: Sprains, Fractures and Severe Bruises

1. **Elevation** of the injured part (above the level of your heart), and ice packs (applied intermittently) on the area of injury will lessen swelling during the first 48 hours. To make an ice pack, place ice in a plastic bag and wrap the bag with a small towel. DO NOT APPLY ICE DIRECTLY ON THE SKIN AS THIS MAY CAUSE FROSTBITE.
2. Occasionally wiggle your fingers or toes to help circulation, but otherwise **REST** the injured part to help prevent or reduce swelling.
3. If the injured part gets more **painful, cold** or **swollen**, turns **blue** or **numb**, is worsening or lasting longer than expected, or if you develop pain in another area (especially your chest or abdomen), call your physician or **return to the Emergency Department.**
4. If you have been advised to use an **elastic bandage (Ace Wrap)**, rewrap if it is either too light or too loose. Remove the elastic bandage before going to sleep, unless it is being used to hold on a splint. **Make sure the splint is not too tight** before you go to sleep.
5. Use a **cane** or **crutches** if so directed.
6. If you have a cast or splint, do not put weight on it unless and until your doctor advises you to. **Serious complications may occur if the cast or splint is too tight.** Watch for and report immediately to your doctor any of the following in your toes or fingers:
    - **Swelling** or increasing **pain**.
    - **Paleness.**
    - **Numbness, tingling** or **coolness** (as compared to the other side).
    - **Change in color** (darkening or blueness).
    - **Loss of movement.**
    - **Rubbing** sensation, **burning** or **soreness** of skin.
7. **X-Rays -** Your X-rays may have had a preliminary reading by the Emergency Physician. They will receive an official reading by the Radiologist in the morning. You can sign out your films after that time, to take to your doctor's office for your follow-up check.

Role-Play 39: Glossary

PO Box 2308, Woburn, MA 01888-0508, **p:** 781-729-3736, **www.EmbracingCulture.com**
PO Box 6401, Manchester, NH 03108, **p:** 1-888-678-CCCS

1. Pathology (diseases, conditions)

2. Laboratory Tests and Diagnostic Procedures

3. Treatment Procedures

4. Idiomatic Expressions (if any)

5. Other (vocabulary in this particular role-play that you feel is important/relevant or that you anticipate problems with)

Role-Play 40: Tendinitis / Bursitis / Arthritis

Tendinitis and Bursitis are inflammatory conditions that may be related to over-use or injury. These conditions generally respond well to rest, warm soaks, and medications. Some patients tend to have recurrent problems. Please follow the instruction outlined below:

1. Occasionally wiggle your fingers or toes to help circulation, but otherwise **REST** the affected part to help prevent or reduce swelling.
2. If possible, **elevation** of the effected part (above the level of your heart), and warm soaks or **packs** (applied intermittently) on the area will reduce pain.
3. If the effected part gets more **painful, cold** or **swollen**, turns **blue** or **numb**, is worsening or lasting longer than expected, or if you develop pain in another area, call your physician or **return to the Emergency Department**.
4. If you have been advised to use an **elastic bandage (Ace Wrap)**, rewrap if it is either too tight or too loose. Remove the elastic bandage before going to sleep, unless it is being used to hold on a splint. **Make sure the splint is not too tight** before you go to sleep.
5. If the doctor has determined that you need **medications**, fill the prescription and use as directed on the bottle.
6. Use a **cane** or **crutches** if so directed.
7. If you have a cast or splint, do not put weight on it unless and until your doctor advises you to do so. **Serious complications may occur if the cast splint is too tight.** Watch for and report immediately to your doctor any of the following signs in your toes or fingers:
   - **Swelling** or increasing **pain**
   - **Paleness – Numbness, tingling** or **coolness** (as compared to the other side).
   - **Change in color** (darkness or blueness).
   - **Loss of movement**
   - **Rubbing** sensation, **burning** or **soreness** of skin.
8. **X-Rays** If you had X-rays, they may have had a preliminary reading by the Emergency Physician. They will receive an official reading by the Radiologist later. You can sign out your films after the final reading to take to your doctor's office for your follow-up check.

Role-Play 40: Glossary

PO Box 2308, Woburn, MA 01888-0508, **p:** 781-729-3736, **www.EmbracingCulture.com**
PO Box 6401, Manchester, NH 03108, **p:** 1-888-678-CCCS

1. Pathology (diseases, conditions)

2. Laboratory Tests and Diagnostic Procedures

3. Treatment Procedures

4. Idiomatic Expressions (if any)

5. Other (vocabulary in this particular role-play that you feel is important/relevant or that you anticipate problems with)

Lesson Eight: Additional Resources
The Skeletal System

COMMON BONE DISORDERS

Below you will find summaries of some common bone disorders.

Illness	Meaning	Target
1. Arthritis	Inflammation of a joint.	
2. Bone Cancer	Cancer originating in the bone is primary bone cancer. Metastatic bone cancer is cancer of a different organ that has spread to the bone. Cancers most likely to spread to bone include thyroid, lung, kidney, prostate, and bladder cancer.	
3. Gout	This is an arthritis, usually sudden with severe pain. It is stimulated by excess uric acid that collects in the synovial fluid in the form of small needles. The clinician collects fluid from the inflamed joint and sees the gouty crystals as small needles in the fluid. It is associated with rich foods and excessive alcohol, but can occur also in times of stress such as an acute hospitalization. It can be treated with anti inflammatory drugs as well as allopurinol, which helps diminish the amount of uric acid available for deposit.	
4. Osteoarthritis	Articular cartilage breaks down leaving bone to press on bone in a synovial joint. This can stimulate inflammatory reactions with painful joints. Eventually a gap in the cartilage reaches the bone and blood vessels grow and a plug made of fibrocartilage fills the gap. Firbrocartilage plugs wear away exposing bone surface.	
5. Osteomalacia	The bones are weakened by the loss of both calcium and phosphorous and this is usually due to shortage of vitamin D. In children this is called rickets.	
6. Osteoporosis	The bone's thinning and becoming more porous with age, which is common in both genders. However as women stop menstruating and have less estrogen, the osteoporosis becomes worse.	
7. Paget's Disease	This disease finds bone broken down at an increased rate and replaced rapidly by abnormal bone. It can occur in the skull, spine, pelvis and leg bones.	

continued

PO Box 2308, Woburn, MA 01888-0508, **p:** 781-729-3736, **www.EmbracingCulture.com**
PO Box 6401, Manchester, NH 03108, **p:** 1-888-678-CCCS

Common Bone Disorders *(continued)*

Illness	Meaning	Target
8. Rheumatoid Arthritis	When the body's own immune system attacks the joint and the joint becomes hot, swollen and tender. This can affect small joints of the body and can cause severe deformation of the joints. Now there are more drugs available to fight this debilitating disease.	

MAIN TESTS AND PROCEDURES

Main Test/Procedure	Meaning	Target
1. Amputation	Partial or complete removal of a limb	
2. Arthrocentesis	Puncture into a joint to remove fluid.	
3. Arthrography	X-ray examination that uses a contrast agent to image a joint.	
4. Arthroscopy	Visual examination of a joint using a fiber-optical scope	
5. Bone scan	Nuclear scanning test to find abnormalities in the bone.	
6. Closed reduction of fractures	Setting a bone without an operation.	
7. Casting	Immobilizing a limb or body part with a special fiber or type of a plaster that snuggles around the limb and solidifies.	
8. Splinting	Immobilizing a limb with a splint. They are ideal for emergency room and first-aid situations, involving fractures or sprains. Splints immobilize the injured area but do not seal it completely, allowing for swelling to happen. Then, when the swelling is resolved, a more permanent cast may be used.	
9. Traction	A pulling force exerted on a fracture by means of a special device that creates the necessary tension to reduce the fracture.	
10. Laminectomy	Excision of part or whole of the lamina of the vertebral bone,	
11. Myelography	X-ray or CT of the spinal column after injection of dye.	
12. Open reduction of fractures	Treatment of bone fractures by the use of surgery.	
13. Sequestrectomy	Surgical removal, or excision, of a sequestrum.	

continued

SKELETAL SYSTEM VOCABULARY

Main Organs and Body Structures:	
Vocabulary Word	**Target Language**
Axial skeleton	
Carpals	
Clavicle	
Coccyx	
Costo	
Cranial bones	
Cranium	
Facial bones	
Femur	
Fibula	
Humerus	
Ischium	
Joints	
Mandible	
Maxilla	
Metacarpals	
Metatarsals	
Osteoclasts	
Osteocytes	
Patella	
Pelvic bone	
Phalanges	
Pelvis	
Pubis	
Radius	
Ribs	
Sacrum	
Scapula	
Short bones	

continued

PO Box 2308, Woburn, MA 01888-0508, **p:** 781-729-3736, **www.EmbracingCulture.com**
PO Box 6401, Manchester, NH 03108, **p:** 1-888-678-CCCS

Main Organs and Body Structures *(continued)*

Vocabulary Word	Target Language
Skull	
Spine	
Sternum	
Tarsals	
Thoracic	
Tibia	
Ulna	
Vertebra	
Vertebral column	

Main Illnesses:

Vocabulary Word	Target Language
Arthritis	
Bone cancer	
Bursitis	
Carpal tunnel	
Dislocation	
Ewing's sarcoma	
Fractures	
Gout	
Herniated disk	
Kyphosis	
Lordosis	
Osteoarthritis	
Osteomalacia	
Osteoporosis	
Osteosarcoma	
Paget's disease	
Rheumatoid arthritis	
Scoliosis	

Main Tests and Procedures:

Vocabulary Word	Target Language
Amputation	
Arthrocentesis	
Arthrography	
Arthroplasty	
Arthroscopy	
Bone scan	
Calcium level	
Closed reduction of fractures	
Casting	
Splinting	
Traction	
Laminectomy	
Myelography	
Open reduction of fractures	
Phosphorus level	
Sequestrectomy	

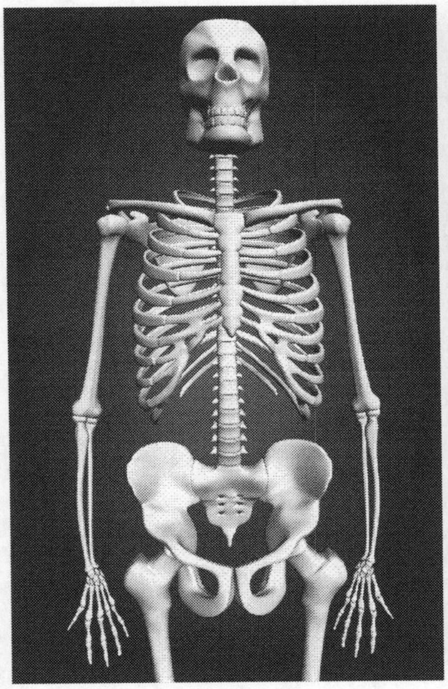
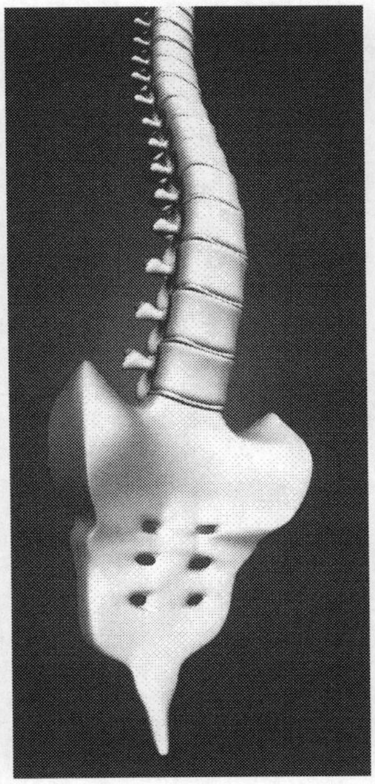
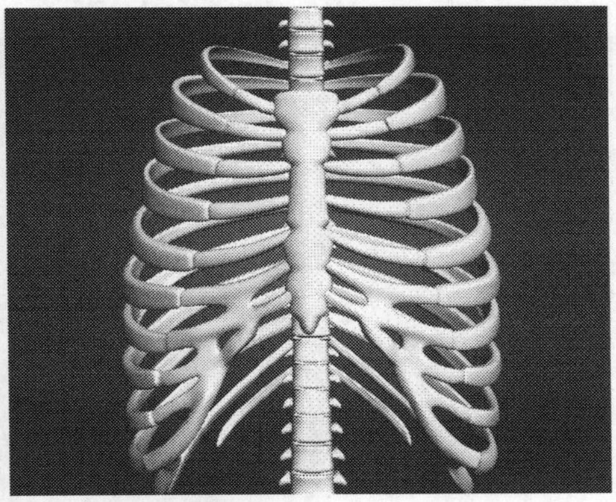
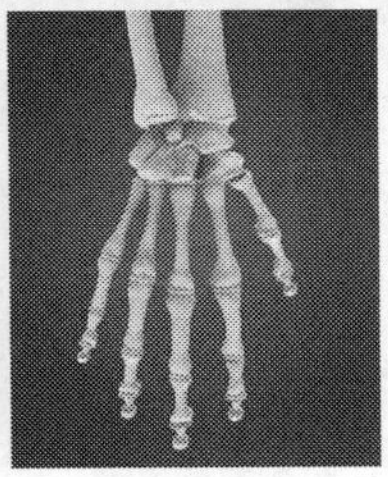

PO Box 2308, Woburn, MA 01888-0508, **p:** 781-729-3736, **www.EmbracingCulture.com**
PO Box 6401, Manchester, NH 03108, **p:** 1-888-678-CCCS

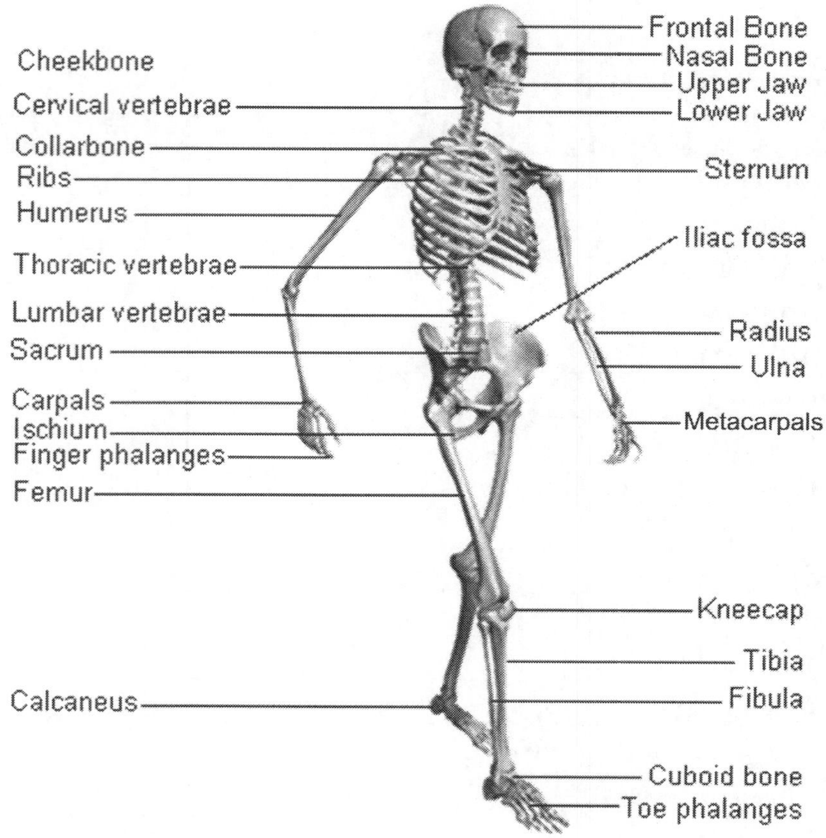
Frontal Bone
Nasal Bone
Upper Jaw
Lower Jaw
Cheekbone
Cervical vertebrae
Collarbone
Ribs
Sternum
Humerus
Iliac fossa
Thoracic vertebrae
Lumbar vertebrae
Radius
Sacrum
Ulna
Carpals
Ischium
Metacarpals
Finger phalanges
Femur
Kneecap
Tibia
Calcaneus
Fibula
Cuboid bone
Toe phalanges

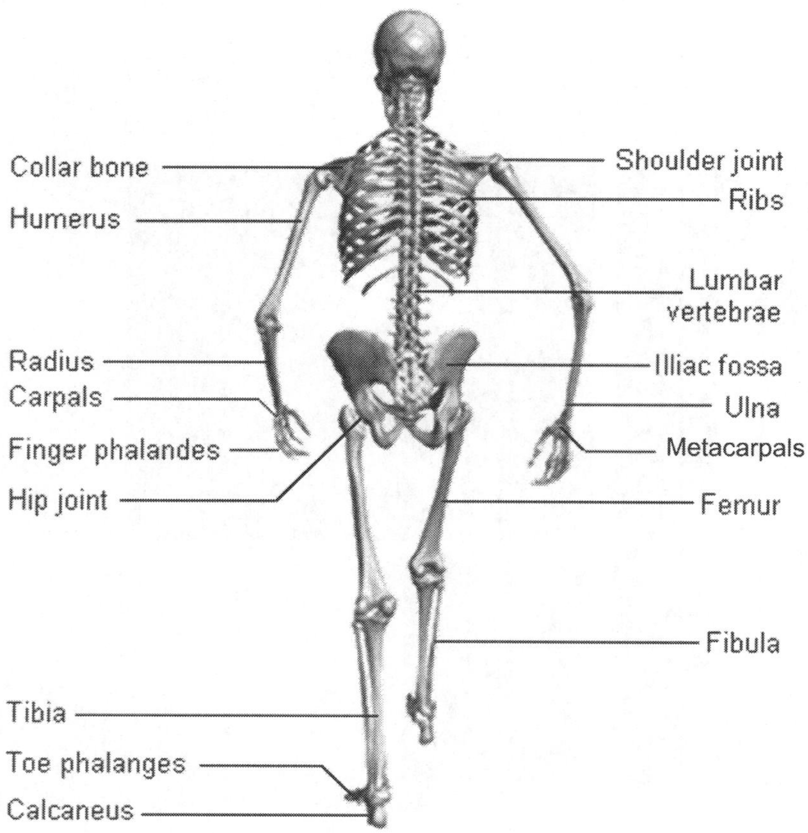
Collar bone
Shoulder joint
Ribs
Humerus
Lumbar vertebrae
Radius
Illiac fossa
Carpals
Ulna
Finger phalandes
Metacarpals
Hip joint
Femur
Fibula
Tibia
Toe phalanges
Calcaneus

Lesson Nine: Role-Play Practice

Understanding Goals

Students will:

- test their knowledge of medical terminology
- test their understanding about illnesses/ conditions studied in previous lessons
- test their understanding of key concepts studied in the course
- practice consecutive interpreting
- practice using memory aids
- apply their understanding of the Standards of Practice

Key concepts are based on the review of:

- Interpreter roles
- Interpreter modes
- CIFE
- Memory aids
- Managing of the flow of the session
- Medical interpreter standards

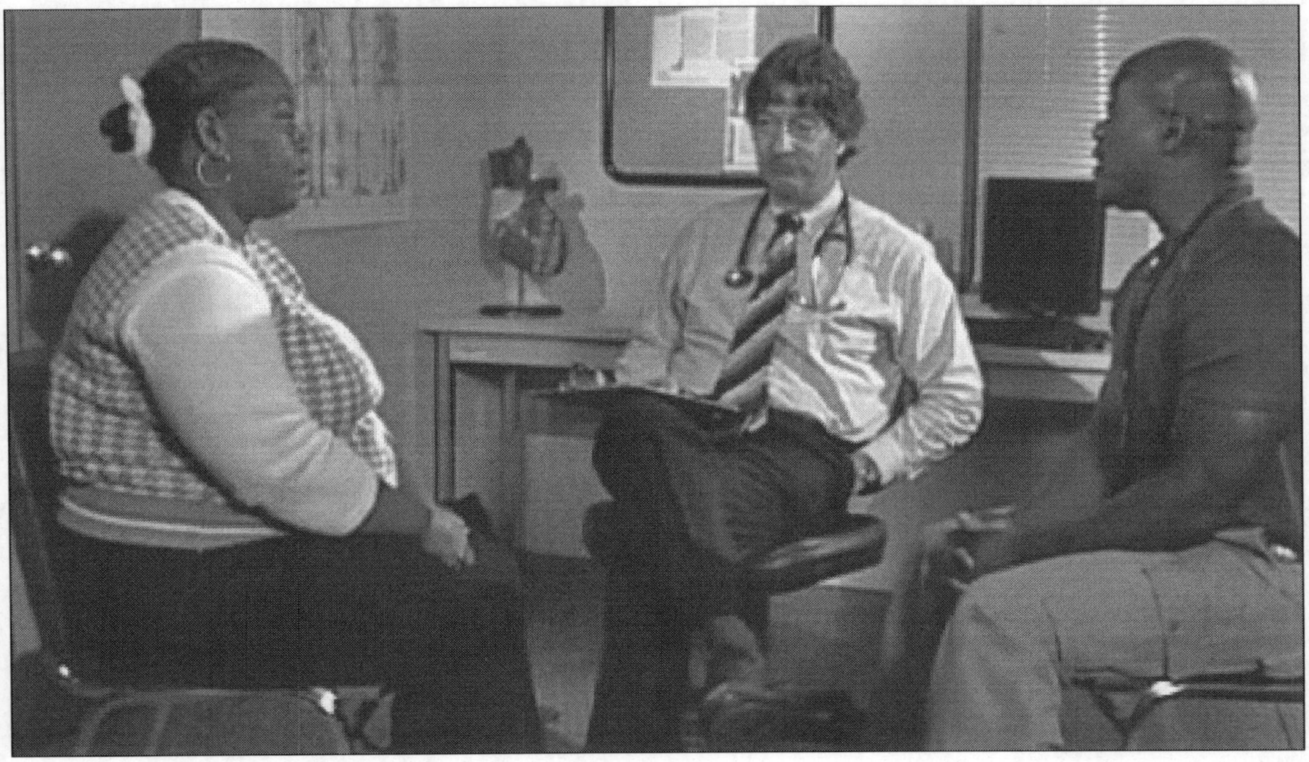

PO Box 2308, Woburn, MA 01888-0508, **p:** 781-729-3736, **www.EmbracingCulture.com**
PO Box 6401, Manchester, NH 03108, **p:** 1-888-678-CCCS

Lesson Nine: Class Activities
Role-Play Practice

Activity 1 – Medical Interpreter Jeopardy Game

- Divide into teams
- All steps will be timed
- We will have two teams on the floor
- Each team will choose a category to answer
- As a team you will have a few seconds to discuss the potential correct answer
- Choose someone in the group to answer
- If your group has the wrong answer or takes longer than time allotted, immediately the other groups will be given a chance to answer questions correctly

A note of caution for all the other groups:
All groups should be equally engaged in sorting correct answers so to quickly replace the one with the wrong answer.

There are nine categories, each category has several questions. Correct answers to Standards of Practice and Word Formation categories will receive double points.

1. Medical Professions
2. Standards of Practice
3. Conditions
4. Diagnostic Tests
5. Treatment and Procedures
6. Word Formation
7. Immunizations
8. Body Parts and Organs
9. Abbreviations

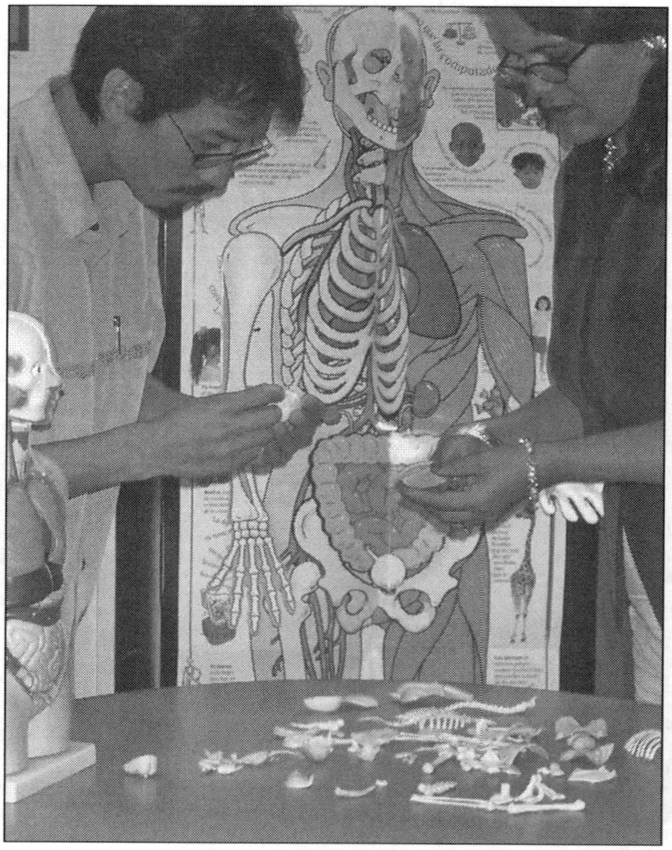

Lesson Nine: Role-Plays
Role-Play Practice

Work individually at first:

- Read the entire role-play
- Get a general sense of its meaning
- Circle the most challenging medical terms
- Apply the Samurai! technique to those terms
- Read the role-play again for a deeper understanding
- Find an accurate equivalent in the target language

Work in a language-specific group of friends, fellow students or colleagues:

- Share your doubts
- Ask for other ways of expressing the same meaning
- Develop a glossary
- Check the dictionary
- Practice the role-plays – remember to do CIFE for all your role-plays
- Have your colleagues observe you and provide feedback on your accuracy and register.
- These colleagues can keep track of any omissions, additions, mistakes or distortions in your interpreting and point these out to you in a follow-up discussion.

Student Interpreter Evaluation

Student Name ______________________ Date ________

Language ______________________

Mode of Interpreting (check one): ☐ Consecutive ☐ Simultaneous

Role-Play/System ______________________

Areas Observed ______________________

Accuracy

Register ______________________

Omissions ______________________

Additions ______________________

Distortions ______________________

Pronunciation ______________________

Speaker's emotions conveyed? ______________________

Explain ______________________

Technique

General flow ______________________

Flow when requesting clarification ______________________

Speed ______________________

Eye Contact ______________________

Distracting Habits ______________________

Ethical Issues

Answered questions for patient? ______________________

Advised patient? ______________________

Vocabulary Expansion Recommendations

____

____

Other Recommendations

____

____

Language Coach Signature ______________________ Date ________

PO Box 2308, Woburn, MA 01888-0508, **p:** 781-729-3736, **www.EmbracingCulture.com**
PO Box 6401, Manchester, NH 03108, **p:** 1-888-678-CCCS

Work individually at first:

- Read the entire role-play
- Get a general sense of its meaning
- Circle the most challenging medical terms
- Apply the Samurai! technique to those terms (using the prefix/root/suffix section of this chapter)
- Read the context again for a deeper understanding of each term
- Find an accurate equivalent for each term in the target language
- Think and note the most appropriate interpreting behaviors according to the Medical Interpreters Standards
- Review your memory aids techniques

Next, work in a language-specific group of fellow students or colleagues:

- Share any doubts that were not resolved in your research
- Exchange definitions for each term and take note of variations in your colleagues' translations
- Check each variation in a dictionary or target language encyclopedia
- Note the terms collected (in glossary format)
- Practice the role-plays. One group member will read the part of the provider in English. A second group member will sight translate the part of the patient. A third group member will act as the interpreter (without a script). Remaining group members will silently evaluate the patient and interpreter's performances, and provide constructive feedback immediately following the role-play.
- Apply the most appropriate interpreting behaviors according to medical interpreters standards
- Apply memory aids techniques (use hand signal to slow down the speaker to a minimum!)

Remember that role-plays are also a look into the mind of a provider; so, the more you practice, the greater your understanding of the concepts behind medical procedure.

Variation: If you are working alone, make use of the audio recordings of this manual's role-plays (for an additional cost), available at www.cccsorg.com. Record your interpretations and play them back with the purpose of post-performance self-evaluation.

Role-Play Practice

Role-Play 41: Hives

Instructions:

1. Do a complete CIFE
2. Apply finger counting in this role-play
3. Use appropriate interpreting mode
4. You can not use your hand signal
5. React appropriately to ethics challenge

A 78-year-old woman went out to dinner at the house of a family member and she developed hives after eating shrimp.

MD: I heard you are feeling pretty miserable. Your daughter just called me and she reported that you have been getting these big hives around your face, arms and on your neck. They seem to be big red blotches that come and go. Is this right?

PT: I had dinner at my son-in-law's parents. They always cook the best shrimp. I love it with cilantro and garlic and wine. It's the best! And I should be used to their cooking by now. Really, I have no idea why I am getting this skin rash.

MD: Are you having any difficulty breathing or did you have any difficulty breathing after you ate the shrimp?

PT: I do not know, I did feel some chest tightness!

MD: Do you have any allergies? Is there anyone in your family with any allergies to food?

PT: No , I do not think so.

MD: I am going to check your lungs. Please take a deep breath, hold it, and breathe out slowly. Again breathe in, a big breath, hold it and breathe out. Your lungs sound perfect!

PT: Do not tell me that now I can't eat any more shrimp. I did feel a bit of a ticklish feeling in my throat. I got some water and I went outside for some fresh air and my breathing got better. I went home and I noticed the skin rash right here (pointing to her neck, face and arms).

(**MD to the Interpreter**: There is a good reason why our people do not eat shrimp!)

MD: I have a feeling that you are developing a low allergy to the shrimp. I would like for you to schedule an appointment with the allergy clinic. There are people who all of a sudden develop these types of allergies, and they can just manifest with your symptoms or sometimes the symptoms can even become life threatening. I am going to give you Benadryl for the hives. Take one pill four times a day. Please go to the emergency room nearest you right away if you are having difficulty breathing. And don't eat shrimp until we get the results of the test. Here is the referral to the allergist.

continued

PO Box 2308, Woburn, MA 01888-0508, **p:** 781-729-3736, **www.EmbracingCulture.com**
PO Box 6401, Manchester, NH 03108, **p:** 1-888-678-CCCS

Role-Play 41 *(continued)*

Questions:

1. What should the interpreter do when a provider makes a side remark?

2. How did you manage the finger-counting technique?

3. Were you able to complete CIFE in a timely matter?

Additional Comments:

Role-Play 41: Glossary

continued

1. Pathology (diseases, conditions)

2. Laboratory Tests and Diagnostic Procedures

3. Treatment Procedures

4. Idiomatic Expressions (if any)

5. Other (vocabulary in this particular role-play that you feel is important/relevant or that you anticipate problems with)

PO Box 2308, Woburn, MA 01888-0508, **p:** 781-729-3736, **www.EmbracingCulture.com**
PO Box 6401, Manchester, NH 03108, **p:** 1-888-678-CCCS

Role-Play 42: Conjunctivitis

Instructions:
1. Do a complete CIFE
2. Apply the memory aid that suits you best in this role play
3. Use consecutive mode
4. You can only use your hand signal one time
5. React appropriately to ethics challenge

A 15-year-old girl arrives at the outpatient clinic with conjunctivitis.

MD: So, I heard you've had a lot of itching in one of your eyes today. Your mother called me and said you weren't feeling so good.

PT: A few days ago I started to notice that I was scratching my right eye for no particular reason. The itching has been increasing and today I woke up with a discharge from my eye. Just look how swollen and red my eye looks! I am having difficulty opening it.

MD: This looks like a classic case of conjunctivitis. This is contagious for the first 24 hours after your start the treatment with this ointment. The ointment will relieve the pain and reduce the inflammation or redness.

PT: What am I going to do about school?

MD: Today and tomorrow just rest. Please wash your hands every time you touch your eye and avoid any physical contact with other people. This is extremely contagious, and I am sure you got it from someone else you know.

PT: Is my vision going to stay blurry for a long time?

MD: Perhaps for the next twenty-four hours and after each time you place the ointment in your eye. I will show you how to best place the ointment, watch. With your left hand place one finger on your right upper eyelid and place the other finger on your lower right lid. Keep your eyelids wide open and give the tube of ointment one nice squeeze when it is over the inside part of your eyelid. Blink your eyes twice, and then rest them. Avoid touching or rubbing your right eye.

MD to the Interpreter: Wow, did you smell that curry? The hygiene with these people is not so good. I am wondering if they wash their hands after cooking their curry dishes.

continued

Role-Play 42 *(continued)*

Questions:

"Wow, did you smell that curry? The hygiene with these people is not so good. I am wondering if they wash their hands after cooking their curry dishes."

This comment was made at the end of the session when the patient was not present.

1. Should you ignore it? Support your answer with the Standards of Practice.

2. Describe your memory aids

3. Which mode(s) did you use and why?

Additional Comments:

Role-Play 42: Glossary

continued

PO Box 2308, Woburn, MA 01888-0508, **p:** 781-729-3736, **www.EmbracingCulture.com**
PO Box 6401, Manchester, NH 03108, **p:** 1-888-678-CCCS

1. Pathology (diseases, conditions)

2. Laboratory Tests and Diagnostic Procedures

3. Treatment Procedures

4. Idiomatic Expressions (if any)

5. Other (vocabulary in this particular role-play that you feel is important/relevant or that you anticipate problems with)

Role-Play 43: Ulcer

Instructions:

1. Do a complete CIFE.
2. Apply the memory aid that suits you the best in this role-play.
3. Use consecutive mode.
4. React appropriately to ethics challenge.

A man comes to the emergency room complaining of "chest pain."

MD: Can you describe your pain?

Patient: I have a terrible burning in my chest.

MD: Where exactly is this burning sensation? Can you point to where you feel the most pain?

Patient: Right here (points to mid-chest) and here (points to stomach).

MD: Does the burning sensation intensify an hour or so after meals, if you miss a meal or after you drink alcohol or eat fatty or spicy foods?

Patient: Yes, in all of those cases it does, but it's much worse at night.

MD: It sounds like, at the very least, you have acid indigestion and heartburn. Often, when people eat too much heavy or greasy food or drink too much alcohol or coffee, the stomach produces extra acid which causes the discomfort or burning feeling you've been having. Some people mistake the chest pain for a heart problem rather than indigestion. But if the pain gets worse when you are lying down, it is probably heartburn. Frequent or lasting indigestion is often a warning sign of an ulcer, but without an endoscopy, it will be hard to tell whether you have an ulcer or not.

Patient: What is an ulcer?

MD: An ulcer is a chronic sore in the stomach or small intestine caused by too much acid. It may cause a continual dull or sometimes sharp pain in the pit of the stomach.

continued

PO Box 2308, Woburn, MA 01888-0508, **p:** 781-729-3736, **www.EmbracingCulture.com**
PO Box 6401, Manchester, NH 03108, **p:** 1-888-678-CCCS

Role-Play 43 *(continued)*

Questions:

Keep in mind that some patients describe their anatomy differently than medical providers, such as pointing to their stomach while complaining of their chest pain.

1. In this situation, should the interpreter interfere and ask for clarification?

2. Describe your memory aids.

3. How often did you use your hand signal?

Additional Comments:

Role-Play 43: Glossary

continued

1. Pathology (diseases, conditions)

2. Laboratory Tests and Diagnostic Procedures

3. Treatment Procedures

4. Idiomatic Expressions (if any)

5. Other (vocabulary in this particular role-play that you feel is important/relevant or that you anticipate problems with)

PO Box 2308, Woburn, MA 01888-0508, **p:** 781-729-3736, **www.EmbracingCulture.com**
PO Box 6401, Manchester, NH 03108, **p:** 1-888-678-CCCS

Role-Play 44: Cataracts

Instructions:

1. Do a complete CIFE.
2. Apply the memory aid that suits you the best in this role-play.
3. Use consecutive mode.
4. You can only use your hand signal one time.
5. React appropriately to ethics challenge.

Mrs. Esquival is a 77-year-old woman from El Salvador who takes care of her grandchildren during the day. Her daughter and son-in-law each work two jobs and so her help is very necessary to the family. Lately, she has been having trouble with her vision. Her grandson, Enrique, noticed it and urged her to see an eye doctor. During a recent trip to the health center when her grandson had conjunctivitis, the precocious 8-year-old talked his grandmother into going to the eye doctor, who fortuitously had an open slot for her.

MD: Hello, Mrs. Esquival. My assistant tells me that you are having trouble with your eyes. Can you tell me what the problem is?

Mrs. E: Well, it started last year. I had more and more difficulty seeing at night. I do not drive, but when in the car at night, I had trouble reading signs. Now it seems like I am looking through a film of water on my eyes.

MD: OK, do you have problems with pain in your eyes or headaches?

Mrs. E: No.

MD: OK, let's examine your eyes and see what's happening.

(Examines the eye with the slit lamp machine and takes a pressure reading of each eye.)

MD: Mrs. E. I am happy to tell you that the pressure inside your eyes is normal and so you don't have glaucoma. But the lenses in both of your eyes are showing that you have cataracts.

Mrs. E: What is a cataract? Is it dangerous?

MD: A cataract is a change that occurs inside the lens of the eye. The lens is normally transparent, allowing light to enter and focus itself on the back of the eye; however, a cataract is a loss of transparency of the lens. It affects night vision and eventually makes day-to-day activities such as reading or watching TV very difficult. Some say, just like you did, that it is like trying to see through a mist, or a room filled with water. The name cataract comes from Latin and means waterfall.

Mrs. E: Is there a medicine that I can take to get rid of this? Can I get glasses to fix it?

MD: Well, I can give you some glasses that will help you, but the way to fix this is for you to have surgery. You are an excellent candidate for this. We would do one eye at a time, extracting the lens and implanting an artificial lens in the eye. Your vision will be better than it has been for ten years.

continued

Role-Play 44 *(continued)*

Mrs. E: Is it expensive?

MD: Well, I see you are covered under your daughter's health insurance and it is completely covered by the insurance.

Mrs. E: How long would I be in the hospital? I have to take care of my grandchildren and our house.

MD: Well, the surgery is done without admission to a hospital. It is a day surgery. You would have to rest, but you could be taking care of Enrique again in three days. Of course, you can't lift heavy weights greater than 10 pounds for at least two weeks.

Mrs. E: Is it painful?

MD: It is uncomfortable at first, but it is rarely painful.

Mrs. E: Well, I know I need to do this because I need to be useful to my family. I will do it.

MD: OK, we'll start with your right eye. My assistant will schedule an appointment for you when you leave. I won't give you glasses right now because your prescription will change after you have had the surgery. Since it will be performed within the next two weeks, I think you'll be fine in the meantime. We'll examine you again after the surgery.

Mrs. E: OK, thank you very much.

MD: Of course, anytime.

Mrs. E: Thank you.

MD: Thank you.

Mrs. E (to the interpreter): If my daughter has questions, can she call you?

continued

PO Box 2308, Woburn, MA 01888-0508, **p:** 781-729-3736, **www.EmbracingCulture.com**
PO Box 6401, Manchester, NH 03108, **p:** 1-888-678-CCCS

Role-Play 44 *(continued)*

Questions:

1. How would you have handled this request?

2. Describe how your memory aids helped you managing the flow and assisted you with conveying accuracy of the message.

Additional Comments:

Role-Play 44: Glossary

continued

1. Pathology (diseases, conditions)

2. Laboratory Tests and Diagnostic Procedures

3. Treatment Procedures

4. Idiomatic Expressions (if any)

5. Other (vocabulary in this particular role-play that you feel is important/relevant or that you anticipate problems with)

PO Box 2308, Woburn, MA 01888-0508, **p:** 781-729-3736, **www.EmbracingCulture.com**
PO Box 6401, Manchester, NH 03108, **p:** 1-888-678-CCCS

Role-Play 45: Nutrition

Instructions:

1. Do a complete CIFE.
2. Apply the memory aid that suits you the best in this role-play.
3. You can not use your hand signal.
4. Use the interpreting mode that best suits this triadic encounter.
5. React appropriately to ethics challenge.

Tom is seeing his doctor today because he has been feeling tired a lot lately, even though he gets plenty of sleep. Along with feeling tired, he often lacks the energy to play sports with his friends during recess.

Doctor: Good morning, Tom. What brings you into my office today?

Tom: I feel tired all the time. I always feel like napping or sleeping.

Doctor: Do you get enough sleep? How many hours do you usually sleep at night?

Tom: I get plenty of sleep; at least 8 hours a night.

Doctor: Well, what about your eating habits? Do you eat three well-rounded meals each day?

Tom: Not really. For breakfast, I usually have a bowl of Lucky Charms before school. Then at lunch, I have like a slice of pizza or a cheeseburger with French fries. For dinner, Mom usually makes spaghetti or sloppy joes or something like that.

Doctor: Do you eat enough fruit and vegetables every day, like a banana with your cereal or some salad with Mom's spaghetti?

Tom: Not really. I don't really like vegetables. Fruits are OK, but I don't eat very much. Do French fries count as vegetables?

Doctor: No, French fries don't count. Have you heard of the food pyramid, Tom?

Tom: Yeah, it's like a triangle with a bunch of little boxes. You're supposed to eat what it says to stay healthy or something like that, right?

Doctor: That's right, Tom. It's put out by the Department of Agriculture and it lists the types of foods we should eat every day to stay balanced and healthy. According to the food pyramid, we're supposed to eat 6-11 servings of breads and cereals, 2-3 servings of milk, yogurt, and cheese, 2-3 servings of meat and nuts, 3-5 servings of vegetables and 2-4 servings of fruit. It seems like you get plenty of bread, milk and meat, but how many servings of vegetables and fruits do you eat every day?

continued

Role-Play 45 *(continued)*

Tom: I'm not sure, but I don't think it's that much. Is that why I feel tired all the time, because I don't eat my fruits and vegetables?

Doctor: Well, that's probably part of the reason why. In general, when our bodies aren't balanced with the right amount of food and exercise, we tend to lack energy and feel tired. That's probably why you feel the way you do.

Tom: So, if I started to eat more fruits and vegetables, then I'd feel better?

Doctor: You'll probably start to feel better, but you also have to eat healthier in general. Like instead of having French fries all the time, maybe you can have rice pilaf or a baked potato instead. It's best to cut down on fried foods and sweets.

Tom: What were you also saying about exercise? Will that help too?

Doctor: Yes, getting regular exercise will build up your energy level. So, the combination of eating right and exercising regularly will definitely help you feel better.

Tom: I had no idea that the foods I ate would make such a big difference in how I felt. So, even though I'm not the biggest fan of fruits and vegetables, I'm going to start eating more of them so that I'll have more energy from now on. And if I ever forget how many servings I'm supposed to eat, I'll just look at the food pyramid and find out.

The interpreter to the mother: I feel so bad for you and your son, my son also has diabetes and it is challenging because you know how kids are with sweets and birthday parties? God bless you!

continued

PO Box 2308, Woburn, MA 01888-0508, **p:** 781-729-3736, **www.EmbracingCulture.com**
PO Box 6401, Manchester, NH 03108, **p:** 1-888-678-CCCS

Role-Play 45 *(continued)*

Questions:

1. Were the interpreter's comments appropriate?

2. How could the interpreter have shown empathy towards the mother?

3. Describe your memory aids.

4. Describe your interpreting mode and explain why you have chosen it.

Additional Comments:

continued

Role-Play 45: Glossary

1. Pathology (diseases, conditions)

2. Laboratory Tests and Diagnostic Procedures

3. Treatment Procedures

4. Idiomatic Expressions (if any)

5. Other (vocabulary in this particular role-play that you feel is important/relevant or that you anticipate problems with)

PO Box 2308, Woburn, MA 01888-0508, **p:** 781-729-3736, **www.EmbracingCulture.com**
PO Box 6401, Manchester, NH 03108, **p:** 1-888-678-CCCS

Role-Play: 46 Herpes Zoster

Instructions:

1. Apply all the appropriate interpreting tools and standards that best suits this role-play.

Isabel is a 65-year-old Mexican immigrant. She went to her cousin's house in the country last week for a grand celebration. Everything went well until Isabel tripped up the stairs going into the church auditorium where everyone sat in long rows eating and talking about their work in the local factory. The next day, she noticed some itching on her back. Within two days, there was a long line of blisters on her left posterior thorax running from her spine to right under her left breast. It had become a burning pain. Isabel went to her Physician Assistant.

PA: Hello. What would you like to accomplish today?

Isabel: Well, I went to my cousin's house last week and I got this bad rash.

PA: Did you go out in the woods?

Isabel: No, I went to a party at the church. I fell. I was embarrassed, but I didn't hurt my back. Now I have this rash. It has blisters and it's very painful.

PA: OK, so you didn't walk in a wooded area.

Isabel: No.

PA: Let's examine you.

(Examines Patient)

PA: Well, this is a classic Herpes Zoster.

Isabel: Herpes! You can't be serious. I haven't had sex in five years.

PA: But this is Herpes Zoster, also called shingles. It is the same virus that causes chicken pox. After you get chicken pox, the virus goes into the nerve and stays there for a long time doing nothing. It's almost as if it were hibernating. If you suffer stress or get over-tired, or sometimes for no reason at all, the virus can "turn on" and cause a painful rash. I can give you a medicine that you can take that will diminish the length of time the active rash will be present. Sometimes though, the pain can continue long after the rash goes away. We won't know if that's true for you for about a week or two. Here is the medicine and here is an oatmeal bath that you should take twice a day to help with the rash. I'll also prescribe a pain medication that will help with the pain. Please call me in one week so I can know how you're doing.

Client to Interpreter: Can you please tell me how to get to the Pharmacy? And can you write down in English the name of that cereal? Thanks so much.

continued

Role-Play 46 *(continued)*

Questions:

1. What would you do as a professional interpreter?

2. Did you do a complete CIFE?

3. Describe your memory aids.

4. Describe your main interpreting mode.

Additional Comments:

continued

PO Box 2308, Woburn, MA 01888-0508, **p:** 781-729-3736, **www.EmbracingCulture.com**
PO Box 6401, Manchester, NH 03108, **p:** 1-888-678-CCCS

Role-Play 46: Glossary

1. Pathology (diseases, conditions)

2. Laboratory Tests and Diagnostic Procedures

3. Treatment Procedures

4. Idiomatic Expressions (if any)

5. Other (vocabulary in this particular role-play that you feel is important/relevant or that you anticipate problems with)

Role-Play 47: Mr. Vieira's Knees

Instructions:

1. Do a complete CIFE.
2. Apply the memory aid that suits you the best in this role-play.
3. You can only use your hand signal one time.
4. Use consecutive mode.
5. React appropriately to ethics challenge.

Mr. Vieira works in a computer manufacturing company. He speaks little English, but has learned how to assemble circuit boards for the company. He has done so well that he is the night supervisor for his shift and gets all the overtime he wants. In his free time, he loves to work on his home, doing repairs, renovations and odd jobs.

Mr. Vieira comes to his doctor's office for an appointment. The interpreter meets him in the waiting room. As the interpreter introduces herself, Mr. Vieira seems a little embarrassed. He tells the interpreter he would never have come to see the doctor, but the pain in both of his knees is so bad that it impedes his ability to walk. He is having difficulty climbing stairs at work, which is a problem, since he needs to supervise two floors and make sure that the circuit boards are moving quickly from station to station.

In the exam room, the medical assistant asks Mr. Vieira to take his pants off and she gives him a johnny to wear. The physician comes in.

MD: Hello Mr. Vieira. What brings you in today?

MR. V: I have bad pain in both of my knees. It's so bad I cannot walk. And if I can't walk, I can't work.

MD: How long have you had this pain?

MR. V: About two weeks now.

MD: Have you missed work because of it?

MR. V: No, but if it doesn't get better, I may have to take vacation time.

MD: Do you have sick time?

MR. V: I do not want to take it. I'm never sick.

MD: Did you twist or hit your knees recently?

MR. V: No. But I did put in a tile floor in my kitchen, three weeks ago. They started to hurt about halfway through the job. It got so bad I couldn't work on the floor unless I had some tequila first. It was so painful.

MD: Have your knees ever buckled or given way?

continued

PO Box 2308, Woburn, MA 01888-0508, **p:** 781-729-3736, **www.EmbracingCulture.com**
PO Box 6401, Manchester, NH 03108, **p:** 1-888-678-CCCS

Role-Play 47 *(continued)*

MR. V: No.

MD: Are they hot, tender or swollen?

MR. V: Yes, they feel hot and swollen right in front.

MD: When you were working on the floor, did you do a lot of kneeling?

MR. V: Yes.

MD: Did you use kneepads or knee cushions?

MR. V: No.

MD: OK. Let's see your knees

(MD examines the patient)

MD: Well, Mr. Vieira, I've examined your knees. You do not have a fracture of the femur or of the tibia. Your patella is in the correct place. However, in the front of both your patella, you have inflammation of the bursa. It is called "pre-patellar" bursitis. It can also be called carpenter's knee or housekeeper's knee, because people who work on their knees can have this kind of inflammation. I am going to give you an anti-inflammatory pill that will fight the pain and inflammation. You must take it twice a day on a full stomach. You must also do an ice massage on both knees three times a day. I'll give you an ace wrap for both knees.

MR. V: When can I return to work?

MD: You can return to work tomorrow if you start the pills and the ice massage later today. Avoid kneeling for about the next 4 weeks. When you begin to kneel, you should get basketball knee guards to protect your knees.

MR. V: Are you sure I don't have a fracture or growth? I don't want to end up like my brother who died of lung cancer, which had spread to the bones.

MD: You have a swelling of the front of the knee, or the pre-patellar bursa. It is not in the joint itself.

MR. V: I don't know. Can I have an x-ray?

MD: Sure. We'll do one now.

MR. V: Thank you. I feel better already.

Patient to the interpreter: This doctor at first did not seem that nice. They always think that Latinos don't want to work. Where are you from? How long have you been in this country? Are you married?

continued

Role-Play 47 *(continued)*

Questions:

1. How would you have handled this comment by the patient?

2. Describe your memory aid (aids).

3. How did you manage the consecutive mode and maintain 100% accuracy?

Additional Comments:

Role-Play 47: Glossary

continued

PO Box 2308, Woburn, MA 01888-0508, **p:** 781-729-3736, **www.EmbracingCulture.com**
PO Box 6401, Manchester, NH 03108, **p:** 1-888-678-CCCS

1. Pathology (diseases, conditions)

2. Laboratory Tests and Diagnostic Procedures

3. Treatment Procedures

4. Idiomatic Expressions (if any)

5. Other (vocabulary in this particular role-play that you feel is important/relevant or that you anticipate problems with)

Role-Play 48: Fahim's Tenderness

Instructions:

1. Do a complete CIFE.
2. Apply the memory aid that suits you the best in this role-play.
3. Use consecutive mode.
4. You can only use your hand signal one time.
5. React appropriately to ethics challenge.

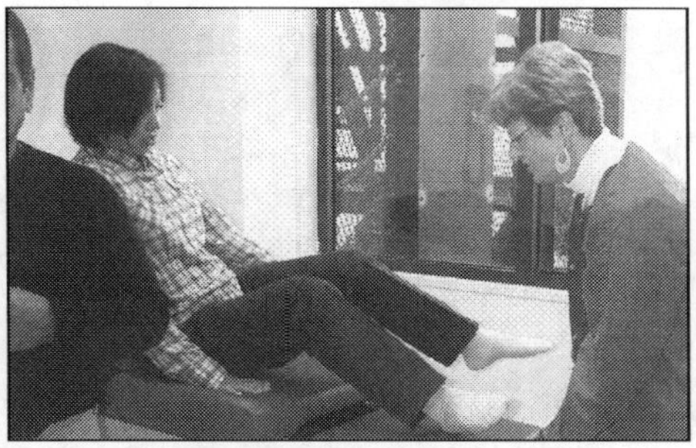

Fahim is an 18-year-old from Morocco. She is an attractive young woman who lives with her extended family in Manchester. She is in her last year of high school and works at T.J. Maxx in the evenings. She has learned a lot of English in the 8 months since she and her family moved here. Fahim is frightened and when she is frightened her English comes more slowly. So she's asked for an interpreter.

In the waiting room, she tells you that she's nervous because she's never been to an American doctor. At first, you are apprehensive, but when you see that her appointment is with the female nurse practitioner, you breathe a sigh of relief.

Nurse: Hello, I am Diane. How can I help you?

PT: I have terrible pains in my stomach.

Nurse: How long have you had these pains?

PT: For about three weeks.

Nurse: Can you show me exactly where it hurts?

(Patient looks embarrassed and does not respond.)

Nurse (to interpreter): Did you ask her to show me where it hurts?

PT: Well, it hurts down there.

Nurse: In your lower stomach?

PT: Yes, I have stomach pain and a bad smelling liquid down there.

Nurse: Do you mean from your vagina?

PT: Yes.

Nurse: Have you recently had sexual intercourse?

(Patient looks embarrassed and does not answer.)

Nurse: Fahim, I'm going to examine you. First, I'll take your temperature and blood pressure. Then I'll take a speculum and put it in the opening of the vagina. We'll take a culture and a Pap smear from your uterus. After that, I'll feel your uterus, ovaries and cervix with my hand. Then we can discuss what we find. I know this is your first time and I'll go slowly and you can tell me at any time if you are uncomfortable. OK?

continued

PO Box 2308, Woburn, MA 01888-0508, **p:** 781-729-3736, **www.EmbracingCulture.com**
PO Box 6401, Manchester, NH 03108, **p:** 1-888-678-CCCS

Role-Play 48 *(continued)*

PT: OK

(Later, after the exam)

Nurse: Well, we've found that you have cervicitis and a tender uterus, called endometritis. I am going to put you on two antibiotics that will help. The culture we took may not come back with any results, but if it does, I'll let you know. In the meantime, I'll give you some Motrin for the abdominal pain. You must rest for at least five days. Please call me if your pain intensifies. But I believe you'll be fine.

Questions:

There were no other interpreters available on the phone or face-to-face.

1. If you were a male interpreter, would you have accepted this interpretation request? Why/Why not?

2. Describe your memory aid (aids).

3. How did you manage the consecutive mode and maintain 100% accuracy?

Additional Comments:

continued

Role-Play 48: Glossary

1. Pathology (diseases, conditions)

2. Laboratory Tests and Diagnostic Procedures

3. Treatment Procedures

4. Idiomatic Expressions (if any)

5. Other (vocabulary in this particular role-play that you feel is important/relevant or that you anticipate problems with)

PO Box 2308, Woburn, MA 01888-0508, **p:** 781-729-3736, **www.EmbracingCulture.com**
PO Box 6401, Manchester, NH 03108, **p:** 1-888-678-CCCS

Role-Play 49: Leo's Lung Carcinoma

Instructions:

1. Do a complete CIFE.
2. Apply the memory aid that suits you the best in this role-play.
3. Use consecutive mode.
4. You can not use your hand signal.
5. React appropriately to ethics challenge.

Leo is a 56-year-old male. He complains of breathlessness, hoarseness, cough and hemoptysis (coughing up blood, from Greek, "Haima," meaning "blood" and "ptysis," meaning "spitting"). He has also lost a significant amount of weight over the last three months.

MD: Leo, it's good to see you again. What brings you to the clinic today?

Leo: (wheezing) I can't breathe, I'm hoarse. I can't eat...I don't know what to do.

MD: Hmm, you say you can't eat...why is that?

Leo: I have no appetite, and I feel so weak.

MD: For how long has this been going on?

Leo: For a few months now...I was going to come sooner, but I thought it would pass.

MD: Are there any other symptoms that you've experienced in conjunction with the hoarseness, loss of appetite and labored breathing?

Leo: I've had a persistent cough for a few weeks now. I've been coughing up blood.

MD: Are you still smoking, Leo?

Leo: Yes, but I can quit at any time.

MD: I see that you are quite pale and that you're wheezing even when at rest.

(MD examines Leo)

MD: You appear to have clubbing in your fingers. See how the tips are enlarged and the nails curved back?

Leo: I noticed that, but thought it was because of the type of work I do. I work in house cleaning, you know.

MD: Actually, clubbing is caused by low blood oxygen levels and can be a symptom of a variety of serious conditions. Another thing I noticed is that your chest is barrel-shaped and your movements diminished on the right side. When I listen to your chest, I don't hear any breathing sounds over the right middle lobe. I'd like to run some tests to further investigate the matter

(Later, after examination)

MD: Leo, the tests reveal the presence of malignant squamous cells.

continued

Role-Play 49 *(continued)*

Leo: What are squamous cells?

MD: Squamous cells are flat cells, usually found in epithelial tissue, where the body meets the outside environment. These cells can turn cancerous. I'd like you to go for a bronchoscopy so we can determine the nature of these cells.

(Later, after bronchoscopy)

MD: Leo, the bronchoscopy revealed a grayish-tan tumor spreading out from your right middle bronchus and obstructing it. The biopsy revealed that the tumor is cancerous. Thankfully, lung cancer is the most preventable of cancers, and surgical resection can be potentially curative in patients like you. Let's talk about your treatment options.

Questions:

The interpreter interprets all the words but s/he omitted the word "cancer," because s/he felt that it was not well received culturally. In addition, she felt that she needed not only to protect the patient, but also to preserve the patient-provider relationship.

1. Comment on the interpreter's actions.

____

____

____

2. Describe your memory aid (aids).

____

____

____

3. How did you manage the consecutive mode and maintain 100% accuracy?

____

____

____

Additional Comments:

____

____

____

PO Box 2308, Woburn, MA 01888-0508, **p:** 781-729-3736, **www.EmbracingCulture.com**
PO Box 6401, Manchester, NH 03108, **p:** 1-888-678-CCCS

Role-Play 49: Glossary

1. Pathology (diseases, conditions)

2. Laboratory Tests and Diagnostic Procedures

3. Treatment Procedures

4. Idiomatic Expressions (if any)

5. Other (vocabulary in this particular role-play that you feel is important/relevant or that you anticipate problems with)

Role-Play 50: Mrs. De Jesus' Eyes

Instructions:

1. Do a complete CIFE.
2. Apply the memory aid that suits you the best in this role-play.
3. You can not use your hand signal.
4. Use consecutive mode.
5. React appropriately to ethics challenge.

Mrs. De Jesus was an incredible 78-year old woman who had emigrated from the Azores over 10 years ago. She was a "pillar of her community." She had worked two jobs and had gone to church every night for 25 years. Her children loved her and swarmed to her bedside when they heard that she had fallen and broken her hip. She suffered an open reduction and closed internal fixation of the hip fracture.

The surprise came after the surgery when she became confused. She began to see bugs on the wall and dead relatives in her hospital room. The doctors were worried. They wanted to know why she was acting this way.

An attending physician, Mrs. De Jesus' daughter and the interpreter meet with Ms. De Jesus at her bedside.

MD: Ms. De Jesus, how are you feeling?

Patient: Excellent! I always love to fish. When my husband died, I learned to fish in the ocean.

MD: I am going to ask you some memory questions. Is that alright?

Patient: I need to be finished by June.

MD: What day is it?

Patient: It is Sunday.

MD: Well, actually, it is Saturday.

Patient: The pretty angel is sitting here in my room.

MD: Do you know what month it is?

Patient: I was born in July.

MD: What is today's date?

Patient: April 24th.

MD: Mrs. De Jesus, are you seeing things you know aren't here?

Patient: I have seen a little dog in the corner of the room. (She laughs)

continued

PO Box 2308, Woburn, MA 01888-0508, **p:** 781-729-3736, **www.EmbracingCulture.com**
PO Box 6401, Manchester, NH 03108, **p:** 1-888-678-CCCS

Role-Play 50 *(continued)*

MD: Do you hear people speaking to you when there is no one around?

Patient: No, but I do listen to the radio at night.

MD: Can you spell the word "world" backwards?

Patient: I can, but I don't care to say it.

MD: Who is the new President of the United States?

Patient: I have no idea. Who is the Bishop of Braga?

MD: (to Mrs. De Jesus' Daughter) Has she been confused like this before?

Daughter: No! Never.

MD: Does she use alcohol?

Daughter: She drinks a little wine every day and sometimes brandy or aguardente (fire water used in many of the Portuguese speaking countries). She used to work two jobs. She earned a lot of money. She hasn't had to work for a while. She stays at home now.

MD: Well, her blood pressure, pulse, and temperature are all elevated. I think she is going through withdrawal from alcohol. We will treat her with Ativan. She also has difficulty with her eye movements and she does not walk well. It looks like she may have a form of confusion called Wiernicke's encephalopathy. It is a kind of vitamin deficiency that occurs with poor diets or with alcohol consumption. We'll treat her with injections of a vitamin called Thiamine.

Daughter: I am so surprised. She took care of us all our lives. She never missed a day of work. Now, at this age, she is having trouble with drinking?

MD: We will get her through this. I will run blood tests for other kinds of delirium and we will send her for a CT scan of the brain just to make sure she has no irregularities there.

Daughter: Will she get well?

MD: I am hoping she will. If she cannot get her mind to calm down, she won't be able to learn from the physical therapists. She also will need to be on blood thinners. There is also a risk of falling if she does not recover judgment and safety awareness.

Daughter: Oh my God! I hope she gets better.

Patient: My, that angel is handsome!

continued

Role-Play 50 *(continued)*

Questions:

Interpreting for a mental health patient can be challenging at times.

What was challenging for you as an interpreter?

Describe your memory aid (aids).

How did you manage the consecutive mode and maintain 100% accuracy?

Additional Comments:

continued

PO Box 2308, Woburn, MA 01888-0508, **p:** 781-729-3736, **www.EmbracingCulture.com**
PO Box 6401, Manchester, NH 03108, **p:** 1-888-678-CCCS

Role-Play 50: Glossary

1. Pathology (diseases, conditions)

2. Laboratory Tests and Diagnostic Procedures

3. Treatment Procedures

4. Idiomatic Expressions (if any)

5. Other (vocabulary in this particular role-play that you feel is important/relevant or that you anticipate problems with)

Role-Play 51: SARS

Instructions:
1. Do a complete CIFE.
2. Apply the memory aid that suits you the best in this role-play.
3. Use consecutive mode.
4. React appropriately to ethics challenge.

A young immigrant family has just returned from visiting their native country, China. The family took all the preventive protections. As soon as they were informed of the dangers of SARS, they made sure that all their family members wore facemasks in public places. They also decided to cut their visit short and travel to Boston as soon as they were able to settle a refund for their tickets with the airlines.

A few days after their arrival from Beijing, they noticed some possible signs of SARS in their ten-year-old son, Aaron. The family pediatrician was contacted and the entire family ended up being checked. This case is with Aaron and Mr. Wong, his worried father.

MD: I received your call and I understand your concern, especially after all the media attention regarding this new illness called Severe Acute Respiratory Syndrome or SARS. Tell me more about the onset of Aaron's symptoms.

Mr. Wong: We were so good about keeping the masks on the children every time we went out of the house. My family always washed their hands and made sure not to go into public places that were not well aired, such as the subway and small restaurants. I hope Aaron does not have SARS. I have noticed that my neighbors are not as friendly. They seem scared and have kept their kids from playing with our kids since our return.

MD: I can imagine how this illness must be putting so much stress on the Asian population in the USA. The good news is that we have been able to treat all the SARS cases in the USA, and no one has died yet of SARS. Unfortunately people have started associating race with the illness, but the truth is that anyone, regardless of race, who travels to China, Hong Kong, Singapore, Canada and Malay could have reason to worry if they develop the sudden symptoms of a cold or a respiratory infection. But a diagnosis would only come after a medical examination.

Mr. Wong: My wife first noticed that Aaron was complaining of all kinds of pains and aches all over his body. At first, he did not have either a fever or a cough. We believed that the aches and pains had to do with the long trip back to Boston; and also with all the stress of trying to get the tickets changed.

MD: Aaron, I am going to check your temperature and listen to your lungs. The good thing is that now you are in my care and I will make sure that we will take care of you no matter if you have SARS or not. As you breathe in and out, I will give you a Kleenex to cover your mouth so this way your father and I may prevent some of the possible germs from passing through.

continued

PO Box 2308, Woburn, MA 01888-0508, **p:** 781-729-3736, **www.EmbracingCulture.com**
PO Box 6401, Manchester, NH 03108, **p:** 1-888-678-CCCS

Role-Play 51 *(continued)*

MD: Your temperature is just about 100.4. Let me see how your lungs sound. I can hear some crackles. You seem pretty congested and your difficulty breathing appears to be from a combination of nasal congestion and pneumonia. I am so glad that your parents brought you in. I am going to give you some medications, but I will need your cooperation in protecting you and your family. Before I make this diagnosis I will ask that you wear this mask and come with me to the X-Ray Department for an X-ray in order to confirm the pneumonia.

MD: Mr. Wong and Aaron, I am so glad that you did not wait too long before calling me. It appears that Aaron's symptoms are similar to the ones of SARS. I will send a specimen to the lab in Washington. Meanwhile I am going to need Aaron's and everyone in the family's cooperation with the following infection control precautions:

- Frequent hand washing and use of alcohol hand swabs
- No sharing of dishes, food, or drinks
- No school until ten days after the symptoms disappear
- Stay home; avoid public outings for Aaron or any other family member who has shown any of the SARS symptoms.
- Wear a surgical mask

Mr. Wong: Should my son stay in the hospital? I will stay with him. I do not want my neighbors to be afraid of my family. Can I call my wife?

MD: If it makes it easier for your family, I can arrange for Aaron to be hospitalized. This can be a bit scary. He would be in a room by himself and all the staff will be wearing gloves, gowns and masks, the same type of precautions we would take with any potentially infectious disease. Aaron, would you like to get a TV in your room? Do you have any questions? I will visit you every day. You are so healthy that I am sure you are going to get rid of this viral infection. And when you grow up, you'll laugh when you think back on this scary moment.

Here is the flyer with a list of some of the symptoms that your family should look for. You all did a great job by bringing Aaron in so quickly after the onset of the illness.

continued

Role-Play 51 *(continued)*

Questions:

As soon as the provider realized that the patient might have a contagious disease, s/he took all the necessary precautions, but did not inform the interpreter that s/he needed to follow the same contagious disease precautions.

1. How would you have handled this situation?

2. What difficult/challenging with this interpretation?

3. What memory aids did/could you use to help you?

Additional Comments

continued

PO Box 2308, Woburn, MA 01888-0508, **p:** 781-729-3736, **www.EmbracingCulture.com**
PO Box 6401, Manchester, NH 03108, **p:** 1-888-678-CCCS

Role-Play 51: Glossary

1. Pathology (diseases, conditions)

2. Laboratory Tests and Diagnostic Procedures

3. Treatment Procedures

4. Idiomatic Expressions (if any)

5. Other (vocabulary in this particular role-play that you feel is important/relevant or that you anticipate problems with)

Role-Play 52: Substance Abuse/ High Blood Pressure

Instructions:

1. Do a complete CIFE
2. Apply the memory aid that suits you the best in this role-play
3. Use consecutive mode
4. React appropriately to ethics challenge

Mr. Nestor Calderon is a 35-year-old Latino male who comes for a physical exam and is found to have borderline blood pressure. His father died of a heart attack at 45 and his mother has diabetes and hypertension and she takes multiple medications. Mr. Calderon has three children and works as a foreman in a local curtain factory. He also works part-time doing remodeling work for friends and family. He came to the United States as a teenager and left high school to work. He learned English at night and then got a GED high school equivalency diploma while working fulltime. He has completed enough course work to get an associates degree in business at Bunker Hill Community College. Mr. Calderon is concerned about his blood pressure. He has returned to see the doctor three times now, and each time his blood pressure is high. Initially, the doctor did blood tests and an EKG, which were normal. Then Mr. Calderon was asked to decrease sodium (Na) in his diet and lose weight. He lost five lbs. and returned with his blood pressure still high.

MD: I'm very pleased you've lost weight but unfortunately, your blood pressure is still elevated.

NC: I've done everything, Doctor, and I still have the problem. Maybe it's time for a pill.

MD: You know. I asked you if you smoked, but one thing I never asked you was if you use alcohol?

NC: You mean do I drink alcohol?

MD: Yes.

NC: Well, yes.

MD: How much do you drink each day?

NC: Only one or two beers. I drink Colt 45.

MD: What size bottles?

NC: Oh you know, the large size. I'm thirsty when I come home from work.

MD: Have you ever felt you needed to cut down your use of alcohol?

NC: Well, when I first left high school, for a while I was drinking every night, but I woke up feeling nasty so I stopped for a while. That way I could concentrate on my work and soon I was doing ok.

MD: Do you feel annoyed if someone asks you about your drinking?

continued

PO Box 2308, Woburn, MA 01888-0508, **p:** 781-729-3736, **www.EmbracingCulture.com**
PO Box 6401, Manchester, NH 03108, **p:** 1-888-678-CCCS

Role-Play 52 *(continued)*

NC: No, but sometimes I am pretty peeved if they ask me about drinking and I know they do it too.

MD: Do you feel guilty about drinking or something you do when you drink?

NC: Well, when I was young, I would party and I woke up with a friend's girlfriend. My wife would kill me if she knew, even though this happened before we were married.

MD: Have you ever taken a drink in the morning to take the edge off or as an "eye opener?"

NC: Yes, but mostly when I was young and not married. You know, now, if I am not working, I'm in church. I can't play around anymore and I don't want to, but I like my beer after work.

MD: Well, a minute ago you asked me for a pill and I can easily do that, but I think we should wait a bit and here's why. I would hate to give you a pill to counteract the effect of another medicine. And I think that your daily intake of alcohol may be leading you to have high blood pressure. Do you think you could stop drinking for six weeks and we'll take your blood pressure and see if there's an improvement?

NC: Hey man, do you think I'm an alcoholic?

MD: Well, I don't know. But it may be that your use of alcohol is causing this problem. We should try a six-week alcohol holiday and see what the effect is, ok?

NC: Fine. For six weeks I could go without sex if I had to.

MD: This means that from the time you leave this office, to the next time you arrive in six weeks you will not have one drink or swallow of alcohol. Do you agree?

NC: Absolutely.

MD: See you in six weeks.

(Six weeks later)

MD: Hello Mr. Calderon, I see that your blood pressure is still a little high. How do you feel?

NC: Fine, Doc.

MD: Were you able to stay off alcohol?

NC: Look, Doc. alcohol is not my problem. I cut down but we had the Super Bowl and I was really thirsty after work. What's up with this? You think I got a problem?

MD: Well, this is important information. You agreed to an alcohol holiday, yet you were unable to do it. So, alcohol may be a problem for you. Is there anybody in your family who might have a problem with alcohol?

NC: Well, my father would come home and get drunk and we wouldn't see him 'cause he'd sit in his room drinking. After he died, my mother was always drunk. Now, she doesn't drink. She goes to church and the church people help her out.

continued

Role-Play 52 *(continued)*

MD: Well, Mr. Calderon. I know you are concerned about your blood pressure. Alcohol every day can make the body tolerant and during the next day after consistent drinking the body goes through a mini withdrawal until the next drink calms it down. That may be why it feels so good to drink after work. I'd like you to meet a friend of mine. His name is Charlie and he runs an alcohol education group which meets on Friday mornings for six weeks; and there he'll teach you about alcohol and your body.

NC: It's not AA, is it?

MD: No. It's an educational group. But sometimes AA turns out to be a real help.

NC: Well, I'll go if you think it will help. All of this, just because I get thirsty.

(Provider leaves the room)

The interpreter notices that the patient is stressed and tells him: These American Providers are so rigid about drinking; my father and uncles are just like you. They drink when they are thirsty. They work hard and they have a house. What is the big deal about drinking a little bit?

The Patient: I know, do you know another doctor that likes Latinos better? I believe that this doctor could give me the right medication and leave my drinking alone.

The Interpreter: Yes, I will call you at home. Can you just write your number down? I will help you. Perhaps you want to join my church.

Questions:

Comment on the interpreter's actions.

____

____

____

Knowing that the patient spoke English for his daily activities, how did you feel about being his interpreter?

____

____

____

continued

PO Box 2308, Woburn, MA 01888-0508, **p:** 781-729-3736, **www.EmbracingCulture.com**
PO Box 6401, Manchester, NH 03108, **p:** 1-888-678-CCCS

Role-Play 52 *(continued)*

Describe your memory aids.

How did you manage the consecutive mode and maintain 100% accuracy?

Additional Comments:

Role-Play 52: Glossary

continued

1. Pathology (diseases, conditions)

2. Laboratory Tests and Diagnostic Procedures

3. Treatment Procedures

4. Idiomatic Expressions (if any)

5. Other (vocabulary in this particular role-play that you feel is important/relevant or that you anticipate problems with)

PO Box 2308, Woburn, MA 01888-0508, **p:** 781-729-3736, **www.EmbracingCulture.com**
PO Box 6401, Manchester, NH 03108, **p:** 1-888-678-CCCS

Role-Play 53: Circumcision

Instructions:

1. Do a complete CIFE
2. Apply the memory aid that suits you the best in this role-play
3. Apply interpreting mode that best suits this triadic encounter
4. React appropriately to ethics challenge

Mr. Serra was born in Brazil. He is 51 years old. He married when he was 18 years old. He had two children and his wife died early on. He raised his two children in Brazil and brought them to the United States. He has worked for twenty years for the same cleaning firm. His children are grown and married and he has four grandchildren, although he appears younger than his years. Being a serious man, he never found another woman since his wife died. Even though he has had dates, nothing ever came of them. He felt that he had to be there for his children. Last year, when his youngest finished college, Mr. Serra began to date a woman from his church. She was 10 years younger than Mr. Serra and although she was also very serious about church and her work, she had what Mr. Serra called "a malandra" (flirtatious and cute) smile. He has now come to his primary care provider with a problem.

MD: Mr. Serra, welcome back. What brings you to the office today?

Mr. S: I have a problem. It is embarrassing.

MD: What seems to be the problem?

Mr. S: When I try to make love, my penis becomes so painful that it is difficult to finish.

MD: How long have you had this problem?

Mr. S: It began around ten years ago, but it has not been a real problem until this year when I began to see this woman. She is wonderful and she is patient with me, but I think there is something wrong.

MD: I think I recall that you are not circumcised. Is that correct?

Mr. S: Yes.

MD: Yes, and I remember that you have a phimotic foreskin.

Mr. S: What is that?

MD: When I did your physical a few years ago, we talked about how the foreskin of your penis had a diminished diameter at the distal end, so it was difficult to retract the foreskin behind the glans of the penis.

Mr. S: I remember you told me to pull it back and wash it at least once a day. I have done that, but now making love is more painful. I can become erect but any extra movement is painful. Can you help me?

MD: Let me examine you and see what it looks like now.

continued

Role-Play 53 *(continued)*

(Examines patient)

MD: Mr. Serra, your phimosis has become even smaller. I imagine that with an erection, the foreskin binds the penis and makes it painful.

Mr. S: Yes, and sometimes after the erection is over, I cannot bring the foreskin over the penis again until I shower and use soap to bring it forward.

MD: I see. That can lead to a paraphimosis which in turn can lead to a possible infection and a strangling of the distal portion of the penis. The good news is that with a circumcision, this can be fixed. It is a relatively simple operation that removes the foreskin. It can sometimes be complicated with bleeding and infection but that is very rare.

Mr. S: Circumcision? Isn't that what they do to baby boys?

MD: Yes, but you would be surprised how common it is in adult men. I will refer you to Dr. Sherman. He is the urologist here in the clinic. I think you will be very pleased with how quickly he will be able to get you back to functioning without pain.

Mr. S: OK, I will go see him. I think it will be worth it.

Questions:

Female circumcision is illegal in the USA.

How would you have handled the interpretation for a female patient who was having difficulty giving birth due to a circumcision done in her native country?

Describe your memory aid (aids).

How did you manage the interpreting mode that you chose and still maintain 100% accuracy?

Additional Comments:

PO Box 2308, Woburn, MA 01888-0508, **p:** 781-729-3736, **www.EmbracingCulture.com**
PO Box 6401, Manchester, NH 03108, **p:** 1-888-678-CCCS

Role-Play 53: Glossary

1. Pathology (diseases, conditions)

2. Laboratory Tests and Diagnostic Procedures

3. Treatment Procedures

4. Idiomatic Expressions (if any)

5. Other (vocabulary in this particular role-play that you feel is important/relevant or that you anticipate problems with)

Role-Play 54: Colon Cancer

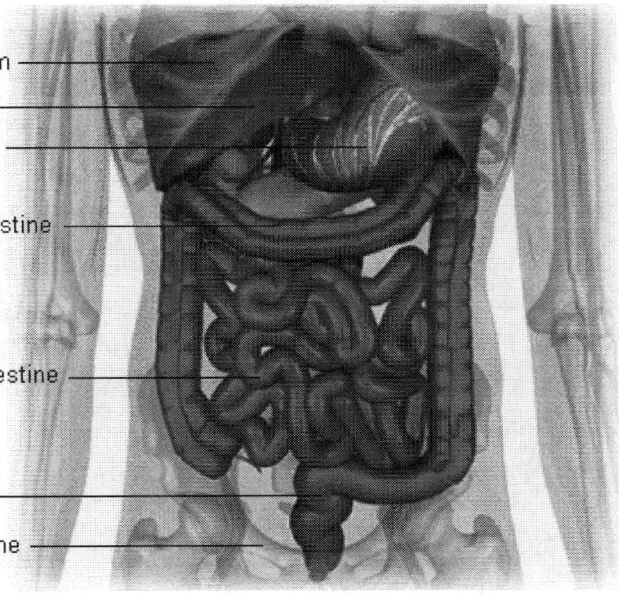

Instructions:

1. Do a complete CIFE.
2. Apply the memory aid that suits you the best in this role-play.
3. Use consecutive mode.
4. React appropriately to ethics challenge.

MD: So, Mr. Chavez, I received your FOBT or the stool card, and it showed positive for blood in your stool.

PT: Doctor, can you talk in a way that I can understand you? What is this FOBT?

Interpreter to Patient: It is to check your stool, you know?

MD: Oh, I am sorry with my medicalese. It is the stool test that I gave you to take home 6 months ago after your check up, when you then told me that you had some family history of colon cancer; and because you are over 50 … and you are a bit overweight and you love to eat red meat and fatty foods and you drink alcohol often enough that … I just wanted to have you on my radar as a precaution.

PT: OK, but tell me about this FOBT.

MD: It stands for Fecal Occult Blood Test and we give it to patients in your situation; it is used to check for hidden or occult blood. Sometimes a person bleeds from a cancerous polyp which is not always detected by the naked eye.

PT: I got it, so now that you have told me that I am fat and ugly what can I do for you doctor? (laughs)

MD: Oh .. no, I did not say you were ugly, I am just concerned and I have a few questions for you. Are you ready?

PT: For you doctor I am always ready! (big smile)

MD: Have you noticed a change in your bowel habits?

PT: Yes, for some time my poop seems to come out very thin and it used to be wide and pretty big.

MD: Any diarrhea?

PT: Sometimes I get it; more often than before.

MD: Any feeling that after you move your bowels you are still full and need to empty again?

PT: Sometimes, but more often now.

continued

PO Box 2308, Woburn, MA 01888-0508, **p:** 781-729-3736, **www.EmbracingCulture.com**
PO Box 6401, Manchester, NH 03108, **p:** 1-888-678-CCCS

Role-Play 54 *(continued)*

MD: Any blood in your stools?

PT: No.

MD: Any blood on the toilet paper after you wipe yourself?

PT: No.

MD: Any blood on your underwear?

PT: Oh, I do not know, perhaps my wife will know about this. She is the woman in charge of all our laundry at home.

MD: Do you feel bloated or any abdominal cramps?

PT: Sometimes I pass .. excuse me doctor.. a lot of gas.

MD: More now than in the past?

PT: Perhaps.. yes… I was just thinking that my wife seems to be nagging me about the smell in the car every time we drive together.

MD: Good. Let me tell you what we are going to do in order to rule out any malignancies in your colon or rectum.

PT: Doctor what is my colon…my gut?

MD: Yes, it is your large intestine…the part between your appendix and rectum and small intestine..the section between your stomach and the appendix. I am worried about a problem with your colon and less with your rectum, but we will check both.

I am going to examine you and check your abdomen, your vital signs, such as fever, blood pressure. I will check your weight which you seemed to have lost quite a bit!

PT: Finally as I get older I am losing the weight, too bad that I could not do it earlier on, but I guess that age just brings thinness (laughing).

MD: I know it is confusing, all these years I have told you to lose weight, change your eating habits, eat more fiber, less fatty foods, but still I do not want you to lose weight just out of the blue, when you have not even worked to lose it.. but, let's see. After my examination I am going to send you for a series of tests.

PT: OK, I am ready. I have just retired and I want to see the grandchildren…although lately I have been feeling pretty tired.

MD: OK, we are going to help you and we will schedule a series of blood tests: one to check your blood count to see if you are anemic and then, we will send you for a colonoscopy.

PT: A colonoscopy?

Interpreter to the patient: It is an exam of your intestines!

MD: A very nice radiologist and a very helpful technician will be gently inserting a long and very flexible thin tube with a light, through your anus, all the way up through your gut or intestines. We just want to check for polyps and if we find them we will biopsy or extract them.

continued

Role-Play 54 *(continued)*

PT: OK, and If I need to go the bathroom during the test?

MD: Do not worry. The lab will give you all the instructions and we are equipped to deal with any accident… (smiles).. You need to understand that this occult blood business may turn to be nothing or we may need to proceed with more tests such as Barium enema and a few others.

PT: OK doctor.

Questions:

How would you have handled the patient's requests for clarification?

Describe your memory aid (aids).

How did you manage the consecutive mode and maintain 100% accuracy?

Additional Comments:

continued

PO Box 2308, Woburn, MA 01888-0508, **p:** 781-729-3736, **www.EmbracingCulture.com**
PO Box 6401, Manchester, NH 03108, **p:** 1-888-678-CCCS

Role-Play 54: Glossary

1. Pathology (diseases, conditions)

2. Laboratory Tests and Diagnostic Procedures

3. Treatment Procedures

4. Idiomatic Expressions (if any)

5. Other (vocabulary in that particular role-play that you feel is important/relevant or that you anticipate problems with)

Role-Play 55: Visit with a Family Planning Counselor

Instructions:

1. Do a complete CIFE.
2. Apply the memory aid that suits you the best in this role-play.
3. Use appropriate Interpreting modes for this session.
4. React appropriately to ethics challenge.

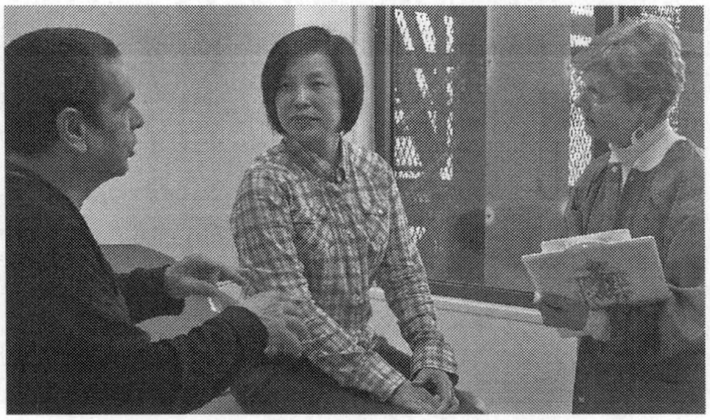

FPC: Your PCP referred you to Family Planning so that we can further discuss birth control options.

PT: I know she told me about a pill that's a combination of two hormones. And she told me that I need to take a pill every day if I don't want to get pregnant.

FPC: Before I explain about the pill, did your provider ever share information on other birth control methods?

PT: Yes, she did tell me about the diaphragm, but that is not going to work for me! It's kind of gross to touch yourself down there (pointing downwards); and she said you have to wait several hours after intercourse before you remove it. Oh no, that's not for me!

FPC: There are other forms of birth control where you do not have to touch your private parts. One example is the contraceptive patch. It contains the same two types of hormones as the pill; but with the patch, you get a little more estrogen than with the pill.

PT: My doctor told me that the patch might even be good for my acne and for my PMS. But I don't trust the patch. It could fall off at any time. I think I should stick with the pill. It's what all my friends are taking.

FPC: The patch does stick well to your skin, but if you like, we can further discuss how the pill works. The two hormones that you were correctly referring to are estrogen and progestin. Although estrogen is present in men and women, in women it suppresses the secretion of the follicles and inhibits ovulation.

PT: What are follicles?

FPC: If you look at these drawings you can see the follicles. They are small cells that contain the eggs in your ovaries.

PT: I get it! You are a good teacher. But what is progestin? Does it stop the eggs from growing?

continued

PO Box 2308, Woburn, MA 01888-0508, **p:** 781-729-3736, **www.EmbracingCulture.com**
PO Box 6401, Manchester, NH 03108, **p:** 1-888-678-CCCS

Role-Play 55 *(continued)*

FPC: At birth, you have all the eggs your body will ever produce, but they are dormant. Your ovaries release them during your menstrual cycle; but back to progestin. Progestin is a female hormone produced by the ovaries after ovulation that prepares the uterine lining for pregnancy.

PT: But I don't want to be pregnant!

FPC: Yes, of course. In this case, progestin is used in combination with estrogen to prevent pregnancy by suppressing ovulation.

PT: Okay. So, whether I get pregnant or not depends on the doses of the hormones?

FPC: Correct. Together these two hormones work to prevent the egg from being released from the ovary. That way, the egg will not get fertilized. The hormones can also make the mucus in your cervix thick so that the sperm does not get through to reach the egg.

PT: Interesting. So, what are the possibilities of me getting pregnant if I take the pill?

FPC: The pill is considered an effective birth control method if used appropriately. For every 100 women correctly using the pill, only eight may get pregnant in a year.

PT: What are the side effects of the pill?

FPC: Some women may have less pain and bleeding with their periods but also you may notice some changes in your body like nausea, vomiting, and breast pain or larger breast size. Some women report less desire for sex, headaches, changes in the period, and even mood changes.

PT: What about my weight?

FPC: Some women gain weight, but others do not notice any weight change at all. If you do begin to notice changes in any of your normal bodily functions, let your PCP know right away. Some side effects can be regulated with different dosages and different pills.

PT: My doctor already asked me about heart problems and blood clots. I told her that I never had any of those problems. I'm a very healthy person. I never smoke and I am at a regular weight for my size. My doctor gave me a clean bill of health.

FPC: There are certain health conditions that would preclude taking the pill. Do you have any of the following?

- Current liver diseases
- History of blood clot, stroke, heart attack or heart disease
- Diabetes for more than 20 years or diabetes with kidney or eye problems
- Abnormal vaginal bleeding
- Cancer of the breast, uterus, or other cancers

PT: No, none of that.

continued

Role-Play 55 *(continued)*

FPC: Good. I just have to inform you of all the possibilities. But you are right; your doctor would not have referred you for the pill if she did not think you were healthy. Now, when you take the pill, look out for the following symptoms:

- Shortness of breath
- Pain in your chest
- Sudden changes in your vision
- Very heavy vaginal bleeding
- New leg pain
- Lower stomach pain
- New or worse headaches
- New or worse depression
- A new lump in your breast
- Sudden nausea, vomiting, dizziness, faintness, numbness or weakness in the arms or legs
- Missing two periods in a row or one period after not taking the pill correctly, or if you think you are pregnant

PT: Don't worry. I will call the clinic right away if I experience any of those symptoms. Thank God I have my health!

FPC: The pharmacy will provide you with a one-month supply of pills with up to six refills. The provider would like to see you every six months in the beginning to make sure that everything is all right with you.

PT: Okay.

FPC: *(opens the pill box and shows it to the patient)* You will be taking one pill at the same time every day for 28 days. Each week of pills is a different color. On week four, you will be getting your period.

PT: OK. So, I should never stop the pill, not even during my period?

FPC: Right. The last week you are just taking a placebo pill that does not have any hormones, but this keeps you in the habit of taking the pill. When are you expecting your period?

PT: In a few weeks.

FPC: And what are you doing now to protect yourself?

PT: I am using the rubber, you know, the condom. After meeting with you, I am going upstairs to check with my doctor about when to start taking the pill.

FPC: Now, if you miss two or more pills in the first, second or third week, it is very important that you use a condom and call your health center to find out if you need to take EC.

PT: But what if I only miss one pill?

FPC: Take the missed pill as soon as you remember and get back to your regular schedule by following the instructions that come with the birth control pack. You can always call my office with questions about the pill.

continued

PO Box 2308, Woburn, MA 01888-0508, **p:** 781-729-3736, **www.EmbracingCulture.com**
PO Box 6401, Manchester, NH 03108, **p:** 1-888-678-CCCS

Role-Play 55 *(continued)*

PT: Okay.

FPC: Before you leave my office today, let's go over the informed consent form. Would you prefer that I read it or do you want to read it yourself?

PT: I can read it at home. I forgot my glasses today.

FPC: Then let me go over it with you. The first paragraph informs you that you chose your birth control freely and that you consent to the medical treatment and procedures. The second paragraph states that you received a full explanation of all the birth control options and that you understand that sexual abstinence is the most effective method of birth control. The third states that you accept and understand the potential side effects of the pill and what can happen if you stop taking the pill.

PT: Oh, don't worry. I'm not going to sue you.

FPC: Going over this informed consent form gives us an opportunity to make sure we do not miss any information. By signing, you are also agreeing that you understand that smoking while on the pill may cause serious health problems and that you understand that the pill does not provide protection from sexually transmitted diseases.

PT: I can sign it.

PT: (looking at the interpreter) You did a good job! I am going to send my sister here and you can tell her what I am taking so she can ask for the same prescription. By the way, remember Maria from the bakery? I think she's HIV positive. I saw her leave here the other day, and she was crying. Then, I heard two medical assistants talking about her. They speak our language, you know. They were saying something about Maria.

continued

Role-Play 55 *(continued)*

Questions:

1. How would you have answered the patient's questions?

2. How would you have handled the breach of HIPAA policies?

3. Which interpreting modes did you use the most and why?

Role-Play 55: Glossary

PO Box 2308, Woburn, MA 01888-0508, **p:** 781-729-3736, **www.EmbracingCulture.com**
PO Box 6401, Manchester, NH 03108, **p:** 1-888-678-CCCS

1. Pathology (diseases, conditions)

2. Laboratory Tests and Diagnostic Procedures

3. Treatment Procedures

4. Idiomatic Expressions (if any)

5. Other (vocabulary in this particular role-play that you feel is important/relevant or that you anticipate problems with)

Lesson Nine: Homework
Role-Play Practice

1. Practice the role-plays that you were not able to complete in class.

2. Gather all the information from your role-play glossaries for this class and the following glossary table:

English

Conditions	Diagnostic Tests
1	
2	
3	
4	
5	
6	
7	
8	
9	
10	
11	
12	

Treatments and Procedures	Other
1	
2	
3	
4	
5	
6	
7	
8	
9	
10	
11	
12	

continued

PO Box 2308, Woburn, MA 01888-0508, **p:** 781-729-3736, **www.EmbracingCulture.com**
PO Box 6401, Manchester, NH 03108, **p:** 1-888-678-CCCS

3. Translate English glossary and categories into your Target Language

Target Language

Conditions	Diagnostic Tests
1	
2	
3	
4	
5	
6	
7	
8	
9	
10	
11	
12	

Treatments and Procedures	Other
1	
2	
3	
4	
5	
6	
7	
8	
9	
10	
11	
12	

4. Finding your learning pulse. Moving forward with your interpreting skills
Write a brief letter to your teacher about your skills as an interpreter by describing your strengths and weakenesses as well as the areas you feel you need room to improve. End the letter with what you are planning to do to enhance your skills.

Lesson Ten: Reproductive System

Understanding Goals

Students will:

- review learned concepts
- practice the Samurai! Technique
- learn about the top ten sexually transmitted diseases in the U.S.
- learn about the male and female reproductive systems
- sharpen their consecutive interpreting skills through role-play practice

Key concepts:

- STD (sexually transmitted diseases)
- Reproductive System

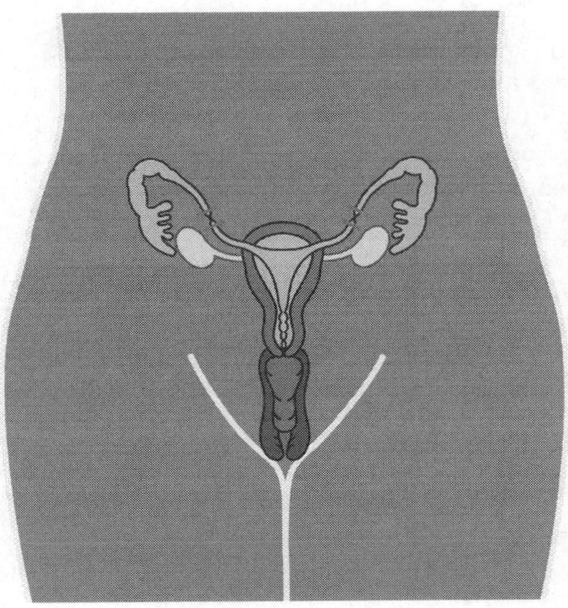

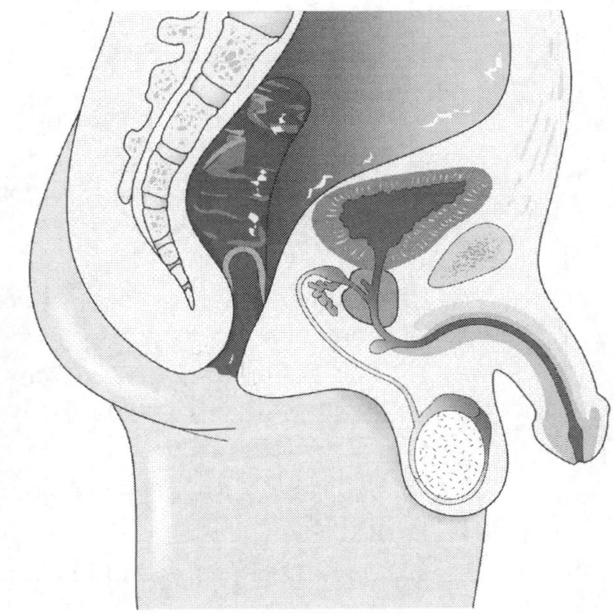

Quiz

THE ART OF MEDICAL INTERPRETATION®

Lesson Ten: Quiz
Reproductive System

TEST YOUR KNOWLEDGE OF SEXUALLY TRANSMITTED DISEASES (STDS)
Mark each item "True" or "False."

1. You always know when you have an STD.
   ○ True ○ False
2. The majority of infections occur among people 35-50 years of age.
   ○ True ○ False
3. People who get an STD have a lot of sex partners.
   ○ True ○ False
4. Approximately 9 million new infections occur in the United States each year.
   ○ True ○ False
5. Chlamydia and gonorrhea can result in infertility in women if left untreated.
   ○ True ○ False
6. All STDs can be cured.
   ○ True ○ False
7. STDs are preventable.
   ○ True ○ False
8. You can have no symptoms, yet be infected with an STD; and therefore be able to pass it on to someone else.
   ○ True ○ False
9. Some STDs can be transmitted from a pregnant woman to her unborn child.
   ○ True ○ False
10. There are at least 10 different STDs.
    ○ True ○ False
11. STD statistics often show an unequal gender distribution usually with more males infected than females.
    ○ True ○ False
12. Most of the time, STDs cause no symptoms.
    ○ True ○ False
13. It is estimated that as many as 1 in 10 Americans has genital herpes.
    ○ True ○ False
14. More than half of the U.S. population will have an STD at some point in their lifetime.
    ○ True ○ False
15. Parental consent is needed before you are treated for a sexually transmitted disease if you are under 18 years of age. ○ True ○ False
16. The Center for Disease Control and Prevention found that at least 1 in 8 teenage American girls has a STD. ○ True ○ False
17. All genital infections are a result of sexual contact. ○ True ○ False
18. You cannot get an STD more than once. ○ True ○ False
19. If the signs of an STD go away, you are cured. ○ True ○ False
20. One in ten people in the United States has an STD. ○ True ○ False

Lesson Ten: Class Activities
Reproductive System

Sexually Transmitted Diseases

According to the CDC, sexually transmitted diseases (STDs) cause over $7 billion to be expended annually for treatment. STDs can affect the sex partners, fetus, and newborn infants. STDs are grouped into three categories:

1. STD:Category One

STDs that produce inflammation of the urethra, epididymis, cervix, or fallopian tubes. Gonorrhea and Chlamydia are the most common STDs in this category. Both diseases can be treated and cured with antibiotics, once diagnosed.

2. STD: Category Two

STDs that produce sores on the external genitals. Genital herpes is the most common disease in this class, affecting more than 25 million individuals in the US each year. Symptoms of herpes can be treated by antiviral drugs, but the infection cannot be cured. Syphilis is a bacteria-induced infection, and can, if left untreated, cause serious symptoms and death. However, the disease is curable with antibiotics.

3. STD: Category Three

This class of STDs includes viral diseases that affect organ systems other than those of the reproductive system. AIDS and hepatitis B are in this category. Both can be spread by sexual contact or blood. Infected individuals may appear symptom-free for years after infection.

REFLECTION

Was this information surprising to you? Why/why not?

____

____

____

____

____

____

____

PO Box 2308, Woburn, MA 01888-0508, **p:** 781-729-3736, **www.EmbracingCulture.com**
PO Box 6401, Manchester, NH 03108, **p:** 1-888-678-CCCS

Human Reproduction and Development

Human reproduction employs internal fertilization, and depends on the integrated action of hormones, the nervous system, and the reproductive system. Gonads are sex organs that produce gametes, eggs and sperm. Male gonads are the testes, which produce sperm and male sex hormones. Female gonads are the ovaries, which produce eggs and female sex hormones.

The Male Reproductive System

Testes (testicles) are suspended outside the abdominal cavity by the scrotum, a pouch of skin that keeps the testes outside of the body at an optimal temperature for sperm development.

Seminiferous tubules are inside each testis, and are where sperm is produced by meiosis. About 250 meters (850 feet) of tubules are packed into each testis. Spermatocytes inside the tubules divide by meiosis to produce spermatids that in turn develop into mature sperm.

Spermatogenesis

Sperm production begins at puberty and continues throughout life, with several hundred million sperm being produced each day. Once sperm form they move into the epididymis, where they mature and are stored.

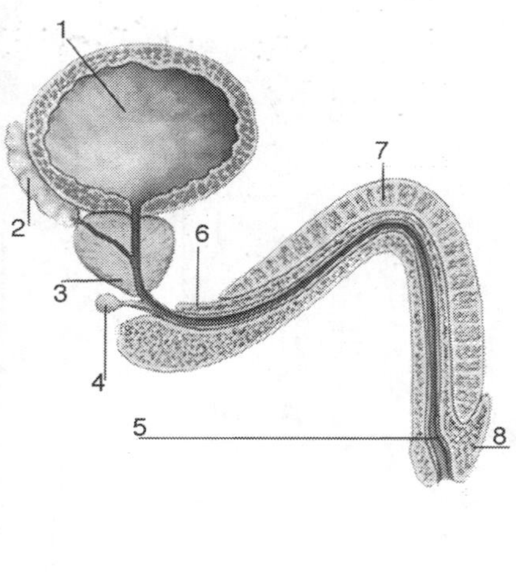

Male Sex Hormones

The hypothalamous produces gonadotropin-releasing hormone (GnRH) which stimulates the anterior pituitary to produce follicle stimulating hormone (FSH) and luteinizing hormone (LH). LH stimulates cells in the seminiferous tubules to secrete testosterone,which has a role in sperm production and developing male secondary sex characteristics. FSH acts on cells to help in sperm maturation. Negative feedback by testosterone controls the actions of GnRH.

Sexual Structures

Sperm passes through the vas deferens and connects to a short ejaculatory duct that connects to the urethra. The urethra passes through the penis and opens to the outside. Secretions from the seminal vesicles add fructose and prostaglandins to sperm as they pass.

The prostate gland secretes a milky alkaline fluid. The bulbourethral gland secretes a mucus-like fluid that provides lubrication for intercourse. Sperm and secretions make up semen.

EXERCISE

Label the diagram of the male reproductive system below:

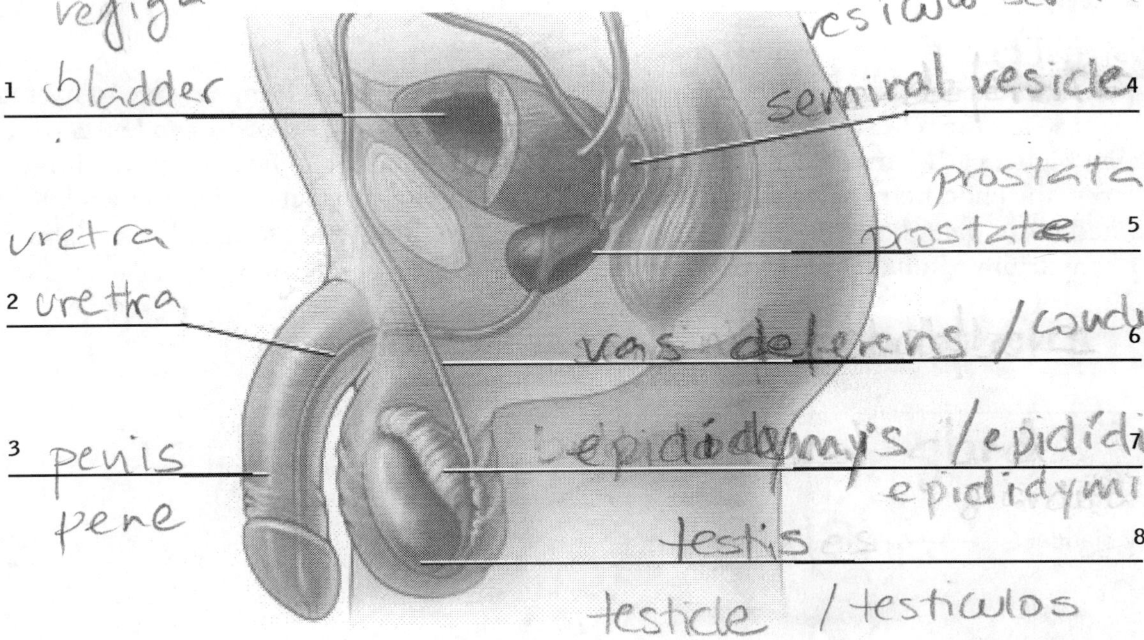

PO Box 2308, Woburn, MA 01888-0508, **p:** 781-729-3736, **www.EmbracingCulture.com**
PO Box 6401, Manchester, NH 03108, **p:** 1-888-678-CCCS

The Female Reproductive System

The female gonads, ovaries, are located within the lower abdominal cavity. The ovary contains many follicles composed of a developing egg surrounded by an outer layer of follicle cells. Each egg "oocyte" begins oogenesis as a primary "oocyte." At birth each female carries a lifetime supply of developing oocytes, each of which is in Prophase I. A developing egg (secondary oocyte) is released each month from puberty until menopause, a total of 400-500 eggs.

Women who are of reproductive age go through a cycle of fertility that is designed to produce an egg that can be fertilized every 28 days. This cycle either results in menstruation or pregnancy. For most women, this cycle lasts 28 days but can be as short as 24 or as long as 35. The cycle can be understood to have four phases: menstrual, follicular, ovulatory and luteal.

Menstrual Phase

This phase begins on day one of the menstrual cycle and usually lasts from day one to five. It will occur when the released egg is not fertilized. Both progesterone and estrogen levels which had been higher earlier in the cycle have decreased. Without these two hormones, the lining of the uterus, the endometrium, which has become rich with blood vessels to support an embryo implanted in the wall, begins to disintegrate and is released out of the uterus. This sloughing of the endometrium results in menstrual bleeding and can last one to five days.

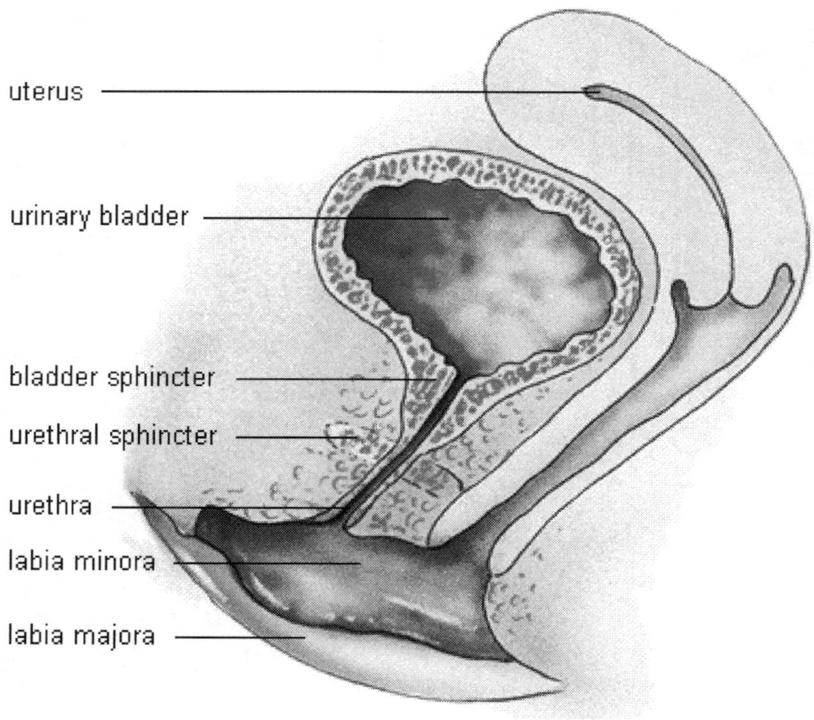

Follicular Phase

During this phase which will run from day 1 through day 13, the pituitary gland releases a hormone called follicle stimulating hormone (FSH). FSH stimulates multiple groups of cells in the ovary to develop. One becomes dominant and this one will eventually release the egg into the fallopian tube. As the follicle develops, it can release estrogen which begins to help the lining of the uterus (the endometrium) to thicken and develop blood vessels which will later increase in thickness to support the development of the attached embryo.

Ovulatory Phase

This phase occurs between day 10 and day 18 and is heralded by a surge of hormone called luteinizing hormone. This helps the dominant follicle develop and release the egg into the fallopian tube. This release is called ovulation and it averages around day 14. Once the egg is released and in the fallopian tube, the woman is at her most fertile phase of the cycle. Couples wishing to get pregnant will do tests in late follicular phase looking for the surge in luteinizing hormone. Having sexual intercourse at this point, helps the chances of fertilization and then implantation.

Luteal Phase

This is usually between day 15-28 of the menstrual cycle. The follicle that released the egg continues to develop and becomes what is called a "luteal body." This collection of cells releases progesterone which helps the endometrium develop even more depth and blood vessel supply. When the released egg is not fertilized, the progesterone and estrogen both decline leading to the disintegration and sloughing of the endometrium which causes the act of menstruation which brings us back to the Menstruation Phase which is the beginning of the next reproductive cycle.

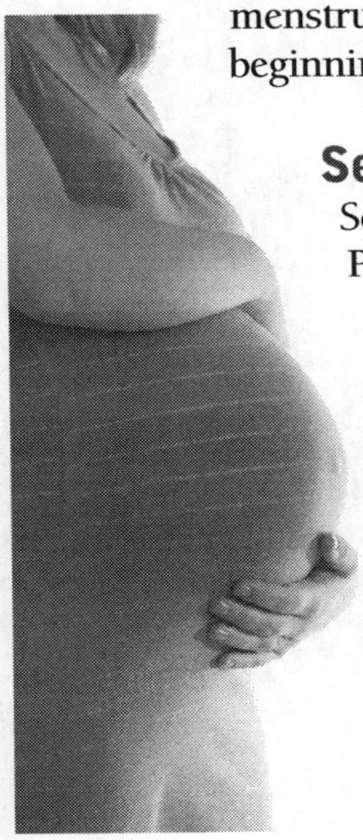

Secretory and Proliferative Phases

Some authorities will describe the Reproductive Cycle in terms of Secretory Phase and Proliferative Phase. The Secretory Phase is usually felt to be day 1-14 and includes menstruation and follicular phase. It is characterized by the "secretion" of hormones which support ovulation and the development of the supportive endometrium. Once ovulation occurs, then the proliferative phase occurs which includes the ovulatory and luteal phase and is characterized by the proliferation of glands and blood vessels in the endometrium.

PO Box 2308, Woburn, MA 01888-0508, **p:** 781-729-3736, **www.EmbracingCulture.com**
PO Box 6401, Manchester, NH 03108, **p:** 1-888-678-CCCS

External Genitals

The female external genitals are collectively known as the vulva. The labia minora is a thin membrane of folded skin just outside the vaginal opening. The labia majora cover and protect the genital area. A clitoris, important in arousal, is a short shaft with a sensitive tip covered by a fold of skin.

EXERCISE

Label the diagram of the female reproductive system below:

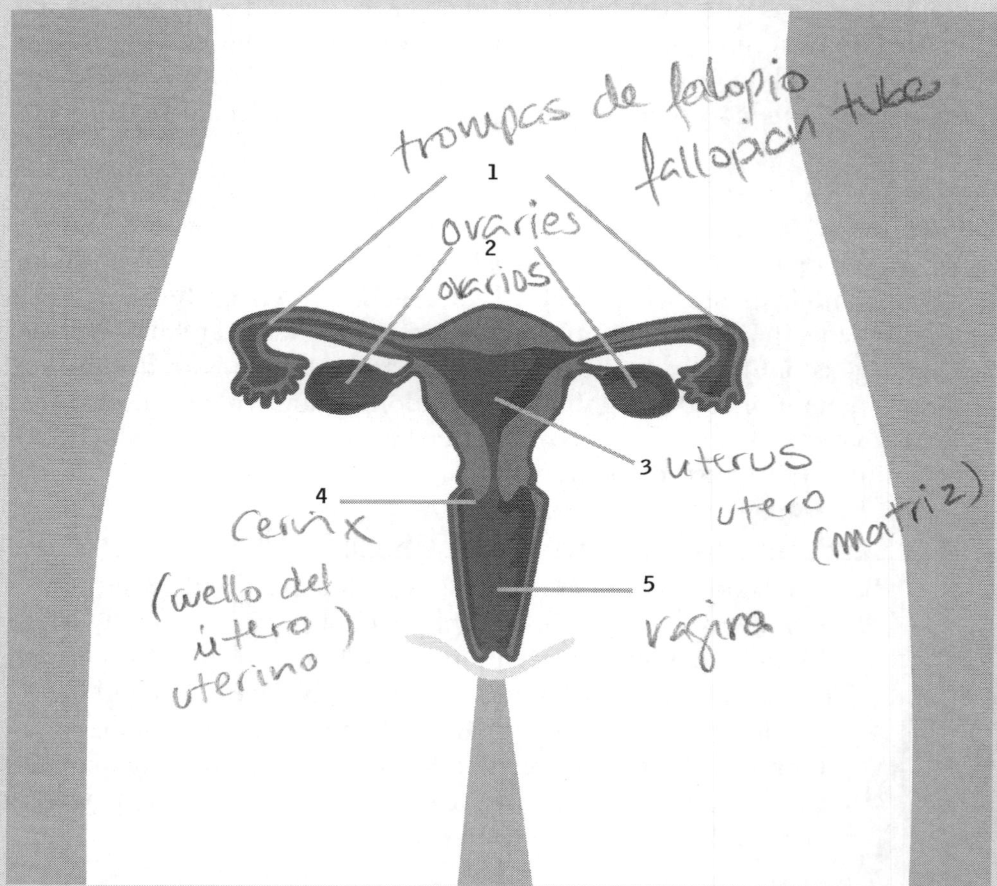

Breasts— connected with reproductive system

PREGNANCY

Watch the video "Invaders – Body Snatchers" from the *Body Story* DVD to learn how the body of a woman reacts to her "invader" – a growing fetus. Use the space below to take notes on what you see or what you find interesting.

Fertilization/Implantation – how are they different?

Fetus/Embryo – how are they different?

womb

PO Box 2308, Woburn, MA 01888-0508, **p:** 781-729-3736, **www.EmbracingCulture.com**
PO Box 6401, Manchester, NH 03108, **p:** 1-888-678-CCCS

Human Development

The female vagina receives the penis in sexual intercourse and sperm is injected by the penis into the vagina. The sperm goes into an opening in the cervix in the vagina, which then leads up through the uterus into the fallopian tube.

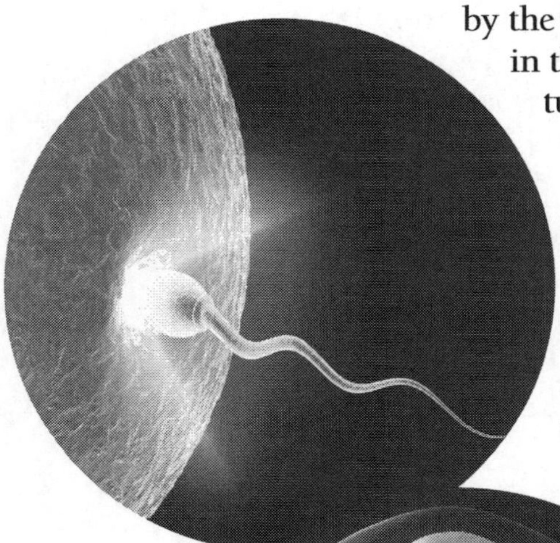

Fertilization, the fusion of the sperm and egg, usually occurs in the upper third area of the fallopian tube. Thirty minutes after ejaculation, sperm is present in the tube, having traveled from the vagina through the uterus and into the oviduct. Sperm traverses this distance by the beating of its flagellum. Of the several hundred million sperm released in the ejaculation, only a few thousand reach the egg.

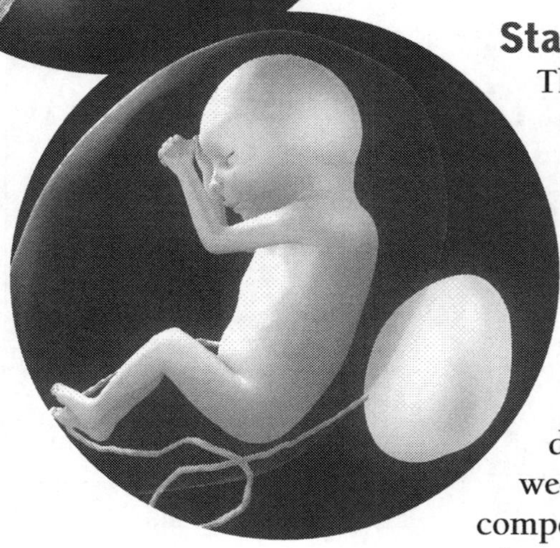

Stages

The period of time from fertilization to birth (usually 9 months) is divided into trimesters, each about three months long. During pregnancy the zygote undergoes 40 to 44 rounds of mitosis, producing an infant containing trillions of specialized cells organized into tissues and organs.

The First Trimester

Three embryonic tissue layers form. Cellular differentiation begins to form organs during the third week. After one month the embryo is 5 mm long and composed mostly of paired somite segments. During the second month most of the major organ systems form while limb buds develop. The embryo becomes a fetus by the seventh week. Beginning the eighth week, the sexually neutral fetus activates gene pathways for sex determination, forming testes in XY fetuses and ovaries in XX fetuses. External genitalia develop.

The Second Trimester

The fetus increases in size during this trimester, and bony parts of the skeleton begin to form. Fetal movements can be felt by the mother.

The Last Trimester

During this trimester the fetus increases in size. Circulatory and respiratory systems mature in preparation for breathing outside the body. Fetal growth during this time uses large parts of its mother's protein and calcium intake. Maternal antibodies pass to the fetus during the last month, conferring temporary immunity.

BIRTH

Birth is a process of positive facilitated by hormonal positive feedback. During birth the cervix dilates to allow passage of the fetus. Uterine contractions propel the fetus through the birth canal, usually headfirst. Hormonal control of the birth process involves the release of oxytocin and prostaglandins, which are stimulated by uterine contractions, which stimulate more hormones that cause more contractions.

First Stage of Birth

The first stage of birth lasts from beginning of contractions to the full (10 cm) dilation of the cervix. Membranes of the amniotic sac rupture, releasing amniotic fluid thus lubricating the vagina.

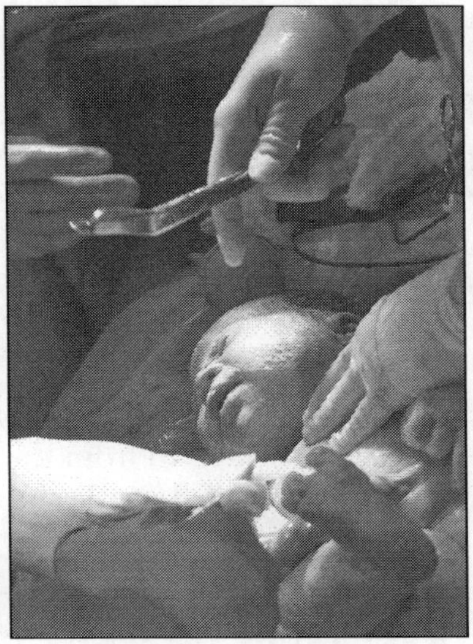

Second Stage of Birth

Strong uterine contractions of a minute in duration separated by two to three minute intervals propel the fetus down the birth canal. Abdominal muscles relax in synchrony with the uterine contractions.

Third Stage of Birth

After delivery of the baby, the umbilical cord is clipped and cut. The placenta (or afterbirth) is expelled through the vagina.

Milk Production

Breasts develop the capability for milk secretion about the mid point of pregnancy. Secretion of milk does not occur until delivery, and the release of prolactin. Sucking by the infant causes production of oxytocin to promote release of milk into the ducts emptying into the nipple. Nursing mothers maintain certain hormone levels and uterine size returns to normal much faster than non-nursing mothers.

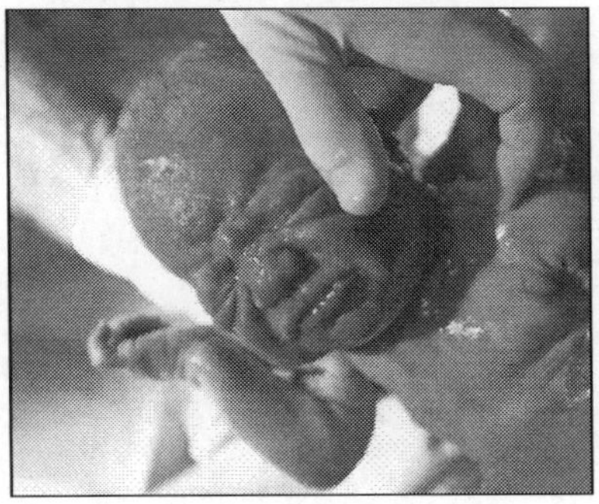

PO Box 2308, Woburn, MA 01888-0508, **p:** 781-729-3736, **www.EmbracingCulture.com**
PO Box 6401, Manchester, NH 03108, **p:** 1-888-678-CCCS

CONTRACEPTION

Various contraceptive methods have been developed, none of which is 100% successful at preventing pregnancy or the transmission of STDs. Abstinence is the only completely effective method.

Methods

1. Physical prevention (most effective) includes vasectomy and tubal ligation. Vasectomy: The vas deferens connects the testes with the urethra. In a vasectomy, the vas deferens is cut and sealed to prevent the transport of sperm. In tubal ligation, the fallopian tube is cut and ends tied off to prevent eggs from reaching the uterus.

2. Oral contraceptives (birth control pills) usually contain a combination of hormones that prevent release of FSH and LH and ultimately estrogen inhibiting development of the follicle so that no oocytes are released. Time-release capsules (Norplant) can be implanted under the skin and offer long-term suppression of ovulation. RU-486, the so-called morning after pill, interferes with implantation of the blastula into the uterine wall. Its use as a contraceptive is very controversial.

3. Barrier methods employ physical (condom, diaphragm) or chemical (spermicides) means to separate the sperm from the egg. Male condoms are fitted over the erect penis; female condoms are placed inside the vagina. Only latex condoms prevent the spread of STDs.

Diaphragms cap the cervix and block passage of the sperm into the uterus. Spermicidal jellies or foams kill sperm on contact and must be placed in the vagina prior to intercourse.

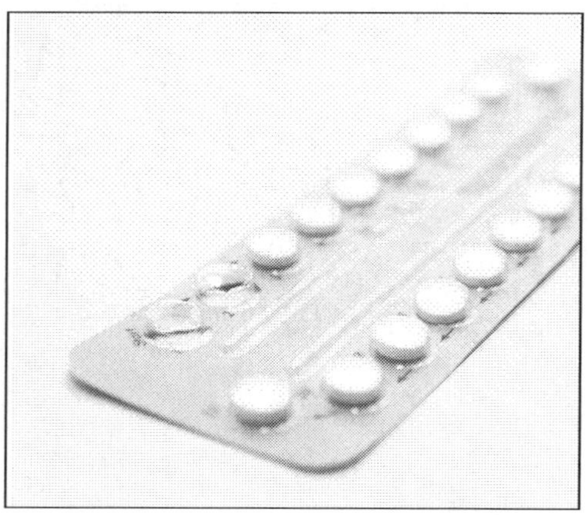

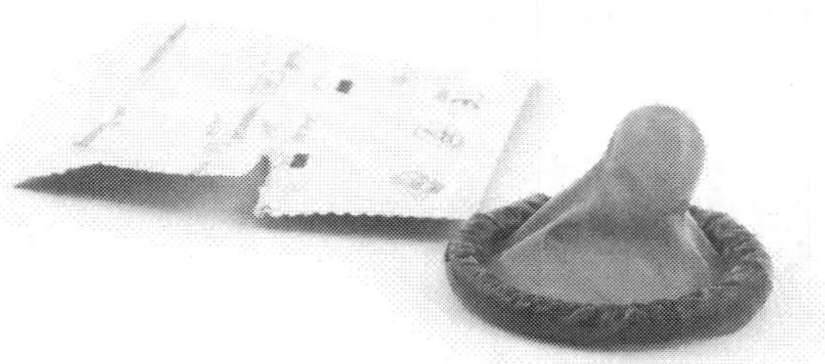

Do you remember the different contraception methods? How many are you able to name? Translate them into your Target Language.

Contraception methods	Target Language

Reproductive Technologies Can Enhance Fertility

About 1 in 6 couples are infertile due to physical conditions preventing gamete production, implantation, or fertilization.

Blocked fallopian tubes (often from untreated STDs) are the leading cause of infertility in females.

Low sperm count, low mobility, or blocked ducts are common causes of male infertility.

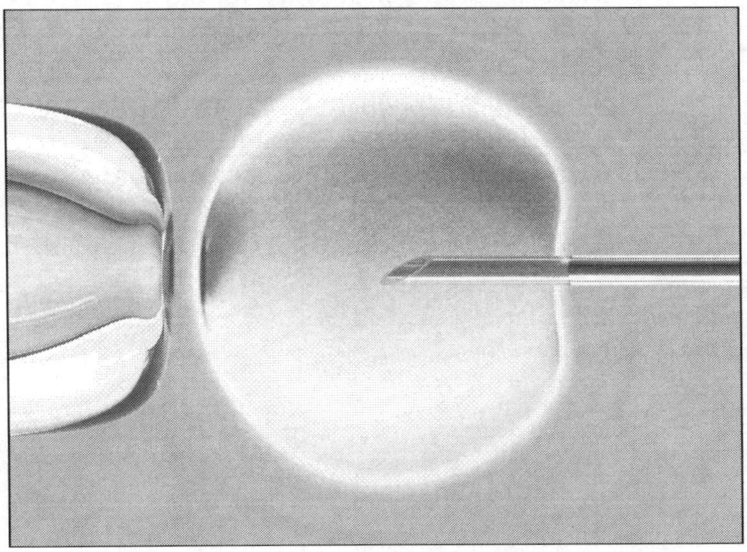

Hormone therapy can cause increased egg production. Surgery can open blocked ducts. About 40% of the cases are due to male problems, 40 % are due to female problems and the remaining 20% are caused by some unknown agent(s). In vitro fertilization (test-tube babies) is a widely used technique to aid infertile couples.

PO Box 2308, Woburn, MA 01888-0508, **p:** 781-729-3736, **www.EmbracingCulture.com**
PO Box 6401, Manchester, NH 03108, **p:** 1-888-678-CCCS

Most Common Illnesses:

1. Ovarian Cancer

The Center for Disease Control reports that ovarian cancer is the seventh most common cancer and the fifth most likely to lead to death. The National Cancer Institute estimated for the year 2009 that there were at least 21,550 new diagnosed cases of ovarian cancer and that more than half of these women would die of this cancer. Women with family history of breast, endometrial or colon cancer seem to have an increased risk. Ovarian cancer is more common among women over 50 , but it can also occur among women in their forties or younger.

2. Breast Cancer

The Center for Disease Control web page reports that, as well as ovarian cancer, family history and age may be influential variables in the prediction of breast cancer. Mammographies and self-breast examination may detect breast cancer at its early stages. An estimated 192,370 new invasive cases of breast cancer were expected to occur among women in the United States during 2009. Although breast cancer is an illness mainly associated with women, men can also suffer from breast cancer.

According to www.cancer.gov, the following are the main risk factors for breast cancer:

- Older age
- Menstruating at an early age
- Older age at first birth or never having given birth
- Personal history of breast cancer or benign (non cancer) breast disease
- A mother or sister with breast cancer
- Treatment with radiation therapy to the breast/chest
- Dense breast tissue as seen on a mammogram
- Hormone use (such as estrogen and progesterone)
- Drinking alcoholic beverages
- Caucasian race

There are four main stages of breast cancer. These stages will indicate how spread the cancer cells may be throughout the body. The stages run from the least advanced to the most advanced.

Stages	Meaning
Stage O	(carcinoma in situ) (two types: ductal and lobular)
Stage I	(no larger than 2cm not spread outside the breast)
Stage IIA	(no larger than 2cm, but has spread to the axillary lymph nodes) or (between 2cm and 5cm but has not spread)
Stage IIB	(between 2cm and 5cm but has spread to the axillary lymph nodes) or (larger than 5cm but has not spread)
Stage IIIA	(smaller than 5cm but has spread to the axillary lymph nodes and they are attached to each other) or (larger than 5cm but has spread to the axillary lymph nodes and they are attached to each other)
Stage IIIB	(spread to tissue near breast, the skin or chest wall, including ribs and muscles in the chest) or (spread lymph nodes inside the chest wall along the breastbone)
Stage IV	(spread to other organs of the body, most often the bones, lungs, liver or brain) or (spread to lymph nodes in the neck, near the collarbone)

Four Main Types of Treatments for Breast Cancer:

1. **Surgery:**
    - **Lumpectomy** removal of the lump and a small amount of tissue
    - **Partial segmental mastectomy** only the part of the breast with the cancer gets removed plus some surrounding tissue
    - **Total mastectomy** removal of the entire breast and some of the lymph nodes for a biopsy.
    - **Modified radical mastectomy** removal of the entire breast, many of the lymph nodes, the lining over the chest and at times part of the chest wall.
2. **Radiation Therapy** A form of treatment with a very strong X-ray or other types of radiation to kill cancer cells.
3. **Chemotherapy** The treatment via special drugs that stops the cancer from growing
4. **Hormone Therapy** A form of treatment that prevents hormones from interacting and puts a barrier to the growth of the cancer cells

PO Box 2308, Woburn, MA 01888-0508, **p:** 781-729-3736, **www.EmbracingCulture.com**
PO Box 6401, Manchester, NH 03108, **p:** 1-888-678-CCCS

EXERCISE

Choose the answer that best completes the statement.

1. Ovarian cancer is the Seventh most common cancer and the fifth form of cancer most likely to lead to death.
   a. First
   b. Fifth
   c. Seventh
   d. Fourth

2. Family history and Age may be influential variables in the prediction of breast cancer.
   a. Profession
   b. Education
   c. Age
   d. Birth order

3. Main risk factors for breast cancer may include:
   a. Older age
   b. Menstruating at an early age
   c. Older age at first birth or never having given birth
   d. All of the above

4. There are FOUR main stages of breast cancer.
   a. Two
   b. Nine
   c. Four
   d. Six

5. Treatments for breast cancer may include
   a. Mastectomy
   b. Lumpectomy
   c. Radiation therapy
   d. All of the above

6. Treatment via special drugs that stops the cancer from growing is called:
   a. Osteotherapy
   b. Radiation therapy
   c. Chemotherapy
   d. Occipital drug course

Illnesses/Conditions

More Illnesses or Conditions (consult the Additional Resources Section for more information on these conditions)

1. Amenorrhea
2. Balanitis
3. Cervicitis
4. Chlamydia
5. Crabs (pubic lice)
6. Cryptorchism
7. Dysmenorrhea
8. Ectopic Pregnancy
9. Endometriosis
10. Fibroids
11. Genital herpes
12. Gonorrhea
13. HPV (Human Papillomavirus)
14. Impotence
15. Menorrhagia
16. Orchitis
17. Pelvic inflammatory disease
18. Prostatic carcinoma
19. Prostatitis
20. Syphilis
21. Testicular carcinoma
22. Trichomoniasis
23. Urethritis
24. Vaginal Candidiasis (yeast infection)

PO Box 2308, Woburn, MA 01888-0508, **p:** 781-729-3736, **www.EmbracingCulture.com**
PO Box 6401, Manchester, NH 03108, **p:** 1-888-678-CCCS

EXERCISE

A. Group the illnesses/conditions in the following table as they pertain to men or women:

Illnesses/Conditions	Female ♀	Male ♂
1. Amenorrhea		
2. Balanitis		
3. Cervicitis		
4. Chlamydia		
5. Crabs (pubic lice)		
6. Cryptorchism		
7. Dysmenorrhea		
8. Ectopic Pregnancy		
9. Endometriosis		
10. Fibroids		
11. Genital herpes		
12. Gonorrhea		
13. HPV (Human Papillomavirus)		
14. Impotence		
15. Menorrhagia		
16. Orchitis		
17. Pelvic inflammatory disease		
18. Prostatic carcinoma		
19. Prostatitis		
20. Syphilis		
21. Testicular carcinoma		
22. Trichomoniasis		
23. Urethritis		
24. Vaginal Candidiasis (yeast infection)		

When unfamiliar with the disease/condition, what technique did you use to find out if it was a "female disease" or a "male disease"? If your answer was the Samurai! Technique, you are correct!

EXERCISE

B. What do the following root words refer to?

Root Word	Refers to the...	Target
1. balan/o		
2. cervic/o		
3. colp/o		
4. hyster/o		
5. mast/o		
6. metri/o		
7. oophor/o		
8. orch/o		
9. prostat/o		
10. salping/o		
11. scrot/o		
12. urethra/o		
13. uter/o		
14. vas/o		

PO Box 2308, Woburn, MA 01888-0508, **p:** 781-729-3736, **www.EmbracingCulture.com**
PO Box 6401, Manchester, NH 03108, **p:** 1-888-678-CCCS

EXERCISE

C. **Using your knowledge of word formation, match the medical terms for the female reproductive system in column I with its meaning in column II**

	Column I	Column II
______	1. endometriosis	A. breast inflammation
______	2. ectopic pregnancy	B. absence of menstrual flow
______	3. amenorrhea	C. excessive discharge of blood (from the uterus) between menstrual periods
______	4. mastitis	D. painful menstrual flow
______	5. menorrhagia	E. type of tissue that lines the uterus is found in sites other than the uterus
______	6. dysmenorrhea	F. the embryo develops outside the uterus

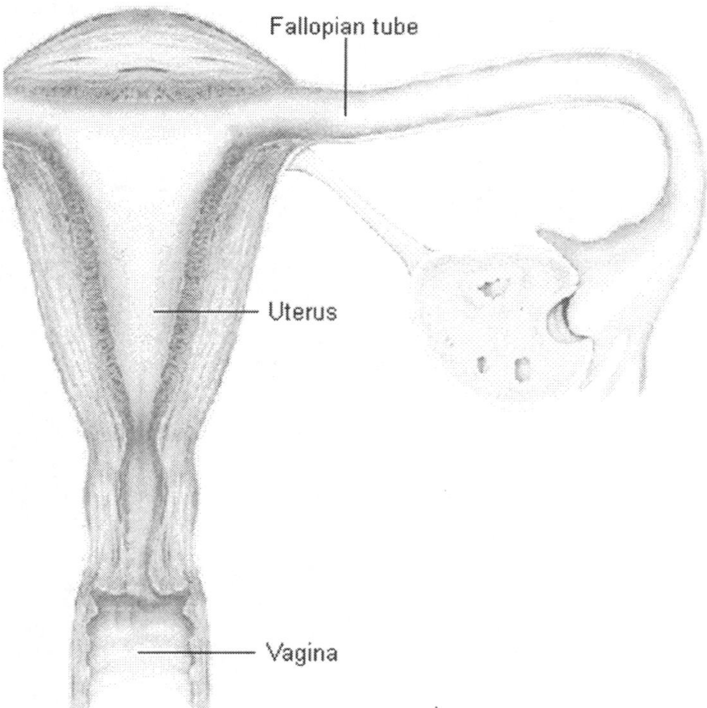

EXERCISE

D. Using your knowledge of word formation, match the test or treatment procedure for the female reproductive system in column I with its meaning in column II

	Column I	Column II
_______	1. amniocentesis	A. removal of a fallopian tube
_______	2. cauterization	B. X-ray imaging of the breast
_______	3. spinal tap	C. ultrasound examination of organs in the hip region
_______	4. hysterectomy	D. surgical removal of the uterus
_______	5. mammography	E. a test to look at a sample of cells taken from a woman's cervix
_______	6. myomectomy	F. measurement of HCG levels
_______	7. pelvic ulltrasonography	G. surgical removal of fibroids from the uterus.
_______	8. pregnancy test	H. fallopian tubes are tied to prevent pregnancy
_______	9. pap smear	I. use of heat to destroy abnormal tissue
_______	10. salpingectomy	J. surgical puncture to remove amniotic fluid that surrounds the fetus
_______	11. tubal ligation	K. visual imaging of the vagina
_______	12. epidural	L. regional anesthesia that frees a laboring woman from pain
_______	13. colposcopy	M. procedure to look at the fluid that surrounds the brain and spinal cord (cerebrospinal fluid)

PO Box 2308, Woburn, MA 01888-0508, **p:** 781-729-3736, **www.EmbracingCulture.com**
PO Box 6401, Manchester, NH 03108, **p:** 1-888-678-CCCS

EXERCISE

E. Using your knowledge of word formation, match the medical terms for the male reproductive system in column I with its meaning in column II

	Column I	Column II
_______	1. balanitis	A. inflammation of the urethra
_______	2. cryptorchism	B. inflammation of the penis
_______	3. orchitis	C. cancer of the prostate gland
_______	4. prostatic carcinoma	D. malignant tumor of the testis
_______	5. testicular carcinoma	E. undescended testicle
_______	6. urethritis	F. inflammation of a testis

F. Using your knowledge of word formation, match the test or treatment procedure for the male reproductive system in column I with its meaning in column II

	Column I	Column II
_______	1. DRE	A. examination of the prostate gland with finger palpation through the rectum
_______	2. orchidectomy	B. surgical procedure to cut and close off the tubes (vas deferens) that deliver sperm from the testes
_______	3. orchiopexy	C. surgical procedure to remove tissue from the prostate using an instrument inserted through the urethra
_______	4. prostatectomy	D. removal of a testicle
_______	5. semen analysis	E. a procedure to move an undescended testicle into the scrotum
_______	6. TURP	F. test to measure the amount and quality of a man's semen and sperm
_______	7. vasectomy	G. removal of the prostate gland

Lesson Ten: Homework
Reproductive System

1. Go over your notes for today's class and read section "Additional Resources"
2. Read and practice ALL role-plays for this lesson
3. Continue developing your glossary
4. Translate the illnesses/conditions for this topic into your TL

Illness/Condition	Target Language
1. Balanitis	
2. Breast cancer	
3. Ovarian cancer	
4. Amenorrhea	
5. Cervicitis	
6.Chlamydia	
7. Circumcision	
8. Crabs (pubic lice)	
9. Cryptorchism/Cryptorchidism	
10. Dysmenorrhea	
11. Ectopic Pregnancy	
12. Endometriosis	
13. Fibroids	
14. Genital herpes	
15. Gestational Diabetes	
16. Gonorrhea	
17. HPV (Human Papillomavirus)	
18. Impotence	
19. Incontinence	
20. Menorrhagia	
21. Orchitis	
22. Pelvic inflammatory disease	
23. Prostatic carcinoma	
24. Prostatitis	
25. Syphilis	
26. Testicular carcinoma	
27. Trichomoniasis	
28. Urethritis	
29. Vaginal Candidiasis (yeast infection)	

PO Box 2308, Woburn, MA 01888-0508, **p:** 781-729-3736, **www.EmbracingCulture.com**
PO Box 6401, Manchester, NH 03108, **p:** 1-888-678-CCCS

5. Translate the tests/treatment procedures for this topic into your TL:

Tests and Procedures	Target Language
1. amniocentesis	
2. cauterization	
3. spinal tap	
4. hysterectomy	
5. mammography	
6. myomectomy	
7. pelvic ultrasonography	
8. pregnancy test	
9. pap smear	
10. salpingectomy	
11. tubal ligation	
12. epidural	
13. colposcopy	
14. DRE	
15. orchidectomy	
16. orchiopexy	
17. prostatectomy	
18. semen analysis	
19. TURP	
20. vasectomy	

Lesson Ten: Role-Plays
Reproductive System

Work individually at first:
- Read the entire role-play
- Get a general sense of its meaning
- Circle the most challenging medical terms
- Apply the Samurai! technique to those terms
- Read the role-play again for a deeper understanding
- Find an accurate equivalent in the target language

Work in a language-specific group of friends, fellow students or colleagues:
- Share your doubts
- Ask for other ways of expressing the same meaning
- Develop a glossary
- Check the dictionary
- Practice the role-plays remember to do CIFE for all your role-plays
- Have your colleagues observe you and provide feedback on your accuracy and register.
- These colleagues can keep track of any omissions, additions, mistakes or distortions in your interpreting and point these out to you in a follow-up discussion.

Student Interpreter Evaluation

Student Name ______________________ Date

Language ______________________

Mode of Interpreting (check one): ☐ Consecutive ☐ Simultaneous

Role-Play/System ______________________

Areas Observed ______________________

Accuracy

Register ______________________

Omissions ______________________

Additions ______________________

Distortions ______________________

Pronunciation ______________________

Speaker's emotions conveyed? ______________________

Explain ______________________

Technique

General flow ______________________

Flow when requesting clarification ______________________

Speed ______________________

Eye Contact ______________________

Distracting Habits ______________________

Ethical Issues

Answered questions for patient? ______________________

Advised patient? ______________________

Vocabulary Expansion Recommendations

____

____

Other Recommendations

____

____

Language Coach Signature ______________________ Date

) Box 2308, Woburn, MA 01888-0508, **p:** 781-729-3736, **www.EmbracingCulture.com**
) Box 6401, Manchester, NH 03108, **p:** 1-888-678-CCCS

Role-Play 56: Chlamydia

	Pronunciation	Additions	Omissions	Mistakes
DR: Linda, the Nurse Practitioner, just told me about your call this morning. I am glad that we could squeeze you in for an appointment today. What can I do for you?				
PT: I have been living here with the kids and without my husband for most of the summer, but about 3 weeks ago after a very short visit from my husband to this country, I began to notice an abnormal discharge from my vagina. Although I am not urinating more often I must have a urinary tract infection. It burns when I urinate and this is new to me.				
DR: Hmm. Are you running a fever?				
PT: I guess so. I feel a bit warm, and I am having some abdominal pain.				
DR: I see. You're pointing to the lower part of the abdomen…any pain during intercourse?				
PT: Not at the time I had it … but my husband went back to our country so I am not sure how to answer this question. But my back is killing me and I never ever had back problems.				
DR: Any changes at work or at home? Like stress? Or lifting weights?				
PT: No, I am used to having my husband back and forth. He is trying to sell our house and he is helping his mother with her store.				
DR: Have you asked your husband if he is also experiencing any of the symptoms like a burning pain when urinating or a discharge from his penis or unusual itching around the opening of the penis? Or some swelling of his testicles?				
PT: No, but I will ask him. I hope he is not messing around when I am not with him. I just do not want to get a venereal disease!				
DR: It will be good for you to ask him. But anyway I am going to do a pelvic exam and I will swab your cervix to rule out chlamydia.				
PT: OK, but what is chlamydia?				

continued

Role-Play 56 *(continued)*

	Pronunciation	Additions	Omissions	Mistakes
DR: It is a sexually transmitted disease caused by a bacterium called *chlamydia trachomatis* that can be treated with antibiotics but often it gets missed; it is considered a silent illness. Women are generally not aware of their symptoms. The good thing is that if you test positive for chlamydia, we can treat you and your husband before it does any serious damage, especially to your reproductive system. Chlamydia can damage the fallopian tubes, the uterus, and in some cases, due to oral sex, the throat and the mouth or in the cases of anal sex, the rectum.				
PT: OK, but if you are going to treat me, my husband is not around and I am not sure what he is doing when I am not with him.				
DR: Perhaps you want to ask him to see a doctor and let him know of the potential diagnosis and the seriousness if he does not get treated. To be sure you may want to abstain from intercourse with him until you know for sure he has taken the medications.				
PT: OK.				
DR: All sexual partners should have the treatment and this message needs to be passed to your husband and any other partners.				
PT: I have no one except my husband. I will follow the treatment but with my husband I cannot guarantee it.				
DR: Perhaps you want to schedule an appointment with both of you the next time he comes to the USA?				
PT: OK.				
Break It Down	☐	☐	☐	☐

☐ **CIFE with patient** ☐ **CIFE with provider** ☐ **FLOW** ☐ **REGISTER**

Role-Play 56: Glossary

______________ ______________ ______________

______________ ______________ ______________

______________ ______________ ______________

continued

PO Box 2308, Woburn, MA 01888-0508, **p:** 781-729-3736, **www.EmbracingCulture.com**
PO Box 6401, Manchester, NH 03108, **p:** 1-888-678-CCCS

1. Pathology (diseases, conditions)

2. Laboratory Tests and Diagnostic Procedures

3. Treatment Procedures

4. Idiomatic Expressions (if any)

5. Other (vocabulary in this particular role-play that you feel is important/relevant or that you anticipate problems with)

Role-Play 57: Vaginitis

A 19-year-old female comes in with complaint of vaginal symptoms.

		Pronunciation	Additions	Omissions	Mistakes
PT:	I have been having a lot of vaginal itching and soreness for the past week.				
MD:	Have you ever had this problem before?				
PT:	No, this is the first time.				
MD:	Have you noticed any discharge or odor?				
PT:	Yes, there is a lot of whitish-yellow discharge on my underwear. I feel like taking a shower three times a day.				
MD:	Are you sexually active?				
PT:	No, not in the past year.				
MD:	Do you routinely take any medications, or have you recently been on an antibiotic?				
PT:	No, I am not taking any medications, just vitamins.				
MD:	Have you spent much time in a wet bathing suit?				
PT:	I was just on vacation so I spent entire days at the beach.				
MD:	Do you tend to eat a lot of sweets or fresh fruit everyday?				
PT:	I tend to have more ice cream and fruit in the summer, especially on vacation. Why?				
MD:	Your symptoms are suggestive of a vaginal yeast infection. Yeast is a spore that tends to grow when the conditions are right. The right conditions are a warm, moist place with extra sugar. During the summer, many women develop yeast infections due to a diet that is high in sugar, and the time spent in a bathing suit.				
MD:	One more question before I examine you. Have you had any fever, chills, frequent urination, or pain in the vaginal area?				
PT:	No, I feel fine except for the itching and soreness down there.				
MD:	I will need to do a pelvic exam to determine what the cause of your discomfort is. Have you ever had a pelvic exam before?				

continued

PO Box 2308, Woburn, MA 01888-0508, **p:** 781-729-3736, **www.EmbracingCulture.com**
PO Box 6401, Manchester, NH 03108, **p:** 1-888-678-CCCS

Role-Play 57 *(continued)*

		Pronunciation	Additions	Omissions	Mistakes
PT:	Yes, I was seen for my first pap smear in November of last year.				
MD:	Did you have any discomfort with that exam?				
PT:	It wasn't fun, but it was okay.				
MD:	All right, during this exam I need to put a small amount of discharge on a slide. I will be able to look at the discharge under the microscope and see the cause of your discomfort.				
(Exam is done and confirms yeast or monilial vaginitis)					
MD:	Yeast is the cause of your symptoms. This is a very common type of vaginitis.				
PT:	How do I get rid of it and will it come back?				
MD:	There are medications available over-the-counter such as "Monistat" or "Gynelotrimin." These are vaginal creams that you insert in the vagina at night. The medication is inserted using a tampon-like applicator. It works best to use it at bedtime, as the cream will leak out in the morning when you are standing. You will need to use a panty liner the next day.				
PT:	That sounds really messy. Isn't there anything else to treat this with?				
MD:	There is a pill known as 'Diflucan' which is taken as one dose. It is simple but it is also good to treat a vaginal infection locally with one of the yeast creams. The Diflucan will take up to 48 hours for you to get relief because the pill needs to work its way into your system.				
PT:	I would really prefer the pill this time.				
MD:	I will give you a prescription that you can take right away. You should also avoid excess sweets, layers of clothing or spending too much time in a wet suit. If you do develop the same symptoms again, you may treat this yourself with one of the over-the-counter medications for yeast.				
PT:	Thank you.				
	Break It Down	☐	☐	☐	☐

☐ **CIFE with patient** ☐ **CIFE with provider** ☐ **FLOW** ☐ **REGISTER**

continued

Role-Play 57: Glossary

1. Pathology (diseases, conditions)

2. Laboratory Tests and Diagnostic Procedures

3. Treatment Procedures

4. Idiomatic Expressions (if any)

5. Other (vocabulary in this particular role-play that you feel is important/relevant or that you anticipate problems with)

PO Box 2308, Woburn, MA 01888-0508, **p:** 781-729-3736, **www.EmbracingCulture.com**
PO Box 6401, Manchester, NH 03108, **p:** 1-888-678-CCCS

Role-Play 58: Male Genital Herpes

	Pronunciation	Additions	Omissions	Mistakes
PT: (Showing his genitals) Doctor, I am so afraid that I got a bad disease. Look at all the blisters I have gotten right around my penis.				
DR: Yes, the blisters and sores around your penis and scrotum look like genital herpes, but let me take a sample and send it to the lab. We also will need a few blood tests to see if you have HSV.				
PT: OK. I am in so much pain! And now I am going to have trouble finding a sexual partner...I am marked forever! I cannot forgive myself.				
DR: Let's take a deep breath and before you panic, there are a few things that we will need to do before I actually diagnose genital herpes. This sexually transmitted disease is serious but it can be treated with an antiviral medication such as Valtrex.				
PT: Is it curable?				
DR: No, it's not curable, but it can be managed if you learn how to live with it and protect yourself and your sexual partner or partners.				
PT: You said it is serious. How serious?				
DR: It is transmitted through sexual intercourse and women who get herpes can have serious complications when giving birth; it can be fatal for the baby. So, you need to wear a condom especially when you first notice the blisters. But you may not always be able to protect your sexual partner, because the latex from the condom may not always cover the ulcers or sores.				
PT: Is this the same as canker sores that I have had since I am a young boy?				
DR: No, canker sores or lesions are a form of stomatitis or an inflammation of the mouth. Cold sores, however, are from a different variation of the herpes virus. Like cold sores, genital herpes is both painful and contagious.				
PT: OK, I get it now! I thought that canker and cold sores were the same.				

continued

Role-Play 58 *(continued)*

		Pronunciation	Additions	Omissions	Mistakes
DR:	One is an inflammation in the inside of your mouth and we are not sure if it is viral or not. The other is a virus transmitted by saliva and is on the outside of your mouth. In the past, we treated Genital herpes with Acyclovir 200 mg po 5 doses x 7 days but now we have an easier medication, called Valacyclovir or Valtrex where you only have to take it twice a day for 10 days.				
PT:	OK.				
	Break It Down	☐	☐	☐	☐

☐ **CIFE with patient** ☐ **CIFE with provider** ☐ **FLOW** ☐ **REGISTER**

Role-Play 58: Glossary

continued

PO Box 2308, Woburn, MA 01888-0508, **p:** 781-729-3736, **www.EmbracingCulture.com**
PO Box 6401, Manchester, NH 03108, **p:** 1-888-678-CCCS

1. Pathology (diseases, conditions)

2. Laboratory Tests and Diagnostic Procedures

3. Treatment Procedures

4. Idiomatic Expressions (if any)

5. Other (vocabulary in this particular role-play that you feel is important/relevant or that you anticipate problems with)

Role-Play 59: Herpes Progenitalis

A 16-year-old female comes in with a complaint of a painful rash in the vaginal area.

	Pronunciation	Additions	Omissions	Mistakes
PT: I am having so much pain I can hardly walk or sit.				
MD: How long have you had this pain and how did it start?				
PT: I first noticed some bumps down there when I was in the shower two days ago. They felt a little sore, but then today I couldn't even touch the area.				
MD: Are you sexually active with anyone?				
PT: I have only been with my boyfriend for a few months.				
MD: Have you had intercourse with him and do you use condoms?				
PT: Yes, but not since I developed this rash. We stopped using condoms because we didn't like the way they felt.				
MD: Have you had more than one partner?				
PT: No, he is the first boy I have had sex with.				
MD: Are you having any other symptoms like fever, chills, or burning with urination?				
PT: I felt really lousy during the night like I have a flu. It has also started to hurt when I pee so I am afraid to drink too much.				
MD: I will need to examine you to diagnose the cause of your symptoms. Have you ever had a pelvic or gynecological exam?				
PT: No, I have not been to a gynecologist before.				
MD: I will explain everything and help you relax for this exam. It is important that I am able to at least look at the genital area to see this rash. Then we will decide if I need to do an internal exam.				
PT: Will this hurt?				
MD: I will make every effort to cause you as little discomfort as necessary.				
MD: This rash looks like a herpes infection. I will need to do a culture to be certain, which means I will be touching a few of the lesions with a Q-tip. It will be uncomfortable when I touch the lesions but it will be very quick.				
PT: How would I have gotten herpes?				
MD: Herpes progenitalis is a sexually transmitted disease that you only get from another person during sex.				

continued

PO Box 2308, Woburn, MA 01888-0508, **p:** 781-729-3736, **www.EmbracingCulture.com**
PO Box 6401, Manchester, NH 03108, **p:** 1-888-678-CCCS

Role-Play 59 *(continued)*

		Pronunciation	Additions	Omissions	Mistakes
PT:	Do you mean that I got this from my boyfriend?				
MD:	If he is the only person you have had sex with, then he probably has the virus and transmitted it to you.				
PT:	Is there an antibiotic I can take to get rid of this?				
MD:	There is a medication called "Acyclovir" that I will give you to start today. It is a 200 mg tablet that you need to take five times a day for five days. It works by shortening the course of this outbreak, but it does not get rid of the virus. This virus lives in your system and can cause repeated outbreaks. Whenever you notice the beginning of another outbreak, you should start this medication immediately to reduce the severity of your symptoms.				
PT:	How often will this happen again?				
MD:	Outbreaks can be close together or far apart. If the culture confirms herpes, then I would recommend suppressive treatment. That means that you may take a dose of Acyclovir or another medication called Valtrex on a daily basis. This treatment will reduce your chance of a reoccurrence and it will reduce transmission to any other partners you may have in the future.				
PT:	When will I feel better?				
MD:	It will take a week to ten days to feel completely better. I will also give you a prescription for Tylenol with codeine which will help the pain. It is important to rest, drink fluids, take the acyclovir and keep the area clean and dry. You can also soak in a lukewarm bath to soothe the area. I would like to see you in one week to check on how you are doing and to review your culture results. I realize that this is a lot of information and I will be happy to review this again when you are feeling better.				
	Break It Down	☐	☐	☐	☐

☐ CIFE with patient ☐ CIFE with provider ☐ FLOW ☐ REGISTER

Role-Play 59: Glossary

______ ______ ______

______ ______ ______

______ ______ ______

continued

1. Pathology (diseases, conditions)

2. Laboratory Tests and Diagnostic Procedures

3. Treatment Procedures

4. Idiomatic Expressions (if any)

5. Other (vocabulary in this particular role-play that you feel is important/relevant or that you anticipate problems with)

PO Box 2308, Woburn, MA 01888-0508, **p:** 781-729-3736, **www.EmbracingCulture.com**
PO Box 6401, Manchester, NH 03108, **p:** 1-888-678-CCCS

Role-Play 60: Birth Control Consult

A 15 y.o. female and her 17 y.o. boyfriend are here to discuss options for birth control.

		Pronunciation	Additions	Omissions	Mistakes
NP:	How can I help you today?				
PT:	Well, we wanted to talk about birth control.				
BF:	And…we don't want her parents to know we are here.				
NP:	It is very responsible of you both to come in together as a couple because it is an important decision that affects each of you. I can also reassure you that this visit is confidential. There is a law that enables a teenager under the age of 18 to seek care for birth control and for sexually transmitted disease screening and treatment. Under this law, you are considered a mature minor who can make a decision about your contraceptive needs without your parent's consent.				
BF:	That is good to know.				
NP:	At this point in time, have you been sexually active together?				
PT:	Yes, we have been together for four months.				
NP:	Have you used anything to prevent pregnancy and sexually transmitted diseases?				
PT:	Well, we have been using condoms but we are worried about getting pregnant because it has slipped off during sex.				
NP:	Do you know about emergency contraception?				
PT:	No, what is that?				
NP:	Emergency contraception is a birth control pill in a higher dose that you take after a condom accident, which is the term used when a condom slips off or breaks. It is two doses, taken 12 hours apart, that can help prevent a pregnancy from happening. It works best when taken as soon as possible after a condom accident but can be taken up to 5 days after intercourse. When you are using condoms for birth control, it is a good idea to have a prescription for Plan B on hand. Plan B is the common name for emergency contraception.				
NP:	Do you have an idea of what you would like to use for birth control?				
PT:	I have thought about the pill, but I really don't know much about it and I am worried about gaining weight.				
NP:	Let me give you an overview of the methods available to you and the key things to consider in making your decision. There are barrier methods, which include condoms, the diaphragm and the cervical cap along with the use of a spermicide.				

continued

Role-Play 60 *(continued)*

		Pronunciation	Additions	Omissions	Mistakes
BF:	What is spermicide?				
NP:	Spermicide is a chemical that stops the sperm from reaching the egg. It is a cream or jelly that is put in the vagina, inside the diaphragm or cap, or is part of the condom. There is one known as contraceptive film that is a small thin square which looks like saran wrap. It can easily be kept in a pocket or wallet and placed in the vagina prior to intercourse.				
PT:	I don't know what a diaphragm is.				
NP:	The diaphragm and the cap are both devices that you need to place in the vagina prior to sex. They cover the cervix and hold spermicide in place so that sperm is unable to get inside of the uterus to find an egg. Each of these methods needs to be used every time you have intercourse. Barrier methods have almost no side effects but they are less effective in preventing pregnancy than the hormonal methods. The condom also protects you against sexually transmitted diseases and when used with the diaphragm your protection against pregnancy is close to 100%.				
PT:	I don't think I want to deal with barrier methods and I am not comfortable putting things in my vagina. What are our other choices?				
NP:	The hormonal methods are the most effective in preventing pregnancy. There are quite a few options in this group. The pill is very popular because it is easy and allows for spontaneity. That means that you do not have to stop to use a barrier method prior to having intercourse. However, I still recommend using a condom to prevent STD's.				
BF:	Right, we learned about that in health class.				
NP:	You need to remember to take a pill everyday at approximately the same time. As with all medications, there are side effects to the pill. Since the pill was invented, the dosage of hormones has been lowered to the least amount necessary to prevent you from releasing an egg, which is how the pill works. With the low dose pills, the side effects have been reduced. The pill also has a risk of causing development of a blood clot. This risk occurs more often in women who smoke and are over the age of 35. In a teen that does not smoke and has no history of blood clots, the pill is very low risk. It is actually riskier for you to be pregnant than to take the pill.				
PT:	But there are side effects, right?				

continued

PO Box 2308, Woburn, MA 01888-0508, **p:** 781-729-3736, **www.EmbracingCulture.com**
PO Box 6401, Manchester, NH 03108, **p:** 1-888-678-CCCS

Role-Play 60 *(continued)*

		Pronunciation	Additions	Omissions	Mistakes
NP:	The minor side effects that are common include mood changes, weight gain of 2-3 pounds, acne, and breakthrough bleeding. The benefits include regular menstrual cycles, lighter periods, less cramping, less anemia, less acne, and a decreased risk of ovarian cancer.				
PT:	I heard about the patch. How does that work?				
NP:	The patch is a form of the pill. You wear it on your arm, back or lower hip and it is changed weekly. There is also the vaginal ring, which is placed in the vagina for 3 weeks then removed for one week during which you have a period. These two options reduce the need to remember to take a pill everyday and keep the hormonal level in your system more constant. Do you think you would be able to remember to take a pill everyday?				
PT:	I am not sure. I don't always remember to take my daily multivitamin.				
NP:	There is another very effective hormonal method known as Depo-Provera, which does not require you to remember to take something everyday. This is a medication that is a form of progesterone that is given as an injection every three months. It is extremely effective in preventing pregnancy. It does cause irregular periods and in 50% of women, the menstrual period stops completely while they are taking the medication.				
PT:	Is that safe? It doesn't sound natural not to have a period. Doesn't the blood build up?				
NP:	Yes, it is safe. Depo-Provera prevents ovulation, which is the release of an egg, and prevents the build up of a thick uterine lining. If there is no lining, then there is no need for a period to shed the lining. Depo-Provera can cause a weight gain of about 5lbs per year.				
PT:	I really don't like the idea of shots or of gaining weight.				
NP:	There is another option called the IUD or intrauterine device. This is a 'T' shaped object that is inserted inside of the uterus during a pelvic exam. There are two IUD's available today. One is the Paraguard, which works for 10 years and has no hormones in it. The other is the Mirena which has progestin in it and lasts for 5 years. The progestin thins the uterine lining and thickens cervical mucous so the sperm cannot even reach the egg. The Paraguard makes the lining unfavorable for an egg to implant.				

continued

Role-Play 60 *(continued)*

		Pronunciation	Additions	Omissions	Mistakes
PT:	I really don't like the idea of an object inside of me for that long. This is a lot of information and I am not sure I can decide today. What would you suggest?				
NP:	It is a good idea to take your time and discuss what the best option for you is. I will give you handouts on each of the methods so that you can take your time reviewing your choices. Once you decide, you can come back and I will review that method in detail. In the meantime, I would recommend continuing to use condoms and I will give you a prescription for plan B to use as emergency contraception. I will also need to do an exam prior to starting any hormonal method.				
PT:	That sounds like a good idea for now. Can we schedule another appointment with you for this?				
NP:	I would be happy to see you again for an exam and to get you started on any of the methods I have gone over. Here is my card in case you have any questions or concerns that you may think of after you leave.				
	Break It Down	☐	☐	☐	☐

☐ **CIFE with patient** ☐ **CIFE with provider** ☐ **FLOW** ☐ **REGISTER**

Role-Play 60: Glossary

continued

1. Pathology (diseases, conditions)

2. Laboratory Tests and Diagnostic Procedures

3. Treatment Procedures

4. Idiomatic Expressions (if any)

5. Other (vocabulary in this particular role-play that you feel is important/relevant or that you anticipate problems with)

Role-Play 61: Choosing the Birth Control Pill

Teenager returns with decision to try oral contraceptives.

		Pronunciation	Additions	Omissions	Mistakes
NP:	Hello again. What have you decided?				
PT:	I talked to my friends and my sister. They are all using the pill. It sounds like something I would like to try. My sister takes Levlen, and she hasn't gained any weight on it.				
NP:	There are a lot of pills to choose from and the one your sister is on is fine to start with. Basically, we need to find a pill that matches your system so that you are not having any unwanted side effects. Even though you are sisters, your systems are different. I would like to explain just how the pill works to prevent pregnancy and to review some basic information about your menstrual cycle. The first day of your period is called cycle day 1. During the period, the hormones of your cycle are at baseline and the lining of the uterus is shedding. After the first 7 days your estrogen level begins to rise which matures an egg and thickens the lining in the uterus to get ready for a pregnancy. Once the egg is released, progesterone comes into your system and keeps the lining in place while waiting for a pregnancy. If there is no pregnancy, the hormone levels drop and that is your body's signal to have a period.				
PT:	How should I take the pills?				
NP:	When you are on birth control pills, you will take your first pill on the first day of your period or on the first Sunday of your period. You must start by cycle day 7. Each pill contains both estrogen and progesterone. By giving your body these hormones, it stops the normal rise in estrogen and prevents the release of an egg. It also produces a thin uterine lining which can make your period very light. This is one of the benefits of the pill. It lightens your period, which reduces cramps and your risk of developing anemia or a low iron level. Because the pills today are very low dose, it is important to take the pill at the same time every day. If you forget a dose, the hormone level will drop and your body will think it is time for a period and start to shed the lining. This is known as breakthrough bleeding. This can also happen during the first 1-3 cycles while your body adjusts to the pill.				

continued

PO Box 2308, Woburn, MA 01888-0508, **p:** 781-729-3736, **www.EmbracingCulture.com**
PO Box 6401, Manchester, NH 03108, **p:** 1-888-678-CCCS

Role-Play 61 *(continued)*

		Pronunciation	Additions	Omissions	Mistakes
PT:	Does this happen a lot?				
NP:	It will happen whenever you miss taking one or more of your pills. Try to choose a time when you will best remember to take your pill. For many young women, I have advised them to set an alarm on their cell phone to remind them to take their pill.				
PT:	Oh, that is a good idea for me. I always have my cell with me.				
NP:	Whenever you miss a pill, take it as soon as you remember. If it is the next day you should take both doses together. Some women may feel a little nausea when they take two doses together but it passes. If you begin to bleed due to a missed dose, just continue taking the rest of the pills as planned. If you double up as I mentioned, you should still be protected against pregnancy, but if you miss more than 2 doses in a row, your protection drops. By using a condom with the pill, you will be protected against pregnancy and sexually transmitted diseases.				
PT:	This is a lot of information.				
NP:	Most of what I have explained will be in the handouts. I have added the information about the normal menstrual cycle so that you understand the pill cycle better. When you open the pack of pills, the first 3 weeks are the active pills. That means that they have hormones in them. The last week of the pack are known as placebos or sugar pills that have no hormones in them. When you take that week of pills, the hormone level in your system will drop and you will have a period. It may be very light, even as little as light spotting. If you miss a period completely, you should do a home pregnancy test just before you start your next pack.				
PT:	What are the side effects?				
NP:	The most common minor side effects may include bloating, irritability, acne, and breakthrough bleeding. If you have side effects that you do not like, we will change the pill to one that matches your system better.				
PT:	Last time, you said something about blood clots.				

continued

Role-Play 61 *(continued)*

	Pronunciation	Additions	Omissions	Mistakes
NP: The major risk is the development of a blood clot. Signs of a blood clot include sudden severe calf pain, chest pain, shortness of breath, and visual changes. If you experience any of these, stop your pills and call the doctor immediately. There is also the risk of developing an elevation in your blood pressure so we would like to see you in 3 months to check your blood pressure and see how you are doing on this pill.				
PT: So, when can I get started?				
NP: It is a good idea to do a pelvic exam prior to starting the pill. We will also check your blood pressure and weight as part of the exam. Then you may start with your next period. You will be protected against pregnancy after the first week of pills are taken but we encourage everyone to continue using condoms all the time.				
PT: I don't have enough time today for an exam and I am also a little nervous about a pelvic exam.				
NP: It is ok to schedule an appointment for the exam before you are due for your next period. I will explain everything I am going to do and give you tips on how to relax for the exam.				
PT: I would like to schedule an appointment soon so I can get started this month.				
NP: That is a good idea.				
Break It Down	☐	☐	☐	☐

☐ **CIFE with patient** ☐ **CIFE with provider** ☐ **FLOW** ☐ **REGISTER**

Role-Play 61: Glossary

continued

PO Box 2308, Woburn, MA 01888-0508, **p:** 781-729-3736, **www.EmbracingCulture.com**
PO Box 6401, Manchester, NH 03108, **p:** 1-888-678-CCCS

1. Pathology (diseases, conditions)

2. Laboratory Tests and Diagnostic Procedures

3. Treatment Procedures

4. Idiomatic Expressions (if any)

5. Other (vocabulary in this particular role-play that you feel is important/relevant or that you anticipate problems with)

Role-Play 62: Emergency Contraception

A 17-year-old female comes to the health center with complaint of a missed period.

	Pronunciation	Additions	Omissions	Mistakes
PT: I am late for my period and I am worried that I may be pregnant.				
MD: Do you have a period every month?				
PT: My period does not come on the same day each month.				
MD: Do you ever skip a month?				
PT: Sometimes I miss a month, but that is rare.				
MD: When was your last period? Was it normal or was it lighter than you are used to?				
PT: I think it was around May 15th, and it was the same as usual.				
MD: That would be almost 6 weeks ago. Are you sexually active and do you use any form of birth control?				
PT: I have a boyfriend and I do not take anything.				
MD: Do you ever use condoms to prevent pregnancy and sexually transmitted diseases?				
PT: We used condoms in the beginning but we have been together for a long time so we stopped.				
MD: Are you having any symptoms of pregnancy such as breast tenderness or nausea?				
PT: No, I feel the same, just worried.				
MD: Have you been ill this past month or very stressed?				
PT: No, I've been fine but I am really scared that I might be pregnant.				
MD: It is possible to miss a period and not be pregnant. We will need a urine sample to do a pregnancy test. If it is positive, I will help you review your choices about what to do. When was the last time you had intercourse or sex without using a condom?				
PT: It has been two weeks since we were together.				
(Urine sample tested negative)				
MD: I have good news for you. Your pregnancy test was negative today. If it has truly been two weeks since you last had sex, then we can rely on this test to be accurate.				
PT: I am so relieved but why haven't I had a period?				

continued

PO Box 2308, Woburn, MA 01888-0508, **p:** 781-729-3736, **www.EmbracingCulture.com**
PO Box 6401, Manchester, NH 03108, **p:** 1-888-678-CCCS

Role-Play 62 *(continued)*

	Pronunciation	Additions	Omissions	Mistakes
MD: There are a number of reasons for a period to be late or missed. First, we need you to keep track of your periods on a calendar or chart. Many teens have menstrual cycles that are longer than 30 days so they can miss a full calendar month.				
PT: Oh, I see. February is a short month so that could be missed.				
MD: That is correct. Also, in times of high stress such as final exams, or going away to college, a young woman may miss a cycle. Here is a chart for you to start keeping track of your cycles. The first day you bleed is considered cycle day one. Each month, mark an X on the days of your period. Always bring this chart with you so we can see what your cycle is like. It is also important that you and your partner use condoms or another form of birth control to prevent pregnancy. If the condom slips off or breaks, there is a form of emergency contraception called "Plan B."				
PT: What is that?				
MD: Plan B is a birth control pill in a higher dose that is taken twice, twelve hours apart. It is available in the pharmacy without a prescription for women over 18. It is most effective if you start the medication as soon as possible after intercourse when a condom breaks or slips off.				
PT: Are there any side effects?				
MD: This form of emergency contraception has little to no side effects. The most common side effect is a mild nausea that you may experience when you wake up in the morning.				
PT: How will I know if it works?				
MD: If you get your period when you expect it, then you will know it worked. If your period is late, you will need to do a pregnancy test. I will give you a prescription for Plan B to use as a back-up to the condom. I would also like you to take this pamphlet on birth control options that we can discuss at another visit.				
Break It Down	☐	☐	☐	☐

☐ CIFE with patient ☐ CIFE with provider ☐ FLOW ☐ REGISTER

continued

Role-Play 62: Glossary

1. Pathology (diseases, conditions)

2. Laboratory Tests and Diagnostic Procedures

3. Treatment Procedures

4. Idiomatic Expressions (if any)

5. Other (vocabulary in this particular role-play that you feel is important/relevant or that you anticipate problems with)

PO Box 2308, Woburn, MA 01888-0508, **p:** 781-729-3736, **www.EmbracingCulture.com**
PO Box 6401, Manchester, NH 03108, **p:** 1-888-678-CCCS

Role-Play 63: Gestational Diabetes

A 30-year-old visits her OB/GYN in her 24th week of pregnancy with symptoms of increased thirst, tiredness and frequent urination.

	Pronunciation	Additions	Omissions	Mistakes
MD: Can you tell me more about your concerns?				
Patient: I am feeling this incredible thirst. No matter how much I drink, I still have this unsatisfied feeling! I am urinating a lot more, and I am not sure if this has anything to do with the increased drinking. I am feeling tired.				
MD: Hmm…Let me review your fasting blood glucose test. The normal range for glucose is 126 or under and I see that your glucose level is 200. Pretty high! Do you have anyone in your family with a history of gestational diabetes?				
Patient: Gestational Diabetes? Is that a bad disease?				
MD: It is not a bad disease, but if you have developed this condition, you will have to be supervised very carefully and you will have to visit the nutritionist and the diabetologist for consults and again for some additional follow-up appointments. Gestational Diabetes happens to women who do not already have diabetes. Around the 24th week, we sometimes see high blood glucose levels. The hormones that pregnant women normally produce to help the baby grow, at times, and we do not understand why, block the production of the insulin. This can sometimes lead to the birth of an abnormally large baby.				
Patient: Perhaps this is what happened to my mother when she was pregnant with my brother. I guess he grew too big inside the womb and she had to be medically supervised very closely.				
MD: Now this is making more sense! Your mother must have had the same condition. I am not too worried but we need to watch this pregnancy. You are not overweight and your last baby was only 7 pounds at birth.				
Patient: So doctor, God will help us both. I will pray and light my candle.				

continued

Role-Play 63 *(continued)*

	Pronunciation	Additions	Omissions	Mistakes
MD: Hmm…It is important that you believe in helping yourself. Here are the potential signs of trouble that I will be watching for throughout this pregnancy: the size of the baby, and your glucose levels right before giving birth, so the baby does not have to struggle with getting your levels and therefore producing extra insulin, which could possibly make the baby's insulin levels to go down too much.				
Patient: Please just take care of my baby and me. I am getting sicker as I listen to what can go wrong. Maybe you can talk to my husband the next time he comes with me. Look, I am sweaty and shaky! This is all nerves. I am sorry doctor, but men like to have the fun and we women suffer the consequences.				
MD: I understand this is overwhelming and as long as you meet with the nutritionist right after this appointment, take the insulin and check your sugar levels before and after a meal, I can wait to meet you husband next week.				
Patient: I get so nervous when I do not have my husband with me.				
MD: I understand, but we all will be working together to help you and your baby. The good thing is that when this pregnancy is over you will not have to take any more insulin and the diabetes will be gone. Let's live one day at a time. I will see you next week.				
(the following week)				
MD: How are you doing with the insulin and the diet regimen?				
Patient: It is a lot of work! I do not like the idea of needles but I will do anything to have a healthy baby.				
MD: I know, sometimes it can be difficult, especially when you already have a young child. Let me examine you. (Examines her legs.) I see a bit more swelling in your legs. Did you notice it? I am going to gently press and let go. Please let me know if I am hurting you.				

continued

PO Box 2308, Woburn, MA 01888-0508, **p:** 781-729-3736, **www.EmbracingCulture.com**
PO Box 6401, Manchester, NH 03108, **p:** 1-888-678-CCCS

Role-Play 63 *(continued)*

	Pronunciation	Additions	Omissions	Mistakes
Patient: I get a bit swollen, but my belly is pretty big and I am drinking so much fluid that the water has to go someplace in the body.				
MD: I understand. Let me check your blood pressure. Have you noticed any of the following symptoms in the past two weeks: headaches, nausea, vomiting, abdominal pain, and blurred vision?				
Patient: No, but sometimes I get a bit dizzy. Otherwise I am fine. Why?				
MD: As I told you earlier, we need to check for possible complications from your gestational diabetes. You have elevated blood pressure and a significant edema in your legs. We just need to keep an eye on it.				
Patient: Am I, and the baby, going to be ok?				
MD: I am a bit concerned with the possibility of preeclampsia. I am going to ask you to have your blood pressure checked every day until I am comfortable with the numbers. Perhaps I might have to give you an additional medication. We are watching and in some ways we expect some of these complications with gestational diabetes.				
Break It Down	☐	☐	☐	☐

☐ **CIFE with patient** ☐ **CIFE with provider** ☐ **FLOW** ☐ **REGISTER**

Role-Play 63: Glossary

continued

1. Pathology (diseases, conditions)

2. Laboratory Tests and Diagnostic Procedures

3. Treatment Procedures

4. Idiomatic Expressions (if any)

5. Other (vocabulary in this particular role-play that you feel is important/relevant or that you anticipate problems with)

PO Box 2308, Woburn, MA 01888-0508, **p:** 781-729-3736, **www.EmbracingCulture.com**
PO Box 6401, Manchester, NH 03108, **p:** 1-888-678-CCCS

Role-Play 64: Pap Smear

Selena came for a check up. She would like to get birth control and her friends have told her that in order to get birth control pills, she would have to have a check up and a pap smear. Selena is 17 years old and she has never had a pap smear before.

		Pronunciation	Additions	Omissions	Mistakes
NP:	Hello. What brings you in today?				
S:	I came because I would like to get birth control pills and I would like to have a Pap smear.				
NP:	OK, have you ever had a pelvic examination and Pap smear before?				
S:	No.				
NP:	Have you ever been on birth control pills before?				
S:	No.				
NP:	Are you sexually active?				
S:	What does that mean?				
NP:	Are you having sexual intercourse now?				
S:	Yes.				
NP:	Are you having unprotected intercourse?				
S:	The first time, my boyfriend and I did not use anything. But since then, we have been using condoms.				
NP:	When did you have unprotected intercourse?				
S:	Three months ago.				
NP:	When was your last menstrual period?				
S:	I finished it yesterday.				
NP:	From the first day of your period, to the first day of the next period, how many days occur?				
S:	28.				
NP:	How long does the bleeding last?				
S:	5 days.				
NP:	Have your 28 day cycles been regular?				
S:	Yes. I am like a clock.				
NP:	Have you ever been pregnant?				
S:	Oh no! You know, this is my first boyfriend, and we just started to, you know, three months ago.				
NP:	OK, today we'll do a pelvic examination and a Pap smear. Because your cycle is normal, I doubt you are pregnant, but we will do a urine pregnancy test. If it is negative and your pelvic exam is ok, I can start you on birth control pills.				
S:	Do my parents have to give permission?				
NP:	No, not at your age, but it would be best if we did let your mother know. Is that ok with you?				

continued

Role-Play 64 *(continued)*

		Pronunciation	Additions	Omissions	Mistakes
S:	OK. I do have a question. What is a Pap smear?				
NP:	During the pelvic exam, I'll take a long cotton swab and a small wooden spatula and take samples from the mouth of your cervix. There is an area of transition from one cell type to another. It is in this area that cervical cancer can get its start. We look at the cells under the microscope and can tell if there is cancer or pre-cancerous inflammation. This is an excellent way to find cancer early and prevent problems.				
S:	How often should I have the test?				
NP:	Well, if you are sexually active, we recommend it every year. But, you could safely do it every other year after having two in a row that were negative. So, now let's do the exam...				
	The NP leaves the room and the patient gets undressed from the waist down. She puts on a johnny and the medical assistant puts a paper sheet over her lap. The NP comes in again.				
NP:	OK, Selena. Now lie back and put your feet into the stirrups on the sides of the examination table. Let your knees fall apart. I now am going to touch your labia and examine them.				
	I am going to spread them apart and put this speculum into your vagina. I have warmed it so you shouldn't feel cold. Just the pressure of the speculum opening.				
	There, that's good. Now I am going to open the speculum. As I do it, why don't you take a deep breath.				
	Good, don't forget to breathe. Do you feel any pain?				
S:	No, I am fine.				
NP:	Your cervix looks healthy. Now I am going to put the swab into your cervix. Now I am going to take this wooden spatula and run it around the outside of the mouth of the cervix.				
	Good. Now I am taking the speculum out. Now I am going to put my fingers into the vagina and feel your cervix, your uterus and your ovaries. It should not hurt. You may feel a little discomfort. There will be some pressure.				
S:	OK. This feels fine. Is my uterus big? You don't think I'm pregnant?				

continued

PO Box 2308, Woburn, MA 01888-0508, **p:** 781-729-3736, **www.EmbracingCulture.com**
PO Box 6401, Manchester, NH 03108, **p:** 1-888-678-CCCS

		Pronunciation	Additions	Omissions	Mistakes
NP:	No. Everything appears fine. We'll get the urine test and if it also shows you're not pregnant, we can then prescribe the pill for you. Is your mother here?				
S:	Yes, she's in the waiting room.				
NP:	Do you mind if I speak with her after we know the results of the test?				
S:	That would be fine. When do I find out about the Pap smear?				
NP:	The results come back in one to four weeks. I'll send a card with the results.				
S:	Thank you.				
	Break It Down	☐	☐	☐	☐

☐ **CIFE with patient** ☐ **CIFE with provider** ☐ **FLOW** ☐ **REGISTER**

Role-Play 64 Glossary

continued

1. Pathology (diseases, conditions)

2. Laboratory Tests and Diagnostic Procedures

3. Treatment Procedures

4. Idiomatic Expressions (if any)

5. Other (vocabulary in this particular role-play that you feel is important/relevant or that you anticipate problems with)

PO Box 2308, Woburn, MA 01888-0508, **p:** 781-729-3736, **www.EmbracingCulture.com**
PO Box 6401, Manchester, NH 03108, **p:** 1-888-678-CCCS

Role-Play 65: Mr. Baptiste's Prostate

Mr. Baptiste has been in the United States for 15 years. He is 60 years old. He and his wife work long hours and they are proud that their children all have gone to college here. His wife is a Registered Nurse (RN). She has begun to study for her Nurse Practitioner degree. She encouraged Mr. Baptiste to go see his primary care physician for a check up. The PCP found something wrong with his prostate and ordered a special blood test. Mr. Baptiste was not bothered by this, but his wife was very concerned. He is now back for the follow-up visit with his PCP.

	Pronunciation	Additions	Omissions	Mistakes
MD: Hello, Mr. Baptiste. I have the results from your blood test.				
Mr. B: Hello, doctor. My wife is very concerned about these results and I've become a little worried too.				
MD: Well, you know that when I examined your prostate, I found a small nodule on the right posterior lobe. I didn't think much of it, but to make sure I ordered the PSA, which is the prostatic specific antigen. If it is elevated above 4, then it means that we need to think about a biopsy. Your PSA was 16. This is elevated.				
Mr. B: Does this mean I have prostate cancer?				
MD: It does not actually mean you have prostate cancer. But, as it is elevated and you have this discrete hardening in the right lobe, it means we have to do a biopsy to be sure.				
Mr. B: I am not sure what a biopsy is. To be honest, I don't even know what the prostate is.				
MD: The prostate is a gland that surrounds the tube that goes from the bladder to the penis. It is a gland that makes the fluid that sperm swims in. In many men above the age of 50, the prostate enlarges and makes it difficult for the urine to flow. Often it causes men to have to get up several times at night to urinate as well. Prostate cancer occurs in many men. It can be found in the prostates of men who have died of other causes. In fact, it is very common. We don't know why some men can have cancer in the prostate and it stays there, while other men have prostate cancer that moves on to affect the bones. If we do a biopsy on you, and we do find prostate cancer, then we'll have to do a CT scan of your pelvis as well as a bone scan to make sure it has not spread beyond the prostate. If it is contained, then we would probably suggest surgery.				
Mr. B: Well, what is a biopsy?				

continued

Role-Play 65 *(continued)*

	Pronunciation	Additions	Omissions	Mistakes
MD: Oh yes. The urologist takes a small probe and puts it in the rectum and visualizes the prostate with an ultra sound. He then sees if he can visualize any areas of hardening. These hardened areas are called nodules. A biopsy is when he uses the probe to take a small piece of tissue from there. He then sends the tissue to a pathologist who examines it under a microscope and determines whether or not there is cancer.				
Mr. B: You said that in some people the cancer never leaves the prostate. If that is true, and the bone scan and CT scan are normal, why would you recommend surgery?				
MD: That is a great question. We don't know whose cancer will progress and whose will stay in the prostate. In a young healthy man like you, we would recommend a radical prostatectomy because it is the best way of assuring that the cancer will be cured. In 15% of these operations though, men end up with incontinence or impotence.				
Mr. B: Oh, no!				
MD: But in older men, say in their late 70's or 80's, if we find cancer in the prostate that has not spread, we often advise watchful waiting—that means no surgery. This is because the act of surgery is more hazardous than the possibility that the cancer will spread.				
Mr. B: This is all pretty complicated. In my case, do you think I have cancer?				
MD: Well, I don't know. But I do believe we need to move forward with a biopsy, because the PSA is elevated and you have a nodule.				
Mr. B: When can I see the urologist?				
MD: I'll have my medical assistant set up an appointment for you as soon as possible.				
Mr. B: Thank you.				
Break It Down	☐	☐	☐	☐

☐ **CIFE with patient** ☐ **CIFE with provider** ☐ **FLOW** ☐ **REGISTER**

Role-Play 65: Glossary

_______________ _______________ _______________

_______________ _______________ _______________

continued

PO Box 2308, Woburn, MA 01888-0508, **p:** 781-729-3736, **www.EmbracingCulture.com**
PO Box 6401, Manchester, NH 03108, **p:** 1-888-678-CCCS

1. Pathology (diseases, conditions)

2. Laboratory Tests and Diagnostic Procedures

3. Treatment Procedures

4. Idiomatic Expressions (if any)

5. Other (vocabulary in this particular role-play that you feel is important/relevant or that you anticipate problems with)

Role-Play 66: Mr. Serra's Circumcision

Mr. Serra was born in Brazil. He is 51 years old. He married when he was 18 years old. He had two children and his wife died early on. He raised his two children in Brazil and brought them to the United States. He has worked for twenty years for the same cleaning firm. His children are grown and married and he has four grandchildren. He is young appearing but has always been a serious man. He never found another woman in all the time since his wife died. He has had dates, but nothing ever came of them. He felt he had to be there for his children. Last year, when his youngest finished college, Mr. Serra began to date a woman from his church. She was 10 years younger than Mr. Serra and although she was also very serious about church and her work, she had what Mr. Serra called "a malandra smile." He has now come to his primary care provider with a problem.

	Pronunciation	Additions	Omissions	Mistakes
MD: Mr. Serra, welcome back. What brings you to the office today?				
Mr. S: I have a problem. It is embarrassing.				
MD: What seems to be the problem?				
Mr. S: When I try to make love, my penis becomes so painful that it is difficult to finish.				
MD: How long have you had this problem?				
Mr. S: It began around ten years ago, but it has not been a real problem until this year when I began to see this woman. She is wonderful and she is patient with me, but I think there is something wrong.				
MD: I think I recall that you are not circumcised. Is that correct?				
Mr. S: Yes.				
MD: Yes, and I remember that you have a phimotic foreskin.				
Mr. S: What is that?				
MD: When I did your physical a few years ago, we talked about how the foreskin of your penis had a diminished diameter at the distal end, so it was difficult to retract the foreskin behind the glans of the penis.				
Mr. S: I remember you told me to pull it back and wash it at least once a day. I have done that, but now making love is more painful. I can become erect but any extra movement is painful. Can you help me?				
MD: Let me examine you and see what it looks like now.				
(Examines patient)				

continued

PO Box 2308, Woburn, MA 01888-0508, **p:** 781-729-3736, **www.EmbracingCulture.com**
PO Box 6401, Manchester, NH 03108, **p:** 1-888-678-CCCS

Role-Play 66 *(continued)*

	Pronunciation	Additions	Omissions	Mistakes
MD: Mr. Serra, your phimosis has become even smaller. I imagine that with an erection the foreskin binds the penis and makes it painful.				
Mr. S: Yes, and sometimes after the erection is over, I cannot bring the foreskin over the penis again until I shower and use soap to bring it forward.				
MD: I see. That can lead to a paraphimosis which in turn can lead to a possible infection and a strangling of the distal portion of the penis. The good news is that with a circumcision, this can be fixed. It is a relatively simple operation that removes the foreskin. It can sometime be complicated with bleeding and infection but that is very rare.				
Mr. S: Circumcision? Isn't that what they do to baby boys?				
MD: Yes, but you would be surprised how common it is in adult men. I will refer you to Dr. Sherman. He is the urologist here in the clinic. I think you will be very pleased with how quickly he will be able to get you back to functioning without pain.				
Mr. S: OK, I will go see him. I think it will be worth it.				
Break It Down	☐	☐	☐	☐

☐ **CIFE with patient** ☐ **CIFE with provider** ☐ **FLOW** ☐ **REGISTER**

Role-Play 66: Glossary

continued

1. Pathology (diseases, conditions)

2. Laboratory Tests and Diagnostic Procedures

3. Treatment Procedures

4. Idiomatic Expressions (if any)

5. Other (vocabulary in this particular role-play that you feel is important/relevant or that you anticipate problems with)

PO Box 2308, Woburn, MA 01888-0508, **p:** 781-729-3736, **www.EmbracingCulture.com**
PO Box 6401, Manchester, NH 03108, **p:** 1-888-678-CCCS

Role-Play 67: Nadia's Fear

Nadia Arcos is 60 years old. She arrived from Guatemala in April of 1995. She has 7 children and most of them immigrated to the US fifteen years ago. Nadia did not want to leave her home, but her husband could no longer work and their children pressured them to immigrate.

Some time ago, Nadia began to experience some difficulty moving her right arm, but ignored the pain and kept up with the household chores. Then, her arm got swollen, and her daughter Maria noticed it. She instantly told her mother that she would have to go to the clinic.

Nadia got upset and said that she wasn't dying and would not go to a clinic. She believes that thinking bad things might make them come true. Because she had given birth to all 7 children at home with no doctors present, she felt that she could manage any type of pain. Her herbal teas had always cured everything. Her daughter took her to the doctor anyway.

	Pronunciation	Additions	Omissions	Mistakes
(NP enters room) Hi. My name is Nancy. I am going to check your temperature, blood pressure, arm and breast.				
(Nurse begins preliminary tests.)				
NP: Since this is your first time at the clinic, we'll need to run some blood tests. Please wait while I call the technician to draw some blood.				
LATER... (Doctor comes in)				
MD: Good evening, Mrs. Arcos. I'm Dr. Katz. Your chart says you've had some swelling in your right arm. Have you seen your primary care physician for this problem?				
Nadia: No. I don't have a doctor in this country.				
MD: Really? How long have you been here?				
Nadia: My husband and I came to New Hampshire when there was no more work in Guatemala. It's been about 8 years since we came here.				
MD: Oh. So you've been here since 1995?				
Nadia: Yes, we came in December of '95.				
MD: And you've not been to the doctor since then?				
Maria: Oh, my mother is a funny woman. I don't think she's ever been to a doctor, not even in Guatemala.				
MD: Mrs. Arcos, why don't you like to go to the doctor?				

continued

Role-Play 67 *(continued)*

	Pronunciation	Additions	Omissions	Mistakes
Nadia: I've always been very strong. I had 7 children at home.				
MD: Seven? That's quite a handful! Well, let's try to get some background information on you. Do you smoke?				
Nadia: No.				
MD: You said you have 7 children. How old were you when you had your first child?				
Nadia: I was fifteen.				
MD: Umm, has anyone in your family had breast cancer?				
Nadia: My sister had breast cancer. She got very sick after she went to the doctor and died three months later. My father was fine too before he went to the doctor. People get sick in the hospital.				
MD: My condolences. Sometimes, though, if we wait for a long time before going to the doctor, we could get very sick, and if we continue to procrastinate, we could become so sick that medicine can do very little for us. It was very wise of you to come today!				
On a subsequent visit…				
MD: Mrs. Arcos, thank you for coming in today. We've received your test results and I'd like to discuss them with you.				
Nadia: Am I sick?				
MD: Well, we've found some lumps in your breast and the tests indicate that they might be cancerous. Just to be sure, we'd like to run a new series of tests as soon as possible.				
Break It Down	☐	☐	☐	☐

☐ **CIFE with patient** ☐ **CIFE with provider** ☐ **FLOW** ☐ **REGISTER**

Role-Play 67: Glossary

_______________ _______________ _______________

_______________ _______________ _______________

_______________ _______________ _______________

_______________ _______________ _______________

continued

PO Box 2308, Woburn, MA 01888-0508, **p:** 781-729-3736, **www.EmbracingCulture.com**
PO Box 6401, Manchester, NH 03108, **p:** 1-888-678-CCCS

1. Pathology (diseases, conditions)

2. Laboratory Tests and Diagnostic Procedures

3. Treatment Procedures

4. Idiomatic Expressions (if any)

5. Other (vocabulary in this particular role-play that you feel is important/relevant or that you anticipate problems with)

Lesson Ten: Additional Resources Reproductive System

Landmarks

The stages of life are noted by the acquisition of social, physical, and mental skills.

Infancy and Childhood

Infancy lasts from birth until age two. Infant reflexes concern finding the nipple; suckling can occur minutes after birth, and the rooting reflex is a tactile clue for the infant to turn its head toward a touch. During the first year the infant passes through a series of developmental stages.

Childhood begins at two and lasts until puberty. Physical growth is accompanied by increasing development of motor and language skills. Play, make-believe, and increased memory and attention span also occur.

Adolescence and Adulthood

Growth accelerates during puberty. Boys increase in height by 3-5 inches per year, girls 2-4 inches. The heart doubles in size, and hormones stimulate sexual maturity. Growth ends during the end of adolescence, and aging starts during the late twenties. Life expectancy (47 and 50 years for males and females in 1900; 75 and 81 in 2008) has increased.

ILLNESSES/CONDITIONS

Copied or adapted from the Centers for Disease Control (www.cdc.gov), www.medlineplus.gov, and "Human Diseases" by Marianne Neighbors and Ruth Tannehill-Jones, a Delmar Thomson Learning publication.

Illnesses and Conditions	Meaning
Balanitis	An inflammation of the tip (glans) of the penis due to a fungus infection, sexually transmitted diseases, allergy to fabric. Men who are circumcised have lower incidents of getting this bacteria.
Amenorrhea	The absence of any menstrual flow in a woman who has not yet menstruated by the age of 16. There are many possible causes of primary amenorrhea, including drastic weight reduction, malnutrition, extreme obesity, chronic illnesses, genital abnormalities present since birth (absence of the uterus or vagina, vaginal septum, cervical stenosis, imperforate hymen), hypoglycemia and testicular feminization. Treatment will depend on the cause. Primary amenorrhea caused by developmental abnormalities (which may result when the parts of the female reproductive system did not form properly before birth) may require hormonal supplementation, surgery, or both. If the amenorrhea cannot be corrected, it is sometimes possible to create a pseudomenstruation with medications to help the young woman feel more like her friends or family.

continued

PO Box 2308, Woburn, MA 01888-0508, **p:** 781-729-3736, **www.EmbracingCulture.com**
PO Box 6401, Manchester, NH 03108, **p:** 1-888-678-CCCS

ILLNESSES/CONDITIONS *(continued)*

Illnesses and Conditions	Meaning
Cervicitis	An inflammation of the cervix, usually caused by infection. However, in a few cases it may be attributed to chemical exposure or a foreign body, such as a pessary (a device inserted into the vagina to support the uterus), cervical cap, or diaphragm. The condition may also be caused by an allergy to contraceptive spermicides or to latex in condoms. In cases of cervicitis attributed to foreign objects, infection is still frequently the cause, but the presence of the foreign object may make the cervix more susceptible to infection. Cervicitis is very common, affecting more than half of all women at some point during their adult lives. Increased risk is associated with intercourse at an early age, high-risk sexual behavior, multiple sexual partners, and a history of sexually transmitted disease.
Chlamydia	A bacterial infection that may go asymptomatic in some infected individuals until dangerous complications occur. In others, it may cause discharge (from the penis or vagina), burning and itching with urination in males and burning and itching of the genital area in females. Treatment with antibiotics is effective. Untreated females may develop PID (pelvic inflammatory disease, and both sexes may develop infertility/sterility.
Circumcision	Male circumcision is the surgical removal of some or all of the foreskin (or prepuce) from the penis. Those men who are circumcised seem to have a lower incident of STDs and HIV infections. There are three different clamps that can be used when circumcising infants. They are Gomco. Plastibell and the Mogen. Not every religion supports circumcision in males. Female circumcision, illegal in the USA, is considered a form of mutilation of the women's genitalia. However many young females for cultural and or religious reasons go through this procedure in their native country or in the USA. Female genital cutting can be done partially or fully. This may cause PID (Pelvic Inflammatory Disease). Women who are circumcised report suffering from pain when having intercourse, seem to have difficulty giving birth by the vaginal canal. Most will need a cesarean birth and report other sexual difficulties.
Crabs (pubic lice)	Small, six-legged creatures that invade the genital hair region and infest it with their eggs. These lice can also infest armpit hair and eyebrows, but they are drawn to the pubic region. Lice infestation is a common sexually transmitted condition and is found mostly in adolescents. Transmission generally occurs during sexual activity, but it can occur through physical contact with contaminated objects such as toilet seats, sheets, and blankets. Some women have acquired it while trying on swimming suits at a store. The presence of pubic lice is heralded by moderate to severe itching in the area covered by pubic hair. This itch is frequently worse at night. Because the crab louse requires human blood to survive, it buries its head inside a pubic hair follicle. It excretes a substance into the skin that causes the itching. Pubic lice are best treated with a prescription wash.

continued

ILLNESSES/CONDITIONS *(continued)*

Illnesses and Conditions	Meaning
Cryptorchism (or Cryptorchidism)	A condition of a small percentage of infant males where one or both testicles does not move from the abdomen into the scrotum by birth. Testicles begin inside the abdominal cavity and push through to the scrotal sac. Approximately 3 percent of male newborns have an undescended testicle at birth and up to 30 percent of premature males will have at least one undescended testicle. By age one, 80% of all undescended testes will have descended to the scrotum. If the condition is not treated, it can increase the patient's chances of getting testicular cancer or becoming sterile.
Dysmenorrhea	Menstrual periods that are accompanied by either sharp, intermittent pain, or dull, aching pain, usually in the pelvis or lower abdomen. There are two general types of dysmenorrheal conditions. Primary dysmenorrhea refers to menstrual pain that occurs in otherwise healthy women. This type of pain is not related to any specific problems with the uterus or other pelvic organs. Secondary dysmenorrhea is menstrual pain that is attributed to some underlying disease process or structural abnormality either within or outside the uterus. Birth control pills may be prescribed to alleviate menstrual pain. Surgery may be necessary for women who are unable to obtain adequate pain relief or pain control. Procedures may range from removal of cysts, polyps, adhesions, or fibroids, to complete hysterectomy in cases of extreme endometriosis. Prescription medications may be used for endometriosis. For pain caused by an IUD, removal of the IUD and alternative birth control methods may be needed.
Dyspareunia	A condition of pain during sexual intercourse that may affect men and women alike; and may be related to physical or psychological conditions. In women, some physical causes include an intact hymen, vaginal deformity, insufficient lubrication, STD, sensitivity to spermicide, PID, bladder infection, and endometriosis. In men, physical causes may include penile deformity, STD, an abnormally tight foreskin, prostatitis and epididymitis.
Ectopic Pregnancy	A condition in which the fertilized egg implants itself in the abdomen outside the uterus. It most commonly occurs in one of the fallopian tubes and is called a tubal pregnancy. The most serious complication is intraabdominal hemorrhage. For example, if the fetus starts to grow in the tube, it can rupture the tube and thereby rupture the artery supplying the ovary. If this artery ruptures along with the tube, there can be serious, life-threatening loss of blood.

continued

ILLNESSES/CONDITIONS *(continued)*

Illnesses and Conditions	Meaning
Endometriosis	A condition in which the endometrium, tissue that normally lines the uterus, grows in other areas of the body, causing pain, irregular bleeding, and frequently infertility. The tissue growth typically occurs in the pelvic area, outside of the uterus, on the ovaries, bowel, rectum, bladder, and the delicate lining of the pelvis, but it can occur in other areas of the body as well. Treatment with medications may focus on several strategies. Analgesic therapy, treating the discomfort of the disease only, may be indicated for women with mild to moderate premenstrual pain, with no pelvic examination abnormalities, and with no immediate desire to become pregnant. "Pseudopregnancy" (a state resembling pregnancy) may be achieved through hormonal drug regimens. This approach was developed in response to the observed regression of endometriosis during pregnancy. Pseudopregnancy can be induced using oral contraceptives containing estrogen and progesterone. This takes 6 to 9 months and relieves most of the symptoms, but does not prevent scarring and adhesion left by the disease. Progesterone medications by themselves are another effective hormonal treatment for endometriosis. Possible side effects of these agents – including depression, weight gain, and breakthrough spotting, may be a problem for some patients. "Pseudomenopause" (a state resembling menopause) was developed as a means of treatment because of the observation that endometriosis regresses after menopause. Danazol, a weak androgenic (male characteristic) hormonal drug may be used to reduce natural levels of estrogen and progesterone to low levels.
Fibroids	A benign growth of smooth muscle in the wall of a woman's uterus; hence they are called uterine fibroids. They may grow as a single tumor or a cluster of small growths. They can cause increased menstrual bleeding, pelvic pain and frequency of urination. One in five women over the age of 35 has a uterine fibroid. Fibroids are the leading cause of hysterectomies in the United States.
Genital herpes	A painful, recurring viral infection caused by Herpes Simplex Virus Type II, characterized by multiple blister-like lesions. Severe itching and painful urination are common. In men, the blisters commonly occur on the penis, scrotum and inner thighs; while in women, they commonly appear on the vulva, vagina, inner thighs and rectal area. Genital herpes is highly contagious and is commonly transmitted by sexual intercourse, including oral-genital exposure. Self-infection from the hands is also possible. Herpes disease cannot be cured, and the virus will remain dormant until activated by stress or lowered immunity. Studies have shown that females with genital herpes are significantly more likely to develop cervical cancer.

continued

ILLNESSES/CONDITIONS *(continued)*

Illnesses and Conditions	Meaning
Gestational Diabetes	A condition when a pregnant woman has increased levels of glucose in her blood and her body is unable to produce enough insulin to absorb it. Once the baby is born, this form of diabetes disappears but having the condition makes a woman more likely to develop Type II diabetes later in life. Gestational diabetes usually develops during the second half of the pregnancy and may not present with any symptoms. Gestational Diabetes should be controlled carefully. Reducing the amount of sugary drinks and foods consumed, eating small frequent snacks and exercise are all helpful to control blood sugar. Sometimes gestational diabetes cannot be controlled with just a healthy diet and exercise but will also require insulin. Gestational diabetes can cause a baby to be unexpectedly large, possibly causing difficulties during delivery; and could increase the chance of caesarean birth- an operation to remove the baby from the uterus without its having to go through the birth canal.
Gonorrhea	A bacterial infection that causes inflammation of mucous membranes of the male and female genital and urinary systems. Common symptoms in men include painful and frequent urination and discharge. In women, symptoms may include frequent and painful urination, genital itching, a burning pain and vaginal discharge. Infected individuals who do not show symptoms of gonorrhea may be carriers of the disease, and could transmit it to others. Antibiotic treatment for gonorrhea may be successful, whereas untreated gonorrhea may lead to meningitis and endocarditis.
HPV (Human Papillomavirus)	HPV is the name of a group of viruses that includes more than 100 different strains or types. Over 30 of these are sexually transmitted, and they can infect the genital area, like the skin of the penis, vulva, labia, anus, or the tissues covering the vagina and cervix. Some of these viruses are considered "high-risk" types and may cause abnormal Pap smears and cancer of the cervix, anus, and penis. Others are "low-risk," and they may cause mild Pap smear abnormalities and genital warts. Genital warts are single or multiple growths or bumps that appear in the genital area, and sometimes form a cauliflower-like shape. Most HPV infections have no signs or symptoms; therefore, most infected persons are completely unaware they are infected; yet they can transmit the virus to a partner. There is no "cure" for HPV, although the infection usually goes away on its own. Cancer-related types are more likely to persist.

continued

PO Box 2308, Woburn, MA 01888-0508, **p:** 781-729-3736, **www.EmbracingCulture.com**
PO Box 6401, Manchester, NH 03108, **p:** 1-888-678-CCCS

ILLNESSES/CONDITIONS *(continued)*

Illnesses and Conditions	Meaning
Impotence	The inability of a man to achieve or maintain an erection sufficient enough to complete sexual intercourse. Most men experience impotency at some time in their lives. Impotence, though sometimes caused by psychological factors, is more often caused by physical disorders, such as endocrine disorder affecting testosterone levels; drug or alcohol abuse; neurologic disorders; pelvic surgery; diabetes; arteriosclerosis; and certain medications.
Incontinence	The inability to voluntarily control the flow of urine. There are two major forms of urinary incontinence: one is "stress incontinence." This usually occurs when there is laughter or other maneuvers that put increased intraabdominal pressure on the bladder forcing it to let urine flow. The second form of urinary incontinence is "urge incontinence." This usually is caused by the spasms of the urinary bladder wall forcing urine out of the urethra. This is also called "overactive bladder." When the bladder wall suffers spasms, it produces a sense of urgency, hence the name "urge incontinence."
Menorrhagia	Menstruation at regular cycle intervals but with excessive flow and duration. A normal menstrual cycle is 21-35 days in duration. Bleeding consists of the lining of the unfertilized uterus being sloughed off and extruded, releasing the materials through the cervix. This lasts an average of 7 days, and consists of blood flows between 25 and 80 ml. Clinically, menorrhagia is defined as menstrual bleeding lasting longer than 7 days or total blood loss exceeding 80 ml per cycle.
Orchitis	An acute inflammation of one or both of the testicles most likely caused by a viral mumps infection. It may lead to male infertility and to an atrophy of one or both testicles. Orchitis can result also from other viral infections.
Pelvic inflammatory disease (PID)	An infection of the fallopian tubes and other internal reproductive organs in women. It is a common and serious complication of some STDs. Symptoms of PID vary from none to severe. Women who do have symptoms of PID most commonly have lower abdominal pain. Other signs and symptoms include fever, unusual vaginal discharge that may have a foul odor, painful intercourse, painful urination, irregular menstrual bleeding, and pain in the right upper abdomen (rare). Without treatment, PID can cause permanent damage to the female internal reproductive organs. PID can be cured with antibiotics.

continued

ILLNESSES/CONDITIONS *(continued)*

Illnesses and Conditions	Meaning
Prostatic carcinoma	Most prostate cancers are adenocarcinomas arising in the prostate gland. Non-metastatic prostate cancer is: either clinically localized disease (confined to the prostate gland) or locally advanced disease (spread outside the capsule of the gland but has not spread to organs, other than the seminal vesicles). Metastatic disease is spread beyond the prostate to local, regional, or systemic lymph nodes, or to other body organs (such as bone, liver, or brain). Bone metastases are particularly common. Prostate cancer is the second most common malignancy in men. It is particularly common in older men. Two thirds of those who die from prostate cancer are over 75. When prostate cancer occurs in younger men it is often more aggressive. Relatively few men aged below 50 years are affected, but these men have the highest mortality rate.
Prostatitis	The inflammation of the prostate gland most common in men over 50 years of age. Causes could include urinary tract infection, gonorrhea or others. Symptoms include painful urination, pus in the urine, fever and low back pain. Treatment may include antibiotics like penicillin. Prostatitis generally responds well to treatment.
Syphilis	A serious sexually transmitted bacterial infection, spread by contact with contagious lesions. Bacteria penetrate the skin or mucous membrane and gain access to the vascular system, causing a systemic infection. Antibiotic treatment is very effective and can cure syphilis. There are primary, secondary and tertiary stages of the disease. In the secondary stage, a rash may appear in an area of the body or may spread over the whole body. Tertiary syphilis may manifest itself through aortic aneurysm, heart failure, mental disorders, insanity, deafness, blindness, paralysis and death.
Testicular carcinoma	A cancer occurring in the testes which are found in the scrotum under the penis. Testicles are glands that produce male sex hormones and sperm. Testicular cancer is rare but it is the most common cancer in men between the ages of 15 and 34. It is very treatable even when diagnosed at an advanced stage. It is recommended that young men perform a testicle self-examination every month to find possible cancer containing lumps early on when treatment has the highest chance for success.
Trichomoniasis	A sexually transmitted infection occurring in approximately 10 percent of all sexually active individuals. Most infected persons are asymptomatic, but if symptoms do occur, they may include urethritis, epididymitis and prostatitis in males, as well as vaginal itching and burning and a green frothy discharge in females. Treatment with an anti-parasitic mediation is usually effective.
Urethritis	An infection of the urethra, more prevalent in women, but men can also get infected from this sexually transmitted disease. Often symptoms have some kind of discharge, frequency with urination and pain while urinating. Patients are treated with antibiotics.

continued

PO Box 2308, Woburn, MA 01888-0508, **p:** 781-729-3736, **www.EmbracingCulture.com**
PO Box 6401, Manchester, NH 03108, **p:** 1-888-678-CCCS

ILLNESSES/CONDITIONS *(continued)*

Illnesses and Conditions	Meaning
Vaginal Candidiasis (yeast infection)	A vaginal infection caused most commonly by the fungal organism *Candida Albicans*. Yeast infection may follow a course of antibiotics (particularly tetracycline) that was prescribed for another purpose. Infection is also common among women who use estrogen-containing birth control pills and among women who are pregnant. This is due to the increased level of estrogen in the body. Yeast infections may also occur in association with diabetes or problems that affect the immune system (such as AIDS or HIV). Vaginal candidiasis is not considered a sexually transmitted disease. However, 12% to 15% of men will develop symptoms such as itching and penile rash following sexual contact with an infected partner.

Notes

Lesson Eleven: Respiratory System

Understanding Goals

Students will:

- learn about the structure and function of the respiratory organs
- learn about common disorders of the Respiratory System
- sharpen their consecutive interpreting skills through role-play practice with E.R. situations

Key concepts:

- Respiratory System

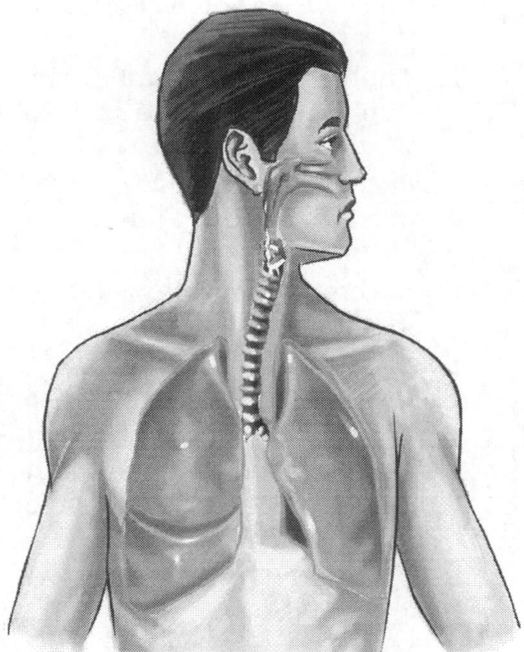

Quiz

THE ART OF MEDICAL INTERPRETATION®

Lesson Eleven: Quiz
Respiratory System

Mark each item "True" or "False."

1. One of the two meanings of respiration is the external act of bringing oxygen into the body, and allowing carbon dioxide and water to leave the body.
   - ○ True ○ False
2. The low register for larynx is voice box.
   - ○ True ○ False
3. The bronchi subdivide into 50-80 tubes called alveoli.
   - ○ True ○ False
4. Each alveolus is surrounded by a net of small blood vessels called capillaries.
   - ○ True ○ False
5. Each lung is covered with two thin membranes called pleural membranes.
   - ○ True ○ False
6. The diaphragm is the big muscle underneath the lungs which contracts and flattens to create a pressure differential between the ambient atmosphere that allows air to rush in.
   - ○ True ○ False
7. Normally, arteries carry deoxygenated blood, and the pulmonary arteries carry oxygenated blood to the lungs.
   - ○ True ○ False
8. The pulmonary vein is the only vein to carry oxygenated blood.
   - ○ True ○ False
9. The deoxygenated blood is carried to the lungs by the pulmonary artery.
   - ○ True ○ False
10. The flu is one of the least common illnesses of the respiratory system.
    - ○ True ○ False
11. Antibiotics are the best treatment against a cold. Other things such as resting and drinking lots of fluids are helpless in the treatment of a cold.
    - ○ True ○ False
12. Pneumonia is when the small bronchioles and alveoli (air sacs) become inflamed and filled with infected fluids.
    - ○ True ○ False
13. In chronic bronchitis and emphysema, the constriction of the small bronchioles is irreversible.
    - ○ True ○ False
14. Cigarette smoking causes 87 percent of all lung cancers.
    - ○ True ○ False
15. When a blood clot forms in the leg and moves to the heart and ultimately into the lung, the clot is called a cardioembolism.
    - ○ True ○ False
16. The Tuberculin test is a test used to determine if someone has developed an allergy to tubercles.
    - ○ True ○ False
17. Flu shots are good just for children and the elderly since they have more vulnerable immune systems.
    - ○ True ○ False

Lesson Eleven: Class Activities
Respiratory System

REVIEW

Do you still remember what the following root words mean?

WORD BANK

bronchial tubes	nose 2X	lung 2X	trachea
alveolus	tonsils	epiglottis	
bronchiole	pharynx	larynx	

ROOT	MEANING
1. alveol/o	alveolus
2. bronch/o	connection / bronchial tube
3. bronchiol/o	bronchiole
4. epiglott/o	epiglottis
5. laryng/o	larynx
6. nas/o	nose
7. rhin/o	nose
8. pharyng/o	Pharynx
9. pneumon/o	lung
10. pulmon/o	lung
11. tonsil/o	tonsils
12. trache/o	trachea

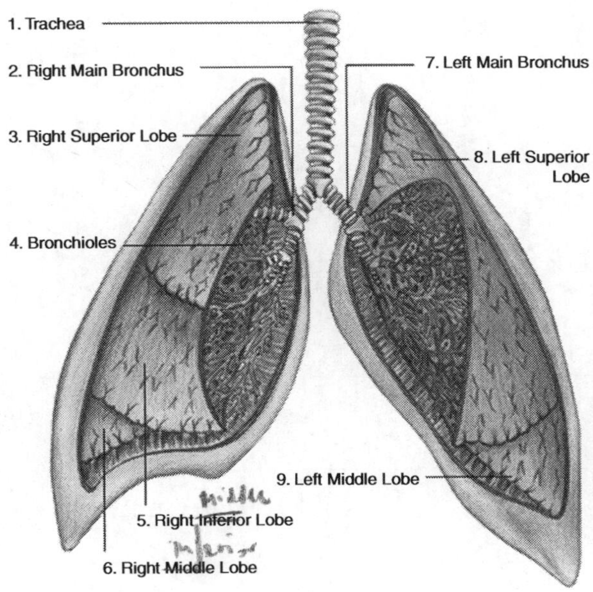

THE ART OF MEDICAL INTERPRETATION®

Class Activities

PO Box 2308, Woburn, MA 01888-0508, **p:** 781-729-3736, **www.EmbracingCulture.com**
PO Box 6401, Manchester, NH 03108, **p:** 1-888-678-CCCS

Intro to the Respiratory System
How much do you know?

1. Label the main organs of the respiratory system in the diagram below.
2. Label the organs in English and your Target Language
3. Trace the path of air from outside the body into the lungs. In the lines below the diagram, explain the path of air into the lungs.

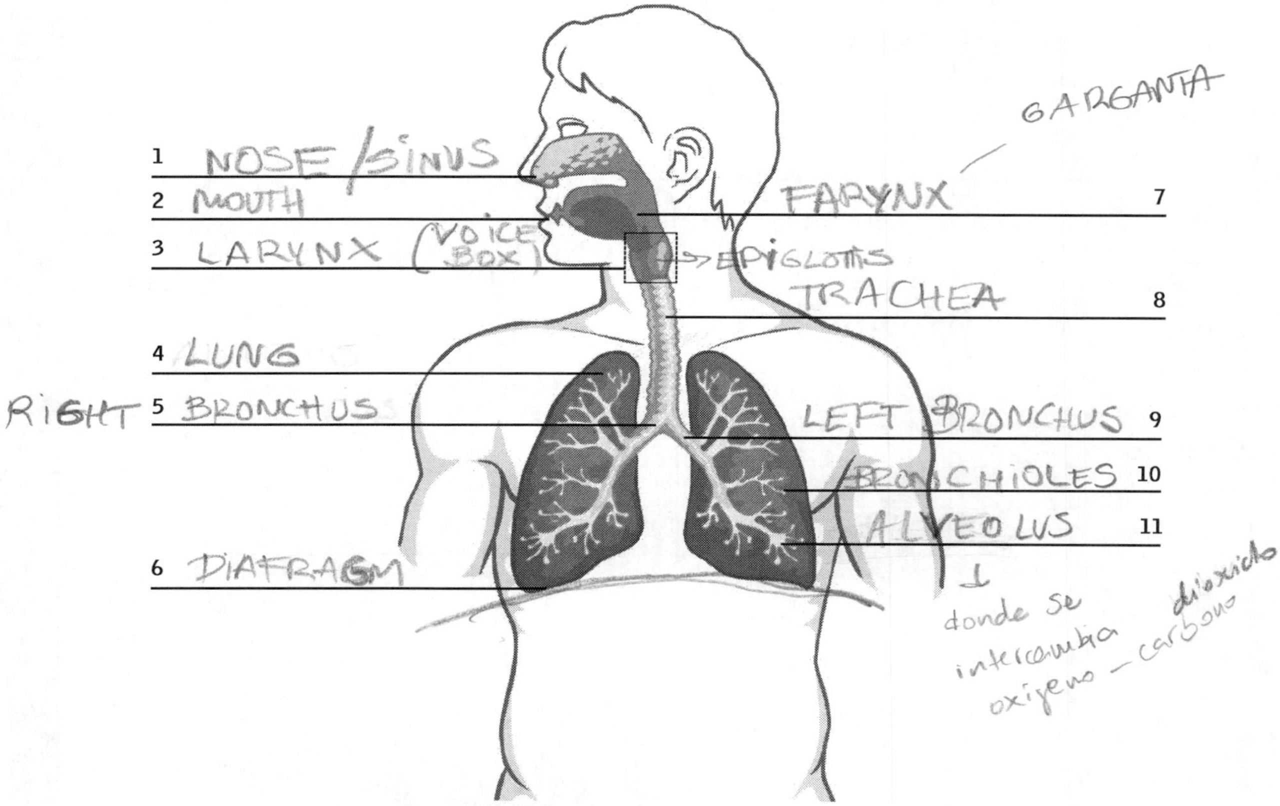

Pleura – covers the lungs (kind of) a sac

Respiratory System

Respiration is a word that has two meanings. The first meaning is in regard to the external act of bringing oxygen into the body, and allowing carbon dioxide and water to leave the body. The second meaning applies to the process within the cell in which carbon and oxygen combine in a chemical process that releases energy and creates water and carbon dioxide. The Respiratory System refers to the part of the body related to the first meaning of bringing oxygen in and carbon dioxide out. The Respiratory System allows the transport of these gases to support the intracellular process that creates the energy we use to fuel our bodily functions. The Respiratory System consists of the air passages, the larynx, the trachea, the lungs, the ribs and intercostal muscles and the diaphragm.

The Organs of the Respiratory System

Nasal Air Passages

Air is inhaled through the nasal passages. The nasal cavity has a sticky mucous membrane that lines the cavity and traps dust; the small surface hairs of the cavity are called cilia. The cilia move particles to the nose for a sneeze or to be blown out. The air in the nasal passages is heated by the warmth of the blood supplying the mucous membranes.

Throat, Larynx and Trachea

From the nasal passages, the air moves into the throat, through the larynx, or voice box, into the hard tube, called the trachea and from each of the twin tubes breaking off from the trachea called bronchi which are in the left and right lung respectively.

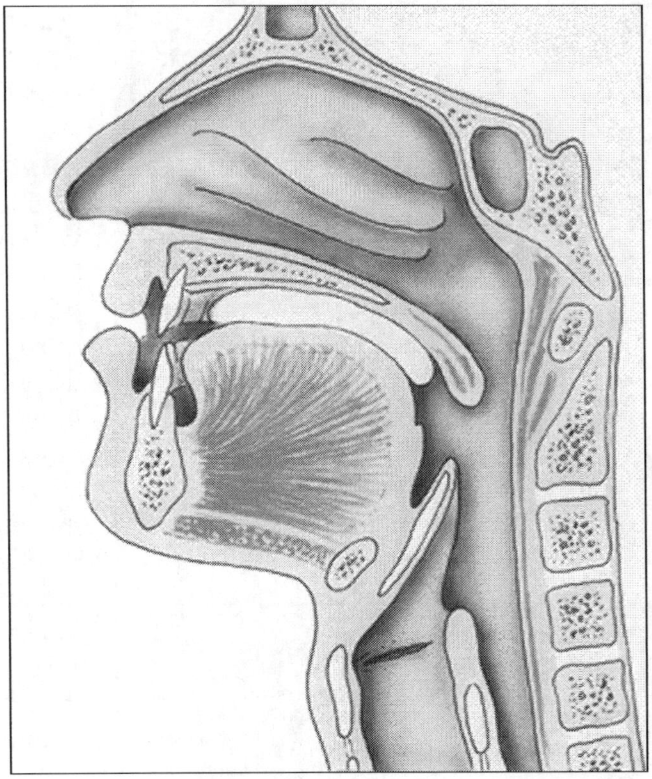

PO Box 2308, Woburn, MA 01888-0508, **p:** 781-729-3736, **www.EmbracingCulture.com**
PO Box 6401, Manchester, NH 03108, **p:** 1-888-678-CCCS

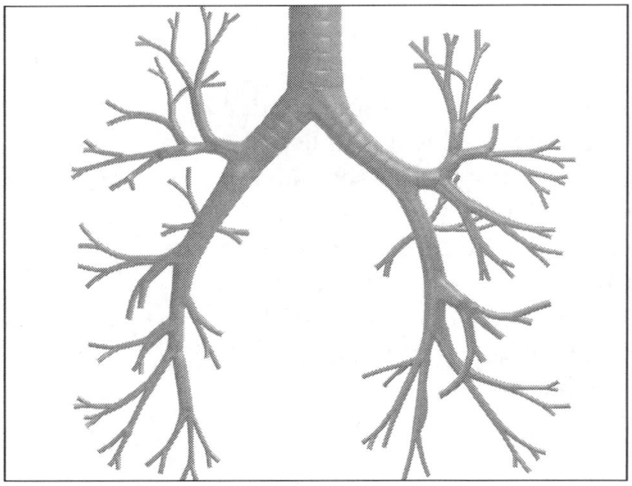

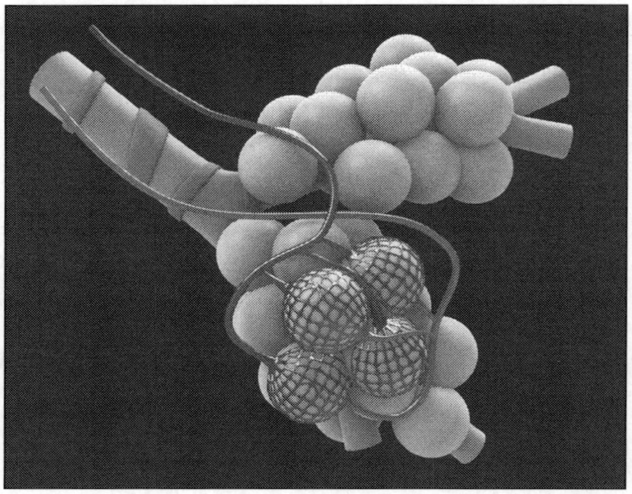

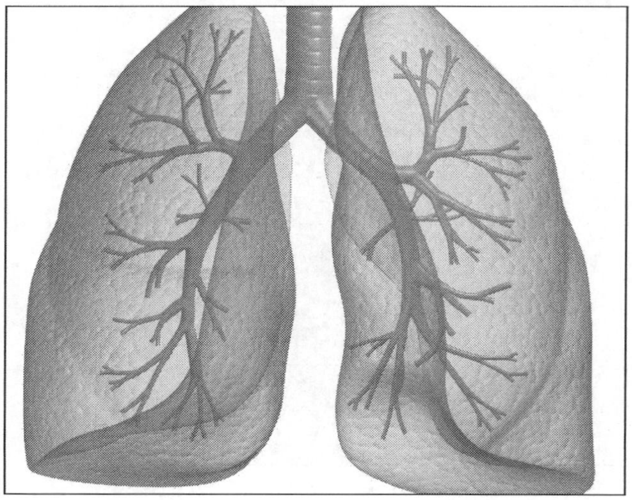

Bronchi

Each bronchus breaks down into progressively smaller tubes called secondary bronchi. There are five secondary or lobar bronchi. Each one supplies a lobe of the lungs (three on the right, two on the left.) The five lobar bronchi break down into tertiary bronchi that are also called segmental bronchi because each one supplies a segment within each lobe. These bronchi further subdivide into 50-80 tubes called bronchioles. There are almost 30,000 bronchioles in each lung.

Alveoli

The bronchioles end in a collection of air sacs called alveoli. A net of small blood vessels called capillaries surrounds each alveolus. It is at this level that oxygen from the air diffuses through the alveolar wall into the blood, and carbon dioxide from the body diffuses into the air sacs to be expelled with an exhalation. On the inside of the alveoli are white cells called macrophages. The macrophages ingest airborne particles like dust, chemicals and or bacteria.

Lungs

Each lung, which is actually quite spongy, is covered with two thin membranes called pleural membranes. The membranes are separated by liquid that acts as a lubricant allowing the membranes to easily slide during breathing. The engine for breathing is the diaphragm, which is the big muscle underneath the lungs. It contracts and flattens and creates a pressure differential between the ambient atmosphere that allows air to rush in. The intercostal muscles help the diaphragm in the process. The vascular supply of the lungs brings oxygenated blood out of the lungs to the heart and deoxygenated blood from the heart to the lungs. Normally blood vessels that carry blood away from the heart are called arteries, and normally the arteries carry oxygenated blood; but the pulmonary arteries carry deoxygenated blood to the lungs and are the only arteries to carry deoxygenated blood. Conversely, blood vessels that carry blood back to the heart are called veins. Most veins carry deoxygenated blood; however, the pulmonary vein carries oxygenated blood back from the lungs to the heart. Hence, the pulmonary vein is the only vein to carry oxygenated blood.

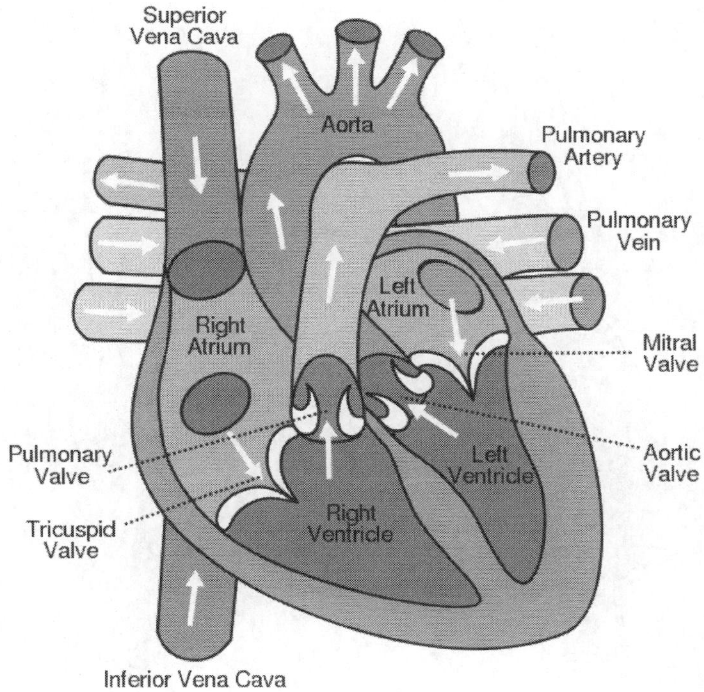

Cardio Respiratory System:

Vessels of the lung bring:

1. Oxygenated blood to the heart (Pulmonary Vein)
2. Deoxygenated blood to the lungs (Pulmonary Artery)

Disorders of the Respiratory System

The flu is one of the most "common" illnesses of the respiratory system. Watch the video "Body Snatchers" from the *Body Story* DVD to learn how our body deals with a flu virus. Use the space below to take notes on what you see or what you find interesting.

PO Box 2308, Woburn, MA 01888-0508, **p:** 781-729-3736, **www.EmbracingCulture.com**
PO Box 6401, Manchester, NH 03108, **p:** 1-888-678-CCCS

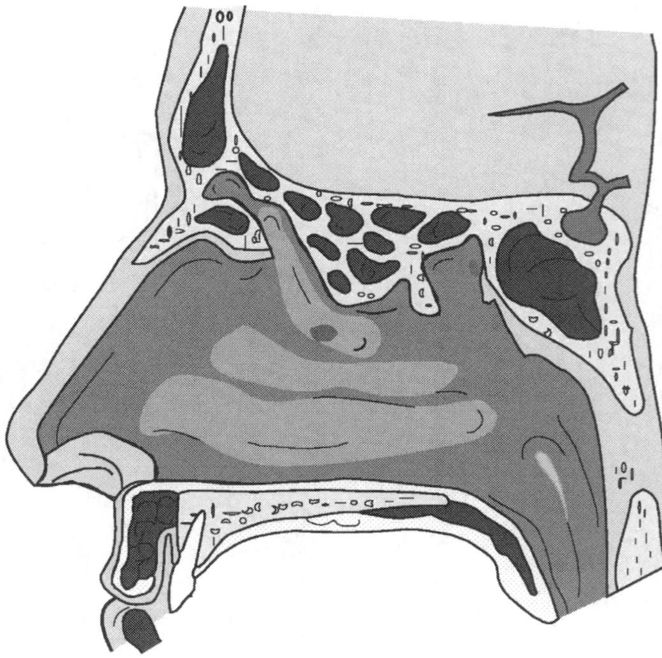

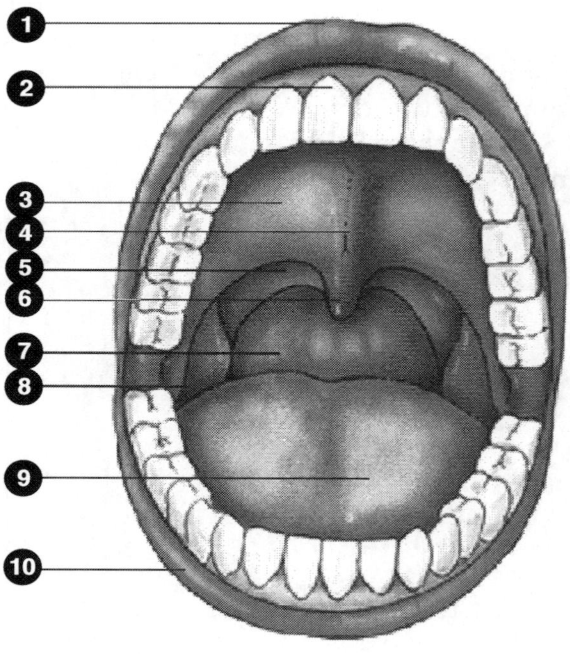

The flu is only one of many respiratory disorders. Let's now learn about some others.

I. Upper Airway Infections:

1. Sinusitis

Sinusitis is an inflammation of the sinuses (hollow air spaces within the bones surrounding the nose) and nasal passages. Symptoms of a sinus infection can include a headache, pressure in the eyes, nose, cheek area, or one side of the head. Treatments include antibiotics, decongestants, and pain relievers.

2. Tonsillitis

It is an infection or inflammation of the tonsils. It can be caused by a virus or the same bacteria that causes strep throat, streptococcus. The main symptom of tonsillitis is a sore throat. The throat and tonsils look red and swollen and the tonsils may have a yellow or white coating on them. Other symptoms are: difficulty swallowing, fever, a hoarse or raspy voice, swollen glands in the neck or jaw, headaches, ear pain, skin rash, vomiting, or abdominal pain.

3. Pharyngitis

Pharyngitis is an inflammation of the pharynx that is often simply referred to as a sore throat. The main symptom is a sore throat. Other symptoms are difficulty speaking or swallowing, tender or swollen lymph nodes (glands) in the neck, fever, headache, and earache.The treatment depends on the underlying cause of the sore throat, but warm salt water gargles, pain relievers, and fluids can be helpful. Antibiotics are prescribed if you are diagnosed with strep throat.

4. Laryngitis

Laryngitis is an inflammation of the larynx. It causes hoarseness, and possibly a temporary loss of use of the voice. Other symptoms may include a dry or sore throat, coughing, and trouble swallowing.

5. The Cold

The common cold is caused by viruses. In fact, any one of up to 200 known cold viruses may be the culprit. It is passed from person to person by droplets sent by coughing or sneezing from one infected person to another. The blood supply brings white blood cells to the infected mucosa and excess fluid is secreted from the nasal mucosa causing a runny nose. Symptoms may spread to the throat and lungs. Antibiotics are useless against a cold. Just treating the symptoms with cold pills, Tylenol, and cough syrup is all one can do. Rest, lots of fluids and more rest will help get rid of a cold.

II. Lung Disease

6. Acute Bronchitis

Inflammation of the bronchi can occur from a cold or with influenza. Most often a virus is the cause; but if fever occurs and sputum looks thick and multicolored, most physicians will treat with antibiotics because it is easy for a viral bronchitis to develop into a super infection from bacteria. Such is the case of the walking pneumonia which is caused by the bacteria called Mycoplasma.

If the patient has chronic obstructive lung disease, bronchiectasis or other lung condition, it is more difficult to fight bacteria; so antibiotics in these cases would easily be given. An acute bronchitis usually affects the large and medium bronchi. The glands in the walls of the bronchi make lots of mucous so it becomes difficult to breathe and catch one's breath. In children, older people or people with chronic lung disease, infection may spread to the smaller bronchioles or even to the lung tissue itself developing into pneumonia.

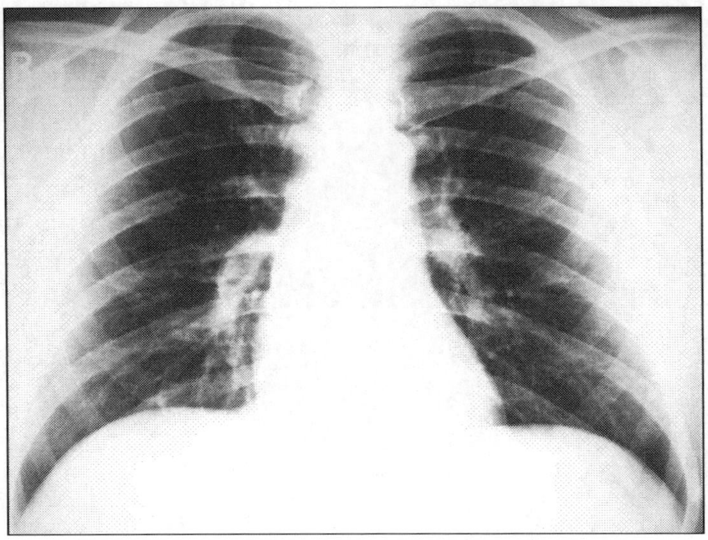

PO Box 2308, Woburn, MA 01888-0508, **p:** 781-729-3736, **www.EmbracingCulture.com**
PO Box 6401, Manchester, NH 03108, **p:** 1-888-678-CCCS

7. Chronic Bronchitis

Chronic irritants such as smoking and other environmental factors cause the bronchi to become irritated and produce large amount of mucous. This fills the bronchial tubes and coughing ensues. The bronchioles constrict and this constriction is not reversible. When someone has a chronic, sputum-producing cough for six or more months, this is called chronic bronchitis.

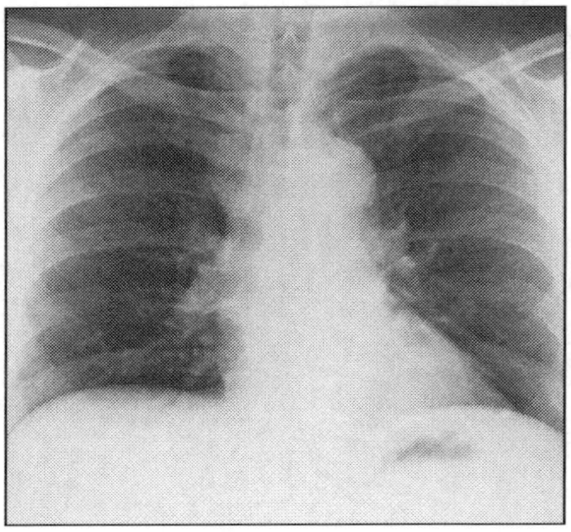

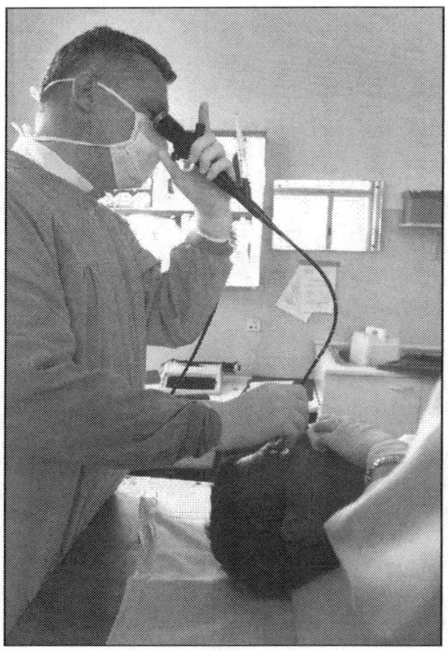

8. Pneumonia

Pneumonia is when the small bronchioles and alveoli (air sacs) become inflamed and filled with infected fluid. One kind of pneumonia is called *lobar*. This affects one or more lobes of the lung. The second kind is called *bronchopneumonia*, which affects patches of lung in one or both lungs. Symptoms include chills, fever, sweating, muscle pain, and headache. A strong shaking chill is usually a sign of lobar pneumonia. The most common cause of lobar pneumonia is a bacterium called "pneumoccocus." Other kinds of bacteria can cause pneumonia, just as viruses, fungi, yeasts or protozoa can. With fluid in the air sacs, gas exchange can diminish, and a patient can have a severe deprivation of oxygen. When a patient already has diffculty supplying oxygen to the body because of chronic emphysema, or the heart has coronary artery disease, the hypoxia (low oxygen) from the pneumonia makes things much worse for the patient.

9. Emphysema

This is a condition in which continuous exposure to cigarette smoke causes the air sacs of the lung to change their shape via stretching and rupturing. The alveoli coalesce into larger, distorted sacs and this gives less area for gas exchange. Sometimes, there is a hereditary tendency for this disease and smoking makes it worse.

10. Asthma

In asthma, the smaller bronchioles become constricted, inflamed and congested with mucus. In chronic bronchitis and emphysema, the constriction is not reversible. In asthma, the constriction is usually reversible with application of medicine. If asthma goes on too long without treatment, or there are multiple toxins causing asthma to continually be active with constriction, asthma can become like chronic bronchitis or emphysema, leading to serious symptoms not easily treated. Asthma is now recognized to be both a product of bronchioles constricting and the production of an inflammatory response in the airways that fills them with mucous, and further makes the bronchiole lumen smaller. Asthma triggers are complex. It is thought there are two kinds, intrinsic and extrinsic. Intrinsic are usually thought of as emotional changes. Extrinsic triggers are thought of as pollutants, or allergens from pollen and molds. Anxiety is a trigger felt to be "intrinsic." Cold weather can also trigger asthma and is extrinsic. Treatment of asthma now consists of inhaled medicine that helps bronchodilate the constriction and a separate medicine to fight the inflammation that causes mucous production. Bronchodilators are designed from adrenaline and anti-inflammatory medicine can be a corticosteroid.

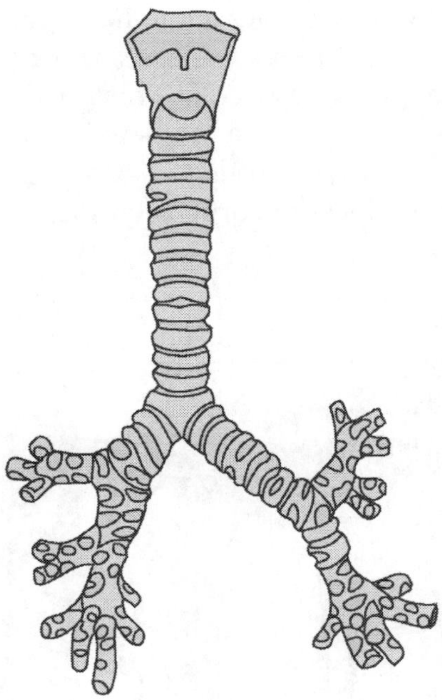

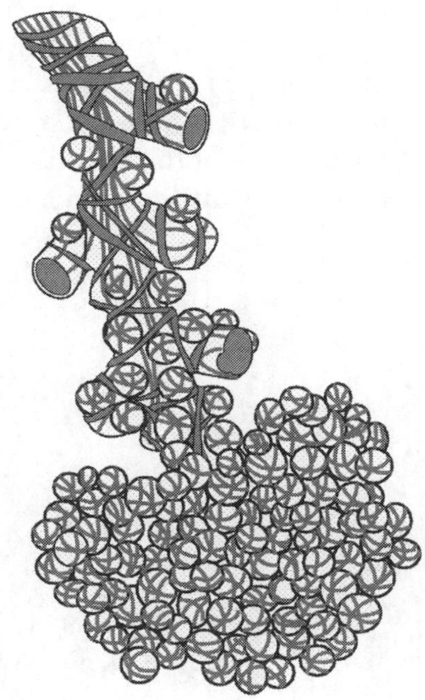

PO Box 2308, Woburn, MA 01888-0508, **p:** 781-729-3736, **www.EmbracingCulture.com**
PO Box 6401, Manchester, NH 03108, **p:** 1-888-678-CCCS

11. Lung Cancer

Cancer is the unrestrained growth of abnormal cells in an organ. These cells can grow locally, and if the mass grows large enough and breaks through various barriers, the abnormal cells can move through the body (metastasize) and grow in other parts of the body. This can happen in the lung. There are many irritants that can cause lung cells to become cancer cells. Cigarette smoking causes 87 percent of all lung cancers. Because now, women are beginning to smoke as much or more than men, the incidence in women is rapidly rising and is more common in women than breast cancer. There are two major forms of lung cancer. The first is so-called small cell. It arises from neuroendocrine cells within the tissue of the lung. It is relatively responsive to chemotherapy. But as in most lung cancer, cures are more successful when surgery is done before the cancer can metastasize. The second form of lung cancer is called large cell cancer. It arises from the glands in the lining of the bronchioles and thus is a true adenocarcinoma. It can be cured with surgery before it spreads. It can respond to chemotherapy but not with the efficacy of small cell.

12. Pulmonary Fibrosis

This is an autoimmune disorder that causes inflammation to attack the walls of the alveoli or air sacs. Scarring occurs in the walls and they become thick and difficult to distend. It takes much more work to move the lungs during the act of breathing, and the thick, scarred walls interfere with gas exchange. The patient becomes breathless in the struggle to move the lungs and get enough oxygen in and CO_2 out. This kind of lung disease is therefore called restrictive disease because the movement of the lung tissue and the gas exchange are restricted. This is in contrast to obstructive disease like asthma and emphysema where the problem is in the obstruction of the airways. In pulmonary fibrosis, there is little to do for treatment other than anti-inflammatory drugs usually in the form of corticosteroids.

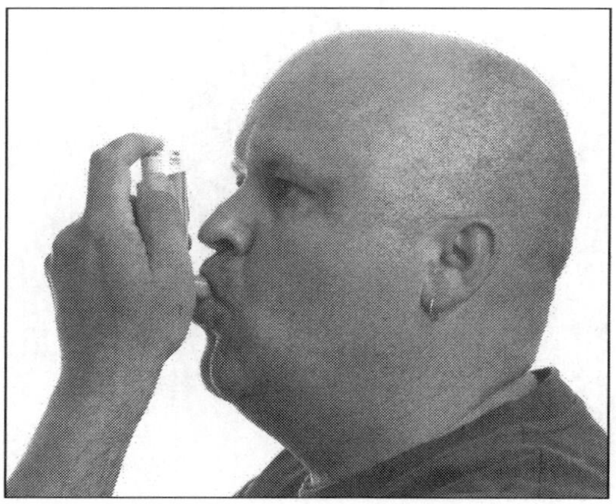

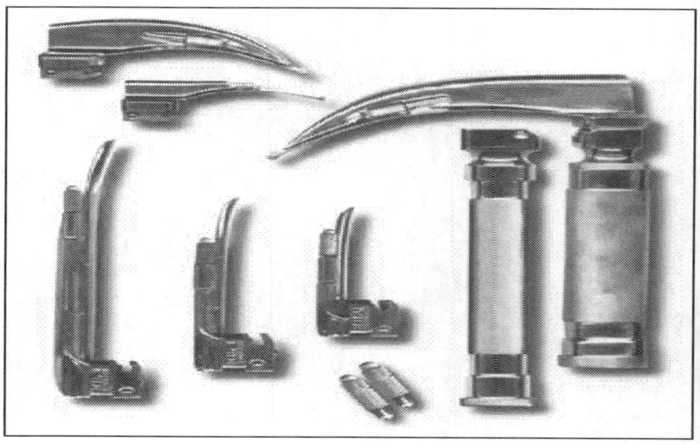

13. Pulmonary Embolism

When a patient is sedentary for a long time, or if the patient has a tendency to clot, or has been on birth control pills, on a prolonged air flight, or has had pelvic, hip or knee surgery, the patient is at risk for a blood clot to form in the leg and move to the heart and into the lung. In the lung, the clot is called a pulmonary embolism.

14. Pneumothorax

A pneumothorax occurs when the lung is punctured or it ruptures. Air then enters the pleural space and the pressure on the lung causes it to collapse. This can happen from trauma, like a car accident, or it can happen when a large bleb of lung pops. Blebs are formed either in people with emphysema from smoking or from an inherited disorder.

III. Dust Diseases

Asbestos, stone dust, and coal dust all are particles in the air that can be inhaled by people, usually workers exposed to these pollutants at work. These particles stimulate an inflammatory response that ultimately results in scarring much the way it occurs in pulmonary fibrosis. This leads to thick, non-distensible lungs with poor oxygen exchange. Thus the patient easily gets short of breath. Inhaling sand particles such as from work of quarry workers or stonemasons leads to **silicosis**. Coal miners can get **pneumoconiosis** and molds from grain or straw can cause **farmer's lung**. Silicosis is the most common occupational disease and it may not cause symptoms for years. It may lead to lung cancer.

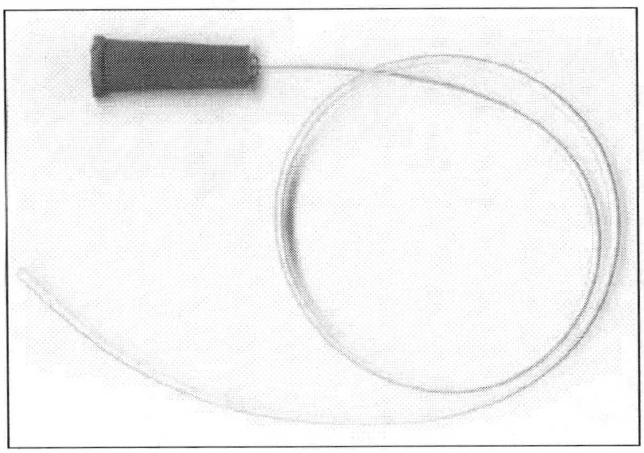

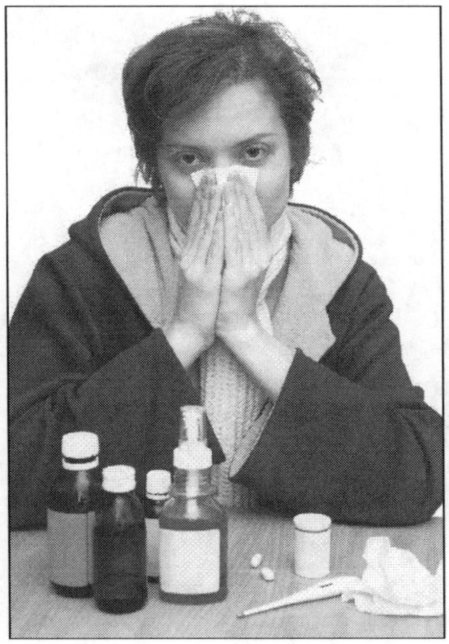

EXERCISES

A. Match each disease to its respective description or symptoms.

Column I		Column II
F	1. Chronic bronchitis	A. This is a condition in which continuous exposure to cigarette smoke causes the air sacs of the lung to change their shape, via stretching and rupturing.
A	2. Emphysema	B. Inflammation of the throat causing a sore throat, fever, pain with swallowing and sometimes an earache.
C	3. Pneumonia	C. When the small bronchioles and alveoli (air sacs) become inflamed and filled with infected fluid.
D	4. Pulmonary Fibrosis	D. Autoimmune disorder that causes inflammation to attack the walls of the alveoli or air sacs.
E	5. Pneumothorax	E. Occurs when the lung is punctured or it ruptures.
B	6. Pharyngitis	F. Chronic irritants such as smoking and other environmental factors cause the bronchi to become irritated and produce a large amount of mucous. This fills the bronchial tubes and coughing ensues.

B. Using your knowledge of the Samurai! Technique and word formation, match the test or procedure in Column I with its description in Column II:

Column I	Column II
D 1. bronchoscopy	A. excision of a lung.
E 2. chest CT scan	B. X-ray image of the chest.
B 3. chest X-ray	C. secretion from the lungs and bronchi is analyzed to look for bacteria that cause infection.
M 4. endotracheal intubation	D. visual examination of bronchial tubes.
H 5. laryngoscopy	E. cross-sectional X-ray images of the chest.
F 6. MRI	F. magnetic waves produce images of the chest in three planes.
I 7. Pulmonary angiography	G. breathing tests using a spirometer.
G 8. PFTs (Pulmonary Function Tests)	H. visual examination of the voice box.
A 9. pneumonectomy (removing)	I. X-ray images of blood vessels in the lung.
C 10. sputum test	J. incision of the chest to remove a lung or portion of a lung.
J 11. thoracotomy	K. surgical procedure to create an opening through the neck into the trachea.
K 12. tracheostomy	L. test used to determine if someone has developed an immune response to the bacterium that causes tuberculosis.
L 13. tuberculin test	M. a tube is placed into the windpipe to open the airway to give you oxygen, medication, or anesthesia.

PO Box 2308, Woburn, MA 01888-0508, **p:** 781-729-3736, **www.EmbracingCulture.com**
PO Box 6401, Manchester, NH 03108, **p:** 1-888-678-CCCS

Lesson Eleven: Homework
Respiratory System

1. Go over your notes for today's class and read section "Additional Resources"
2. Read and practice ALL role-plays for this lesson
3. Continue developing your glossary
4. Translate the Respiratory Disorders into your Target Language:

Respiratory Disorders	Target Language
1. flu	
2. sinusitis	
3. tonsillitis	
4. pharyngitis	
5. laryngitis	
6. the cold	
7. acute bronchitis	
8. chronic bronchitis	
9. pneumonia	
10. emphysema	
11. asthma	
12. lung cancer	
13. pulmonary fibrosis	
14. pulmonary embolism	
15. pneumothorax	

5. **Translate the tests and procedures into your TL:**

Tests and Procedures	Target Language
1. bronchoscopy	
2. chest CT scan	
3. chest x-ray	
4. endotracheal intubation	
5. laryngoscopy	
6. MRI	
7. pulmonary angiography	
8. PFTs (Pulmonary Function Tests)	
9. pneumonectomy	
10. sputum test	
11. thoracotomy	
12. tracheostomy	
13. tuberculin test	

Lesson Eleven: Role-Plays
Respiratory System

Work individually at first:

- Read the entire role-play
- Get a general sense of its meaning
- Circle the most challenging medical terms
- Apply the Samurai! technique to those terms
- Read the role-play again for a deeper understanding
- Find an accurate equivalent in the target language

Work in a language-specific group of friends, fellow students or colleagues:

- Share your doubts
- Ask for other ways of expressing the same meaning
- Develop a glossary
- Check the dictionary
- Practice the role-plays – remember to do CIFE for all your role-plays
- Have your colleagues observe you and provide feedback on your accuracy and register.
- These colleagues can keep track of any omissions, additions, mistakes or distortions in your interpreting and point these out to you in a follow-up discussion.

Student Interpreter Evaluation

Student Name ______________________ Date ______

Language ______________________

Mode of Interpreting (check one): ☐ Consecutive ☐ Simultaneous

Role-Play/System ______________________

Areas Observed ______________________

Accuracy

Register ______________________

Omissions ______________________

Additions ______________________

Distortions ______________________

Pronunciation ______________________

Speaker's emotions conveyed? ______________________

Explain ______________________

Technique

General flow ______________________

Flow when requesting clarification ______________________

Speed ______________________

Eye Contact ______________________

Distracting Habits ______________________

Ethical Issues

Answered questions for patient? ______________________

Advised patient? ______________________

Vocabulary Expansion Recommendations

____

____

Other Recommendations

____

____

Language Coach Signature ______________________ Date ______

THE ART OF MEDICAL INTERPRETATION®

PO Box 2308, Woburn, MA 01888-0508, **p:** 781-729-3736, **www.EmbracingCulture.com**
PO Box 6401, Manchester, NH 03108, **p:** 1-888-678-CCCS

Role-Play 68: Lung Cancer

Augustin is a 56-year-old French-speaking African male. He complains of breathlessness, hoarseness, coughing and hemoptysis (coughing up blood, from Greek, "Haima," meaning "blood" and "ptysis," meaning "spitting"). He has also lost a significant amount of weight over the last three months. Augustin is a refugee in New England. He lives with a few other family members, but he is now unable to care for himself or to help his family. He is afraid that the doctor will give him bad news concerning his health and is planning to go back to his country so as not to be a burden to his family and friends in the United States. But if he goes back, he risks being killed by his country's repressive government.

His family speaks some English and they are reluctant to have a non-native French interpreter. They would rather have a native of their country interpret in the session, but on this given day, that is not an option. The family expects that a native interpreter will filter the cultural appropriateness of the conversation between Augustin and his doctor when they meet alone.

An interpreter arrives just as a doctor who speaks some French is trying his best to communicate with Augustin.

		Pronunciation	Additions	Omissions	Mistakes
MD:	Bonjour Augustin, it's good to see you again. What brings you to the clinic today?				
A:	(Wheezing) I'm having a hard time breathing, doctor. I can't breath, I'm hoarse, I can't eat…I don't know what to do. I just want to go back home.				
MD:	Hmm, you say you can't eat…why is that?				
A:	I have no appetite, and I feel so weak.				
MD:	How long has this been going on?				
A:	For a few months now…I was going to come sooner, but I thought this would pass. I need to work so that my family can survive.				
MD:	I understand you are a good family man, but first you need to take care of yourself. Are there any other symptoms that you've experienced in conjunction with the hoarseness, like a loss of appetite or labored breathing?				
A:	I've had a persistent cough for a few weeks now. And I've been coughing up blood. But I know I am in God's hands.				
MD:	Are you still smoking, Augustin?				
A:	Yes, but I can quit at any time. You know, when your time comes, there is nothing you can do about it. Please do not tell my family if I have something bad, I just want to go back home. At this point in my life it does not matter if I get killed or not!				

continued

Role-Play 68 *(continued)*

	Pronunciation	Additions	Omissions	Mistakes
MD: I see that you are quite pale and that you're wheezing even when at rest. I also understand that you have been giving a lot of thought to your prognosis. Let's examine you and find out what your problem really is.				
(MD examines Augustin)				
MD: You appear to have clubbing in your fingers. See how the tips are enlarged and the nails curved back?				
A: I noticed that, but thought it was because of the type of work I do. I work in a factory cleaning steel nails; you know how it is with all the acids we use.				
MD: Actually, clubbing is caused by low blood oxygen levels and can be a symptom of a variety of serious conditions. Another thing I noticed is that your chest is barrel-shaped and your movements seem diminished on the right side. When I listen to your chest, I don't hear any breathing sounds over the right middle lobe. I'd like to run some tests to further investigate the matter.				
(Later, after examination)				
MD: Augustin, the tests reveal the presence of malignant squamous cells. Would you like to have your family present for the rest of this interview?				
A: No, let's leave them out of this. What are squamous cells?				
MD: Squamous cells are flat cells, usually found in epithelial tissue, where the body meets the outside environment. These cells can turn cancerous. I'd like you to go for a bronchoscopy so we can determine the nature of these cells.				
(Later, after bronchoscopy)				
MD: Augustin, the bronchoscopy revealed a grayish-tan tumor spreading out from your right middle bronchus and obstructing it. We know from the biopsy that the tumor is cancerous. Thankfully, lung cancer is the most preventable of cancers, and surgical resection can be potentially curative in patients like you. Let's talk about your treatment options.				

continued

PO Box 2308, Woburn, MA 01888-0508, **p:** 781-729-3736, **www.EmbracingCulture.com**
PO Box 6401, Manchester, NH 03108, **p:** 1-888-678-CCCS

Role-Play 68 *(continued)*

The interpreter begins to feel very uncomfortable with the doctor's directness and asks the doctor to step outside. But Augustin understands some English and says, "I already knew I had cancer. I am ready for God to take me." Augustin leaves the room crying and the family looks at the interpreter with disdain. In their eyes, the interpreter is the cause of the bad news. The family insists they never want this interpreter (or this doctor) again.

Break It Down ☐ ☐ ☐ ☐

☐ CIFE with patient ☐ CIFE with provider ☐ FLOW ☐ REGISTER

Role-Play 68: Glossary

continued

1. Pathology (diseases, conditions)

2. Laboratory Tests and Diagnostic Procedures

3. Treatment Procedures

4. Idiomatic Expressions (if any)

5. Other (vocabulary in this particular role-play that you feel is important/relevant or that you anticipate problems with)

PO Box 2308, Woburn, MA 01888-0508, **p:** 781-729-3736, **www.EmbracingCulture.com**
PO Box 6401, Manchester, NH 03108, **p:** 1-888-678-CCCS

Role-Play 69: Exercise-induced Asthma

Elder is 24 and plays soccer every Sunday. He runs and cannot keep up with his friends. He notices he is wheezing after exercise, and he is worried he will not be able to keep up with his friends for the New England Amateur World Cup.

	Pronunciation	Additions	Omissions	Mistakes
MD: Hello Mr. Saenz, how can I help you?				
PT: I have been wheezing after I run. I used to have this in high school and now it's back.				
MD: Do you have allergies?				
PT: Not in my country, but since I've been here, my nose drips all the time, especially in the spring and fall.				
MD: Have you seen a doctor for this?				
PT: I saw a primary care doctor who gave me Claritin for my nose. It helped, but I still wheeze when I run.				
MD: Do you have chest pain or palpitations when you run?				
PT: No. I just get out of breath, I wheeze and it is like a band around my chest.				
MD: Do you get these symptoms when you are out in the cold?				
PT: Yes, how did you know?				
MD: Well, this sounds like exercise-induced asthma. This is a special kind of asthma that can occur with exercise or out in the cold. It can be worse in the spring or fall when most people will get allergic symptoms.				
PT: Is there a cure?				
MD: Before we get into that, let's do some tests. My medical assistants will take you to the spirometer to breathe into the machine so we can measure your breathing. It will give me a chance to understand what is happening. We'll also get an X-ray of your chest. Let me listen to your heart and lungs and then we'll do the tests.				
(MD examines patient. MA comes in and takes patient to spirometer. Patient does test, gets a chest X-ray.)				
MD: Well, Mr. Saenz, your CXR is clear. The spirometry shows a pattern that looks typical for what we call mild small airway disease.				

continued

Role-Play 69 *(continued)*

	Pronunciation	Additions	Omissions	Mistakes
PT: Can you help me with my shortness of breath?				
MD: Surely. This is a simple spray. It's an inhaler. Use it twice before you run. Each time you take in a puff, you must hold your breath so that the medicine can be absorbed into your lungs. Then you should have better exercise tolerance.				
PT: What is exercise tolerance?				
MD: It means your endurance and stamina in running will be improved because your lungs will move air in and out more efficiently.				
PT: That's what I need.				
MD: Here is a prescription for the medicine called Albuterol. You may use it before exercise up to four times a day. Some people get a hoarse voice using this medicine. This is temporary. Before you go, you can meet again with the medical assistant who will show you how to do the sprays. Come back in two weeks to tell me how things have been going.				
PT: OK, I 'm ready to try this.				
Break It Down	☐	☐	☐	☐

☐ **CIFE with patient** ☐ **CIFE with provider** ☐ **FLOW** ☐ **REGISTER**

Role-Play 69: Glossary

continued

PO Box 2308, Woburn, MA 01888-0508, **p:** 781-729-3736, **www.EmbracingCulture.com**
PO Box 6401, Manchester, NH 03108, **p:** 1-888-678-CCCS

1. Pathology (diseases, conditions)

2. Laboratory Tests and Diagnostic Procedures

3. Treatment Procedures

4. Idiomatic Expressions (if any)

5. Other (vocabulary in this particular role-play that you feel is important/relevant or that you anticipate problems with)

Role-Play 70: COLD or FLU?

	Pronunciation	Additions	Omissions	Mistakes
Patient: I have been feeling tired and tomorrow is my daughter's birthday.				
Doctor, can you give me something to get me back to normal?				
MD: Hmm, you are looking for a miracle drug! Let me ask a few questions and see what I can do for you. How old is your daughter?				
Patient: She's thirteen going on twenty. She has an older boyfriend. She is a good kid, but you need to always watch out for craziness. A good kid can go bad because of the wrong friends.				
MD: You know, my kids are still young, but I understand that having a teenage girl is always hard for a father. But it is possible to successfully negotiate around friends while keeping the channels of communication open. You pick your fights and give a little, and your family will survive the teenage years!				
Patient: See, she talks with her mom. We are separated and my wife is coming after me for alimony besides the money I already pay for child support.				
MD: The best thing is to leave the money matters to the adults. I wish you all the best. Let's go over your symptoms.				
Patient: OK.				
MD: Do you have a scratchy throat, nasal or ear congestion?				
Patient: I feel that my head is going to explode. You know when you can hear the echo of your own voice in your head? That is the way I feel right now.				
MD: You told me earlier that you felt fatigue. Did I ask you about hoarseness? You sound a bit hoarse. Is it getting better or worse?				
Patient: I guess I have the flu. But then again, maybe I have a cold.				
MD: Your fever is pretty low and your symptoms are not quite as severe as flu symptoms. You know, with the flu, the symptoms can last for a few weeks. Anyway, the treatment for colds and the flu is similar.				

continued

PO Box 2308, Woburn, MA 01888-0508, **p:** 781-729-3736, **www.EmbracingCulture.com**
PO Box 6401, Manchester, NH 03108, **p:** 1-888-678-CCCS

Role-Play 70 *(continued)*

	Pronunciation	Additions	Omissions	Mistakes
Patient: OK.				
MD: Drink a lot of fluids to help your body get rid of the virus. You can buy over-the-counter decongestants like Sudafed, but do not overdo it with the medication. One inexpensive treatment is to gargle with warm salt water. Another recommendation is to stop smoking. It will help you now and in the future. We will discuss the smoking when you are ready. I have a lot of good referrals for you to check the different non-smoking programs in your area.				
Patient: Doctor, can I ask you if you smoke?				
MD: I used to smoke until I started to treat patients with all kinds of bronchitis and lung cancer. For your body aches you can also buy over-the-counter medications such as Tylenol or Aspirin. Call me if your symptoms become a lot worse.				
MD: Symptoms to watch out for include: severe, unusual headaches, and coughing up rusty, gray, green or bloody phlegm. Also, check for fever over 101°.				
Patient: You know, I'm feeling better already. It really helped to talk about my family.				
MD: I am glad you came today. When you are ready to talk some more, I can refer you to a family therapist. By the way, if you do get real chest pain, particularly when you are spitting the phlegm, or if you get an earache with intense pain when swallowing, contact my office right away.				
Patient: OK, Doctor. Should I take one of those flu shots that old people get?				
MD: Flu shots are good for everyone. It's just that children and the elderly have more vulnerable immune systems, and we need to protect them first.				
Patient: I know. I was just joking with you. I like you, Doctor. You make me comfortable and you are not stuck-up, like those doctors who walk around with their noses in the air.				

continued

Role-Play 70 *(continued)*

	Pronunciation	Additions	Omissions	Mistakes
MD: Thanks. Patients like you make a difference, but I am still going to be nagging you about your smoking! Come back in three weeks for a follow-up and then we can talk about various smoking-prevention programs. In the meantime, when you sneeze, wash your hands.				
Patient: OK, Doctor.				
Break It Down	☐	☐	☐	☐

☐ **CIFE with patient** ☐ **CIFE with provider** ☐ **FLOW** ☐ **REGISTER**

Role-Play 70: Glossary

continued

PO Box 2308, Woburn, MA 01888-0508, **p:** 781-729-3736, **www.EmbracingCulture.com**
PO Box 6401, Manchester, NH 03108, **p:** 1-888-678-CCCS

1. Pathology (diseases, conditions)

2. Laboratory Tests and Diagnostic Procedures

3. Treatment Procedures

4. Idiomatic Expressions (if any)

5. Other (vocabulary in this particular role-play that you feel is important/relevant or that you anticipate problems with)

Role-Play 71: Ibuprofen

The following are the instructions on how to take Ibuprofen. Practice **SIGHT INTERPRETATION/TRANSLATION**. Apply all that you know on how to best handle this practice:

IBUPROFEN 800 MG TABLET

MEDICATION

IBUPROFEN 800 MG TABLET

DIRECTIONS

TAKE 1 TABLET BY MOUTH 3 TIMES A DAY FOR 10 DAYS

IMPORTANT NOTE

THIS IS A SUMMARY AND DOES NOT CONTAIN ALL POSSIBLE INFORMATION ABOUT THIS PRODUCT.
FOR COMPLETE INFORMATION ABOUT THIS PRODUCT OR YOUR SPECIFIC HEALTH NEEDS, ASK YOUR HEALTHCARE PROFESSIONAL.
ALWAYS SEEK THE ADVICE OF YOUR healthcare PROFESSIONAL IF YOU HAVE ANY QUESTIONS ABOUT THIS PRODUCT OR YOUR MEDICAL CONDITION.
THIS INFORMATION IS NOT INTENDED AS INDIVIDUAL MEDICAL ADVICE AND DOES NOT SUBSTITUTE FOR THE ACKNOWLEDGEMENT AND JUDGMENT OF YOUR healthcare PROFESSIONAL.
THIS INFORMATION DOES NOT CONTAIN ANY ASSURANCES THAT THIS PRODUCT IS SAFE, EFFECTIVE, OR APPROPRIATE FOR YOU.
IBUPROFEN – ORAL (eye-byou-PRO-fen)

COMMON BRAND NAME(S)

Advil, Motrin, Nuprin

WARNING

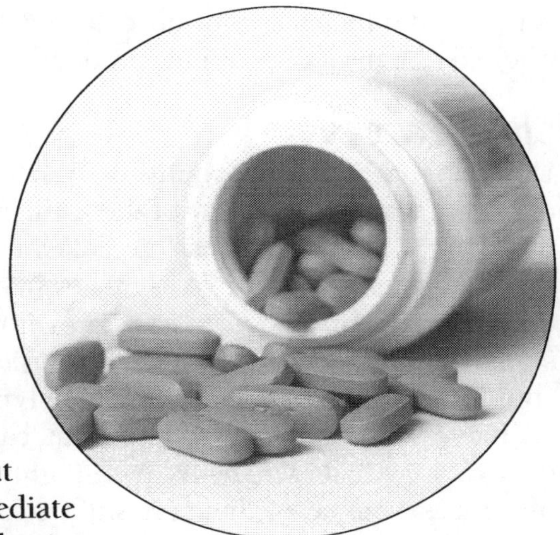

This drug may infrequently cause serious (rarely fatal) bleeding from the stomach or intestines. Also, related drugs rarely have caused blood clots to form, resulting in heart attacks and strokes. This medication might also rarely cause similar problems. Talk to your doctor or pharmacist about the benefits and risks of treatment, as well as other possible medication choices. If you notice any of the following rare but very serious side effects, stop taking ibuprofen and seek immediate medical attention: black stools, persistent stomach/abdominal pain, vomit that looks like coffee grounds, chest pain, weakness on one side of the body, sudden vision changes, slurred speech.

PO Box 2308, Woburn, MA 01888-0508, **p:** 781-729-3736, **www.EmbracingCulture.com**
PO Box 6401, Manchester, NH 03108, **p:** 1-888-678-CCCS

Role-Play 71 *(continued)*

USES

Ibuprofen is a nonsteroidal anti-inflammatory drug (NSAID), which relieves pain and swelling (inflammation). It is used to treat headaches, muscle aches, backaches, dental pain, menstrual cramps, arthritis, or athletic injuries. This medication is also used to reduce fever and to relieve minor aches and pains due to the common cold or flu. This drug works by blocking the enzyme in your body that makes prostaglandins. Decreasing prostaglandins helps to reduce pain, swelling, and fever.

HOW TO USE

Read the Medication Guide provided by your pharmacist before you start using ibuprofen and each time you get a refill. If you have any questions regarding the information, consult your doctor or pharmacist. Take this medication by mouth with a full glass (8 ounces or 240 milliliters) of water unless your doctor directs you otherwise. Do not lie down for at least 30 minutes after taking this drug. If stomach upset occurs while taking this medication, take it with food, milk, or an antacid. The dosage is based on your medical condition and response to therapy. If repeat doses are needed, they are usually given 6 or 8 hours apart; or as directed by your doctor. When ibuprofen is used in children, the dose is based on the child's weight. Read the product instructions to find the appropriate dose for your child's weight. Consult the pharmacist or doctor if you have questions or if you need help choosing the appropriate dosage form. In certain conditions (e.g., arthritis), it may take up to two weeks, taken regularly, before the full benefits of this drug take effect. If you use this medication for migraine headache, and the pain is not relieved or worsens after the first dose, tell your doctor immediately. For nonprescription ibuprofen products: If you are treating yourself or giving this medication to a child for undiagnosed fever or pain, consult the doctor immediately if symptoms do not improve within 24 hours, worsen or last for more than 3 days, or if new symptoms appear. To reduce your risk of stomach bleeding and other side effects, take this medication at the lowest effective dose for the shortest possible time. Do not increase your dose, take it more frequently, or take it for a longer time than prescribed. Do not take the over-the-counter product for more than 10 days unless otherwise directed.

SIDE EFFECTS

Upset stomach, nausea, vomiting, heartburn, headache, diarrhea, constipation, drowsiness, and dizziness may occur. If any of these effects persist or worsen, notify your doctor or pharmacist promptly. If your doctor has directed you to use this medication, remember that he or she has judged that the benefit you receive is greater than the risk of side effects. Many people using this medication do not have serious side effects. Tell your doctor immediately if any of these serious side effects occur: stomach pain, swelling of the hands or feet, sudden or unexplained weight gain, ringing in the ears (tinnitus). Tell your doctor immediately if any of these unlikely but serious side effects occur: vision changes, rapid or pounding heartbeat, easy bruising or bleeding, difficult/painful swallowing. Tell your doctor immediately if any of these highly unlikely but very serious side effects occur: change in amount of urine, severe headache, very stiff neck, mental/mood changes, persistent sore throat or fever. This drug may rarely cause serious (possibly fatal) liver disease. If you notice any of the following highly unlikely but very serious side effects, stop taking ibuprofen and consult your doctor or pharmacist immediately: yellowing eyes and skin, dark urine, unusual/extreme tiredness. An allergic reaction to

continued

Role-Play 71 *(continued)*

this drug is unlikely, but seek immediate medical attention if it occurs. Symptoms of an allergic reaction include: rash, itching/swelling (especially of the face/tongue/throat), severe dizziness, trouble breathing. This is not a complete list of possible side effects. If you notice other effects not listed above, contact your doctor or pharmacist. Contact your doctor for medical advice about side effects. The following numbers do not provide medical advice, but in the US you may report side effects to the Food and Drug Administration (FDA) at 1800-FDA-1088. In Canada, you may call Health Canada at 1-866-234-2345.

PRECAUTIONS

Before taking ibuprofen, tell your doctor or pharmacist if you are allergic to it; or to aspirin or other NSAIDs (e.g., naproxen, celecoxib); or if you have any other allergies. This medication should not be used if you have certain medical conditions. Before using this medicine, consult your doctor or pharmacist if you have: severe kidney disease, aspirin-sensitive asthma (a history of worsening breathing with runny/stuffy nose after taking aspirin or other NSAIDs), recent heart bypass surgery (CABG). Before using this medication, tell your doctor or pharmacist your medical history, especially of: kidney disease, liver disease, poorly controlled diabetes, stomach/intestine/esophagus problems (e.g., bleeding, ulcers, recurring heartburn), heart disease (e.g., congestive heart failure, history of heart attack), high blood pressure, stroke, swelling (edema, fluid retention), dehydration, blood disorders (e.g., anemia), bleeding or clotting problems, asthma, growths in the nose (nasal polyps), history of an allergic reaction with symptoms of lip/tongue/throat swelling (angiodema), any allergies in addition to those listed above. This drug may make you dizzy or drowsy; use caution engaging in activities requiring alertness such as driving or using machinery. Limit alcoholic beverages. This medicine may cause stomach bleeding. Daily use of alcohol and tobacco, especially when combined with this medicine, may increase your risk for stomach bleeding. Limit alcohol and stop smoking. Consult your doctor or pharmacist for more information. This medication may make you more sensitive to the sun. Avoid prolonged sun exposure, tanning booths or sunlamps. Use a sunscreen and wear protective clothing when outdoors. Caution is advised when using this drug in the elderly because they may be more sensitive to the side effects of the drug, especially stomach bleeding and kidney effects. This medication should be used only when clearly needed during the first 6 months of pregnancy. It is not recommended for use during the last 3 months of pregnancy due to the potential for harm to an unborn baby and interference with normal/delivery. Discuss the risks and benefits with your doctor. This medication passes into breast milk. While there have been no reports of harm to nursing infants, consult your doctor before breast-feeding.

continued

Role-Play 71 *(continued)*

DRUG INTERACTIONS

Your healthcare professionals (e.g., doctor or pharmacist) may already be aware of any possible drug interaction and may be monitoring you for it. Do not start, stop or change the dosage of any medicine before checking with them first. This drug should not be used with the following medications because very serious interactions may occur: Cidofovir, Ketorolac. If you are currently using any of these medications listed above, tell your doctor or pharmacist before starting ibuprofen. Before using this medication, tell your doctor or pharmacist of all prescription and nonprescription/herbal products you may use, especially of: anti-platelet drugs (e.g., Cilostazol, Clopidogrel), oral bisphosphonates (e.g., Alendronate), "blood thinners" (e.g., Enoxaparin, Heparin, Warfarin), corticosteroids (e.g., Prednisone), cyclosporine, desmopressin, high blood pressure drugs (including ACE inhibitors such as Captopril, Angiotensin II receptor antagonist such as Losartan, and beta-blockers such as Metoprolol), lithium, pemetrexed, triamterene, "water pills" (diuretics such as Furosemid, Hydrochlorathiazide, Triamterene). Check all prescription and nonprescription medicine labels carefully for other pain/fever drugs (NSAIDs such as Aspirin, Celecoxib, Naproxen). These drugs are similar to ibuprofen so taking one of these drugs while also taking ibuprofen may increase your risk of side effects. Consult your doctor or pharmacist for more details. However, if your doctor has prescribed low doses of aspirin to prevent heart attack or stroke (usually at dosages of 81-325 milligrams a day), you should continue to take the aspirin. Daily use of ibuprofen may decrease aspirin's ability to prevent heart attack/stroke. Talk to your doctor about using a different medication (e.g., Acetaminophen) to treat pain/fever. If you must take ibuprofen, talk to your doctor about possibly taking the ibuprofen dose apart from the aspirin dose. Do not increase your daily dose of aspirin or change the way you take aspirin/other medications without your doctor's approval. This document does not contain all possible interactions. Therefore, before using this product, tell your doctor or pharmacist of all the products you use. Keep a list of all your medications with you, and share the list with your doctor and pharmacist.

OVERDOSE

If overdose is suspected, contact your local poison control center or emergency room immediately. US residents can call the US national poison hotline at 1-800-222-1222. Canadian residents should call their local poison control center directly. Symptoms of overdose may include: severe stomach pain, coffee ground-like vomit, unusually fast or slow heartbeat, trouble breathing, extreme drowsiness, loss of consciousness, or seizures.

NOTES

Do not share this medication with others. Laboratory and/or medical tests may be performed periodically to monitor your progress or check for side effects. Consult your doctor for more details.

Role-Play 71 *(continued)*

MISSED DOSE

If you are prescribed this drug on a regular schedule (not just "as needed") and you miss a dose, take it as soon as you remember. If it is near the time of the next dose, skip the missed dose and resume your usual dosing schedule. Do not double the dose to catch up.

STORAGE

Store at room temperature between 59 and 86 degrees F (15-30 degrees C) away from light and moisture. Do not store in the bathroom. Keep all medicines away from children and pets. Do not flush medications down the toilet or pour them into a drain unless instructed to do so. Properly discard this product when it is expired or no longer needed. Consult your pharmacist or local waste disposal company for more detail about how to safely discard your product.

What do you recall from your sight interpretation/translation?

PO Box 2308, Woburn, MA 01888-0508, **p:** 781-729-3736, **www.EmbracingCulture.com**
PO Box 6401, Manchester, NH 03108, **p:** 1-888-678-CCCS

Lesson Eleven: Additional Resources Respiratory System

RESPIRATORY SYSTEM VOCABULARY

Main Organs and Body Structures:

Word	Target Language
Diaphragm	
Alveolus	
Bronchi	
Bronchiole	
Larynx	
Pleura	
Nose	
Pharynx	
Lung	
Chest	
Trachea	
Epiglottis	
Palatine tonsils	
Nostrils	
Cilia	
Nasal septum	
Paranasal sinuses	
Adam's apple	
Glottis	
Tonsils	
Hilum	
Lobes	
Alveolar ducts	
Mediastinum	

continued

Main Illnesses:

Word	Target Language
Alveolitis	
Anoxia	
Aphonia	
Apnea	
Asbestosis	
Asthma	
Atelectasis	
Bronchiectasis	
Bronchiolitis	
Bronchitis	
Bronchogenic carcinoma	
Bronchospasm	
Croup	
Cystis fibrosis	
Diphtheria	
Dysphonia	
Dyspnea	
Emphysema	
Epistaxis	
Eupnea	
Hyperpnea	
Hypoxia	
Laryngospasm	
Laryngotracheobronchitis	
Oliopnea	
Pansinusitis	
Pertussis	
Pleuralgia	
Pneumoconiosis	
Pneumonia	

continued

PO Box 2308, Woburn, MA 01888-0508, **p:** 781-729-3736, **www.EmbracingCulture.com**
PO Box 6401, Manchester, NH 03108, **p:** 1-888-678-CCCS

Main Illnesses: *(continued)*

Word	Target Language
Pneumopleuritis	
Pulmonary abscess	
Pulmonary edema	
Pulmonary embolism	
Pulmonary fibrosis	
Rhinitis	
Tonsillitis	
Tuberculosis	
Carcinoma of the lung	
COPD (chronic obstructive pulmonary disease)	
Pharyngitis	
Pleuritis	
Sinusitis	
Bronchopneumonia	
Edema	
Homeostasis	
Influenza	
Laryngalgia	
Laryngitis	
Percutaneous biopsy	
Pleuritis	
Pneumonitis	
Pneumothorax	
RDS (respiratory distress syndrome)	
Silicosis	
Tonsillitis	
Pharyngitis	

continued

Main Tests and Procedures:

Word	Target Language
Adenoidectomy	
Auscultation	
Bronchoscopy	
Chest x-ray	
CT scan of the chest	
Endotracheal intubation	
Laryngoscopy	
Lobectomy	
Lung biopsy	
MRI scan of the chest	
Percussion	
Phrenotomy	
Pneumonectomy	
Pulmonary angiography	
Pulmonary function tests (PFTs)	
Radioactive test	
Rhinoplasty	
Sinusotomy	
Sputum test	
Thoracentesis	
Thoracocentesis	
Thoracoplasty	
Thoracotomy	
Tonsillectomy	
Tracheostomy	
Tracheotomy	
Tuberculin test	

PO Box 2308, Woburn, MA 01888-0508, **p:** 781-729-3736, **www.EmbracingCulture.com**
PO Box 6401, Manchester, NH 03108, **p:** 1-888-678-CCCS

Notes

Lesson Twelve: Emergency Room

Understanding Goals

Students will:

- learn about some of the challenges of acute care interpreting
- develop strategies for self-management related to working in the Emergency Room
- learn how to adopt a humanistic approach when giving bad news
- learn about the top 10 reasons for Emergency Room visits
- sharpen their consecutive interpreting skills through role-play practice with ER situations

Key concepts:

- Acute care interpreting
- Emergency Room
- Triage
- The Ethical Interpreter
- Top 10 reasons for ER visits

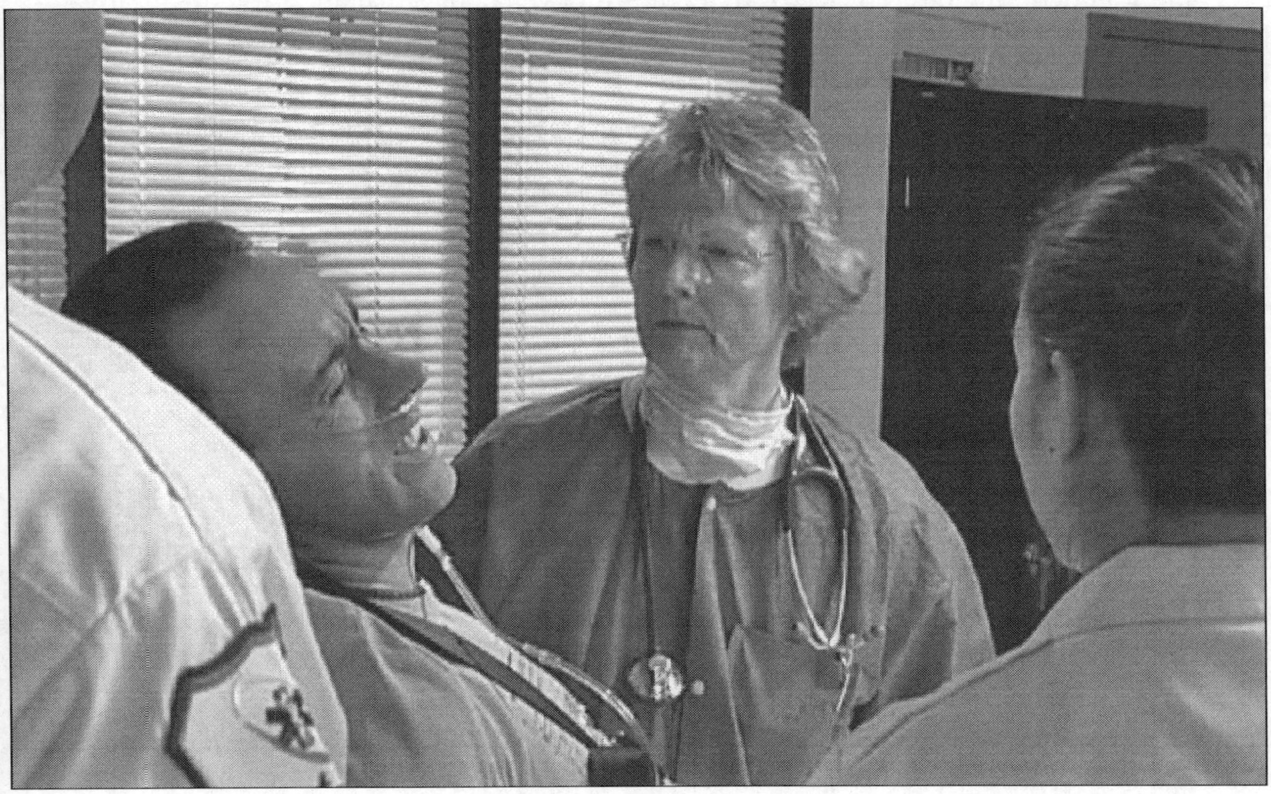

PO Box 2308, Woburn, MA 01888-0508, **p:** 781-729-3736, **www.EmbracingCulture.com**
PO Box 6401, Manchester, NH 03108, **p:** 1-888-678-CCCS

Lesson Twelve: Quiz
Emergency Room

Read the following statements and determine if they are true or false, then circle the appropriate answer next to the statement.

1. The "Emergency Room Interpreter Bill" adopted by the state of Massachusetts, requires all hospitals that provide acute care, either in emergency rooms or in psychiatric services, to use competent interpreters when treating non-English speakers.
   ○ True ○ False

2. When a patient shows up with clear signs of alcohol intoxication and s/he relates to the doctor "I only had 2 six packs of beer," it is okay for the interpreter to interpret "I had 2 six packs of beer," which conveys the same information.
   ○ True ○ False

3. Triage is one of the last stops in an emergency situation, which happens when a provider (usually a nurse) evaluates a patient's condition and classifies it under general categories.
   ○ True ○ False

4. A "crash cart" is a stretcher with wheels used in the ER to pick up patients when they crash on the floor.
   ○ True ○ False

5. A defibrillator is an electrical device with two paddles that are placed on a cardiac arrest patient's chest to discharge electricity through the heart.
   ○ True ○ False

6. An interpreter should show empathy and a humanistic approach in an interview when bad news is being delivered to the patient and/or his relatives.
   ○ True ○ False

7. If the patient or a family member is crying loudly or is exhibiting his/her grief in an agitated manner it is appropriate for the interpreter to sob uncontrollably or to "become" another patient as a way to show empathy.
   ○ True ○ False

8. Nystagmus is the high register for "dancing eyes" or "jerking eyes."
   ○ True ○ False

9. In the United States, alcoholism is defined by the quantity that one drinks, without considering how the drinking affects the person's behavior at work, in the family and socially.
   ○ True ○ False

10. Alcoholism is a curable illness.
   ○ True ○ False

11. Once an alcoholic, always an alcoholic.
○ True ○ False

12. Interpreters should always adhere to their Code of Ethics and should never interpret for police officers in an ER, except when the interpreter is faced with a victim of an abuse such as rape or domestic violence.
○ True ○ False

13. Chest pain is the higher register for angina.
○ True ○ False

14. The pain from lack of blood to the heart is called angina.
○ True ○ False

15. When the heart goes into an irregular rhythm of beating, it is called a dysrrythmia.
○ True ○ False

16. When a patient has a low blood level (not enough for the heart to pump), perhaps caused by terrible bleeding, he is likely to "go into shock."
○ True ○ False

17. CVA stands for Cancero Vascular Accident.
○ True ○ False

18. Symptoms of strep throat and colds are similar.
○ True ○ False

19. The Flu is not contagious and strikes randomly.
○ True ○ False

20. Food poisoning is understood as any disease of an infectious or toxic nature caused by the consumption of food or drink.
○ True ○ False

21. Patients with diabetes mellitus have sweet urine and that is why this form of diabetes is called mellitus, which comes from the Latin word for sweet.
○ True ○ False

22. Type 2 diabetes is the type of diabetes that women get during pregnancy.
○ True ○ False

PO Box 2308, Woburn, MA 01888-0508, **p:** 781-729-3736, **www.EmbracingCulture.com**
PO Box 6401, Manchester, NH 03108, **p:** 1-888-678-CCCS

Lesson Twelve: Class Activities
Emergency Room

On April 14, 2000, the "Emergency Room Interpreter Bill" was adopted by the Commonwealth of Massachusetts. This new law requires all hospitals that provide acute care, either in emergency rooms or in psychiatric services, to use competent interpreters when treating non-English speakers. The bill specifies that whenever an appropriate bilingual clinician is not available, the healthcare facility management must use reasonable judgment in setting up a mix of full time, on call, and electronic interpreting services. This change in Massachusetts state law reflects a growing trend in favor of mandated interpreter services. Increasingly then, interpreters everywhere can expect to be called to emergency rooms and acute psychiatric care facilities. But fear not! Acute care interpreting need not be intimidating! In this lesson, we aim to prepare you for work in the ER.

Do you have a similar law in your state?

____

____

But....are you ready to work as an interpreter?

THINK Consider the following questions:

How do you react to displeasing sights and smells? Do you have a "strong stomach"?

____

____

Do you get dizzy at the sight of blood?

____

____

Are you overcome by the smell of vomit?

____

____

____

Can you control your first-impulse reactions?

____

____

____

Try to imagine yourself as the interpreter in the following real-life situations:

Case #1: An interpreter is called to the emergency ward. She opens the curtain and she sees two police officers and a patient in handcuffs. She starts interpreting for the emergency triage nurse and finds out the patient had been in a fight in jail. All of a sudden, she notices that the patient's fist is closed and he has a bandage over his eye. The nurse asks him to open his fist and as soon as he opens his fist his right eye is in his hand.

Case #2: An interpreter is called to interpret for a patient who had throat cancer surgery. She enters the room. The patient is holding the tracheostomy tube with his finger in order to speak. As he starts speaking, pus starts coming out of the tube. His voice is raspy and he turns to the side to talk to his wife. The interpreter notices that the entire side of his neck is open and s/he could see his entire tongue moving. He was sent to the hyperbolic chamber for oxygen treatment.

Case #3: A patient who speaks English arrives at the ER with chest pain. He waits for several hours and as he is waiting he has a heart attack. He gets rushed into the ER and all of a sudden he starts speaking Portuguese. A Portuguese interpreter is called as he is having a second heart attack. His vital signs are flat, ten doctors are next to him trying to resuscitate him, nurses are rushing back and forth. The patient comes back after being resuscitated and tells the providers he wants to die. His wife gets called. Blood pressure goes down, EKGs are flat, and the patient gets intubated. He gets shocked with the paddles, comes back again and he says he wants to die. The providers ask for his records and he has not signed a DNR and DNI Directive. The attorney gets called and as they wait, the patient goes out again. The medical team decides to numb his chest, open his chest and start squeezing his heart with their hands. There is blood all over, interpreter is in the room standing for 10 hours.

Case #4: Middle-aged woman arrives in a stretcher at the hospital throwing up green pasty bile, holding onto her right side, bending forward, moaning in terrible pain, praying for God's help. All of a sudden, she starts throwing up and she soils her pants with terrible smelly greenish diarrhea. The nurses are very busy and the interpreter stays in between the door and the hallway with the smell of vomit, diarrhea, and the cries and moanings of a patient with uncontrollable pain.

QUESTION

How would you react if you were the interpreter in these situations? Be prepared to share your impressions/reactions with the whole group.

PO Box 2308, Woburn, MA 01888-0508, **p:** 781-729-3736, **www.EmbracingCulture.com**
PO Box 6401, Manchester, NH 03108, **p:** 1-888-678-CCCS

WORKING ON THE EDGE

Acute care interpreting is perhaps the most exciting of interpreting assignments. Since no other hospital department deals with as many different medical conditions, an interpreter stepping into an acute care situation has no way to predict exactly what s/he will face. For this reason, it is imperative that the acute care interpreter be prepared to handle any common emergency situation. Chances are, in your career as an acute care interpreter you will see the after-effects of poisoning, burns, broken bones, heart attacks, convulsions, choking, bleeding, eye contamination, and shock.

It is therefore important that interpreters be proactive by imagining scenarios for different emergencies and assessing possible challenges in self-management. At any time, an interpreter can expect to serve patients who bleed, vomit, cry, have diarrhea, choke, gasp for air, experience psychotic breaks or maintain poor hygiene. Interpreters also witness intubations, birth, gangrenous limbs and belligerent behavior.

An ER Call

For example, an interpreter may be called to an emergency only to encounter a patient throwing up violently. Interpreters need to be prepared to handle such situations. Many have great difficulty controlling an impulse to vomit after watching others vomit.
Here are some helpful tips:

- Do not look at the vomit itself; look up at the ceiling
- Some interpreters squeeze their hands very tightly, and this distracts them from their impulse to vomit
- Others take a few deep, silent breaths
- ________________________________
- ________________________________
- ________________________________
- ________________________________
- ________________________________
- ________________________________
- ________________________________
- ________________________________

Remember though, that even while the interpreter is taking care of him/herself, the accuracy of the interpretation still needs to be 100% complete!

Understanding TRIAGE

The mention of emergency often brings to mind the word "triage." Triage is one of the first stops in an emergency situation. In triage, a provider (usually a nurse) evaluates a patient's condition and classifies it under a general category, such as

- "immediately life threatening,"
- "urgent but not immediately life threatening"
- "less urgent"

These classifications are life-saving tools that allow patients with more serious medical conditions to receive treatment before those with relatively minor problems.

Busy, Busy

Have you ever felt overwhelmed by the bustle of an emergency room? Patients are pretty easy to recognize, but who are all those people in lab coats, scrubs and clogs? Well, most acute care facilities are staffed with attending physicians, nurses and physician assistants. In addition, emergency room technicians may assist with tasks such as checking vital signs and running lab tests, while other support staff handles registration and ER communications.

A crash course in crash carts...

While at this point we won't go into detail describing the whole gamut of emergency room equipment, there is some vocabulary that is sure to pique your curiosity. Ever heard of a "crash cart"? It is a cabinet that houses equipment used primarily to treat cardiac arrest. Among crash cart utensils is the defibrillator, an electrical device with two paddles that are placed on a cardiac arrest patient's chest to discharge electricity through the heart... just one more example of how action-packed acute care can be!

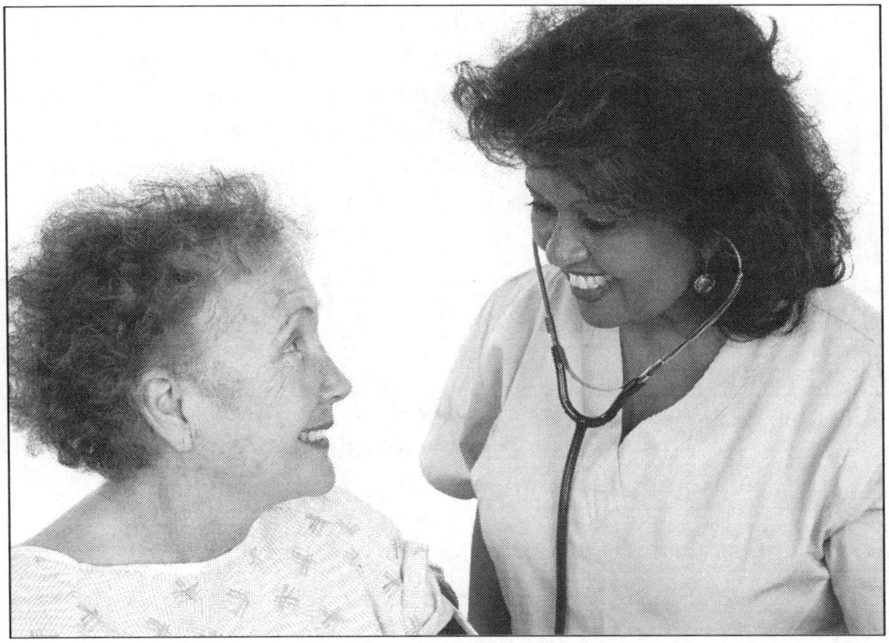

References: HowStuffWorks, Inc. www.howstuffworks.com; NHeLP (National Health Law Program) www.healthlaw.org www.healthlaw.org; Southern Illinois University School of Medicine www.siumed.edu

PO Box 2308, Woburn, MA 01888-0508, **p:** 781-729-3736, **www.EmbracingCulture.com**
PO Box 6401, Manchester, NH 03108, **p:** 1-888-678-CCCS

Giving Bad News

1. Were you ever in a situation where you had to deliver bad news to a close friend or relative?

2. What was difficult about it?

3. How did you deliver the news? Did you do anything differently?

One of the challenges of working in the Emergency Room is the high probability of finding yourself in a situation where you have to interpret for a provider who gives bad news to the family of a patient. Watch the vignette on "Death and Dying" on the CCCS video *"The Healthcare Interpreter's Tools for Successful Communication in the Triadic Encounter – Vol. 2: Interpreting for Sensitive Topics."* As you watch the video, note how the interpreter "behaves" in that session. Use the space below to jot down your ideas.

How did the interpreter show empathy? How did the interpreter show a humanistic approach to the interview?

What would you do as an interpreter if the patient or a family member was crying loudly or was exhibiting their grief in an agitated manner?

____

____

____

____

Grieving varies from individual to individual and culture to culture. It is wise to recommend that the emergency room staff find an empty room with a door, so that when a provider gives bad news the family may privately show their grief, as culturally appropriate. In some cultures, it is not uncommon for patients and/or family members to have some type of seizure when informed of bad news. Others may need to scream or cry out loud. These are important ways for one to express grief, but this public expression can bother ER staff who are not comfortable with vocal expressions of grief. Ideally, the interpreter and the provider should have a mini pre-session where the interpreter could provide some culture coaching regarding the giving of bad news.

Interpreters always ask, "Can I cry if everyone else is crying or if I feel for the patient's family?" Although we ask interpreters to be as unobtrusive as possible when interpreting, it is only human for an interpreter to shed some tears. Keep in mind however that it would be inappropriate for the interpreter to sob uncontrollably, to "become" another patient, or to start sharing his/her own life story. The interpreter's tears are a form of sympathy and humanity, but not an opportunity for the interpreter to get treatment. Be human, but do not become a burden in the session.

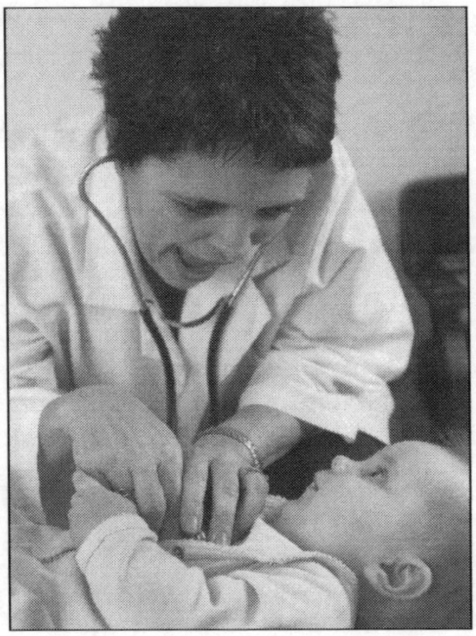

Interpreters need to be very aware of their interpreting role and not become the provider at such difficult times. When the family is distraught and waiting for news in the waiting room, it is quite common for providers to tell the interpreter what to say and ask the interpreter to explain the condition of the patient to the family. An interpreter should politely decline such a role and explain that a provider should always be present, since the interpreter's role is not to explain medicine but to interpret while another party speaks.

PO Box 2308, Woburn, MA 01888-0508, **p:** 781-729-3736, **www.EmbracingCulture.com**
PO Box 6401, Manchester, NH 03108, **p:** 1-888-678-CCCS

Top Ten Reasons for Emergency Room visits:

1. ALCOHOLISM

On occasion a person comes to the emergency room and, because of slurred speech and difficulty walking a straight line (uncoordination), it becomes clear to all that he/she is under the influence of alcohol. Often, showing up regularly and exhibiting consistent belligerence or a poor sense of physical boundaries causes the patient to be well known by emergency room staff. At times, alcoholics can become a source of irritation and thus find themselves the brunt of many jokes. However, when I was a staff interpreter at a community hospital in Massachusetts, a particular patient came for treatment with a bouquet of flowers for his favorite staff! Of course, his docile manner made him loved. Instead of laughing at him, the staff continued to coach him about his illness and refer him to the detox unit.

Alcohol Intoxication

An intoxicated patient must show one or more of the following signs that are not due to a medical cause, occurring after or shortly after alcohol use:

- Slurred speech
- Uncoordinated
- Unsteady gait
- Nystagmus
- Impairment in attention or memory
- Stupor or coma

Alcohol Withdrawal must include two or more of the following symptoms:

- Sweating
- Pulse rate greater than 100
- Increased hand tremors
- Insomnia
- Nausea, vomiting, transient visual, tactile or auditory hallucinations or illusions
- Psychomotor agitation
- Anxiety
- Grand mal seizures

The most common alcoholic does not always manifest symptoms that are easily recognized by the general public. By asking a few discerning questions, a provider will be able to determine if the patient suffers from alcoholism. Some questions directed to the patient could be:

- Can you cut down on drinking for a certain time?
- Do you ever feel you need a drink in the morning?
- Have you ever cut down your drinking?
- Are you annoyed when someone asks do you drink alcohol?
- Do you feel guilty about your drinking?

Known Facts about Alcoholism:

- **Alcoholism affects** people from all socio-economic backgrounds, genders and ages. Whereas alcoholism knows no boundaries, it is more prevalent in certain ethnic groups.
- In the United States, alcoholism is defined, **not by the quantity that one drinks, but by how the drinking affects the person's behavior at work, in the family and socially.** There are alcoholics who have jobs and do not drink every day. There are others who drink intensively at certain times of the year, unable to stop until they are intoxicated (drunk). They are called binge alcoholics. We also recognize that there are "weekend alcoholics," who only drink and get drunk on weekends.
- **Alcoholism is an illness.** Alcoholics do not drink because they are weak or because they necessarily want to drink but because they have a disease. Most individuals have at least one family member that suffers from this illness. Occasionally, as a defense mechanism, people will joke inappropriately about alcoholics and dehumanize them. Alcoholism is an incurable illness, but it is treatable. People can live sober for many years. But, never forget! Once an alcoholic, always an alcoholic!
- **There are many** alcoholics who seek help and support from community groups such as Alcoholics Anonymous (AA). Alcoholics are also urged to find an AA sponsor, and are reminded to take it one day at a time. Although new theories have appeared recently supporting the idea that alcoholics can limit their drinking, the most prevalent clinical belief is that the road to sobriety is staying "dry" (no alcohol intake). The first years of sobriety are quite challenging. Therefore, some patients feel the need to attend daily AA meetings.

Identifying Alcoholism

As previously mentioned, alcoholism is evaluated, not by the quantity or the frequency with which a person drinks, but by how the drinking affects the person's life at work, at home and socially.

There are cultures where people drink a glass of wine with every main meal. We also understand that there are a few countries, such as Germany, where people of all ages can drink beer at any time. Now, we are not assuming everyone in these countries is an alcoholic, but the incidence of alcoholism is very high in France, Portugal, Spain, Ireland and Germany.

PO Box 2308, Woburn, MA 01888-0508, **p:** 781-729-3736, **www.EmbracingCulture.com**
PO Box 6401, Manchester, NH 03108, **p:** 1-888-678-CCCS

Ethical Challenges

It can be difficult for interpreters to show complete impartiality if they conjecture that alcoholism is judged by the quantity of alcohol taken in instead of by how drinking affects a person, his/her family and work. This can result in an almost unconscious siding with a patient and his/her culture. Interpreters who have this misunderstanding regarding alcoholism need to be aware of the dangers of adding or deleting information from the interview.

Not-So-Ethical Request

Unfortunately, it is quite common to have patients in the emergency room who have just had a car accident while driving under the influence. The legal alcohol level in Massachusetts is 0.8%. Often, interpreters interpret for patients who have suffered some type of brain injury and broken bones. It is also common for intoxicated patients to have been involved in violent incidents as victims or as perpetrators. This is when police officers might ask interpreters to interpret for them as well. Our bias is that interpreters hired to cover the emergency medical situation should stick to their roles as medical interpreters. If the interpreter appears to be a conduit for both the health provider and the law enforcer, this could confuse all parties and possibly cause the patient to lose trust in the interpreter. However, interpreters need to ask for policies and guidelines in this and all interpreting matters. It can be intimidating to tell a police officer, "Sorry, I am not allowed to interpret for you because of my job description." Police officers may then ask for your name and title and the name of your supervisor, and suddenly you become the "bad person." Ideally, the entire emergency room staff should be familiar with healthcare institution policies, and the nursing supervisor should be in charge of informing police officers that they need to get their own interpreter. There are always exceptions to the rules, and an interpreter may want to walk through the different possibilities with a supervisor before having to make arbitrary decisions.

Try to think of situations similar to yours and use them as points of reference when you have to decline a not-so-ethical request regarding your role as an interpreter. For example, police officers who are also lawyers or carpenters or electricians will not perform their other jobs while wearing their police officer uniform. This may, in some way, protect the public. If a hospital has a blackout, all the patients might be at some risk, but a police officer/ electrician will not go find his tools, and leave his duties as a police officer in order to fix the electrical problems in the hospital.

Moral Courage

Following a code of ethics is an art, and interpreters must develop moral courage to refuse a job. They may immediately empathize with the request and express the wish to help but also nicely point out that a misguided attempt to help could lead to a drastic and long-term negative impact. For example, if the patient is arrested after medical treatment and the interpreter had done the interpretation for both, healthcare providers and the police, then most likely this patient will associate his/her arrest with the interpreter. By getting involved in police matters, the interpreter may complicate his/her life and find him/herself compromised when it comes to disclosing confidential medical information.

There are exceptions to this directive, however, such as when the interpreter is faced with a victim of an abuse such as rape or domestic violence.

The Ethical Interpreter

A close examination of the MEDICAL INTERPRETING STANDARDS OF PRACTICE developed by the International Medical Interpreters Association and Education Development Center, Inc. reveals the appropriate course of action. According to the Standards, the ethical interpreter has developed the following skills:

- "Can clearly separate own personal values and beliefs from those of the other parties"
- "Is able to withdraw from situations where strongly held personal values and beliefs may interfere with impartiality"
- "Lets the parties speak for themselves and does not takes sides in the conflict"
- "Remains calm in stressful situations or where there is conflict"
- "Focuses on the communication between provider and patient and refrains from interjecting personal issues, beliefs, opinions or biases"
- "Refrains from counseling or advising"

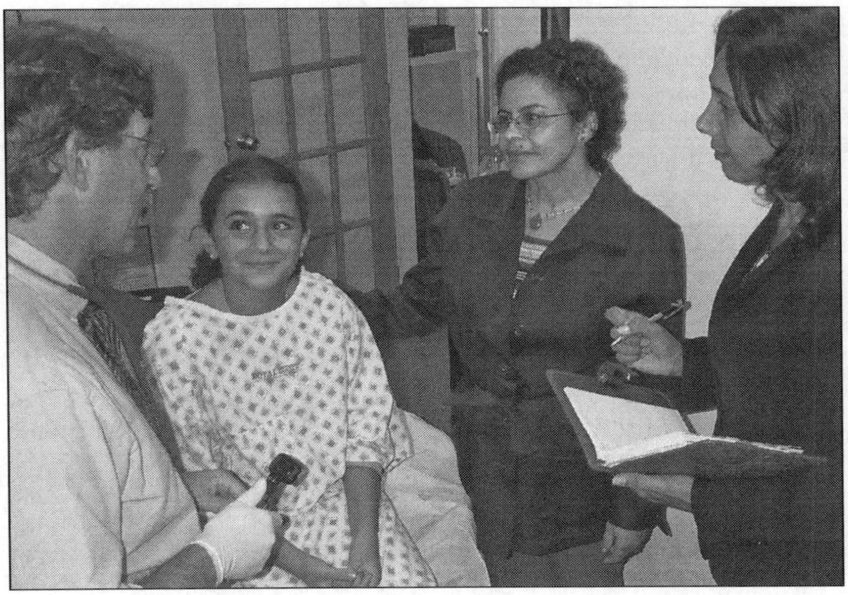

If the acute care interpreter adheres strictly to these standards of practice, s/he will have personally shared in the elevation of the profession and the promotion of equal access to quality medical care.

PO Box 2308, Woburn, MA 01888-0508, **p:** 781-729-3736, **www.EmbracingCulture.com**
PO Box 6401, Manchester, NH 03108, **p:** 1-888-678-CCCS

Role-Play 72: Battle Cry

Ms. S comes to the Emergency Room with a black eye, and a bruised lip. She came from Africa, five years ago and she speaks little English. The emergency room doctor recognizes her because she has been to the ER three times in two months with bruises. Each time there is an explanation of tripping, walking into a swinging door, or falling.

	Pronunciation	Additions	Omissions	Mistakes
MD: Ms. S., this is now the third time I've seen you with bruises. I've done a neuro exam and you are healthy. What is happening?				
S: I'm just unlucky. I trip on my daughter's toys. I fall down the stairs with laundry. I'm just so clumsy these days!				
MD: Sometimes people can have problems at home and they may not feel safe.				
(Patient hesitates. She begins to well up with tears, and just as quickly, she composes herself.)				
S: I am fine. I have a good marriage. I have a good husband. I am fine. My son is fine.				
MD: A minute ago you looked sad. What made you sad?				
S: Nothing.				
MD: You said something about your son? How old is he?				
S: 22. He is fine. He had a hard time.				
MD: What does that mean?				
S: He was drafted into the Army and sent to fight the rebels. They gave him drugs to keep him fighting long hours. He cries and sweats at night. He cannot control himself. He begs me for money for drugs.				
MD: Does he hurt you?				
S: *(Deep sigh and sobs.)* You cannot tell anyone. If my husband finds out, he'll kill the boy! You see, my husband is not the father of my son. They have never gotten along.				
MD: Is your son addicted to drugs?				
S: I think he has been since he came back from the war.				
MD: Has he ever sought help? Have you ever sought help for what he does to you?				

continued

Role-Play 72 *(continued)*

		Pronunciation	Additions	Omissions	Mistakes
S:	He is a good boy. He has gone through so much. If I asked for help, they might hurt him. He does not have papers. Can you help someone who does not have papers?				
MD:	I am sure that there is a part of him that does not want to be hurting you. And it is you who I am worried about right now. We will concentrate on helping you. It will be difficult for you but we can begin there. Are you willing to consider this?				
S:	I am ready.				
	Break It Down	☐	☐	☐	☐

☐ **CIFE with patient** ☐ **CIFE with provider** ☐ **FLOW** ☐ **REGISTER**

Role-Play 72: Glossary

continued

PO Box 2308, Woburn, MA 01888-0508, **p:** 781-729-3736, **www.EmbracingCulture.com**
PO Box 6401, Manchester, NH 03108, **p:** 1-888-678-CCCS

1. Pathology (diseases, conditions)

2. Laboratory Tests and Diagnostic Procedures

3. Treatment Procedures

4. Idiomatic Expressions (if any)

5. Other (vocabulary in this particular role-play that you feel is important/relevant or that you anticipate problems with)

2. ASTHMA

The Centers for Disease Control web page indicates that in the past 10 years the incidence of deaths from asthma increased by 80%. Children seem to be more at risk for this chronic illness, and healthcare institutions are having a difficult time managing the enormous increase.

Approximately 34.1 million Americans have been diagnosed with asthma during their life time. The prevalence of asthma increased 75% from 1980 to 1994. Not only has the prevalence of asthma increased, but the number of deaths as a result of the disease is also alarming. **Recently, the Boston Globe** in Massachusetts had an entire section dedicated to the story of two Latino children who died from asthma as they arrived at Children's Hospital. These were two children whose parents were involved in their care and very knowledgeable on how to treat and manage their children's asthma. One of the youngsters was an asthma poster child for the Department of Public Health.

It is common for providers working in emergency rooms to develop relationships with these patients and their families, since asthma patients may be frequent visitors to the ER. In fact, this chronic illness can flare up when children catch common colds. It appears that in the winter months, more interpreters will have to assist families and their children with acute incidents of asthma.

What is Asthma?

Asthma is a disease that affects your lungs. It is the most common long-term disease of children, but adults have asthma, too. **Asthma** is a condition in which the lung airways are narrowed because of hyper-reactivity of certain stimuli (pollutants, dust mites, stress, etc.) that produce inflammation and/or clog these airways. The narrowing of the airways is thought of as reversible as opposed to emphysema where airway structure is permanently distorted. In asthma, as the airway passages get narrowed, a patient exhibits different levels of breathing difficulty. This chronic illness cannot be cured but it can be treated, and patients themselves can often identify the factors that may trigger asthma attacks, also known as asthma flares.

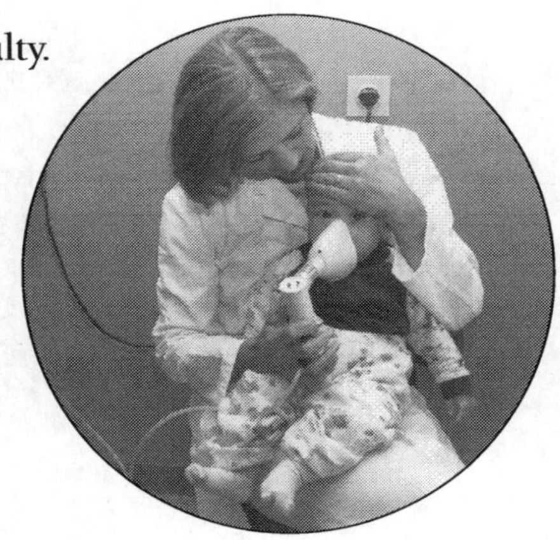

Asthma causes repeated episodes of wheezing, breathlessness, chest tightness, and nighttime or early morning coughing. If you have asthma, you have it all the time, but you will have asthma attacks only when something bothers your lungs.

PO Box 2308, Woburn, MA 01888-0508, **p:** 781-729-3736, **www.EmbracingCulture.com**
PO Box 6401, Manchester, NH 03108, **p:** 1-888-678-CCCS

What Causes Asthma?

Research is being done to establish the multiple correlations between the increase of asthma cases and changes in air and home environment. There is a possibility that the heightened presence of air pollution, due to increased numbers of cars, industrial smoke, and use of pesticides, along with respiratory infections, colds, and life stress, contribute to the increase of asthma. Other factors such as poor housing, rodents, dust mites, and mildew, may also contribute. This chronic illness is the leading cause of hospitalization for young children in this country and it is common for inner city children to be the most affected.

How Is Asthma Diagnosed?

Asthma is diagnosed by the type and timing of the symptoms. It is difficult to diagnose in children under five years old. Wheezing, chest tightness, or paroxysmal cough, especially if triggered by exercise, exposure to smoke or dust, stress or other factors will make a clinician suspect asthma.

A clinician will take a family history as part of the work up. A family history or a personal history of atopy, which includes a history of asthma, allergy or eczema, is suggestive that the symptoms a patient has may well be asthma.

The clinician will listen to a patient's lungs for high-pitched sounds of wheezing, which can suggest asthma. Acute bronchitis or pneumonia can also produce such abnormal sounds but acute illness often is accompanied by fever, chills, malaise. An acute illness such as a cold, bronchitis or pneumonia can cause asthma-like symptoms and findings, and if these are present, this can be because there is an underlying tendency to asthma.

The clinician can give a special kind of breathing test called "FEV1" which is an air flow test on a hand held spirometer. Usually the air flow is measured before a bronchodilator is given and then again after the bronchodilator medicine is taken. An improvement in flow after the medicine is administered is a sign that there is reversible bronchospasm present.

How Is Asthma Treated?

Asthma medicines come in two types - **quick-relief** and **long-term control**. Quick-relief medicines control the symptoms of an asthma attack. If you need to use your quick-relief medicines more and more, say more than two times a week, you should visit your health-care provider to see if you need a different medicine. Long-term control medicines help you have fewer and milder attacks, but they don't help you if you're having an asthma attack. In fact, some of the long term medicines if taken frequently for an attack can cause problems.

Short-term medicines are usually adrenaline derivatives that can open the constricted bronchioles. They are administered in inhalers or nebulizers. Often the simple inhaler is given with a spacer chamber(a medication inhalation apparatus) so that the medicine can be administered effectively. A nebulizer is a machine that takes liquid medicine and changes it into a suspension mist, which is easier and more efficient for patients to self administer. This is especially effective for elderly patients.

Some of the adrenaline based medicines can be given in pill form but currently it is felt that side effects are more common using the pill form than the inhaled or so called "topically" inhaled medicines.

Long-term asthma medicines may be adrenaline based. It is these medicines that if taken too frequently in an acute attack could cause problems with the heart. Often a so called long-term adrenaline based medicine is given in combination with an anti-inflammatory medicine and these are given in an inhaler. They can be given once or twice a day and work on opening bronchioles and fighting the inflammatory reaction in the airways. There is a form of anti-inflammatory medicine called "leukotrienes" which can be given as a pill also with little side effect and this is used more and more in patients. In severe cases, prednisone, which is a cortical steroid, is given either in IV form in acute attacks or as a pill for long-term effect in severe cases. Prednisone is effective in asthma but it can cause bone necrosis, cataracts, gastric ulcers, and increase blood sugar, so its use is for severe cases and the possible side effects need to be clearly spelled out to patients who use these medicines.

The type of medicine for asthma, either short or long-term and the side effects of such medicine, must be considered on a case by case basis. The clinician must help the patient with asthma by selecting the best combination of medicines, explaining their possible side effects and helping patients learn to recognize and avoid triggers that can cause acute attacks. The treatment of asthma involves a careful, close relationship with a provider who can help tailor the best medical and behavioral approaches to the patient's problems.

You can control your asthma and avoid an attack by taking your medicine exactly as your health-care provider tells you to do and by avoiding things that can cause an attack.
Not everyone with asthma takes the same medicine. Some medicines can be inhaled, or breathed in, and some can be taken in pill form. Asthma medicines can have side effects, but most side effects are mild and soon go away. Ask your healthcare provider about the side effects of your medicines.

Adapted and copied from the Centers for Disease Control and Prevention homepage, www.cdc.gov/ASTHMA

An interpreter needs to be experienced in how the nebulizer and the inhaler work. As the therapist is instructing the patient, *it might be helpful to switch to simultaneous interpretation.* Switching from one interpretation mode to another is an art, and it is recommended that interpreters practice making the switch.

PO Box 2308, Woburn, MA 01888-0508, **p:** 781-729-3736, **www.EmbracingCulture.com**
PO Box 6401, Manchester, NH 03108, **p:** 1-888-678-CCCS

Role-Play 73: Teresa's Asthma

Teresa is 12 years old. She has been wheezing, but only when she runs. It has been going on for 6 weeks. School started two weeks ago and she can't run in gym class. She coughs and wheezes. For the rest of the day she is fine, though sometimes her eyes burn and her nose runs.

	Pronunciation	Additions	Omissions	Mistakes
Mother: I am worried about my daughter, she cannot run without coughing or wheezing.				
NP: OK, anything else you're concerned about?				
Mother: Yes, my husband has a heart condition and he can't run or work hard without coughing or having chest pain. Could it be Teresa's heart?				
NP: I doubt this very much because I know Teresa well and I just examined her this summer. But I will check. Teresa, do you have any allergies?				
Teresa: Well, I don't think so.				
NP: How long have you been coughing with exercise?				
Teresa: Since the middle of August. My eyes burn and my nose runs.				
NP: And you cough after running?				
Teresa: Yes, I can get started but then I can't keep up.				
NP: Do you get pain or pressure when you exercise? Does your heart beat too fast or in a funny way?				
Teresa: I don't get pain; but my heart does go fast when I can't breathe or cough.				
NP: Do you also have this cough in cold weather?				
Teresa: Yes. I did last winter, but it went away. That was my first Christmas in Boston. I miss Rio so much.				
NP: Let me examine you.				
(Examines Patient)				
NP: Teresa, does anyone in your family have asthma or hay fever?				
Teresa: No.				
NP: Teresa, your exam and this quick breathing test you did when you came in make it look like you have exercise-induced asthma. Asthma is when the breathing tubes or bronchioles tighten up and get smaller. I think you also have some allergies, probably to ragweed because this is also ragweed season.				

continued

Role-Play 73 *(continued)*

	Pronunciation	Additions	Omissions	Mistakes
Teresa: What is ragweed?				
NP: Ragweed is a specific weed that produces pollen during the months of August and September. I am going to give you some medicine for you to take before you exercise. It is a spray. I am also going to give you some pills and drops for your allergy symptoms. The Medical Assistant will teach you to take your own peak flow at home and how to use the inhaler. I'll see you back in three weeks. You should bring in a record of your peak flow. I think you'll feel a lot better.				

Mother to the interpreter: We are having financial problems. I am so embarrassed to ask you for this very special favor. Do you think that you could loan me a few dollars so that we can take a cab home? I promise that I will pay you back tomorrow.

Break It Down	☐	☐	☐	☐

☐ **CIFE with patient** ☐ **CIFE with provider** ☐ **FLOW** ☐ **REGISTER**

Role-Play 73: Glossary

continued

PO Box 2308, Woburn, MA 01888-0508, **p:** 781-729-3736, **www.EmbracingCulture.com**
PO Box 6401, Manchester, NH 03108, **p:** 1-888-678-CCCS

1. Pathology (diseases, conditions)

2. Laboratory Tests and Diagnostic Procedures

3. Treatment Procedures

4. Idiomatic Expressions (if any)

5. Other (vocabulary in this particular role-play that you feel is important/relevant or that you anticipate problems with)

Role-Play 74: Senhor Alves' Asthma

Senhor Alves was sure he was going to die. He had smoked for thirty years and had never been able to quit the habit. He worked for many years as a bank teller in Ponta Delgada. He came here 15 years ago, but never needed to learn English. He always held jobs in maintenance and construction. Last year, he started work in his cousin's bakery. The staff baker had gone into the hospital with heart failure. Senhor Alves had been his friend and had actually gotten up early on Sunday mornings to help him bake. Now, Mr. Alves has shortness of breath and he thinks he too might have heart failure.

	Pronunciation	Additions	Omissions	Mistakes
MD: Mr. Alves how long have you had shortness of breath like this?				
Senhor: It has never been this bad! Usually, just some shortness of breath going to the bus on the way home from work. I'm afraid that it could be my heart. Tony, the baker, died from heart disease. I don't want to follow in his footsteps.				
MD: Let me examine you.				
(After Exam)				
MD: Well, Mr. Alves. There is no sign of heart trouble. Your EKG and vital signs point away from a lack of oxygen. I hear some wheezing though. Your X-ray has a few markings on it that look like interstitial disease. I think you may have sensitivity to the flour you bake with. It is a kind of asthma.				
(pause)				
Here are some inhalers. Try these out. Let me know if they help. I want you to let me know when and if the symptoms get worse.				
(patient uses inhaler)				
Are you feeling better after the treatment?				
Senhor Alves: Yes. Thank you. But if what you say is true, I will not be able to bake again.				

continued

PO Box 2308, Woburn, MA 01888-0508, **p:** 781-729-3736, **www.EmbracingCulture.com**
PO Box 6401, Manchester, NH 03108, **p:** 1-888-678-CCCS

Role-Play 74 *(continued)*

	Pronunciation	Additions	Omissions	Mistakes
MD: Let's see first. You may be able to work with a mask called a respirator. We can also do hypersensitivity tests to see if there will be problems, especially if you are on the medications.				
Break It Down	☐	☐	☐	☐

☐ CIFE with patient ☐ CIFE with provider ☐ FLOW ☐ REGISTER

Role-Play 74: Glossary

continued

1. Pathology (diseases, conditions)

2. Laboratory Tests and Diagnostic Procedures

3. Treatment procedures

4. Idiomatic Expressions (if any)

5. Other (vocabulary in this particular role-play that you feel is important/relevant or that you anticipate problems with)

PO Box 2308, Woburn, MA 01888-0508, **p:** 781-729-3736, **www.EmbracingCulture.com**
PO Box 6401, Manchester, NH 03108, **p:** 1-888-678-CCCS

3. CARDIOVASCULAR ILLNESSES

I. Chest Pain or Angina

You may be called to interpret for a patient who is experiencing chest pain. Most emergency rooms have a triage nurse who will assess the patient's chest pain before sending the patient back to the waiting room. Medical providers begin by assessing many possibilities, from the most serious possible diagnosis (cardiac arrest) to the least serious, but quite painful, (muscle pain). This process of eliminating diagnostic possibilities is called **differential diagnosis**.

Here are some important questions to determine if a patient is at imminent risk of having a myocardial infarction or a heart attack/cardiac arrest:

Does the pain travel down the patient's left arm?
Does the pain travel to the patient's back?
Is it a shooting pain?
Does the patient feel nauseated?
What type of pain is the patient experiencing?
Is it a pressured pain? (Often, patients say that they feel like a truck or an elephant is on top of their chest.)
Is this a stabbing or sharp pain?
Does the patient have a family member that has suffered from heart disease?
What medications is the patient now taking?
Does the patient experience pain when walking up stairs?
Does the patient have shortness of breath?
What makes the pain worse? What makes it better?
Did the patient take a nitroglycerin pill?
Did it help?
Does the patient get angina (chest pain) even when resting?
Does he/she smoke or drink any alcohol?
Is the patient under stress?

The pain from lack of blood to the heart is called **angina**. If the muscle goes on to die, this process is called **myocardial infarction** or heart attack.

II. Heart Attack/Myocardial Infarction

This is the dying of the heart muscle as a result of lack of oxygen. A small clot blocks off the already small coronary artery and holds blood back from supplying the heart muscle.

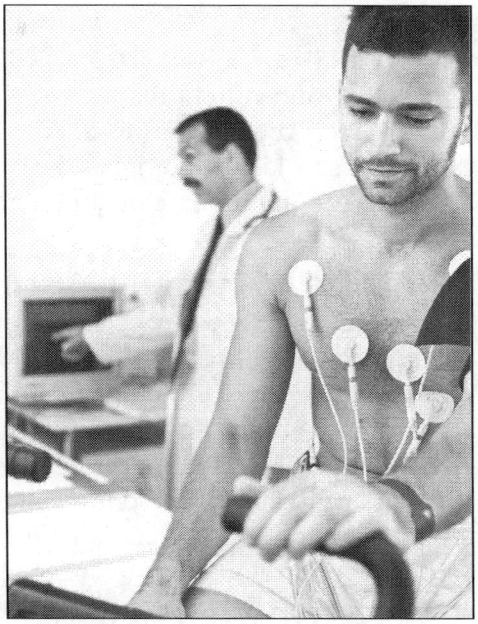

III. Arrhythmia

When the heart beats with an irregular rhythm the irregular rhythm is called an arrhythmia.

IV. Aneurysm

An aneurism is a weakening of an arterial wall so it balloons out. Sometimes, this weakened state can lead to blood cutting into the thick wall of an artery and dissecting the layers of that wall. This is very painful and dangerous.

V. Pulmonary Embolism

A painful and dangerous condition when the blood clots and moves from the heart into the lungs.

VI. Hypertension or High Blood Pressure

A painless condition that slowly adds to the harmful effects of hardening of the arteries and eventually leads to disease in large organs such as the eyes, kidneys, heart or brain.

VII. Endocarditis

An inflammation of the smooth interior lining of the heart, most likely from a bacterial or viral infection.

VIII. Shock

When blood pressure is too low causing a life threatening condition, interpreters may hear providers saying the patient is "going into shock." It may be due to low blood level (not enough for the heart to pump), perhaps caused by terrible bleeding. Victims of violence and car accidents seem to be the ones most prone to arrive at the hospital in shock. These patients should be transported by ambulance.

In the emergency room, the interpreter needs to make sure that he/she is not in the way of ER staff and that the interpreting continues. However, the interpreter may want to ask if the interpreting should continue, especially if the patient has lost consciousness. In such cases, the provider may ask the interpreter to step outside the room. This is when the interpreter might be needed to interpret for family members.

IX. Transient Ischemic Attacks (TIA)

These are intermittent disturbances of the brain as a result of a disturbance of blood supply. Often, interpreters hear providers saying that a patient is having "small strokes." Small pieces of atheromas or fatty material and calcium that is accumulated on the wall of an artery can be pushed into the brain, clogging it and causing these small TIA(s).

X. Stroke or Cerebral Vascular Accident (CVA)

A person can have a stroke or atrophy of brain tissue as a result of poor blood supply and lack of oxygen to the brain. These blockages can be manifested in two main ways: first is *ischemic stroke*, where there is a clot from a fatty tissue from one of the blood vessels or a blood clot, and therefore the blood supply to the brain is cut off. The second possibility is *hemorrhagic stroke*, when blood vessels burst, causing leakage and interrupting blood flow to the brain. When a person's right side of the brain suffers a stroke, the opposite side of the body (the left side) may show paralysis. It is crucial for providers to determine which type of stroke a patient had in order to treat the patient with the appropriate medications. If the stroke is of an ischemic nature, there is a window of three hours to give an anticoagulant called heparin. However, this medication is never given to people with high blood pressure or to patients with cerebral bleeding. In order for a provider to make this **differential diagnosis**, he/she may need to order an MRI, a CT and blood test.

It is common for patients to show up in the emergency room with partial or complete paralysis on one side of their bodies, a twisted mouth, slurred speech or no speech, difficulty swallowing their own saliva, drooling and looking depressed. This is a very traumatic experience for the patient and for family members because it happens all of a sudden and recovery is dependent on the amount of damage done and the patient's general health status. Some patients completely recover, but others will need intensive rehab, and some 20% may die from the stroke.

XI. Peripheral Arterial Disease

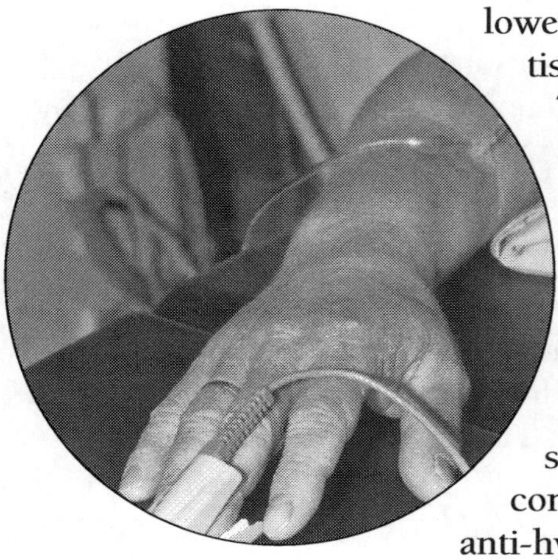

When atherosclerosis affects arteries that supply limbs, especially the lower extremities, there can be skin ulcerations or more serious tissue destruction because of lack of blood supply to the limbs. This is called peripheral arterial disease. (PAD) The process of blockage in the limbs is analogous to the process of blockage in the heart. Some people demonstrate atherosclerosis in one place like the heart, brain, or legs, but it is important to know that if a patient has a blockage in one place, chances are they are developing it in the other parts of the body as well. Treatment of a blockage acutely may require angioplasty, stents or even bypass surgery. Long term treatment includes stopping smoking, control of cholesterol with statin medicines and the use of the anti-hypertensive class of medicine called ACE inhibitors.

Role-Play 75: Mr. Ally's Unstable Angina

Mr. Ally was not happy. Last year, the doctor told him his chest pain was from heart disease. In fact, the pain was getting so bad that Mr. Ally had a catheterization and one of his coronary arteries had to be opened up. They put a tube in the artery called a stent, which could prevent him from having open-heart surgery. After the stent was placed, Mr. Ally had some atrial fibrillation. It immediately went away. Mr. Ally wore two Holter monitors and had an echocardiogram, but the fibrillation did not come back. Mr. Ally's doctor took him off the blood thinner and he has not had to worry about blood thinners or atrial fibrillation since.

Every day, Mr. Ally takes medicine for his blood pressure, one is called a beta-blocker and the other an ace inhibitor. He also takes medicine for his cholesterol, and a coated aspirin. He used to take Nitroglycerin under his tongue for the chest pain. He had not needed it since the stent placement. However, during the past two weeks, he's been taking it again. The pain is back.

	Pronunciation	Additions	Omissions	Mistakes
MD: Hello, Mr. Ally. The medical assistant said your pain is back.				
Mr. Ally: Yes, Doctor. I have had it for two weeks. But I am worried. Instead of coming when I climb stairs or exert myself, the pain comes when I'm at rest.				
MD: Does it go away when you take the nitro?				
Mr. Ally: Yes. But today it came right back.				
MD: Do you have sweating or palpitations with this pain?				
Mr. Ally: No.				
MD: Do you feel faint?				
Mr. Ally: Well, I felt dizzy this morning.				
MD: Let me examine you.				
(Examines patient and does an EKG)				
MD: Well, Mr. Ally. You were very smart to come in. I think you may have re-stenosed your stent. This means that there is either a clot or plaque in the stent and it is difficult to get blood to your heart muscle. I am worried because the left anterior descending coronary artery that has the stent feeds a very important heart muscle. If it is re-stenosed, it could give you problems.Having pain at rest concerns me. I'd like to send you to the hospital now and ask the cardiologists what they think. Is that all right with you?				

continued

PO Box 2308, Woburn, MA 01888-0508, **p:** 781-729-3736, **www.EmbracingCulture.com**
PO Box 6401, Manchester, NH 03108, **p:** 1-888-678-CCCS

Role-Play 75 *(continued)*

	Pronunciation	Additions	Omissions	Mistakes
Mr. Ally: OK. I will drive there right now.				
MD: I'd rather you didn't drive yourself. I am going to call for an ambulance to take you.				
Mr. Ally: Oh doctor, I'm not that sick. I'll drive right over.				
MD: Mr. Ally, driving in Boston during rush hour is a known stress. I'd rather you experience stress under the watchful eye of the emergency room doctor at Brigham and Women's Hospital, not alone on Storrow Drive.				
Mr. Ally: Now you're scaring me.				
MD: I'm sorry. You'll be fine, but I'd like to get you in as soon as possible. You will most likely be admitted. I'll see you there in the morning.				
Mr. Ally: May I borrow your phone? I'll ask my son to come and pick up my car. He can bring my wife, right? Can she ride with me in the ambulance?				
MD: No problem.				
Mr. Ally: Thank you. Does this mean I might need surgery?				
MD: It's a possibility, but if they can do this with stents, they will.				
Mr. Ally: Thank you.				

Client to the Interpreter: Do you think that I am going to die? Please don't tell my wife anything that the doctor said. She is a very nervous person and her nerves can go to her head. Several years ago she went to one of these hospitals for people who suffer from nerves. I'm OK., really!

Break It Down	☐	☐	☐	☐

☐ **CIFE with patient** ☐ **CIFE with provider** ☐ **FLOW** ☐ **REGISTER**

Role-Play 75: Glossary

______________ ______________ ______________

______________ ______________ ______________

______________ ______________ ______________

______________ ______________ ______________

______________ ______________ ______________

continued

1. Pathology (diseases, conditions)

2. Laboratory Tests and Diagnostic Procedures

3. Treatment Procedures

4. Idiomatic Expressions (if any)

5. Other (vocabulary in this particular role-play that you feel is important/relevant or that you anticipate problems with)

PO Box 2308, Woburn, MA 01888-0508, **p:** 781-729-3736, **www.EmbracingCulture.com**
PO Box 6401, Manchester, NH 03108, **p:** 1-888-678-CCCS

Role-Play 76: Sylvestre's Stroke

		Pronunciation	Additions	Omissions	Mistakes
MD:	Mr. Sylvestre, I have reviewed your CT scan.				
S:	Yes, Doctor.				
MD:	It shows that you have had a CVA, a small stroke in the left part of your brain that controls your right side and that is why it is difficult for you to move your right arm and hand.				
S:	I understand.				
MD:	Also, it touched the area on the left side of your brain that controls your speech, which is why initially when you had the stroke, you couldn't speak or move your right side. It immediately got better along with your strength and that bodes well for a speedy recovery.				
S:	Should I also get an MRI?				
MD:	No, I think we're lucky to get all the information we need. I will need to get an EKG, and a special echocardiogram called a transesophageal echo. This stroke occurred at the same time that you had the blood clot in your leg. I want to make sure that you don't have a hole in your heart, which would allow a clot in the leg to travel to the head. We also have to check ultrasounds of your carotids to make sure there is no clot there which could have contributed to the stroke.				
S:	So what if you find a hole in my heart?				
MD:	We'll have several choices. One is to just continue giving you coumadin to thin your blood for the rest of your life. Second, we can arrange for a mesh to be inserted via a catheter to close off the hole. Third, we can have an open-heart surgical repair of the defect.				
S:	I hate surgery.				
MD:	Well, if that's the case, you're in luck, because it is reasonable to continue the coumadin. But it means monthly blood tests and visits with the nurse practitioner.				
S:	Compared with heart surgery, that sounds good. Is the mesh placement dangerous?				

continued

Role-Play 76 *(continued)*

		Pronunciation	Additions	Omissions	Mistakes
MD:	It's a new procedure, fairly well tolerated, but we don't know a lot about how long it lasts or its long-term safety. Why don't we see what the echo shows and then we'll talk some more?				
S:	OK, and I will continue the coumadin. Yes, that's important.				
	Break It Down	☐	☐	☐	☐

☐ **CIFE with patient** ☐ **CIFE with provider** ☐ **FLOW** ☐ **REGISTER**

Role-Play 76: Glossary

continued

PO Box 2308, Woburn, MA 01888-0508, **p:** 781-729-3736, **www.EmbracingCulture.com**
PO Box 6401, Manchester, NH 03108, **p:** 1-888-678-CCCS

1. Pathology (diseases, conditions)

2. Laboratory Tests and Diagnostic Procedures

3. Treatment Procedures

4. Idiomatic Expressions (if any)

5. Other (vocabulary in this particular role-play that you feel is important/relevant or that you anticipate problems with)

4. TRAUMATIC BRAIN INJURY (TBI)

Traumatic brain injury (TBI) results from an external physical force that produces in its victims an altered state of consciousness. It is estimated that one million people a year are treated for TBI in hospital emergency rooms, while over 50,000 die each year as a result of this type of injury.

The risk of TBI is highest among young people and the elderly. Young people are most likely to suffer from vehicular TBI, which accounts for 50% of all traumatic brain injuries. Some major factors in vehicular TBI are inexperienced driving, not using a seat belt, speeding, and substance abuse.

Falls are the leading cause of brain injury in the elderly. There are many reasons why the elderly are most likely to fall. Some take medications that affect perception and balance. Others have pre-existing medical conditions such as visual or orthopedic impairment. Also, an increasing number of elderly persons are exposed to hazardous living conditions.

A third leading cause of TBI is violence, primarily from firearms. It is interesting to note that 2/3 of firearm-related traumatic brain injuries are classified as suicidal in intent.

A TBI patient may be faced with cognitive challenges, such as memory loss, learning blocks, lack of sustained concentration, difficulty carrying on conversation, and impaired judgment. Physical challenges could include the loss of smell or taste, general fatigue, double vision or blindness, seizures, speech impediments and headaches. Emotional impairments might include lack of self-motivation, increased anxiety, depression, mood swings, and impulsive behavior.

According to a new report by the Centers for Disease Control and Prevention, an estimated 5.3 million Americans currently live with disabilities from traumatic brain injuries.

Adapted from the Brain Injury Association of America home page, www.biausa.org.

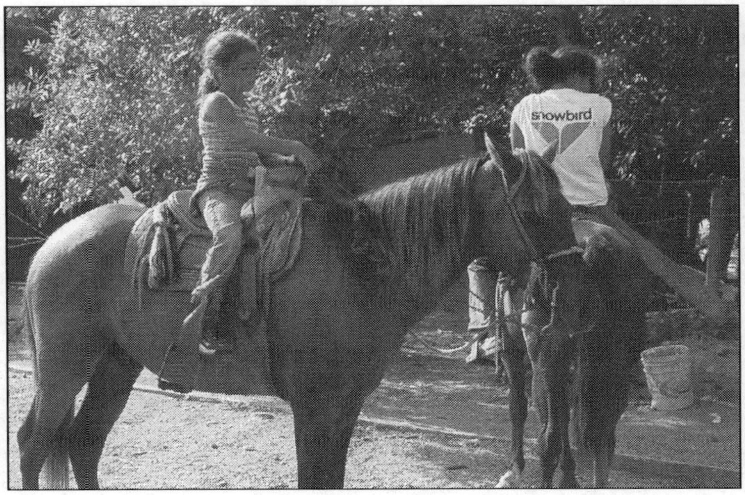

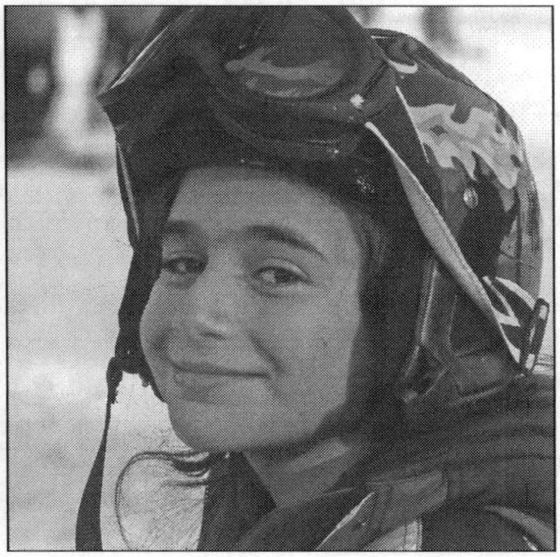

PO Box 2308, Woburn, MA 01888-0508, **p:** 781-729-3736, **www.EmbracingCulture.com**
PO Box 6401, Manchester, NH 03108, **p:** 1-888-678-CCCS

Role-Play 77: TBI Bicycle

A 13-year-old girl has a bicycle accident and is driven to the hospital by ambulance.

	Pronunciation	Additions	Omissions	Mistakes
MD: Carla, can you hear me? Do you know where you are now? Can you feel your toes when I squeeze them?				
(Patient looks somnolent and confused)				
Nurse: Carla, it is very important that you answer us. Do you know what happened to you?				
Patient: I want my sister. Why am I here? What happened? Who are you?				
MD: The ambulance just brought you in to the hospital. A car was turning right at a red light, and because of the rain the driver did not see you. Your bicycle got hit by the front bumper of the car and it appears that you did a summersault and landed with your head on the windshield.				
Patient: I do not know what happened. I was going to pick up some groceries for my mother.				
MD: You know, I need to contact one of your parents. We checked your pockets and we do not have any information on you. A person on the street told the ambulance driver and the police that your name was Carla. You were new in the neighborhood. Are you Carla?				
Patient: Why am I all tied up in this wood and sheets?				
MD: The EMTs (emergency medical technicians) stabilized you so that by moving you onto the stretcher, we wouldn't do more harm to your head injury. It will be a bit uncomfortable, but this is for your own good. I need to know your full name and a telephone number where I can contact your parents.				
Patient: I do not know my mother's telephone number at work.				
Nurse: Is there anyone in your family or neighborhood that can be contacted?				

continued

Role-Play 77 *(continued)*

	Pronunciation	Additions	Omissions	Mistakes
Patient: I only live a few blocks away from the high school, the street is, you know, next to the yellow big house as you turn left at the high school. My grandmother should be home. My house is the white house right next to the blue house.				
MD: I will let the police know and they will send a cruiser there. Does your grandmother speak English?				
Patient: Oh, no.				
MD: I will see what we can do. Meanwhile, I am going to spend some time examining you and we will be sending you for all kinds of tests. I will also be placing this oxygen mask on you, just like a Halloween mask, so that your brain gets all the oxygen it needs to keep you smart.				
Patient: Do I really need this? It feels so cold!				
MD: Oh, yes! You will need the mask until we're all set with the test results.				
Nurse: How are you doing? I am going to take your vital signs, and check your temperature and blood pressure. I will check your eyes and I am going to do a quick neurological exam. This means that I'll need to check your reflexes, ask you to blink your eyes, and to follow my fingers with your eyes. Can you feel me tickling your toes? I'm going to prick you with this pin. Can you feel it? Is it sharp or dull?				
Patient: Yes, I can feel it. It's like a needle.				
Nurse: Good, so now tell me which one you feel is sharper, the right foot or the left?				
Patient: I do not know!				
Nurse: Let's try again. (Pricks patient). The right foot, or the left?				
Patient: This one. (She lifts up the right). I do not know…I guess it is the same.				
MD: The vital signs and the neurological exam went well. We are still a bit concerned because you cannot remember the accident and you have some black and blue bruises on your head and face. We are going to send you for a CT scan (computed tomography). I am looking for possible blood clots and fractures.				
Patient: What is a CT scan?				

continued

PO Box 2308, Woburn, MA 01888-0508, **p:** 781-729-3736, **www.EmbracingCulture.com**
PO Box 6401, Manchester, NH 03108, **p:** 1-888-678-CCCS

Role-Play 77 *(continued)*

	Pronunciation	Additions	Omissions	Mistakes
MD: We also call it "Cat Scan" and it basically scans a series of cross-sectional x-ray images of the head and brain and can show bone fractures. It can also show hematomas, contusions, and brain tissue swelling.				
Patient: I still do not understand it. Are you going to put any needles in me?				
MD: Oh, no, this is painless and I really need you to go through with it. The police found your house and the neighbor knows where your mother's work is.				
Patient: Oh, boy! She's going to kill me!				
Nurse: I will take you to radiology. You will have a CT scan and a few X-rays of your head, back and wrists, just in case you have a fracture.				
Patient: Actually, it's my fingers and knuckles that really hurt.				
Nurse: We'll check on that too. Now remember, we do not want you to move from the stretcher before the CT scan.				
Patient: OK, how do I get to the bathroom?				
Nurse: I just put a catheter in you, so you may go to the bathroom whenever you feel like it.				
(After the CT scan)				
MD: You are a very lucky girl. Despite all the bruising and the fact that you were not wearing your helmet, you only have a small concussion. There is no significant swelling and no hematomas or blood clots. As soon as your mother arrives, we can go over your treatment during the next forty-eight hours and schedule a follow-up visit in three weeks for an MRI.				
Patient: What is a concussion?				
MD: Concussion is a mild bruising of your brain. You need to be watched for any short losses of consciousness. I'm happy that although you do not recall the accident, you can still have a logical conversation with me.				
Patient: I only feel nauseated and a bit dizzy.				
MD: You may get headaches and you may have some difficulty concentrating at school or recalling recent information. With time, most of your memory will return and the other symptoms may improve.				

continued

Role-Play 77 *(continued)*	Pronunciation	Additions	Omissions	Mistakes
(Mother arrives)				
MD: I am so glad that we were able to find you! As you see, your daughter could have had more serious injuries. She got a mild concussion, but still we need to watch her.				
Mother: I have told Carla that she is not allowed to go riding without a helmet. I feel like giving her a big spanking! I am glad she is all right. God really must have been on her side!				
MD: The fact that Carla was not wearing a helmet put her at risk for greater damage to her head and brain. I was worried about the potential for blood clots, but the results of the CT scan were reassuring. She could have had a skull fracture, and if the bone around her brain had broken she might have needed surgery. Or even worse, she could have had what we call the coup/contre-coup, which is a contusion occurring on both sides of the brain. This can happen when an impact causes the brain to hit the opposite side of the skull, damaging both the side initially hit and its opposite side. Not wearing a helmet for almost any kind of sport is a dangerous behavior. Our emergency room staff can help you get a helmet for free. I will ask the social worker to come by before you all leave today.				
Mother: *(Crying)* I work two jobs so that I can support my family and I expect my kids to follow the rules. The rules are for their good. I do not know what else to do with my kids.				
MD: Carla seems to be a very good child. These are the challenges of raising teenagers and I think that you may want to tap into our resources to support you in parenting issues. We will move on from here and this terrible accident can be an opportunity for improvement.				
Mother: Carla, did you hear the doctor? Please pay attention.				

continued

PO Box 2308, Woburn, MA 01888-0508, **p:** 781-729-3736, **www.EmbracingCulture.com**
PO Box 6401, Manchester, NH 03108, **p:** 1-888-678-CCCS

Role-Play 77 *(continued)*

	Pronunciation	Additions	Omissions	Mistakes
MD: There are different types of brain injury and each person can experience different side effects. It all depends on the seriousness of the injury. Although with the CT scan and MRI, (Magnetic Resonance Imaging), we can take a pretty good picture of the status of the injury, we still need to watch the brain activity very carefully. We need to watch for brain edema. This is when the brain tissue gets so swollen as result of the injury that it pushes the other contents of the brain against the skull. Look at this picture of a normal brain.				
Mother and Carla: Hmm.				
MD: See, the brain tissue, the blood vessels and the ventricles look good and healthy. Now take a look at a brain with edema. Show me the difference between one and the other.				
Mother and Carla: Wow!				
MD: What did the two of you notice?				
Mother: The brain tissue is so much bigger. It almost lost the different rounded shapes. It looks like one big mass.				
Carla: In this picture, it looks like one side got all swollen. Is this what can still happen to me?				
MD: Yes, you both are very observant. The brain tissue pushed the contents of the brain against the skull. Here are signs to look for in the next 48 hours: headaches, loss of consciousness, nausea, vomiting, confusion, changes in behavior, fever, and blindness. Mom, you will need to stay home with your daughter. Do you need a letter for work?				
Mother: Yes, doctor. But do you think that she is going to go crazy?				
MD: Brain injuries can be tricky and we can't always predict the long-term impact of each injury. The good thing is that Carla was very lucky and she will go through a series of MRI studies to look for any possible tissue changes.				

continued

Role-Play 77 *(continued)*

	Pronunciation	Additions	Omissions	Mistakes
Carla: What is an MRI?				
MD: An MRI uses magnetic fields to detect subtle changes in brain tissue content and gives us a more detailed image than the CT scan or the X-ray. Your CT scan was pretty good, but I'd still like to send you for an MRI. The MRI machine is like a big tunnel that you lie in and you can choose to listen to music during the exam. You'll need to remove metal objects from your body and pockets during the 45 minutes it takes to run the test.				
Break It Down	☐	☐	☐	☐

☐ **CIFE with patient** ☐ **CIFE with provider** ☐ **FLOW** ☐ **REGISTER**

Role-Play 77: Glossary

continued

PO Box 2308, Woburn, MA 01888-0508, **p:** 781-729-3736, **www.EmbracingCulture.com**
PO Box 6401, Manchester, NH 03108, **p:** 1-888-678-CCCS

1. Pathology (diseases, conditions)

2. Laboratory Tests and Diagnostic Procedures

3. Treatment Procedures

4. Idiomatic Expressions (if any)

5. Other (vocabulary in this particular role-play that you feel is important/relevant or that you anticipate problems with)

5. COLD AND FLU

Colds

Often, interpreters are called into emergency rooms to interpret for patients with scratchy throats, runny noses, sneezing, poor nasal breathing, sinus swelling and headaches. Each year, more than 1 billion US residents get colds. Youngsters average 6 to 10 colds per year. The general adult population averages 2 to 4 colds each year. Colds are one of the main reasons why people miss work. Fortunately, adults over the age of 60 average less than 1 cold per year. Colds are most common in the fall and winter, and symptoms may last 1 to 2 weeks.

More than 200 different viruses cause colds. These viruses cannot be treated with antibiotics. The National Institutes of Health (NIH) report that rhinoviruses seldom produce serious illnesses, and are most common among children. Parainfluenza and respiratory syncytial virus produce mild infections in adults but can trigger severe lower respiratory infections in children. Coronaviruses are responsible for a large percentage of all adult colds. Other more damaging viruses are adenoviruses, coxsackieviruses, echoviruses, and orthomyxoviruses (including influenza A and B).

Symptoms of a cold can also be present in patients with **STREP THROAT**. Although the symptoms of strep throat and colds are similar, strep is caused by a specific type of bacteria called Group A hemolytic streptococci. Strep is not a virus.

A patient usually feels sicker with strep than with a common sore throat, and often has pus on either or both of the tonsils, and swollen, tender lymph nodes in the throat area. It is crucial that a patient who feels that s/he may have strep throat be tested, since certain types of strep may cause serious problems if not appropriately treated. A throat culture or strep test is used to appropriately diagnose strep. Patients may be prescribed an antibiotic and aspirin or Tylenol. However, children and adolescents should not take Aspirin, since it has been known to cause Reye's syndrome, a serious brain and liver disorder.

Flu (Influenza)

Flu is very contagious and strikes suddenly. Patients with the flu complain of general weakness, muscle aches, fever, and headache. It is also common for patients to have a runny nose and sore throat. An untreated flu may cause pneumonia. Influenza is potentially fatal in the elderly, patients with compromised immune systems, young children, and pregnant women.

Influenza is caused by multiple viruses. Public health departments develop flu shots according to the prevalence of certain viruses during a particular flu season. Interpreters will need to be prepared to read flu sheet instructions and consent forms. This is called **sight interpretation**.

PO Box 2308, Woburn, MA 01888-0508, **p:** 781-729-3736, **www.EmbracingCulture.com**
PO Box 6401, Manchester, NH 03108, **p:** 1-888-678-CCCS

Ideally, the provider should be the one reading and the interpreter should be the conduit of the information being read. If an interpreter does use sight interpretation, it is always important that the provider be present at the time of the reading. Interpreters must refrain from explaining to patients their understanding of fact sheets and consent forms. Interestingly, most state departments of public health have flu fact sheets translated into several languages. Interpreters may want to browse the internet for this information.

Role-Play 78: Strep Throat?

Sara, who came from Bosnia six months ago, is 15 years old and learning English. She has been sick for one week. She had been feeling very tired and then developed a sore throat. She had a fever and now it is very painful for her to swallow. Her mother, who works at a factory, let her stay home from school for the week. But now that Sara can't swallow well, her mother is worried and wants the Doctor to check her out.

	Pronunciation	Additions	Omissions	Mistakes
MD: Hello Sara, what brings you into the office today?				
Sara: I have had a sore throat and it is now so bad I				
cannot swallow.				
MD: How long have you been sick?				
Sara: I started feeling tired last week for several days; then a week ago today, I got this sore throat. Four days ago, I got a fever. It has been 99 to 100 degrees Fahrenheit since. The pain has gotten so bad I cannot swallow. And my brother thinks my voice sounds funny.				
MD: Have you had a cough or shortness of breath?				
Sara: No.				
MD: Anyone else you know, have this kind of illness?				
Sara: Well, my boyfriend stayed home from school last week. He had a sore throat and a fever. Now he's better. He didn't have problems with his swallowing or talking.				
MD: Have you had any stomach pain?				
Sara: Well, I have had some pain under my rib.				
(She points to the right side of her thorax)				
MD: Well let's do the exam. First, let me check your ears. I'll take this Otoscope and look inside each of your ears. They look fine.				

continued

Role-Play 78 *(continued)*

	Pronunciation	Additions	Omissions	Mistakes
MD: I will examine your neck and chin in order to see if you have lymph node enlargement. Yes, you have swollen lymph nodes, especially here on the right. (Sara winces with pain.) Sorry, I know it's tender. Hope I didn't hurt you. This gland here, at the angle of your jaw is called the digastric gland. It is swollen and tender. Now let's look in your mouth. The right tonsil is quite enlarged. It also has white exudates or pus on it. The left tonsil is not as bad but is still enlarged. The right one is so large that it is getting in the way when you try to swallow. Now I'll examine your lungs, heart, and abdomen. Hmm, it seems your right upper quadrant of your abdomen is tender. I don't feel an enlarged liver though. Now I'll take a swab of your throat. We'll do two tests. One is a short test for streptococcal bacteria; and the other is a blood test for a complete blood count, liver enzymes and mononucleosis. Come back after these tests are done, the white count and the rapid strep analysis will be done in half an hour.				
(Later)				
PT: Doctor, how are the tests?				
MD: Sara, I believe you have mononucleosis. The test for rapid strep was negative. It is not perfect but very helpful. Your white count was low, which can mean that there is a virus present and your differential or analysis of the white cells shows almost 20% mononuclear cells. I am going to give you an IV now and run some Solumedrol in your vein. This will bring down the swelling of your tonsil so you will be able to swallow and talk. I'll then give you pills of prednisone, to help keep the swelling down, an antibiotic that will fight any bacterial infection, like strep, that may be present along with the virus, and some oxycodone for the pain.				
PT: How long will I take the pills?				

continued

PO Box 2308, Woburn, MA 01888-0508, **p:** 781-729-3736, **www.EmbracingCulture.com**
PO Box 6401, Manchester, NH 03108, **p:** 1-888-678-CCCS

Role-Play 78 *(continued)*

	Pronunciation	Additions	Omissions	Mistakes
MD: The prednisone taper is for ten days. The antibiotics are for ten days. The pain pills you can stop when your throat is better. I will get the remainder of the tests tomorrow and I will call you to tell you the results. In the meantime, if you have difficulty breathing or swallowing you can call my answering service anytime. I'd like for you to stay out of school for the remainder of the week. Also, I think you may have inflammation of your liver from the mono, you should not drink any alcohol.				
PT: I am Muslim and I do not drink alcohol.				
MD: That's good. Also, for the time being, don't use Tylenol until I see how much your liver is involved.				
PT: What should I tell my boyfriend? Is this contagious?				
MD: If he is still sick, he should see his MD for similar tests. If he is now better, that's good.				
Break It Down	☐	☐	☐	☐

☐ **CIFE with patient** ☐ **CIFE with provider** ☐ **FLOW** ☐ **REGISTER**

Role-Play 78: Glossary

continued

1. Pathology (diseases, conditions)

2. Laboratory Tests and Diagnostic Procedures

3. Treatment Procedures

4. Idiomatic Expressions (if any)

5. Other (vocabulary in this particular role-play that you feel is important/relevant or that you anticipate problems with)

PO Box 2308, Woburn, MA 01888-0508, **p:** 781-729-3736, **www.EmbracingCulture.com**
PO Box 6401, Manchester, NH 03108, **p:** 1-888-678-CCCS

6. FOOD POISONING

Food poisoning is understood as any disease of an infectious or toxic nature caused by the consumption of food or drink. The populations most at risk for food poisoning are children, the elderly, and others with impaired immune systems, such as pregnant women, HIV/AIDS patients, and patients diagnosed with Hepatitis.

Patients suffering from food poisoning may arrive at the hospital with different levels of severity. It can take from approximately 6 to 12 hours to several days before a person begins to experience food poisoning symptoms, which include a general feeling of weakness, diarrhea, vomiting, dizziness, and stomach cramps. These symptoms are caused by a bacterial germ, often Staphylococcus, which produces a toxin while growing in food.

Some of the symptoms for food poisoning are similar to other allergen reactions. They vary from mild to deadly:

- hives
- tingling in the mouth
- swelling in the tongue and throat
- difficulty breathing
- abdominal cramps
- vomiting or diarrhea
- eczema or rash
- coughing or wheezing
- loss of consciousness
- dizziness

Food Poisoning: The Most Common Foodborne Illnesses

According to http://www.cdc.gov/ncidod/dbmd/diseaseinfo/foodborneinfections_g.htm#mostcommon

The most commonly recognized food borne infections are caused by the bacteria, Campylobacter, Salmonella and Ecolab 0157:H7 and by a group of viruses called calicivirus also known as Norwalk or Norwalk-like viruses.

1. **Campylobacter** is bacterial causing fever, diarrhea and abdominal cramps. It is the most commonly identified bacterial cause of diarrhea illness in the world. It lives in intestines of healthy birds and most raw poultry meat has Campylobacter on it. Eating uncooked chicken or food contaminated with juices dripping from raw chicken is the most important source of infecti
2. **Salmonella** is found in intestines of birds, reptiles and mammals. It can spread to humans via different foods of animal origin. Usually, the disease includes fever, diarrhea and abdominal cramps. It comes on 6-72 hours after consuming contaminated food. Symptoms can last from 3-5 days. In persons with poor health or weakened immune system, it can invade and cause life threatening infectious days.
3. **E. coli 0157:H7** is found in cattle and other similar animals. Human illness occurs with consumption of food contaminated with small amounts of cow fecies. The illness is often severe and bloody diarrhea and painful abdominal cramps without much fever. In small amount of cases, a complicat ion called hemolytic uremic syndrome can occur weeks after initial presentation. This causes anemia, profuse bleeding and kidney failure.
4. **Calicivirus** or Norwalk-like virus is very common cause of foodborne illness.

   Instead of having an animal reservouir, these viruses tend to transmit person to person.

In addition to disease from direct infection some of the common food borne illness can be caused by a toxin in the food that was produced by a bacterium in the food. Staphylococcus aureas can produce a toxin that causes intense vomiting. Another example of a toxin is the rare, but powerful toxin from clostridium botulinum which produces the toxin producing botulism which can paralyze or make people's muscles contract in agony.

PO Box 2308, Woburn, MA 01888-0508, **p:** 781-729-3736, **www.EmbracingCulture.com**
PO Box 6401, Manchester, NH 03108, **p:** 1-888-678-CCCS

Role-Play 79: Salmonella

		Pronunciation	Additions	Omissions	Mistakes
MD:	How can I help you?				
PT:	I have been very sick for three days. I have a headache, fever and the worse abdominal cramps and diarrhea you've ever seen.				
MD:	Do you have blood in your stool?				
PT:	No, but they are watery.				
MD:	Have you had nausea or vomiting?				
PT:	Yup, last night I was in the bathroom and I was sick from both ends. What a nightmare!				
MD:	Have you done any traveling?				
PT:	No.				
MD:	Have you eaten anything in the past week that could have made you sick or made a friend sick?				
PT:	Well, four days ago, I went to the gym and afterwards my friends and I ate raw eggs in a power drink. Now that you mention it, my lifting partner is sick too, but he didn't get it like I did. He hasn't missed work.				
MD:	Where did you buy the eggs?				
PT:	From a corner store in my neighborhood.				
MD:	You didn't buy them from a farmer's market?				
PT:	No.				
MD:	Do you have a fever?				
PT:	Not now.				
MD:	Let's examine you.				
	(MD examines patient)				
MD:	Well your exam is good but your blood pressure is very low. I think you have become dehydrated. I am going to give you some fluids in an IV over the next few hours and I think you will feel a lot better. The nurse will come in and draw your blood, then put an IV in.				
PT:	Do you think I really need it?				
MD:	Well, don't you feel a little dizzy when you stand?				
PT:	Well, yes.				

continued

Role-Play 79 *(continued)*

	Pronunciation	Additions	Omissions	Mistakes
MD: That means you are dehydrated. You will feel much better after the IV.				
PT: Are you going to give me some medicine for this?				
MD: I don't think so. I think you'll do fine if you drink clear liquids and stay away from dairy. Do you think you could go to the bathroom and give me a stool sample for a culture?				
PT: Absolutely.				
MD: Good. I think you may have gotten salmonella. It is a bacterial diarrheal illness that can be found in poultry, meat and eggs. I won't need to give you an antibiotic unless the culture shows something of concern.				
PT: What about the diarrhea? It is really a pain.				
MD: Well, at night you can take 2mg of Imodium so you can get some sleep. During the day you can drink clear liquids and move your bowels as much as you need to as long as you are getting fluids. Let's get started. After the IV, you are going to feel much better.				
Break It Down	☐	☐	☐	☐

☐ **CIFE with patient** ☐ **CIFE with provider** ☐ **FLOW** ☐ **REGISTER**

Role-Play 79: Glossary

continued

PO Box 2308, Woburn, MA 01888-0508, **p:** 781-729-3736, **www.EmbracingCulture.com**
PO Box 6401, Manchester, NH 03108, **p:** 1-888-678-CCCS

1. Pathology (disease conditions)

2. Laboratory Tests and Diagnostic Procedures

3. Treatment Procedures

4. Idiomatic Expressions (if any)

5. Other (vocabulary in this particular role-play that you feel is important/relevant or that you anticipate problems with)

Role-Play 80: Shigella

A mother and child come to the emergency room with symptoms of dysentery.

		Pronunciation	Additions	Omissions	Mistakes
PT:	My daughter and I have been literally pooping our guts out. We've both been passing this terrible brown water for about four days. We've both been vomiting too, and neither one of us can keep anything down.				
MD:	You look pale. Is there any blood with your diarrhea?				
PT:	Yes, and that is what scares me. Look at my daughter's diaper!				
MD:	Any other recent health-related concerns?				
PT:	Not for me, but my daughter had runny poops about five days ago. She even got a bit of a diaper rash, even though I tried to stay on top of it. But now it looks like we've got the same thing.				
MD:	Did you or your daughter recently eat raw meat or eggs?				
PT:	No, I like my food well done.				
MD:	Any fever?				
PT:	I feel a bit warmer than usual.				
MD:	Your temperature is ninety-nine. Were there any changes in your daily routines? Any recent traveling or visits to unusual places, like a farm or zoo?				
PT:	We went to visit some friends who have a baby around my daughter's age. We were swimming in their pool, and I noticed some poop at the bottom. You know how kids are with swallowing pool water.				
MD:	How long ago was this?				
PT:	Just this past weekend.				
MD:	Did you find out if your friend's baby was suffering from diarrhea?				
PT:	Yes, he has been having diarrhea for several days and now the entire family's got the runs.				
MD:	Let me call the IV nurse and order an antibiotic. Meanwhile I will be taking a swab of the rectal mucus from both of you so I can take a look and also send a stool sample to the lab.				
PT:	Okay, but right now, you're not exactly my favorite person!				

continued

PO Box 2308, Woburn, MA 01888-0508, **p:** 781-729-3736, **www.EmbracingCulture.com**
PO Box 6401, Manchester, NH 03108, **p:** 1-888-678-CCCS

Role-Play 80 *(continued)*

	Pronunciation	Additions	Omissions	Mistakes
MD: Sorry about that. What type of work do you do?				
PT: I work at a local bar a few nights each week.				
MD: Have you been to work since you started with the symptoms?				
PT: No, I was hoping to feel better first.				
(Examines the patient and takes stool samples for wet prep and culture.)				
MD: Most likely, you have a germ called shigella. If so, I'll need to inform the local Department of Public Health. This is a highly contagious bacteria and I will be calling your friends and recommending that they also come to the emergency room tonight.				
PT: I'll make the call, and then you can explain the details.				
MD: OK. I am going to treat both of you with a good antibiotic. After the symptoms clear, wait a few days before going back to bartending. In the meantime, wash your hands very well, especially after changing the baby's diapers and before handling food or her bottle.				
Break It Down	☐	☐	☐	☐

☐ CIFE with patient ☐ CIFE with provider ☐ FLOW ☐ REGISTER

Role-Play 80: Glossary

continued

1. Pathology (diseases, conditions)

2. Laboratory Tests and Diagnostic Procedures

3. Treatment Procedures

4. Idiomatic Expressions (if any)

5. Other (vocabulary in this particular role-play that you feel is important/relevant or that you anticipate problems with)

PO Box 2308, Woburn, MA 01888-0508, **p:** 781-729-3736, **www.EmbracingCulture.com**
PO Box 6401, Manchester, NH 03108, **p:** 1-888-678-CCCS

Role-Play 81: Campylobacter

(A phone conversation)

	Pronunciation	Additions	Omissions	Mistakes
MD: Hello, how can I help you?				
Mother: Dr. Azarof, my daughter has been complaining of pain each time she has a bowel movement. She's been like this for two days.				
MD: Is she running a fever?				
Mother: No, she seems fine all day, playing with her friends and her toys, but she seems to be in terrible pain every time she goes to the bathroom!				
MD: Were there any sudden changes with her diet?				
Mother: No, none that I can think of. We all have been eating the same food and she is the only one having trouble going to the bathroom.				
MD: Do you see any blood?				
Mother: Yes, I see some mucous and blood and then a burst of diarrhea.				
MD: Is the blood bright red?				
Mother: Yes, and it seems not to be mixed with the stool. It almost seems that it is coming along with the mucous.				
MD: Please bring her to my office today. I will examine her and we will send a stool sample to the lab to rule out bacterial infection or parasites.				
Mother: Parasites?				
MD: I will ask the clinical assistant to take care of the appointment for you. Just tell Jane that I told you to come in with your daughter this afternoon as a walk-in patient.				
Mother: OK. Do you think that something bad could have happened to my daughter? She just started at a new school two months ago. It is a reputable school and she seems to like it.				
MD: We'll take a look at all the possibilities, but most likely this is a bug.				
(The family arrives at the clinic)				
MD: So, your mother told me that you been having some trouble with diarrhea. How many times have you moved your bowels today?				
PT: I do not know. I have a bad tummy ache and I feel a big squeeze.				

continued

Role-Play 81 *(continued)*

	Pronunciation	Additions	Omissions	Mistakes
MD: Do you have cramps?				
Mother: Yes, I think that she has cramps. She bends down and holds on to her stomach. Sometimes I give her a pillow to make it more comfortable.				
MD: A pillow or a pill?				
Mother: No, not a pill. Our family tradition is that when the kids go to the bathroom and feel some discomfort I give them a special pillow to hold on to.				
PT: Mom!				
MD: I am glad your mother finds a way to help you out. So, have you been holding onto the pillow a bit more than usual?				
PT: Yes, and I also feel sick in my stomach.				
MD: Have you vomited?				
PT: Yes.				
MD: Are you feeling warm?				
PT: Sometimes.				
MD: How long have you been feeling this way?				
PT: I don't remember exactly, but definitely since Monday.				
MD: OK, so this has been going on for more than 2 days?				
PT: Yes.				
MD: Did you feel this way a few months ago?				
PT: I don't think so.				
MD: Have you done any recent traveling?				
PT: No.				
MD: Did you eat any new foods at school or at home?				
PT: No, I like pizza and pasta - my favorites!				
MD: Good, when you feel better we'll want to see you eating some veggies too! Now I'll step out of the room, and we'll need you to change into this gown.				
PT: Do I have to take everything off?				
MD: No, you can leave your underpants on. I'll be right back.				
(MD returns)				

continued

PO Box 2308, Woburn, MA 01888-0508, **p:** 781-729-3736, **www.EmbracingCulture.com**
PO Box 6401, Manchester, NH 03108, **p:** 1-888-678-CCCS

Role-Play 81 *(continued)*

	Pronunciation	Additions	Omissions	Mistakes
MD: OK. I am going to check your temperature with our new digital thermometer. I'll place it in your ear, and it'll beep when it's ready. Hmm, not bad. Ninety-nine. Let me examine you and then we'll get a stool sample for the lab.				
PT: OK.				
MD: When I press on your tummy, does it hurt?				
PT: Just a bit.				
MD: Does it hurt when I let go of my fingers?				
PT: No.				
MD: Have you had a runny nose or the chills?				
PT: No.				
MD: OK. I believe your diarrhea is caused by a bacteria or a virus. Currently, there is a bacterium in the community causing diarrhea. It is called campylobacter. Most likely you ate or drank something that was carrying this bug. You haven't done any traveling, so I doubt that you have a parasite but we will check a stool sample. Do you think you could move your bowels now and give us a sample?				
PT: You bet I can. I already have to go again! I thought I had the flu.				
MD: I do not think you have the flu, but if you get any worse, tell your mom to call me. Your mother should also call if the cramps get worse or if your fever goes up to 101. I will not give you an antibiotic now, but I will if the culture is positive for campylobacter or if the symptoms do not pass. In the meantime, stay away from dairy products and drink lots of fluids. You can eat toast, rice, and applesauce.				
PT: I like the applesauce idea!				
MD: Mom, your daughter's vital signs are good and she does not seem septic. Her abdominal exam was soft without signs of peritoneal inflammation. I think she probably has viral gastroenteritis.				
Mother: I get confused with "bacterial" and "viral." So if it is viral, does she need to take medications?				

continued

Role-Play 81 *(continued)*

	Pronunciation	Additions	Omissions	Mistakes
MD: Not really, but I am concerned that she did have a slight fever and there is campylobacter going around, so we will get a stool culture and make sure she does not have this bacteria.				
Mother: So, what is the difference between a virus and bacteria causing diarrhea?				
MD: The most common cause of diarrhea is usually a virus. If it is bacteria, and it does not get better in a week or two, then an antibiotic can be helpful. In Salmonella infections, we try not to treat with antibiotics because it can cause the patient to actually carry the bacteria when they are well and this can infect other people.				
Mother: I am glad I have you. Do I need to take any precautions at home?				
MD: Everyone in the family should wash their hands after using the bathroom and before eating or preparing meals. Cook all meats thoroughly and do not eat raw poultry, beef or pork. If you have a pet at home, make sure that everyone washes his or her hands after petting it.				
Break It Down	☐	☐	☐	☐

☐ **CIFE with patient** ☐ **CIFE with provider** ☐ **FLOW** ☐ **REGISTER**

Role-Play 81: Glossary

continued

PO Box 2308, Woburn, MA 01888-0508, **p:** 781-729-3736, **www.EmbracingCulture.com**
PO Box 6401, Manchester, NH 03108, **p:** 1-888-678-CCCS

1. Pathology (diseases, conditions)

2. Laboratory Tests and Diagnostic Procedures

3. Treatment Procedures

4. Idiomatic Expressions (if any)

5. Other (vocabulary in this particular role-play that you feel is important/relevant or that you anticipate problems with)

7. DIABETES

Introduction to Diabetes

Diabetes is a disease of lack of insulin or of decreased sensitivity of organs to insulin. Insulin is the hormone that regulates the use of glucose as an energy source in the body, but insulin's effect on glucose is merely the tip of the iceberg.

The cell needs fuel to make energy for its functions. Insulin is released by the pancreas to help bring glucose into the cells for use in the making of energy. But with diminished amounts or no insulin, or with organs or cells of the body resisting the effect of insulin, the glucose stays in the blood stream and is not utilized.

Diabetes is a Greek word that means "passing through." It's known as an illness that makes a person urinate excessively. When we refer to diabetes, we usually mean **diabetes mellitus**, a form of diabetes in which the level of glucose is high in the blood. When blood sugar is high, sugar is spilled into the urine, and urination increases. The urine is sweet, thus this form of diabetes is called mellitus, which comes from the Latin word for sweet.

Diabetes mellitus appears to have various component causes. There is a tendency for it to run in the family. Obesity, diet and lifestyle also cause diabetes. Some studies indicate that diabetes could be a response to an early viral infection.

Another form of diabetes is called **diabetes insipidus**. With diabetes insipidus, increased urination is due to the kidneys' inability to concentrate the urine. Thus, the urine is dilute or "insipid." In this case, either the body is not producing anti-diuretic hormones, or the kidney is not responding to the anti-diuretic hormones that are present.

Different Forms of Diabetes Mellitus

There are generally thought to be two forms of diabetes mellitus:

Type 1 diabetes often appears during childhood or adolescence. It is common in persons under 30 years of age. When it occurs in young children, it is called juvenile diabetes. Basically, the body stops producing insulin, and the patient becomes dependent on insulin treatment. It is estimated that five to ten percent of all diagnosed diabetics suffer from Type 1 diabetes.

With **Type 2 diabetes**, the body produces some insulin but either the amount is not sufficient, or the body has trouble using the insulin that is produced. It affects ninety to ninety-five percent of all diabetics and most often appears after age 40, although it is sometimes diagnosed in adolescents and younger adults. Type 2 diabetes is linked to obesity and physical inactivity, both of which can be modified to improve health.

PO Box 2308, Woburn, MA 01888-0508, **p:** 781-729-3736, **www.EmbracingCulture.com**
PO Box 6401, Manchester, NH 03108, **p:** 1-888-678-CCCS

Both Type 1 and Type 2 diabetes mellitus can share common symptoms such as weight loss, fatigue, weakness, frequent urination, and constant thirst or hunger. Doctors differentiate between the two types of diabetes mellitus by looking at the age of onset and the patient's ability to produce insulin. The breakdown of a body's insulin producing system may be explained by a high level of antibodies (proteins) that, instead of destroying viruses or germs as programmed, attack the cells that make the insulin or the insulin itself.

Other symptoms common to both Type 1 and Type 2 diabetes mellitus include blurred vision, numbness and tingling, increased infections of the skin, gums, vagina and bladder, and a propensity for coronary artery disease or peripheral vascular disease.

Pregnant women can get a form of diabetes mellitus called "**gestational diabetes**." Gestational diabetes develops in two to five percent of all pregnancies, but disappears when the pregnancy is over. It involves high blood sugar, or hyperglycemia, due to the hormonal changes of pregnancy. Usually when a pregnancy is over, a gestational diabetic returns to her normal state of glucose tolerance. Gestational diabetics have a tendency to develop diabetes in their later years.

It is very important to the health of the fetus that mothers with gestational diabetes maintain a strict control over their blood sugars. When a mother has very high glucose during her pregnancy and passes it into her unborn child, the child starts to produce more insulin. The increase of glucose and the production of insulin may cause the baby to grow to a point where it develops health problems and may greatly increase the likelihood of delivery complications. This condition is known as **macrosomia**.

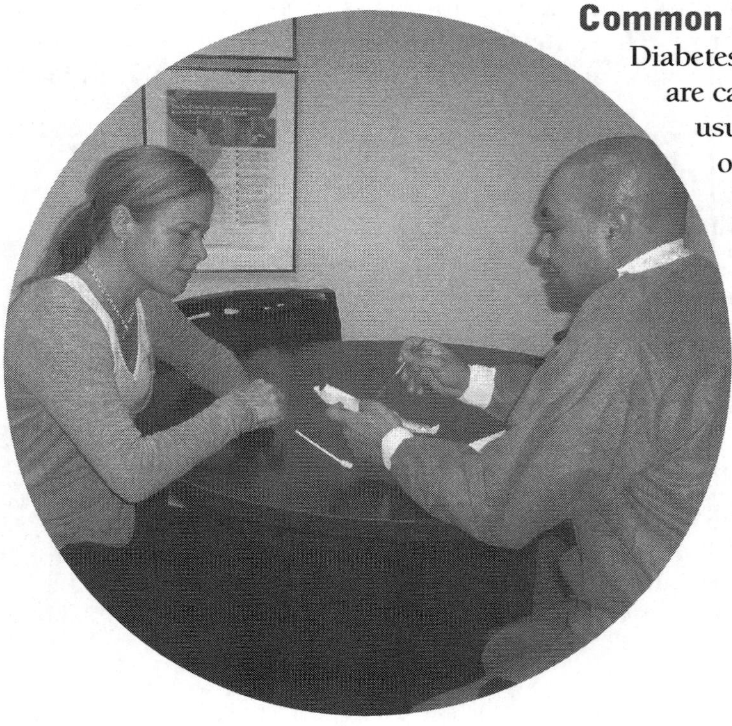

Common Illnesses Stemming from Diabetes

Diabetes mellitus has multiple complications of what are called "end organ" diseases. These diseases are usually the consequence of the effect of diabetes on blood vessels, which often involves hardening of the arteries. Coronary artery disease, strokes, retinal disease, kidney disease, neuropathy and leg ulcers are all examples of these complications.

The following are some diseases linked to diabetes:

- Anorexia and Bulimia
- Cardiovascular Disease
- Coronary Artery Disease(CAD)
- Diabetic Coma
- Diabetic Retinopathy
- Digital Sclerosis
- Foot Conditions
- Gangrene and Amputation
- Gum Disease
- High Blood Pressure
- Impotence for Men
- Kidney Disease
- Lack of Bladder Control
- Nephropathy
- Nerve Damage
- Poor Circulation
- Strokes
- Thrush
- Urinary Tract Infections
- Vaginal Infections
- Vaginal Tightness (Vaginismus)

Diagnosing Diabetes

Diabetes has become one of the most prevalent illnesses in the US. Hospitals and community health centers in collaboration with the American Diabetes Association and other government agencies are developing campaigns to educate the public by sponsoring community health fairs. The main goals are to teach people how to prevent diabetes and to help them recognize the early signs of the disease. Medical providers take careful family and health histories as a part of diabetes screening. If a patient's family has a history of diabetes mellitus, the provider may ask that the patient take a fasting blood sugar test. If the fasting sugar is more than 125, the patient will need further testing.

Diagnostic Criteria for Diabetes

1. Symptoms of Diabetes (thirst, increased urination, unexplained weight loss), plus a random plasma glucose > 200mg/dl.
2. Fasting plasma glucose >126 mg/dl after an overnight (at least 8 hour) fast.
3. Two-hour plasma glucose >200mg/dl during a standard 75g oral glucose tolerance test.

PO Box 2308, Woburn, MA 01888-0508, **p:** 781-729-3736, **www.EmbracingCulture.com**
PO Box 6401, Manchester, NH 03108, **p:** 1-888-678-CCCS

Therapeutic Approaches to Type 2 Diabetes

Type 2 diabetes is an insidious, progressive disease. So, the treatment must also be stepwise and progressive. It should begin with life style interventions and progress to more and more intensive pharmacological interventions.

Life Style Modifications: Diet, Exercise, and Patient Education
The cornerstones of therapy and most cost-effective measures are diet, exercise and patient education. In this regard, Type 2 focuses more on control of obesity.

Physical exercise facilitates weight loss, reduces glucose output by the liver, lowers glucose levels in the blood, decreases risk for macrovascular disease by decreasing serum triglyceride and VLDL cholesterol levels, and raises endorphin levels and improves mood and self esteem. Effects of exercise can persist for up to 48 hours.

It is recommended that diabetics exercise for 20-30 minutes every other day. The elderly must exercise cautiously to avoid hypoglycemia that can trigger heart attack and stroke, especially if they also take oral antidiabetic drugs or insulin regimen.

In many persons, lifestyle modifications can provide glycemic control. However as the disease advances, pharmacological intervention is necessary. The first arm of pharmacotherapy is the category of **oral anti-diabetic drugs**.

The Future of Therapy

- **Insulin Pumps**
  There are insulin pumps that provide both a basilar subcutaneous infusion as well as PRN bolus of insulin, but the amounts and rates given are decided by the patient via capillary blood draw readings.

- **Non-Capillary Glucose Meters**
  There are glucose meters that can take glucose readings from galvanic skin response. These are not terribly accurate but seem effective for helping patients learn if there is asymptomatic hypoglycemia.

- **Pen Injectors**
  Disposable prefilled pen injectors filled with short acting insulin to be used for those doing frequent preprandial injections.

- **Inhaled Insulin**
  There are some studies suggesting that inhaled insulin is just as effective as intramuscular insulin. There are concerns for effect on pulmonary tissues.

- **Pancreas Transplantation**
  Patients undergoing simultaneous pancreas and kidney transplantation have 85% of pancreatic graft survival and 92% chance of renal graft survival. Single pancreatic transplantation should be considered rarely.

- **Islet Cell transplantation**
  Minimally invasive. In Canada, a small number of patients with Type 1 diabetes underwent the procedure and reported insulin independence. Over 20 subjects have undergone percutaneous transhepatic portal vein transplantation islets. All were able to achieve insulin independence, some for more than 2 years of follow-up. Wide acceptance is limited by need for multiple donors and potent long-term immunotherapy.

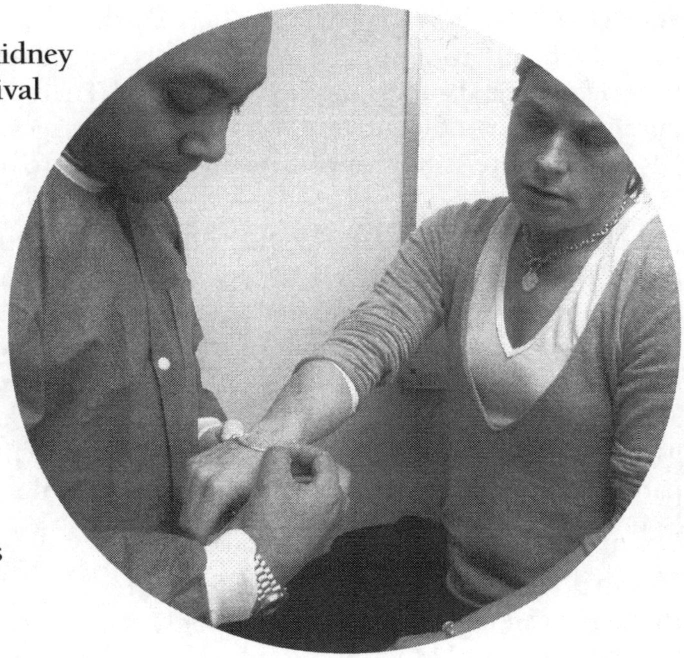

A closer look at a diabetic's daily routine

Glucometer, Test Strips, Insulin and Syringe are all part of Gail's daily routine.

Step 1 Gail gently cleanses the desired testing area – she prefers a simple fingerprick but has also tested blood drawn from her lower arm.

Step 2 Gail quickly pricks her finger to draw a drop of blood for testing.

Step 3 Gail uses the glucometer to measure blood sugar levels.

Step 4 Gail's glucometer reading is 166. She must now take her prescribed insulin dose.

Step 5 Gail fills the syringe with the prescribed insulin dosage. She measures very carefully.

Step 6 Gail chooses a convenient place to inject her insulin dosage. "It doesn't hurt," she says.

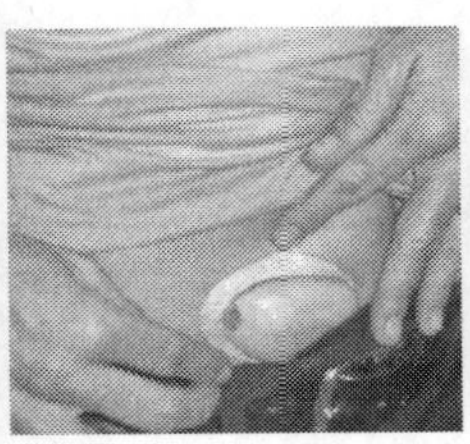
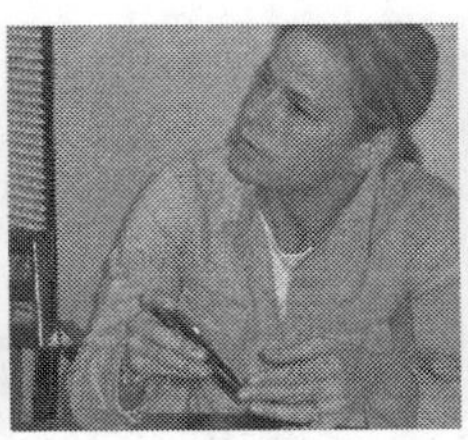
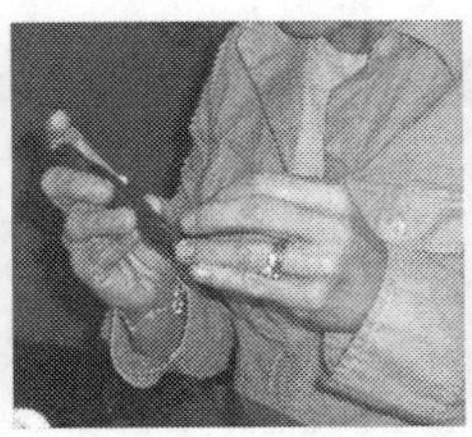
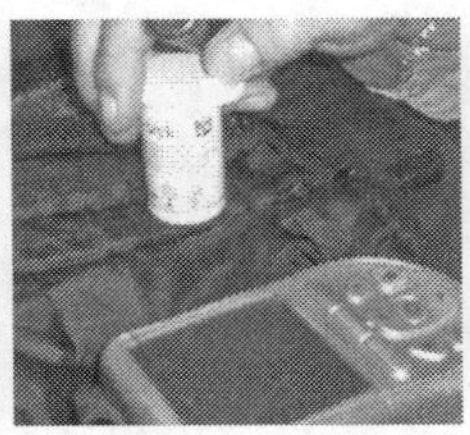
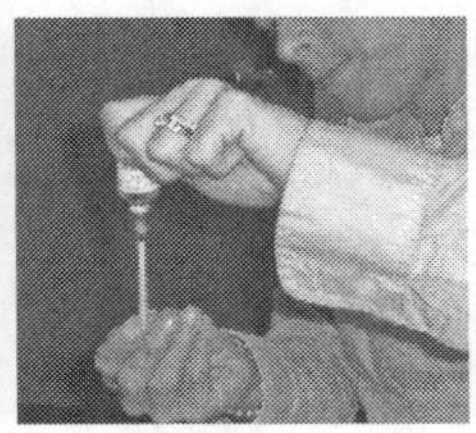

PO Box 2308, Woburn, MA 01888-0508, **p:** 781-729-3736, **www.EmbracingCulture.com**
PO Box 6401, Manchester, NH 03108, **p:** 1-888-678-CCCS

Interpreting for a Patient with Diabetes

As with any interpreting, the interpreter is expected to convey the accurate meaning. Again, *consecutive interpretation* is the ideal mode for a session. There are interpreters however who switch to *simultaneous interpreting* when the provider is explaining dosages, frequency of the medicine, and symptoms. Discuss these possibilities with a supervisor before having to make arbitrary decisions.

Interpreting in Educational and Therapeutic Settings

It is common for interpreters to be asked to interpret for different types of groups or family sessions. In educational groups, for example, a provider might teach different symptoms, explain forms of treatment, or go into the details of administering shots, pricking fingers, reading counts, etc. Diabetic patients may also seek support groups where they can discuss their feelings related to their diagnoses and the aspects of 'living with the illness'. *In group therapy sessions it is recommended that the interpreter use the simultaneous interpretation mode.* Sit next to the patient, placing your chair almost behind the patient, and with a lower voice interpret all the information shared by all group participants and leaders.

Managing the Flow of the Session

Diabetes is an illness that affects not only the patient but also the family. The family of a diabetic needs to be knowledgeable about the side effects of treatment, signs of hyperglycemia and hypoglycemia, the changes in diet, and possible mood and cognitive changes.It is common for family members to speak, all at the same time, as the interpreter is trying to interpret. If this happens, we ask that the interpreter graciously remind the family members of the pre-session agreement. The interpreter will interpret all information shared, but in order for everyone's important message to be heard, the family will have to take turns when speaking.

Any conversation between the interpreter and a second party in the session needs to be conveyed to the other third party. This is managing the flow of an interpreting session. So, if one family member is anxiously trying to explain that his mother still puts sugar in her coffee, while another family member is urgently describing her mother's blurred vision, the interpreter needs to kindly say, "I am sorry, but please speak one at a time so I can be accurate with your information." Another way of handling this situation would be to use hand signals to encourage the parties to pause, slow down or take turns speaking.

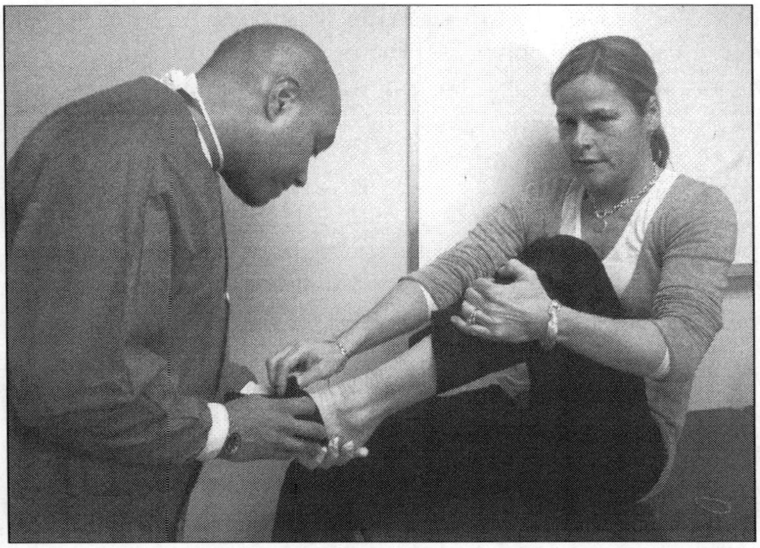

What to expect from a session with a diabetic patient

Some cases involving diabetic patients may represent an emotional challenge for the interpreter. A patient with poor circulation may with time require one or more amputations. It is also common for patients faced with chronic illnesses to want to abandon their treatments and see if they still really suffer from the illness. Interpreters need to be patient, transparent, and avoid using forceful tones or facial expressions. Stories have circulated about interpreters who have taken it upon themselves to "play" provider by exaggerating possible medical conditions. But an interpreter may not add information to an interpretation for any reason, even if the intention is to impress a provider's message more forcefully upon a patient.

If you feel like a patient just isn't going to "get it," the best way to handle the situation is to make some general recommendations to the provider in the pre-session. Encourage the provider to be concrete, and to use plenty of examples. If things still aren't going well during a session, request that the provider step out for a moment to speak with you, or ask him/her for a post-session. If you are uneasy, don't distort anyone's message, but let both parties know what you suspect has gone wrong. Many times, if you stay silent, patients sense the tension and although they may not complain, they are less likely to open up to the provider. Transparency builds trust.

Being a Culture Broker

It is important that interpreters are aware that with any chronic illness such as diabetes, often patients and their families go through different emotional stages no matter what ethnic culture one is from. Providers are trained to handle these situations, but they may lack the knowledge that is particular to the different ethnic cultures regarding certain foods, how they handle bad news, how they look into the past and go over stories of friends and family members who got sick or they look into the future into management and prevention of future diabetes symptoms.

There is a tendency for those who treat patients with a chronic illness to, at times, show some frustration. The provider has knowledge of the possible serious and at times lethal effects of the illness if not managed, and the patient may seem to be denying this possibility and in some ways s/he may act out by not following through with the treatment plan.

PO Box 2308, Woburn, MA 01888-0508, **p:** 781-729-3736, **www.EmbracingCulture.com**
PO Box 6401, Manchester, NH 03108, **p:** 1-888-678-CCCS

For those providers who have not dealt with their own discomfort in working with patients from diverse backgrounds, the denial of the illness may be a trigger point for putting pressure on an interpreter to become a provider and handle the case in a culturally "appropriate way." This is a dangerous invitation, although a bit glorious at first; therefore, interpreters should stick to their roles as culture brokers, and not providers and enforcers of a treatment plan.

When asked by an anxious provider for an intervention, the interpreter could ask the provider: "What would you have done if this were an English speaking patient?" and let the provider answer. Only add any information if in fact needed due to different culture beliefs and rituals . There are many of our patients who do not use spoons, who do not walk or exercise for pleasure, who do not know what pasta and chickpeas are.

Interpreters should be aware that it takes a team to work with a patient who has a chronic illness and does not speak English. The interpreter besides being the conduit of the message spoken is also a coach to the provider, ' behind the scene,' so to speak. We want providers to use the tools they already have by adding a few more culture-specific tips when needed.

A worldwide view of patients who suffer from a lifelong illness is that at first, when they are diagnosed, there is a tendency for denial. So, information is not always completely shared with the provider due to conscious or unconscious motivations.

Later on, due to possible symptoms, blood screenings, family and medical interventions through teaching and coaching, one may minimize it's chronicity by thinking it is not so bad and cutting off with certain diets that may be adverse to good health and habits.

It is not uncommon for those patients who do not have family members with diabetes to only begin to accept the illness after a major medical crisis, such as double vision, confusion, passing out with no explanation and other more serious illnesses. These are the patients that end up in our emergency room and walk-in clinics.

Patients usually begin to accept the illness often after multiple visits to the different medical team members assigned to the case; and with lots of teaching, sometimes a little confrontation along with continual support, one may begin to integrate this new illness and make the necessary life changes in order to maintain good health.

Even when a patient begins to accept the illness, it is understood that there are often feelings of hopelessness, loneliness or even shame. There are certain habits that one needs for physical, social and emotional comfort. For example, in many countries, eating sweets and drinking very sweet beverages reflects one's economic wealth. So, if a provider is not aware of this conflict but the interpreter is, what is the interpreter's role? This would be an opportune time for the interpreter to be a culture broker or a coach with the provider by revealing this possible precious gem of information.

Role-Play 82: Tom's Frequent Urination

A concerned mother brings her 10-year old son, Tom, to see his pediatrician. He has been displaying unusual symptoms, such as frequent urination, abnormal thirst, and fluctuations in appetite for a few weeks now.

	Pronunciation	Additions	Omissions	Mistakes
Doctor: So, how have you been feeling lately, Tom?				
Tom: Well, I've been peeing a lot lately. Sometimes I have to get up in the middle of the night to pee. I even had to ask Mrs. Miller in the middle of class to go to the bathroom.				
Doctor: It sounds like you needed to go pretty bad! Have you noticed anything else out of the ordinary recently?				
Tom: I'm also really thirsty. I have to keep drinking water and Coke because my mouth is dry. Maybe that's why I'm peeing so much.				
Doctor: You might be right, Tom. So you're peeing a lot and drinking a lot. Anything else?				
Tom: No, not really.				
Doctor: All right then. Now let me ask your mom a few questions. Mom, have you noticed anything else about Tom lately?				
Mom: Yes, I have. I've noticed that he's been eating more than before. He seems to always be hungry, even after a meal. Also, he's been having a lot of mood swings. His attitude is different at home and at school. His teacher, Mrs. Miller, even called me last Friday and asked me if Tom was experiencing problems at home. I can tell you that there's nothing wrong at home.				
Doctor: I understand. From what I'm hearing from you and Tom, these symptoms seem to point to Type I diabetes. Does Tom have any relatives who have diabetes?				
Mom: Well, his grandfather on his father's side has it, but I don't really understand what it is.				
Doctor: I'll explain it to you. In general, diabetes is a disease where the body can't break down the foods you eat into sugar for energy. A normal body makes insulin that does that for us, but a diabetic's body either can't make insulin at all, or can't use it properly.				
Mom: What were you saying about Tom possibly having "Type I" diabetes? What is Type I diabetes?				

continued

PO Box 2308, Woburn, MA 01888-0508, **p:** 781-729-3736, **www.EmbracingCulture.com**
PO Box 6401, Manchester, NH 03108, **p:** 1-888-678-CCCS

Role-Play 82 *(continued)*

	Pronunciation	Additions	Omissions	Mistakes
Doctor: There are mainly three types of diabetes: Type I, Type II, and Gestational diabetes. Gestational diabetes only affects certain women during pregnancy, and Type II usually affects older people, many of whom are overweight and don't get much exercise. Because Tom is only 10 and is pretty active, I believe he may have Type I diabetes.				
Tom: How will you know if I really have diabetes?				
Doctor: To find out, we're going to do a few simple tests. One involves taking a drop of blood from your finger. And in another, we're going to need a urine sample.				
Tom: That's good because I already have to pee again.				
Doctor: I'm sure you're both anxious to find out the results, so I'll get right to it. For the first test, we tested the amount of sugar in the blood taken from Tom's finger and found that it was on the high side. The exact reading was 235, while normal readings usually fall between 80 and 150.				
Mom: What about the urine test? How did that come out?				
Doctor: We found a certain amount of ketones in Tom's urine. Ketones are a chemical that the body produces when there is a shortage of insulin in the blood and the body breaks down fat for energy. So the presence of ketones in the urine indicates that something is not quite right. As a result of these findings, it's pretty safe to conclude that Tom has diabetes.				
Tom: So what does that mean? Does this mean I can't eat ice cream anymore?				
Doctor: What's going to happen is that you'll have to start taking insulin injections a few times a day. That's the only way for you to get insulin into your system. In addition to injections, you're going to have to watch what you eat more carefully. Mom, this is probably your area of expertise. I'll have you sit down with a nutritionist and together you'll work out a meal plan to follow. It'll be best to cut sweets out of Tom's diet in the near future. After you're both comfortable with following a regimen, Tom can even have ice cream, but you'll have to work it into his meal plan.				
Tom: I don't like taking shots. The flu shot I took last month hurt a lot!				

continued

Role Play 82 *(continued)*

	Pronunciation	Additions	Omissions	Mistakes
Mom: I'm sure these insulin needles won't hurt as much.				
Doctor: That's right. These needles are much smaller than the one they used for your flu shot. At most, you'll probably only feel a pinch with these.				
Tom: So all I have to do is watch what I eat and take a few shots a day? I guess it's not that bad.				
Mom: There's probably more to it than just that, Tom. What else are we going to have to do?				
Doctor: The single most important thing both of you can do is to learn as much about diabetes as possible. Of course the insulin injections and dieting are important, but when you fully understand what you're doing and why you're doing it, you'll be able to control your diabetes, instead of letting your diabetes control you. Knowledge is the most powerful tool to treat diabetes.				
Tom: But how do I learn about diabetes? They don't teach it in school.				
Doctor: There are many ways to learn more, like reading about it in books and online, as well as talking about it with others. I will have you meet with the nurse practitioner who will teach you a lot about living with diabetes. You'll also learn quite a bit just from your own everyday experiences. You can live a perfectly healthy and normal life with diabetes, but you'll need to know how. You could say that your lesson begins now.				
Tom: I'm going to learn as much about diabetes as I can!				
Mom: You can do it!!				
Break It Down	☐	☐	☐	☐

☐ **CIFE with patient** ☐ **CIFE with provider** ☐ **FLOW** ☐ **REGISTER**

Role-Play 82: Glossary

continued

PO Box 2308, Woburn, MA 01888-0508, **p:** 781-729-3736, **www.EmbracingCulture.com**
PO Box 6401, Manchester, NH 03108, **p:** 1-888-678-CCCS

1. Pathology (diseases, conditions)

2. Laboratory Tests and Diagnostic Procedures

3. Treatment Procedures

4. Idiomatic Expressions (if any)

5. Other (vocabulary in this particular role-play that you feel is important/relevant or that you anticipate problems with)

Role-Play 83: Follow-up Diabetes Visit

Van is seeing his doctor today in follow-up from a visit last week in which he said that he has been feeling very tired, even though he gets plenty of sleep. Along with feeling tired, he often lacks the energy to play sports with his friends during recess. The Doctor did some blood tests and a physical exam.

	Pronunciation	Additions	Omissions	Mistakes
Doctor: Good morning, Van. What brings you into my office today?				
Van: I still feel tired all the time. I always feel like napping or sleeping.				
Doctor: Well, I want you to know that your blood level is good and you do not have anemia; there is no sign of thyroid or liver disease and your kidney functions are excellent. Your exam last week was excellent. I am not seeing any serious medical reasons for your fatigue. However, there are some other issues to review. Do you get enough sleep? How many hours do you usually sleep at night?				
Van: I get plenty of sleep; at least 8 hours a night.				
Doctor: Well what about your eating habits? Do you eat three well-rounded meals each day?				
Van: Not really. For breakfast, I usually have a bowl of Lucky Charms before school. Then at lunch, I have like a slice of pizza or a cheeseburger with french fries. For dinner, Mom usually makes spaghetti or Sloppy Joes, or something like that.				
Doctor: Do you eat enough fruit and vegetables every day, like a banana with your cereal or some salad with Mom's spaghetti?				
Van: Not really. I don't really like vegetables. Fruits are OK, but I don't eat them very much. Do french fries count as vegetables?				
Doctor: No, french fries don't count. Have you heard of the food pyramid, Van?				
Van: Yeah, it's like a triangle with a bunch of little boxes. You're supposed to eat what it says to stay healthy or something like that, right?				
Doctor: That's right, Van. According to the food pyramid, we're supposed to eat 6-11 servings of breads and cereals, 2-3 servings of milk, yogurt, and cheese, 2-3 servings of meat and nuts, 3-5 servings of vegetables and 2-4 servings of fruit. It seems like you get plenty of bread, milk and meat, but how many servings of vegetables and fruits do you eat every day?				

continued

PO Box 2308, Woburn, MA 01888-0508, **p:** 781-729-3736, **www.EmbracingCulture.com**
PO Box 6401, Manchester, NH 03108, **p:** 1-888-678-CCCS

Role-Play 83 *(continued)*

	Pronunciation	Additions	Omissions	Mistakes
Van: I'm not sure, but I don't think it's that much. Is that why I feel tired all the time, because I don't eat my fruits and vegetables?				
Doctor: Well, that's probably part of the reason. In general, when our bodies aren't balanced with the right amount of food and exercise, we tend to lack energy and feel tired. That's probably why you feel the way you do.				
Van: So, if I started to eat more fruits and vegetables, then I'd feel better?				
Doctor: You'll probably start to feel better, but you also have to eat healthier overall. Like, instead of having french fries all the time, maybe you can have rice pilaf or a baked potato. It's best to cut down on fried foods and sweets.				
Van: What were you also saying about exercise? Will that help too?				
Doctor: Yes, getting regular exercise will build up your energy level. So, the combination of eating right and exercising regularly will definitely help you feel better.				
Van: I had no idea that the foods I ate would have such a large effect on how I felt. So, even though I'm not the biggest fan of fruits and vegetables, I'm going to start eating more of them so that I'll have more energy from now on. And if I ever forget how many servings I'm supposed to eat, I'll just look at the food pyramid and find out.				
Break It Down	☐	☐	☐	☐

☐ CIFE with patient ☐ CIFE with provider ☐ FLOW ☐ REGISTER

Role-Play 83: Glossary

continued

1. Pathology (diseases, conditions)

2. Laboratory Tests and Diagnostic Procedures

3. Treatment Procedures

4. Idiomatic Expressions (if any)

5. Other (vocabulary in this particular role-play that you feel is important/relevant or that you anticipate problems with)

PO Box 2308, Woburn, MA 01888-0508, **p:** 781-729-3736, **www.EmbracingCulture.com**
PO Box 6401, Manchester, NH 03108, **p:** 1-888-678-CCCS

Role-Play 84: Mr. Sanchez

Enrico Sanchez is a Spanish speaker. He knew that his mother and father both had diabetes, but he was very happy that for most of his 48 years, he had not had a problem with "azucar." A year ago, he had a two-week period in which he lost weight, yet ate a lot, urinated a lot, was incredibly thirsty, and developed a bad pneumonia. He was told he had high sugar, but it might be made worse by the prednisone he needed in order to breathe well with the pneumonia. His sugar got better when the pneumonia passed and for ten months he did not return to the Doctor. Now he is losing weight again, he is urinating frequently, and there is some pain with urination. He is always thirsty.

	Pronunciation	Additions	Omissions	Mistakes
MD: Hello, Mr. Sanchez, it's good to see you again. I am sorry it has been so long. What brings you in today?				
PT: My wife, Amelia, made me come in, I have been urinating a lot and it burns when I urinate. I am losing weight again. She is worried the sugar has come back.				
MD: How much weight have you lost?				
PT: About 10 kilos since six weeks.				
MD: Have you had a discharge from your penis recently?				
PT: No, but it burns to urinate.				
MD: How long has this been going on?				
PT: About two weeks.				
MD: How is your breathing? Are you still smoking?				
PT: My breathing has been fine; but, yes, I am still smoking.				
MD: How are your bowel movements? Any change in the frequency or shape?				
PT: I've been a little constipated but not very bad.				
MD: Have you seen any blood in your stool, or seen bright black stools?				
PT: No, they are normally brown and I've seen no blood.				
MD: Well, Mr. Sanchez, let me examine you.				
PT: OK.				

(MD examines patient. His medical assistant does a finger stick and measures the blood glucose. The patient also gives a urine sample to the medical assistant.)

continued

Role-Play 84 *(continued)*

	Pronunciation	Additions	Omissions	Mistakes
MD: Your blood pressure is a little low. You're breathing slightly fast. Your temperature is high. And your blood sugar is high. It is 498. Your urine has ketones in it and, under the microscope, I see lots of white cells. Your prostate is mildly tender. Mr. Sanchez, I think you are developing a urinary tract infection and you are also in danger of developing a serious complication of diabetes called diabetic keto-acidosis. I am going to send you to the emergency room at the hospital across the street. If your blood tests suggest acidosis, you will need to be admitted, put on an insulin drip and IV antibiotics.				
PT: I really don't feel that bad.				
MD: Well, I think you must be a very strong person, but now with what I see, you could quickly get very ill. Let's see what the blood shows. I'll give you some Insulin right now and then send you to the emergency room. If your sugar comes down, we might be able to treat you in the emergency room and send you home; but, I think, more likely you'll need to spend a day or two in the hospital.				
PT: Will I need to start to take insulin?				
MD: Yes, I think so. I think for this past year your sugars were up and left you vulnerable to getting infections. Now, you really do need to start insulin. If you go in the hospital, it will also be an opportunity to teach you more about checking your own blood sugar and giving yourself insulin with good technique and the correct dosage.				
Break It Down	☐	☐	☐	☐

☐ CIFE with patient ☐ CIFE with provider ☐ FLOW ☐ REGISTER

Role-Play 84: Glossary

continued

PO Box 2308, Woburn, MA 01888-0508, **p:** 781-729-3736, **www.EmbracingCulture.com**
PO Box 6401, Manchester, NH 03108, **p:** 1-888-678-CCCS

1. Pathology (diseases, conditions)

2. Laboratory Tests and Diagnostic Procedures

3. Treatment Procedures

4. Idiomatic Expressions (if any)

5. Other (vocabulary in this particular role-play that you feel is important/relevant or that you anticipate problems with)

8. ADVERSE DRUG REACTIONS (ADR)

Modern medicines can be like double-edged swords. That is, they have excellent primary effects to ameliorate the symptoms of a disease, or to cure the disease. However, they also have other secondary effects that come along with them which can be as mild as getting a headache, maybe a little itch or as serious as a heart arrhythmia or severe allergic reaction. When a secondary effect is experienced as irritating, harmful or deleterious, it is called an adverse effect. Aspirin, for example, is excellent for headaches and aches and pains. However, it has a secondary effect of making platelets not stick together, causing a patient to have a tendency to bleed easier. This can be an adverse reaction if someone has surgery and does not stop bleeding quickly because the aspirin is in one's system. Antibiotics can cause allergic reactions which can be as mild as an itch or as serious as a complete loss of blood pressure called anaphylactic shock. Finally, in this age of multiple medicines, a person can take one drug which causes another drug to be metabolized slower and in effect cause an "overdose" of the second drug, even though, it is being taken exactly as prescribed. Thus, the adverse effect is only present because of the effect the one drug has on the other drug the patient is taking. It is therefore important that a patient has a primary care clinician who can keep track of all the medicines they are prescribed, or get all medicines from one pharmacy system so the pharmacy's computer can help avoid adverse interactions and thus avoid the creation of doubleedged swords.

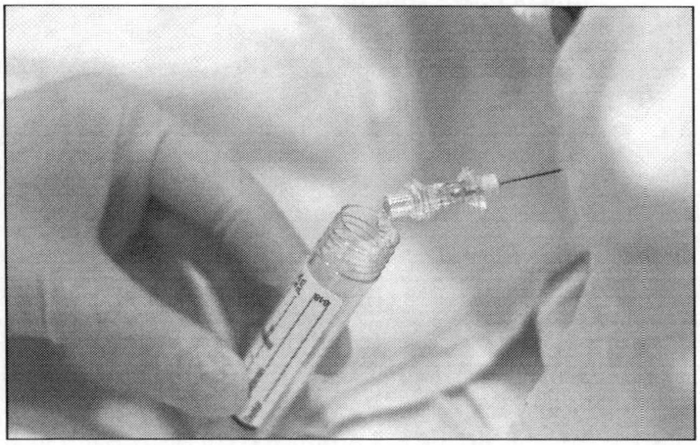

PO Box 2308, Woburn, MA 01888-0508, **p:** 781-729-3736, **www.EmbracingCulture.com**
PO Box 6401, Manchester, NH 03108, **p:** 1-888-678-CCCS

Role-Play 85: Anton's Adverse Reaction

Anton Chekhof is a college student who commutes to school. He has been depressed and he is taking an antidepressant. He lives with his mother and father who are from Russia and have not learned English. He is an all-around athlete and plays football for the school. He comes into the emergency room, agitated, nervous, with a fever of 102 and has jerky movements in his arms and legs. He is quickly confused and not able to communicate with the doctor.

His parents come to the hospital and speak with the emergency room doctor.

	Pronunciation	Additions	Omissions	Mistakes
MD: Well Mr. and Ms. Chekhof, I'm sorry to say that I don't know what is going on with Anton.				
Ms. C: What is happening?				
MD: He is confused and has a fever. He is rigid with some seizure-like movements. I have done a CAT scan which it is normal. I have done a spinal tap and the first cell count is normal. His blood test is normal. I do have a tox screen pending.				
Mr. C: What is a tox screen?				
MD: It's a blood and urine test to see if he has any toxic chemicals or drugs on board.				
Ms. C: He only takes Prozac. He was depressed in the summer.				
MD: Does he take drugs like marijuana or cocaine?				
Ms. C: Not my Anton. He's a good boy. He wants to be a doctor.				
Mr. C: Wait a minute, he had a sore on his leg last week?				
MD: A sore?				
Mr. C: Yes, and he went to the student health service. They said it was that bacteria that is resistant to penicillin.				
MD: Yes, did they say MRSA or methicillin resistant staph aureus?				
Mr. C: I think they did say that. They gave him a new antibiotic. It costs like a car for each pill.				
MD: Was it Linezolid?				
Mr. C: I don't know. He got it from the student health service. They would know. He usually gets his medicine from CVS but the health service said they would pay for it because he got the sore in the locker room.				
MD: Oh, I think I get it. He was on Prozac and he took Linezolid.				

continued

Role-Play 85 *(continued)*

	Pronunciation	Additions	Omissions	Mistakes
Mr. C: What do you get?				
MD: Well, I think Anton is having an adverse drug reaction called Seritonin Syndrome or serotonin toxicity. It is caused by the combination of Linezolid and the Prozac. It usually involves agitation, delirium, fever and seizure like motions called myoclonus.				
Ms. C: Is it dangerous?				
MD: Well, in some cases it has been very dangerous, but I think we can help Anton. We will stop his medications. We will give him muscle relaxants called benzodiazepines and control his fever. I may give him Cyproheptadine which is a serotonin antagonist but right now, with some supportive measures, I think Anton will be fine. Thank you for telling me about the Linezolid. We have other medicines we can use for his MRSA.				
Mr. C: When can we see Anton?				
MD: I am going to go and work with him and I'll come back here in 20 minutes to get you, once I have him feeling better.				
Mr. C: Thank you doctor. We'll be here.				
Break It Down	☐	☐	☐	☐

☐ **CIFE with patient** ☐ **CIFE with provider** ☐ **FLOW** ☐ **REGISTER**

Role-Play 85: Glossary

continued

PO Box 2308, Woburn, MA 01888-0508, **p:** 781-729-3736, **www.EmbracingCulture.com**
PO Box 6401, Manchester, NH 03108, **p:** 1-888-678-CCCS

1. Pathology (diseases, conditions)

2. Laboratory Tests and Diagnostic Procedures

3. Treatment Procedures

4. Idiomatic Expressions (if any)

5. Other (vocabulary in this particular role-play that you feel is important/relevant or that you anticipate problems with)

9. ALLERGIES

According to the CDC, 50 million or more Americans suffer from allergies each year. These allergies can be caused by the open air environment, or home environment such as dust, rodents, type of fabric and detergents one uses. Allergies can be food-related or due to an adverse reaction to a particular medication.

According to the CDC, the most common allergies are the following:

- The most common allergic diseases include: hay fever, asthma, conjunctivitis, hives, eczema, dermatitis, and sinusitis.
- Food allergies – most prevalent in young children and are frequently outgrown.
- Latex allergies – a reaction to the proteins in latex rubber, a substance used in gloves, condoms, and other products.
- Bees, hornets, wasps, yellow jackets, and fire ants can cause insect sting allergies.
- Allergies to drugs, like penicillin, can affect any tissue or organ in the body.

The CDC describes allergies as "an overreaction of the immune system to substances that generally do not affect other individuals." Some of the minor allergic reactions to the allergens may show the following symptoms:

- Sneeze
- Cough
- Itching
- Headaches
- Stuffy nose
- Scratchy throat
- Teary eyes
- Swollen patches
- Hives

Not everyone reacts to the same allergen in the same way. According to the CDC, reactions to the allergens can be upsetting but not life-threatening while others can be severely life-threatening causing anaphylaxis. These symptoms may result in death. According to the CDC, one may feel flush; tingling of the palms of the hands, soles of the feet or lips; light-headedness, and chest-tightness. If not treated immediately with epinephrine or other medications, the allergic reaction can progress into seizures, cardiac arrhythmia, shock, and respiratory distress. This reaction, called anaphylaxis, can result in death.

Interpreters may want to become familiar with the following vocabulary which represents 90% of the food allergies in the emergency room:

- Cow's milk
- Egg
- Peanut
- Tree nuts (for example, walnuts, pecans, almonds, and cashews)
- Fish
- Shellfish (clams, mussels, oysters, periwinkles, scallops. shrimp, prawn, lobster, crayfish, crabs)
- Soybeans
- Wheat

PO Box 2308, Woburn, MA 01888-0508, **p:** 781-729-3736, **www.EmbracingCulture.com**
PO Box 6401, Manchester, NH 03108, **p:** 1-888-678-CCCS

Role-Play 86: Nataly's Reaction to Nuts

Nataly is sixteen years old. She was born in Santo Domingo and appeared to be entirely healthy until she came to the United States four years ago. It was then, when she had some candy, that her tongue immediately began to swell and she had difficulty breathing. Her mother came home from her new job to see that her daughter was doing better and didn't seem to need to go to see a doctor. However, the mother knew that this was not a good situation either; so, she took Nataly to the doctor and then went to an allergist. Nataly took skin tests and was allergic to tree nuts (almonds, cashews and walnuts).

The doctor told her to be careful and avoid eating them. Now, after having had one episode, as benign as it was, Nataly's immune system was revved up and another episode could cause a much more severe immune reaction, even death. He gave her mother a prescription for an epinephrine-injecting syringe for Nathaly to keep with her. Nataly's mother learned how to use it, but time passed and no further incidents occurred.

Today, Nataly went to her friend's Quinceanera. When she had a piece of cake, she suddenly felt that same burning in the back of her throat, swelling of her tongue and headache. This time she heard a funny high-pitched squeak and realized it was her own breathing that was coming in faster and faster gasps. Her friend's mother, recognized the problem and called 911. Nataly went to the emergency room. Her mother was called and ran to the hospital. Nataly's mother is called by the nurse to speak to the Doctor.

		Pronunciation	Additions	Omissions	Mistakes
MD:	I am Dr. Pecard. Are you Nataly's mother?				
M:	Yes, yes, I am, please tell me how she is doing? Is something wrong?				
MD:	Well, she's ok now, and I'll bring you in to see her in a moment, but we did have a few bad moments.				
M:	What do you mean?				
MD:	Well by the time Nataly got here, the EMTs had to give her epinephrine and give her an IV for blood pressure support and put a breathing tube in for her to breath.				
M:	A breathing tube, oh my God, what happened?				
MD:	Nataly had anaphylaxis. This is a severe reaction to a drug or food caused by an allergy to the food. Nataly's friends said she had some birthday cake and started to get sick. Nataly tells me she has a food allergy. I had the cake brought in and it has almonds in it.				
M:	Yes, the doctor told me four years ago that she had allergy to tree nuts. He even gave me a needle to give her if she ate tree nuts. But she hasn't had a reaction since. Oh my God, I haven't renewed the prescription in two years.				

continued

Role-Play 86 *(continued)*

		Pronunciation	Additions	Omissions	Mistakes
MD:	Well, first, you should know that I gave epinephrine and ran steroids in her IV. Her blood pressure never went too low so I didn't have to give her medicines to control her blood pressure. I was actually able to remove the breathing tube right away. I am going to admit her overnight, but I think she'll be able to go home tomorrow morning.				
M:	Can I see her now?				
MD:	Of course, we can go in now, but before Nataly goes home tomorrow, you both are going to learn how to do something.				
M:	What's that?				
MD:	I want to make sure you both know how to use an epipen.				
M:	I knew but I will learn again. Nataly will learn too. And we will make sure she never eats another almond.				
	Break It Down	☐	☐	☐	☐

☐ **CIFE with patient** ☐ **CIFE with provider** ☐ **FLOW** ☐ **REGISTER**

Role-Play 86: Glossary

continued

PO Box 2308, Woburn, MA 01888-0508, **p:** 781-729-3736, **www.EmbracingCulture.com**
PO Box 6401, Manchester, NH 03108, **p:** 1-888-678-CCCS

1. Pathology (diseases, conditions)

2. Laboratory Tests and Diagnostic Procedures

3. Treatment Procedures

4. Idiomatic Expressions (if any)

5. Other (vocabulary in this particular role-play that you feel is important/relevant or that you anticipate problems with)

10. BROKEN BONES

(Already covered in lesson 8)

Lesson Twelve: Homework
Emergency Room

1. Go over your notes for today's class and read section "Additional Resources"
2. Read and practice ALL role-plays for this lesson
3. Continue developing your glossary by adding new terms
4. Research vocabulary related to equipment typically used in the ER. List all the words you found and provide the target language equivalent.

Equipment used in the Emergency Room (ER)

English	Target Language

THE ART OF MEDICAL INTERPRETATION®

Homework

PO Box 2308, Woburn, MA 01888-0508, **p:** 781-729-3736, **www.EmbracingCulture.com**
PO Box 6401, Manchester, NH 03108, **p:** 1-888-678-CCCS

Lesson Twelve: Additional Resources
Emergency Room

Medical Procedures and Tests

Word	Meaning	Target
Auscultation	Listening with a stethoscope for abnormal heart sounds	
Barium X-ray studies	X-ray study to detect ulcers, tumors or other abnormalities	
Blood pressure measurement	Test for high or low blood pressure	
Blood tests	Measurement of substances in the blood to evaluate organ function, diagnose and monitor various disorders	
Computed tomography (CT)	Computer-enhanced X-ray study to detect structural abnormalities	
Echocardiography	Study of heart structure and function using sound waves	
Electrocardiography	Study of the heart's electrical function	
Electroencephalography (EEG)	Study of brain's electrical function	
Intravenous urography	X-ray study of the kidneys and urinary tract after intravenous injection of a radiopaque substance	
Magnetic resonance imaging (MRI)	Magnetic imaging test for any structural abnormality	
Occult blood test	Test for blood in the stool	
Ophthalmoscopy	Direct visual inspection to detect abnormalities at the back of the eye	
Positron emission tomography (PET)	Radioactive imaging to detect function abnormality of the brain and heart	
Pulmonary function tests	Tests to measure the lungs' capacity to hold air, to move air in and out of the body, and to exchange oxygen and carbon dioxide	
Skin allergy tests	Tests for allergies	
Spinal tap	Test for abnormalities of spinal fluid	
Spirometry	Test of lung function involving blowing into a measuring device	
Stress test (exercise tolerance)	Test of heart function with exertion	
Thoracentesis	Removal of fluid from the chest with a needle to detect abnormalities	
Ultrasonography (ultrasound scanning)	Ultrasound imaging to detect structural or functional abnormalities	
Urinalysis	Chemical analysis of urine specimen to detect protein, sugar, ketones, and blood cells	
Venography	X-ray study to detect blockage of a vein	

continued

Body Parts:

Word	Meaning	Target
Brain	Part of the central nervous system contained within the cranium, comprising the prosencephalon, mesencephalon, and rhombencephalon.	
Endocrine glands	Organs that secrete hormones which are released into the circulatory system and which influence the metabolism. The glands include the pituitary, thyroid, parathyroid, adrenal, the pineal body, and the gonads.	
Eye	The organ of vision, composed of three coats: the sclera and cornea, the choroid, and the retina.	
Gallbladder	The pear-shaped reservoir for the bile on the posteroinferior surface of the liver, between the right and the quadrate lobe. Primary functions are to store, concentrate and secrete bile into the small intestine by a series of ducts. The gallbladder and these ducts are called the biliary system.	
Head	The upper, anterior, or proximal extremity of a structure or body. It contains the brain and the organs of special sense.	
Heart	The viscus of cardiac muscle that maintains the blood circulation. It is divided into four cavities: two atria and two ventricles.	
Intestines	The portion of the alimentary canal extending from the pyloric opening of the stomach to the anus. The small intestine consists of three sections: the duodenum, the jejunum, and the ileum. The large intestine consists of ascending, transverse, and descending sections.	
Kidneys	Either of the two organs in the lumbar region that filter the blood, excreting the end-products of body metabolism in the form of urine, and regulating the concentrations of hydrogen, sodium, potassium, phosphate, and other ions in the extracellular fluid.	
Liver	A large gland of a dark red color situated in the upper part of the abdomen on the right side. Its functions include the storage and filtration of blood, the secretion of bile, the excretion of bilirubin and other substances, and numerous metabolic functions.	
Lung	The organs of respiration; they occupy the lateral cavities of the chest, separated from each other by the heart and mediastinal structures.	
Neck	A constricted portion, such as the part connecting the head and trunk of the body, or the constricted part of an organ.	

continued

PO Box 2308, Woburn, MA 01888-0508, **p:** 781-729-3736, **www.EmbracingCulture.com**
PO Box 6401, Manchester, NH 03108, **p:** 1-888-678-CCCS

Body Parts: *(continued)*

Word	Meaning	Target
Pancreas	A large, elongated, racemose gland situated transversely behind the stomach, between the spleen and the duodenum.	
Skin	The outer covering of the body, consisting of the corium, or dermis, and the epidermis and resting upon the subcutaneous tissues.	
Spine	A strong but flexible support that holds the head and body upright and allows the upper body to bend and twist. It is made up of three main types of vertebrae: cervical, thoracic and lumbar.	
Spleen	Large, gland-like organ situated in the upper part of the abdominal cavity on the left side and lateral to the cardiac end of the stomach. Disintegrates red blood cells, sets hemoglobin free, and serves as a reservoir of blood.	
Stomach	The musculomembranous expansion of the alimentary canal between the esophagus and the duodenum. It consists of two chambers: an upper portion (cardiac end) called fondus, and a pyloric end called antum.	

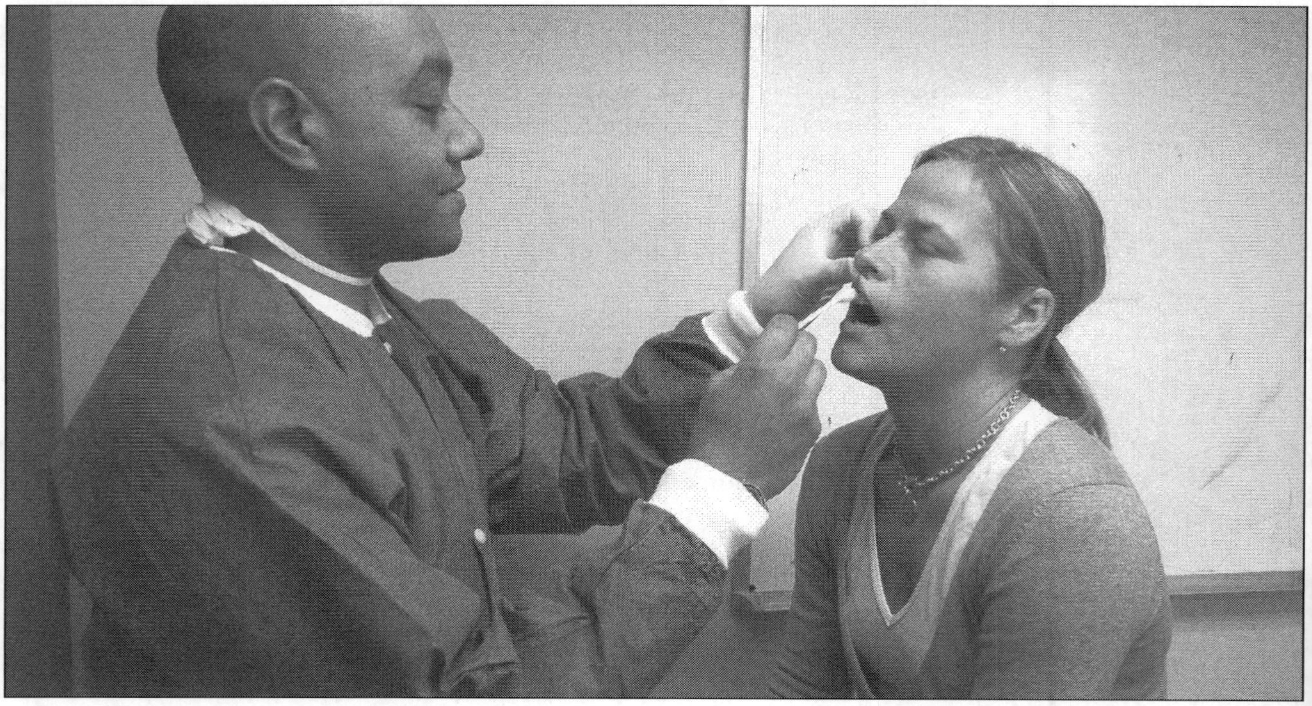

Lesson Thirteen: Interpreting in Mental Health Encounters

Understanding Goals

Students will be able to:

- understand what mental illness is
- learn about different types of mental illness
- understand substance abuse as a type of mental illness
- identify the best interpreting modes for mental health sessions
- become familiar with basic mental health vocabulary

Key Concepts

- Mental Illness
- Substance use, abuse, and dependency
- Mental Status Exam
- Affect
- Suicide Ideation vs. Suicide Attempt
- Safety Contract

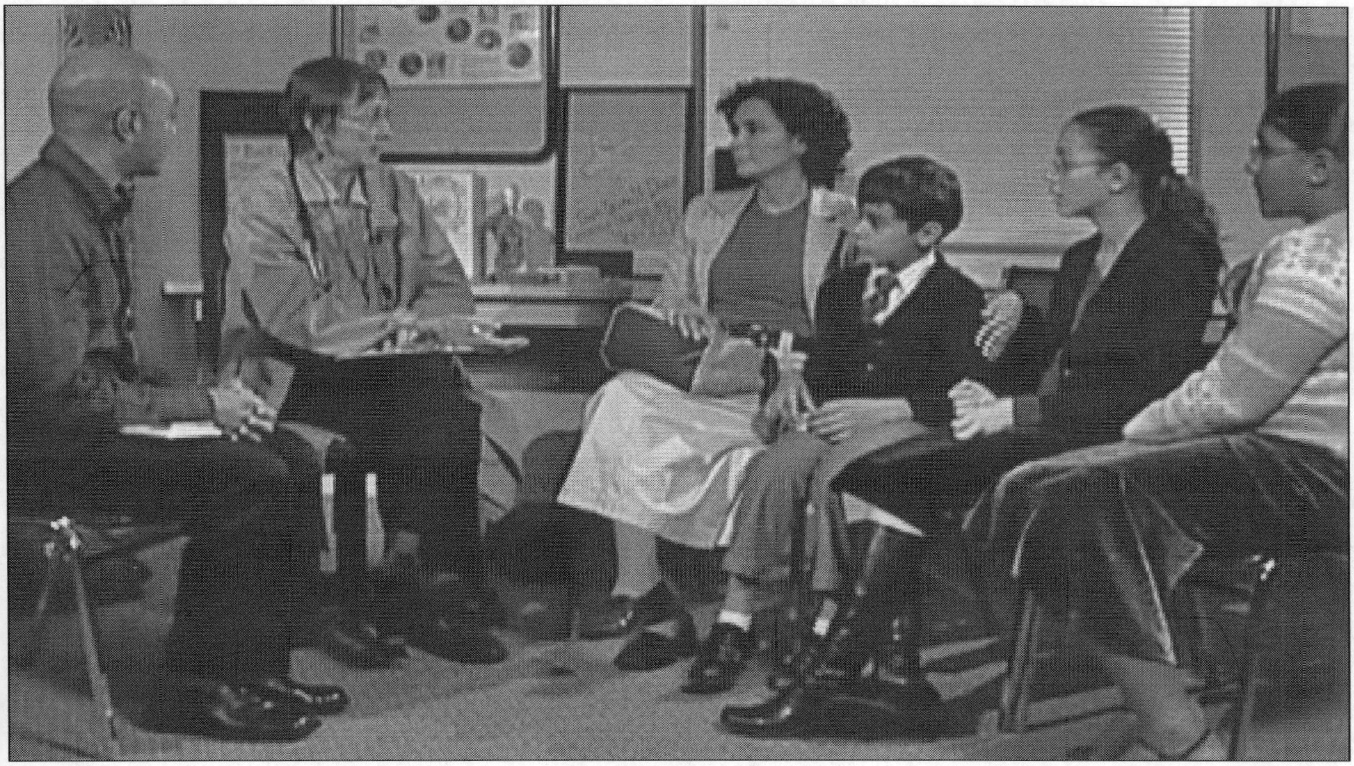

Lesson Thirteen: Quiz
Interpreting in Mental Health Encounters

Read the following statements and determine if they are true or false, then circle the appropriate answer next to the statement.

1. A great majority of mental health encounters happen in primary care or in the emergency room.
   O True O False
2. Interpreters working in hospitals other than mental health institutions, never find themselves interpreting for patients with mental health issues.
   O True O False
3. According to the CDC, ethnic minorities are more likely to seek professional help for mental health issues.
   O True O False
4. To be a good mental health interpreter, one must have some understanding of how mental illness is defined and classified in the clinical world perspective.
   O True O False
5. The current version, DSM-IV TR, defines mental illness as a "clinically significant behavioral or psychological syndrome or pattern that occurs in an individual and that is associated with present distress, pain or disability or with significant risk of suffering pain, disability or an important loss of freedom."
   O True O False
6. The terms "use," "abuse" and "dependency" could be used indistinctly.
   O True O False
7. Drug abuse is "the use of illicit drugs or the abuse of prescription or over-the-counter drugs for purposes other than those for which they are indicated or in a manner or in quantities other than directed."
   O True O False
8. In the United States, if you exceed your use of drugs, but this does not impact the individual, his or her loved ones, his or her work and other functioning in life then it is not considered substance abuse.
   O True O False
9. It is considered substance "dependency" when a person, within a 12-month period of having an adverse reaction to a particular substance, discontinues the use of the substance.
   O True O False
10. An over-the-counter drug medication is that in which a doctor's prescription is not required.
    O True O False
11. CAGE is the place where mental health patients with alcoholism issues will be taken to be treated.
    O True O False
12. Interpreters decide on the mode of interpretation to use in a mental health setting based on the patient coherency and on the type of treatment the patient or family is receiving.
    O True O False
13. The consecutive mode is not the most appropriate for those patients who are coherent and are able to organize their thoughts.
    O True O False
14. If a patient says, "I only take a drink once in a while," is OK for the interpreter to render his/her interpretation into the target language as, "I drink once in a while."
    O True O False

Lesson Thirteen: Class Activities
Interpreting in Mental Health Encounters

A great majority of mental health encounters happen in primary care or in the emergency room. According to the Bazelton Center for Mental Health Law, 25% of all primary care encounters involve a diagnosable mental illness and 50% of mental health problems are still not being diagnosed properly. The World Health Organization is recommending that all medical providers "screen for mental health issues, assess and furnish care to those with mild or moderate disorders or whose severe mental health disorders are stable."

Thus, even if interpreters decide not to interpret in traditional mental health settings, they will certainly find themselves interpreting for patients with mental health issues. For example, in her assessment of a patient with possible memory impairments, a family doctor may conduct memory testing through the interpreter. Or, an ER doctor may see a patient presenting with suicidal ideation, one who is experiencing his first psychotic break, or one who suffers from substance abuse issues. In all of these situations, the interpreter will be practicing mental health interpretation. As you receive your interpreter training, it is wise to ask yourself, "Am I ready to interpret in mental health settings?"

EXERCISE 1

1. When you think of the term "mental health," what is your first reaction?

____

____

2. How would you describe a person who suffers from a mental illness or disorder?

____

____

3. What kind of behaviors do you expect from that individual?

____

____

PO Box 2308, Woburn, MA 01888-0508, **p:** 781-729-3736, **www.EmbracingCulture.com**
PO Box 6401, Manchester, NH 03108, **p:** 1-888-678-CCCS

Society's Views on Mental Illness

Mental illness is prevalent in today's society. According to the Centers for Disease Control (CDC), "One in two Americans has a diagnosable mental disorder." The reality, then, is that all of us, as individuals, have been impacted to some extent by someone who suffers from a mental illness or by our own mental health issues.

Unfortunately, our society's take on mental illness has caused the subject to remain taboo in many circles. When we or someone we love suffer from a mental illness, we generally do not talk about it is as much as we would talk about any other type of chronic illness. Often, insurance companies do not pay for certain types of outpatient psychiatric visits. So, the mentally ill are likely to live in silence and isolation. The U. S. Centers for Disease Control estimates that less than half of the adults suffering from mental illness get help, and that only one third of the children get help. The CDC also asserts that ethnic minorities are less likely to seek professional help for mental health issues.

Those who suffer from mental illness are often forgotten and feared by society. Mental Health interpreters can be the linguistic and cultural bridge between the provider and the patients' worlds. But no matter how good we are as interpreters in terms of facilitating communication from one language to another, in mental health interpreting we encounter extra "weight" – the stigma attached to the seeking of mental health treatment and the shame a patient often feels when there is a third person in the session.

EXERCISE 2

1. Is mental illness openly discussed in the communities you will serve as an interpreter? Please explain.

____

____

____

____

2. How might the communities you will serve as an interpreter generally view a patient who seeks mental health treatment?

____

____

____

____

3. List three or more factors that might influence a patient's decision to seek mental health treatment.

____

____

____

____

How Mental Illness is Defined and Classified

To be an effective mental health interpreter, one must have some understanding of how mental illness is defined and classified in the clinical world perspective. In the 1840s, there was only one category of mental illness, "idiocy/insanity." Since then, there have been many attempts worldwide to collect and to standardize guidelines on how to assess and treat patients who suffer from a mental illness. It has taken many generations of doctors and researchers to arrive at today's definition of what constitutes a mental illness or disorder.

In the early 1960s, the Mental Health Program of the World Health Organization (WHO) became actively engaged in improving the diagnosis and classification of mental disorders. At that time, WHO convened a series of meetings actively involving representatives of different disciplines and various schools of thought in psychiatry from around the world. Numerous proposals to improve the classification of mental disorders resulted from the WHO consultation process, and these were used in drafting the Eighth Revision of the International Classification of Diseases (ICD-8). Since then, the ICD has undergone additional revisions.

The 1970s were marked by significant international interest in improving psychiatric classification worldwide with a view to improving diagnostic reliability. One notable achievement was the American Psychiatric Association's Third Revision of the Diagnostic and Statistical Manual (DSM), which incorporated operational criteria into its classification system.

In the last thirty years, the DSM has undergone multiple revisions. The current version, DSM-IV TR, defines mental illness as a "clinically significant behavioral or psychological syndrome or pattern that occurs in an individual and that is associated with present distress, pain or disability or with significant risk of suffering pain, disability or an important loss of freedom."

PO Box 2308, Woburn, MA 01888-0508, **p:** 781-729-3736, **www.EmbracingCulture.com**
PO Box 6401, Manchester, NH 03108, **p:** 1-888-678-CCCS

Both the ICD-10 and DSM-IV TR recognize several categories of mental disorders, including, but not limited to, personality and behavioral disorders; organic mental disorders; substance-related disorders; schizophrenia, schizotypal and delusional disorders; mood disorders; neurotic, stress-related and somatoform disorders; as well as mental retardation and learning disorders.

EXERCISE 3

1. What is WHO, and what involvement has it had in the history of the definition and classification of mental health disorders?

____

____

____

____

____

2. What is the ICD-10? What is the DSM-IV TR? How are they similar?

____

____

____

____

____

3. Why do you think both publications have undergone repeated revision? Explain.

____

____

____

____

____

Substance-Related Mental Disorders

Interpreters working in medical and mental health settings will eventually facilitate between a provider and a patient with a substance-related disorder. For that reason, interpreters need to understand the difference between the terms "**use**," "**abuse**" and "**dependency**."

DEFINE

1. USE

   ____

   ____

2. ABUSE

   ____

   ____

3. DEPENDENCY

   ____

   ____

Nearly all of us "**use**" substances from time to time. For example, some individuals like to have a glass of wine with an evening meal. Others may smoke an occasional cigarette. A good number of people all over the world start each day with a cup of coffee. All of these situations are examples of "substance use." But what is the difference between the "use" and "abuse" of a substance?

Medline's medical encyclopedia has defined drug **abuse** as "the use of illicit drugs or the abuse of prescription or over-the-counter drugs for purposes other than those for which they are indicated or in a manner or in quantities other than directed." From a legal perspective, then, we see that any use of an illegal drug is considered "abuse," as is any use of a legal substance in excess of or apart from what the doctor or manufacturer has indicated.

PO Box 2308, Woburn, MA 01888-0508, **p:** 781-729-3736, **www.EmbracingCulture.com**
PO Box 6401, Manchester, NH 03108, **p:** 1-888-678-CCCS

From a medical perspective, however, substance abuse is a bit more complex. In the United States, it is characterized, not by the quantity of a substance a person uses, but by how it impacts the individual, his or her loved ones, his or her work and other functioning in life. Although substance abusers have different ranges of behaviors, a common pattern is the denial or minimization that one has a problem, which often leads to the breaking of promises, and the covering up of behaviors. Such dynamics are perceived by the general society as a flaw with someone's character. This perception in fact can create very dysfunctional dynamics within the individual, loved ones and society, where at times one feels shame so one covers up a behavior or enables the intake of substance as long as the individual is hiding it. Substance abuse is an illness that in fact impacts all, not just the individual.

As with the legal perspective, excessive use of certain substances is clearly considered abuse. Any interpreter regularly working in an Emergency Department has likely seen patients who suffer from alcohol intoxication. These patients have recently ingested too much alcohol and are experiencing a sudden change in behavior and thinking processes. At that moment, the patient has abused a substance, but from that single event we cannot determine if the patient has a substance-related disorder.

In order to diagnose a substance-related disorder, U.S. medical and mental health providers will look for a pattern of substance use within a 12 month-period that shows significant impairments or distresses as illustrated by one or more of the following:

1. Recurrent substance use resulting in a failure to fulfill major role obligations at work, school, or home
2. Recurrent substance use in situations in which it is physically hazardous
3. Recurrent substance-related legal problems
4. Continued substance use despite having persistent or recurrent negative effects of the substance

Substance "**dependency**" is a serious form of mental illness. With substance dependency, a person, within a 12-month period of having an adverse reaction to a particular substance, will continue to use the substance. One can observe a pattern of repeated intoxications and, with certain substances, withdrawals. With dependence, there is a craving or desire to take or use the substance, or an inability to stop using the substance.

EXERCISE 4

1. **Match each term to its corresponding definition:**

_____ 1. substance use	a. harmful to one's health or wellbeing
_____ 2. substance abuse	b. medication for which a doctor's prescription is not required
_____ 3. substance dependency	c. medication for which a doctor's prescription is required
_____ 4. intoxication	d. recurring use of a substance with inability to stop this behavior
_____ 5. illegal drug	e. result of ingestion of a substance that causes a change in behavior or thinking processes
_____ 6. prescription drug	f. substance that is prohibited by law
_____ 7. over-the-counter drug	g. the ingestion, injection or inhalation of a substance
_____ 8. hazardous	h. to misuse a substance (in quantity or purpose)

2. List four signs in a patient's life or relationships that he or she may have a substance-related disorder.

____

____

____

____

____

____

PO Box 2308, Woburn, MA 01888-0508, **p:** 781-729-3736, **www.EmbracingCulture.com**
PO Box 6401, Manchester, NH 03108, **p:** 1-888-678-CCCS

Detecting a Substance-Related Disorder

Oftentimes, signs of a substance-related disorder are first noticed by a primary care provider. To further investigate, the provider may ask the patient a series of questions designed to detect problems with substance abuse or dependency.

One example of a standard set of questions used by providers is the CAGE questionnaire, designed to detect alcoholism in adult patients during a primary care encounter. CAGE asks the following questions:

- Have you ever felt you should Cut down on your drinking?
- Have people Annoyed you by criticizing your drinking?
- Have you ever felt bad or Guilty about your drinking?
- Have you ever had an "Eye opener" (drink) first thing in the morning to steady your nerves or to get rid of a hangover?

The patient's responses on the CAGE are scored 0 or 1, with a higher score being an indication of alcohol problems. A total score of 2 or greater is considered clinically significant.

EXERCISE 5

(Role-Play Practice)

Your teacher will divide the class into target-language specific groups for role-play practice. Two of your colleagues will be assigned to play the respective roles of provider and patient. The provider will ask the patient the questions listed above in the CAGE questionnaire. Practice interpreting these questions in your target language. Then, discuss alternative interpretations with your colleagues.

Topics for discussion

1. How would you interpret the phrase "cut down on your drinking?"
2. What possible interpretations could you use to transmit the concept of being "annoyed?"
3. How many different ways can the concept of "guilt" be transmitted in your target language?
4. What is an "eye opener" and how could you best interpret this term in your target language?

Interpreting Modes for Mental Health Interpretation

Mental Health Interpreters need to feel comfortable switching back and forth between consecutive and simultaneous modes of interpretation. The mode you choose will depend on if the patient is coherent and on the type of treatment the patient or family is receiving.

The **consecutive mode** is the most appropriate for those patients who are coherent and are able to organize their thoughts. In consecutive interpretation, the interpreter waits for the speaker to complete an idea and then conveys it as soon as the speaker is finished, while keeping the same language register and order of thoughts. Interpreters may find that consecutive interpretation is appropriate for some family sessions where each member takes a turn speaking and for individual evaluations and one-on-one treatment sessions.

In consecutive interpretation, *accuracy* is essential. For example, if a patient says, "I only take a drink once in a while," the interpreter must say "I only take a drink once in a while" and not, "I drink once in a while." The omission of the word "only" nullifies a diagnostic tool useful to providers looking for information to help the patient.

Similarly, if a patient says, "I sometimes think about ending it all," the interpreter should be careful not to say, "I'm thinking of ending it all." To a provider, one statement may indicate *suicidal ideation* (thoughts), while the other may be indicative of a *suicidal intent* (plan). In like manner, the statement, "I feel like hurting myself" is different from "I hurt myself." Patients with acute suicidal intent may be hospitalized for their own safety. In cases of long-term suicidal risk, many mental health professionals ask the patient to enter into a "safety contract," a verbal or written agreement that the patient will contact them or seek other help before acting on a suicidal impulse.

The **simultaneous mode** (speaking at the same time as the speaker) is best applied when a patient's thinking is disorganized. Also, this mode works well with the type of treatment where the counselor is using a confrontative type of questioning regarding the substance abuse, the facts about the abuse and how it has affected a patient's life.

Simultaneous interpreting is also used where there is more than one language spoken in a group therapy setting. In such settings, the interpreter may want to sit next to and slightly behind the patient while simultaneously interpreting in a low tone of voice. The purpose of interpreting in an undertone is to not disturb the speaker or other group therapy participants, while keeping the patient informed of the communication. However, when it is the non-English speaking patient's turn to speak, the interpreter will switch to a louder interpretation, either simultaneous or consecutive, so that the group therapy participants can easily hear the patient. The interpreter's choice of simultaneous or consecutive interpreting depends largely on the patient's ability to pace him or herself.

PO Box 2308, Woburn, MA 01888-0508, **p:** 781-729-3736, **www.EmbracingCulture.com**
PO Box 6401, Manchester, NH 03108, **p:** 1-888-678-CCCS

There are moments in the clinical encounter where the patient does not speak logically, or the patient's speech is slurred and therefore unclear. This is perhaps one of the very few times where interpreters may resort to **summarization**, a dangerous mode because the interpreter can miss important information. When using summarization, the interpreter must inform the clinician that he or she has switched to this mode of interpretation. In such a situation, the patient would likely not understand the concept of summarization due to his or her state of mind, so an explanation to the patient would not be necessary.

As part of an evaluation and registration process, or upon discharge from a detox center or emergency room, the interpreter might be asked to perform a **sight interpretation** of a self-assessment tool or referral contact sheet. Ideally, the provider will read the questions or instructions out loud and the interpreter will interpret using the consecutive mode. In the event that the provider does not make him or herself available, and the interpreter is required to assist the patient or family member complete an intake questionnaire or medical history, the interpreter must refrain from answering the intake questions or from explaining them to the patient. We recommend that the interpreter circle the questions or statements on the form that the patient does not understand, and ask the patient to refer to those items as he or she meets with the provider.

EXERCISE 6

(Role-Play Practice)

Role-Play 87: Group Therapy

This role-play represents a mental health group therapy session.
For this exercise, we will need seven volunteers.

Setting Up...

1. Sit in a circle.
2. Choose one group member to be the therapist.
3. Choose one group member to be the interpreter.
4. The other five members will each take a number (1 to 5).
5. Group member #1 will speak only in the target language. All other group members will speak in English. The interpreter will sit next to and slightly behind Member #1.

Role-Play 87 *(continued)*

Therapist: Welcome to our support group. We will be having a great Interpreter for the _____ language. At first it may sound strange, but soon you will get used to it and it will seem like the interpreter is not here.

You all are here because you all share a story. I am Linda and we will be spending 60 minutes once a week for about 15 sessions. There are a few rules. Members need to speak for themselves and will need to wait for their turn to speak.Information is confidential and it cannot be shared outside the group. The interpreter will have to follow the same expectations as all of us in regard to confidentiality.

Every group member will have an equal opportunity to speak and to be an active participant in this group. If you do not feel safe, you need to share this with the group or you can let me know at the end of the group. I do not discuss group dynamics with anyone outside the group. I would like it if we can start with the introductions. Can you please share your name with the group?

Member #1: I am Maria and I am here because I am having a hard time with my husband *(gets interrupted by Member #2)*

Member #2: *(Interrupting Member #1)* Dear, we all are here because we are having a hard time. Oops, I'm not supposed to speak yet! Sorry, but I have a hard time watching someone cry over a man.

Therapist: Maria, is there anything you want to say to… *(Looking at Member #2)* …and you are?

Member #2: I am Christina.

Therapist: At this point, let's try our best not to interrupt each other. Christina, can you introduce yourself?

Member #4: This feels like kindergarten to me. Is this a support group? You seem a bit bossy, like, "Here are the rules and you kids need to behave" *(Gets interrupted by Member #2)*.

Member #2: *(Interrupting Member #4)* I am so sorry, but if I do not speak up now I'll end up walking away. I am here because I am having some trouble with my stepchildren. I feel that I have done everything I can to please them to welcome them into our new family and they treat me like I am no one – *(Gets interrupted by Member #5)*.

Member #5: *(Interrupting Member #2)* I know that feeling. Oops, I interrupted you. Sorry.

continued

PO Box 2308, Woburn, MA 01888-0508, **p:** 781-729-3736, **www.EmbracingCulture.com**
PO Box 6401, Manchester, NH 03108, **p:** 1-888-678-CCCS

Topics for Discussion

1. Which modes did the interpreter use in this setting?
2. Was there a point at which the interpreter switched modes?
3. Might the number of speakers or the flow of conversation influence the interpreter's choice of modes? Explain.
4. What other modes of interpreting might have been appropriate in this setting? Provide specific examples.

Role-Play 87: Glossary

continued

1. Pathology (diseases, conditions)

2. Laboratory Tests and Diagnostic Procedures

3. Treatment Procedures

4. Idiomatic Expressions (if any)

5. Other (vocabulary in that particular role-play that you feel is important/relevant or that you anticipate problems with)

PO Box 2308, Woburn, MA 01888-0508, **p:** 781-729-3736, **www.EmbracingCulture.com**
PO Box 6401, Manchester, NH 03108, **p:** 1-888-678-CCCS

Role-Play 88: Family Therapy

This role-play represents a family therapy session. It will require four participants: provider, interpreter, and two students representing a husband and wife.

Counselor: Good morning and welcome to the behavioral health department. May I ask what has brought you in today?

Mrs. A: Doctor, I'm concerned for my husband's health.

Counselor: What concerns you?

Mrs. A: My husband is a good man who has worked very hard all of his life to provide for his family but now I'm afraid he won't live long enough to enjoy what he has worked so long for.

Counselor: Is your husband in poor health?

Mrs. A: He is getting worse.

Counselor: What exactly is the problem?

Mrs. A: I'm afraid that he is drinking too much wine. All the time now, all he does is stay home and drink wine.

Counselor: Is this true, Mr. A.?

Mrs. A: Not entirely. I do enjoy a glass of wine now and then but I think my wife is exaggerating.

Mrs. A: That's not true, doctor. My husband has so much wine in him, he doesn't know what's true or not. I come home from work and he is yelling at me asking me where I was and who I was with. He knows I was working but the alcohol makes him crazy.

Mrs. A: She goes out and doesn't tell me anything. I'm supposed to take care of myself. What kind of man does she think I am?

Counselor: Mr. A., do you mind if I ask you a few questions about your use of wine?

Mrs. A: Sure, ask me anything you want to.

Counselor: Can you tell me how much you drink throughout the course of the day?

Mrs. A: Just a few glasses of wine, nothing much more.

Counselor: Would you finish the bottle before the end of the day?

Mrs. A: Oh sure, but you have to remember, I've been drinking for a long time.

Counselor: And you do that everyday?

Mrs. A: Well…maybe not everyday.

Mrs. A: Doctor, it's everyday. Everyday, the man drinks a whole bottle of wine. I am so concerned for him.

continued

Role-Play 88 *(continued)*

Mrs. A: See how she gets? She makes a mountain out of a molehill!

Counselor: Mr. A, has anyone else ever told you that you might have a problem with drinking too much wine?

Mrs. A: No, nobody else.

Mrs. A: Doctor, his children tell him all the time. They want him to stop drinking, but he doesn't listen.

Counselor: Mr. A., is that true?

Mrs. A: They're as bad as she is. No one wants to see me having any fun.

Counselor: What about the doctor? Has he said anything to you?

Mrs. A: No, except for my family no one says anything to me about my wine.

Counselor: Why do you think your family brings it up to you?

Mrs. A: I don't know.

Counselor: Is it possible that they think you're hurting yourself with alcohol and they don't want to see that happen?

Topics for Discussion

1. Which modes did the interpreter use in this setting?
2. Was there a point at which the interpreter switched modes?
3. Might the emotion of the speaker influence the interpreter's choice of modes? Explain.
4. What other modes of interpreting might have been appropriate in this setting? Provide specific examples.

continued

PO Box 2308, Woburn, MA 01888-0508, **p:** 781-729-3736, **www.EmbracingCulture.com**
PO Box 6401, Manchester, NH 03108, **p:** 1-888-678-CCCS

Role-Play 88: Glossary

continued

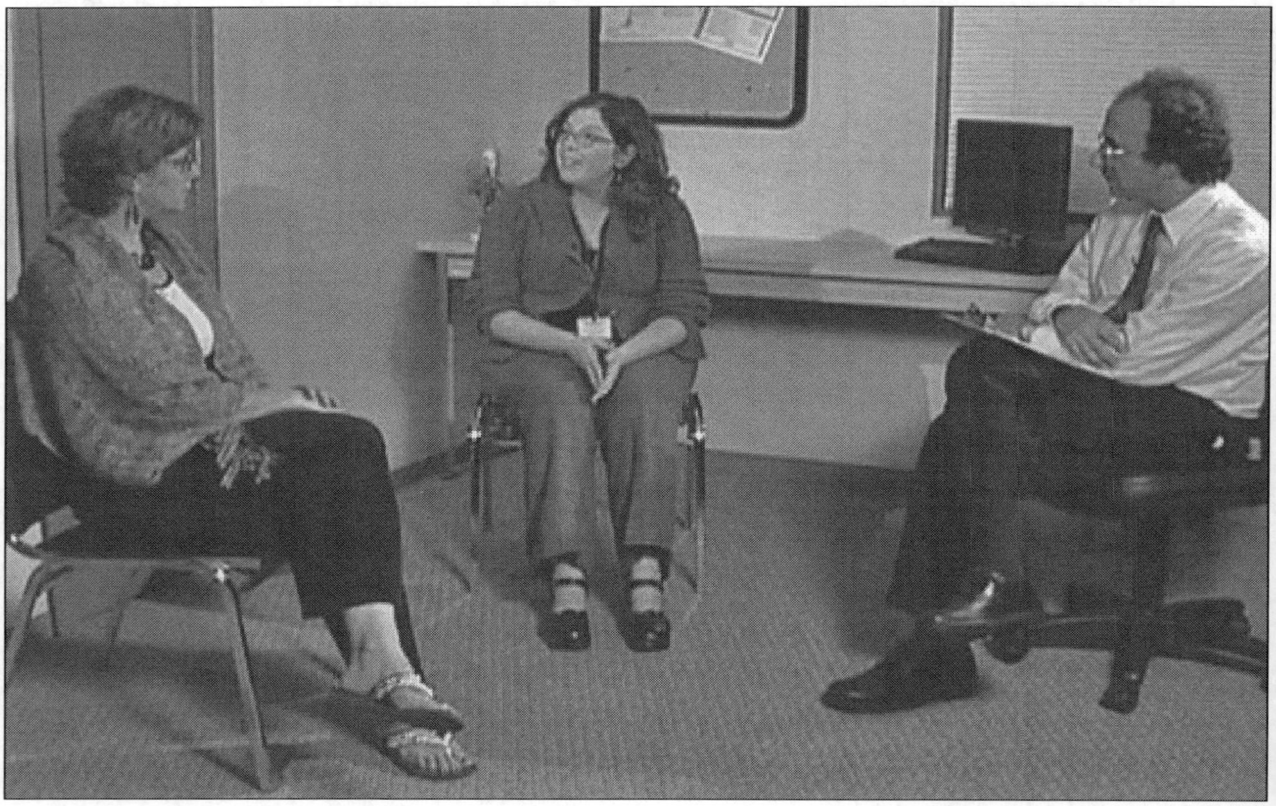

1. Pathology (diseases, conditions)

2. Laboratory Tests and Diagnostic Procedures

3. Treatment Procedures

4. Idiomatic Expressions (if any)

5. Other (vocabulary in that particular role-play that you feel is important/relevant or that you anticipate problems with)

PO Box 2308, Woburn, MA 01888-0508, **p:** 781-729-3736, **www.EmbracingCulture.com**
PO Box 6401, Manchester, NH 03108, **p:** 1-888-678-CCCS

Asking for clarification in the mental health encounter

Interpreters can only interpret as much as they understand. If a patient's thought and speech is disorganized and lacks logic, it is the interpreter's responsibility to ask the provider to ask the patient to explain the term or phrase. However, in mental health settings, too many interruptions and requests for clarification may disrupt the clinician or the patient's thinking.

The number of interpreter requests for clarification from a patient may depend on the treatment setting and on the patient's ability to be coherent. But if the interpreter does not get the meaning of the message, the clinician will also not get it. Thus, requests for clarification are of vital importance.

To avoid excessive requests for repetition, the interpreter might choose to do some note taking or to switch from the consecutive to the simultaneous mode. When it is absolutely necessary to request clarification, the effective interpreter will repeat back in the source language the last word the patient or clinician said in order to capture missed information.

For example, the clinician might say, "I understand that in the past 3 months you have taken an eye opener and that your shakes disappear after you do this. Tell me more about your work." The interpreter might interpret, "I understand that in the past 3 months you have taken an eye opener…" As the interpreter senses that he or she has lost some information, the interpreter looks at the clinician and says, "eye opener, and that your…?" The clinician, now fully aware of exactly how much information the interpreter had relayed, completes the sentence and renders an appropriate interpretation. This technique is called **anchoring**.

When a patient is incoherent, clarification might not always be possible. In this case, it may be best to interpret to the provider exactly what you are hearing from the patient; even if it does not appear to make sense. Both the patient's general way of speaking and specific wording can provide diagnostic clues to the provider.

In mental health treatment sessions, providers often use **echoing**; the repetition or reframing of a patient's key words or thoughts as a technique for demonstrating empathy, connecting with the patient, and helping the patient develop insight.

When a provider is echoing or reframing, the interpreter should mirror the provider's choice of words. Often, the provider chooses a specific word with the purpose of deescalating a potentially dangerous interaction. Other times, the provider implements a word or phrase with the purpose of eliciting a certain reaction. The interpreter should be careful that the interpreted message is equivalent in its effect upon the patient.

Mental health providers often make use of "therapeutic silence," a technique of pausing after a question or comment to observe a patient's reaction. In this silence, the patient is able to reflect on both the provider's choice of words and on his/her own response to the provider.

Interpreters must be careful to not "fill" these moments of silence with the noise of interpretation, and thus dilute their effect. In a pre-session with the mental health clinician, agree on a signal that will indicate when a provider wishes the interpreter to replicate the silence in the target language.

EXERCISE 7

(Role-Play Practice)

In the following role-play, the patient is unable to speak coherently. Practice interpreting to the provider exactly what you hear from the patient.

Role-Play 89:

MD: Ms. De Jesus, how are you feeling?

Patient: Excellent! I always love to fish. When my husband died, I learned to fish in the ocean.

MD: I am going to ask you some memory questions. Is that alright?

Patient: I need to be finished by June.

MD: What day is it?

Patient: It is Sunday.

MD: Well, actually, it is Saturday.

Patient: The pretty angel is sitting here in my room.

MD: Do you know what month it is?

Patient: I was born in July.

MD: What is today's date?

Patient: April 24th.

MD: Mrs. De Jesus, are you seeing things you know aren't here?

Patient: I have seen a little dog in the corner of the room. (She laughs)

MD: Do you hear people speaking to you when there is no one around?

Patient: No, but I do listen to the radio at night.

MD: Can you spell the word "world" backwards?

Patient: I can, but I don't care to say it.

MD: Who is the new President of the United States?

Patient: I have no idea. Who is the Bishop of Braga?

continued

PO Box 2308, Woburn, MA 01888-0508, **p:** 781-729-3736, **www.EmbracingCulture.com**
PO Box 6401, Manchester, NH 03108, **p:** 1-888-678-CCCS

Role-Play 89 *(continued)*

Topics for Discussion

1. What was it like to interpret for this patient?
2. What did you perceive as the greatest challenges to accuracy?
3. Why was it important for the provider to hear exactly what the patient was saying?
4. What might the patient's responses have indicated to the provider?

Role-Play 89: Glossary

continued

1. Pathology (diseases, conditions)

2. Laboratory Tests and Diagnostic Procedures

3. Treatment Procedures

4. Idiomatic Expressions (if any)

5. Other (vocabulary in that particular role-play that you feel is important/relevant or that you anticipate problems with)

PO Box 2308, Woburn, MA 01888-0508, **p:** 781-729-3736, **www.EmbracingCulture.com**
PO Box 6401, Manchester, NH 03108, **p:** 1-888-678-CCCS

Finding your center as an interpreter

What if you, the interpreter, have had some type of experience with mental health or substance abuse issues involving yourself or a loved one? Clinicians and family members have also had similar experiences. Though each case is different, most carry underlying themes of counter transference, anger, wanting to be helpful but feeling helpless, lonely or betrayed. An interpreter must be in touch with these feelings and revisit his or her unpleasant experiences without becoming an imposition on the session.

In cases of substance abuse, it is common for drugs to take over an addict's life and the lives of innocent family members, creating a spectrum of conflicting feelings and raising expectations that are often broken. There are times during sessions where interpreters begin to recognize in themselves behaviors that had not previously surfaced. Suddenly, the interpreter is listening to an internal voice but not to the voices of the other parties in the session. Vital information is inadvertently omitted.

Part of finding your center as an interpreter is to revisit a specific situation in which you were the patient, the family member, or the friend. By replaying the scenario in your mind and re-experiencing the loaded feelings, you, in a way, desensitize yourself so that if the feelings suddenly re-arise in an interpreting session, you are not caught off guard and do not lose your focus.

One interpreter reports that she has a family member who is an alcoholic but has not yet accepted the fact. In the past 10 years, the family member's life has become a mire of stories made up to cover her losses at work and her inability to maintain an independent social life. But because she has so many assets, is intelligent and does not look like a homeless person, family and friends have enabled her drinking by minimizing her lies. When the interpreter assisted patients who are alcoholics, she was constantly reminded of her family member, and this made it hard for her to interpret. What did the interpreter do to change the situation?

The interpreter reports that she began to set limits in her personal life in regard to her relationship with the family member. She stopped being the enabler by being loving but firm when expressing to the family member how her behavior has broken trust and has hurt her feelings. Thus, by addressing these issues in her personal life, she was able to resolve previously unspoken feelings towards alcoholics and alcoholism. Now, when she interprets for a substance abuser, she no longer feels the frustration she once felt and she is able to maintain her composure and to interpret without prejudice. She has "found her center" as an interpreter.

Finding one's center is not as easy as many interpreters affirm in trainings. Often, we hear, "It's not a big deal! I just convey what people say. I simply disconnect and do my job." Interpreter trainers must worry about interpreters who believe that transparency is effortless. We are all human. We all have feelings. Lines of professionalism are crossed every day as interpreters distracted by personal feelings get lost fighting these feelings and subsequently sacrifice their accuracy in the triadic encounter.

Finding one's center involves being able to recognize the humanity in each of us. It is a state of mind in which the interpreter acknowledges, but is not overwhelmed, by personal feelings. The interpreter "stores" or "parks" the feelings, revisiting them only after the session is finished.

Another potential pitfall in the mental health encounter are alliances between the patient and the interpreter. These can happen because of our own feelings towards the illness and because of how we perceive the clinician should react to the situation. For example, if you are interpreting in an outpatient setting, you may experience some of the "fuzziness" that comes with a clinician's efforts to establish rapport (therapeutic relationship) with the patient. However, if you are in an emergency room and the patient is a chronic visitor with substance abuse issues, you may feel that the provider does not attempt to develop any type of rapport with the patient. In this case, the provider's job is to assess the level of intoxication and to plan for the patient's sobriety. The provider may even appear to treat the patient in an aggressive or confrontational way in an attempt to break the patient's denial. These actions might be understood by the novice interpreter as unfair, and the interpreter may begin to develop positive feelings about the "poor" patient and negative feelings about the "bad" doctor.

Many times, patients will appear quite sad during parts of a session, and it is common for patients to cry. While it is natural for an interpreter to feel sorry for the patient, guard against a misguided display of sympathy. Many interpreters have offered the patient a tissue, or whispered words of encouragement. Such action, in many ways, would weaken the effect of the therapy. Follow the provider's cues, and never take it upon yourself to interject with an offer of assistance that does not originate with the provider.

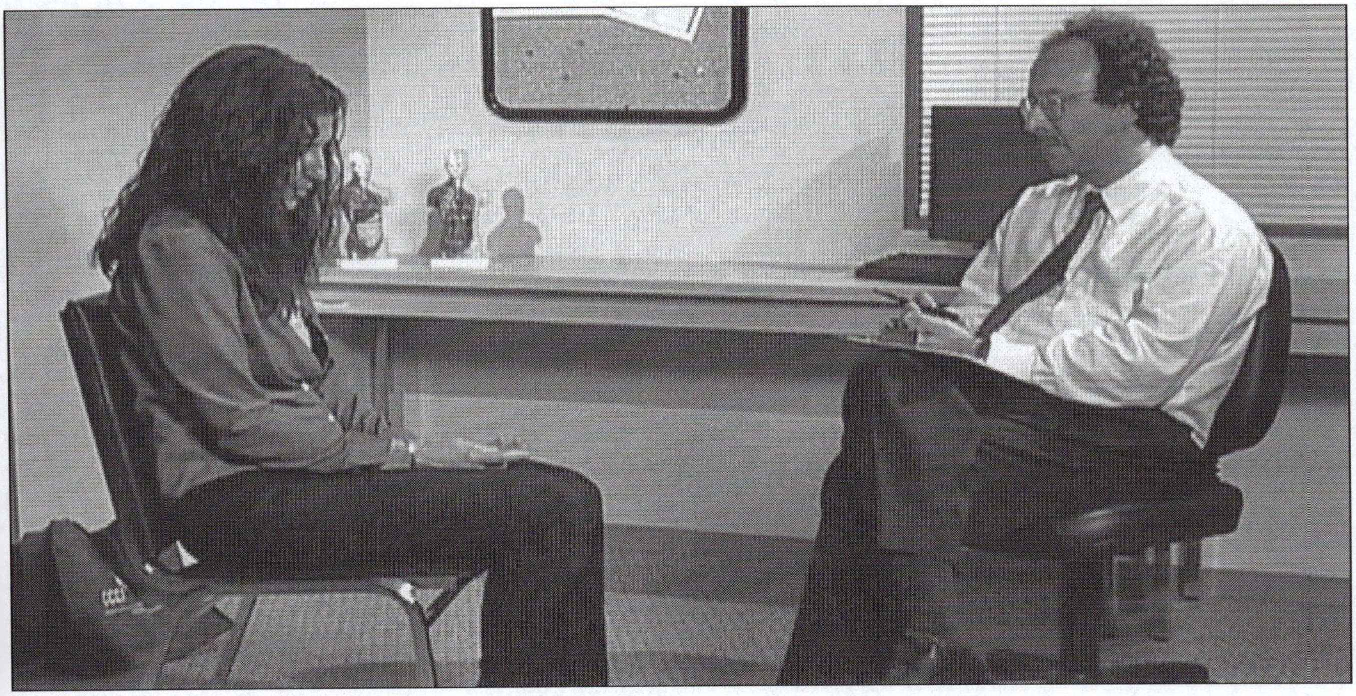

PO Box 2308, Woburn, MA 01888-0508, **p:** 781-729-3736, **www.EmbracingCulture.com**
PO Box 6401, Manchester, NH 03108, **p:** 1-888-678-CCCS

EXERCISE 8

What would you do in the following situations? What standard of practice supports your decision? Are there ways in which similar situations might be avoided in the future?

1. Provider is confrontative with substance abuser and you are uncomfortable with this style of questioning.

____

____

____

2. Patient begins to cry during a treatment session and the provider does not reach out to offer a Kleenex.

____

____

____

3. Patient reminds you of your grandfather, who drank away the family fortune. You don't like to think of your grandfather.

____

____

____

4. You begin to get the feeling that the provider doesn't like the patient, and you feel bad for the patient.

____

____

____

5. Patient was a victim of a violent crime and is experiencing post-traumatic symptoms. This reminds you of an experience in your life. You begin to feel very sad while interpreting in the session.

____

____

____

The Mental Status Exam

Mental Status Examination is the methodical observation of an individual's general behavior and evaluation through specific questions and exercises with the purpose of better understanding his/her thinking process and content. Such evaluations are conducted both in mental health assessment and treatment sessions, as well as in routine medical examinations, primarily involving elderly patients or those suspected of experiencing early dementia.

The Mini-Mental Status Examination offers a quick and simple way for medical providers to quantify cognitive function and screen for cognitive loss. It tests the individual's orientation, attention, calculation, recall, language and motor skills.

Watch the video *Mental Status Exams for Patients with Early Dementia*, from the collection "The Healthcare Interpreter's Tools for Mental Health Interpreting," volume 2. Use the space below to take notes on what you see or what you find interesting.

PO Box 2308, Woburn, MA 01888-0508, **p:** 781-729-3736, **www.EmbracingCulture.com**
PO Box 6401, Manchester, NH 03108, **p:** 1-888-678-CCCS

Topics for discussion

1. Are there portions of the mini mental status examination that might not be culturally relevant for the populations you serve? Provide specific examples. (Note: some examples may include cultural views on time and place, limited English proficiency, illiteracy, cultural taboos, etc.)

2. In the examples you cite in question #1, what level of cultural brokering might be appropriate for each, and how would you share this information with the provider?

3. Should the interpreter ask the provider if names of objects should be translated exactly or if he/she can exchange them for items that are more culturally relevant?

4. Should proverbs be literally interpreted?

5. How would you interpret the following proverbs?

   Proverb 1: *A rolling stone gathers no moss.*

   Proverb 2: *People in glass houses shouldn't throw stones*

How is the Mental Status Exam structured?

Each section of the test involves a related series of questions or commands. The individual receives one point for each correct answer. The individual can receive a maximum score of 30 points. A score below 20 usually indicates cognitive impairment.

The following are some standard questions in the mini mental status exam. Practice interpreting them with your colleagues.

- **Orientation to Time**
  What is today's date?
  What is the month?
  What is the year?
  What is the day of the week today?
  What season is it?
- **Orientation to Place**
  Whose home is this?
  What room is this?
  What city are we in?
  What county are we in?
  What state are we in?
- **Immediate Recall**
  Provider asks if he/she may test patient's memory. Provider then says three words (such as "ball," "flag," "tree") clearly and slowly, about 1 second for each. After provider has said all three words, patient is asked to repeat them – the first repetition determines the score (0-3):
- **Attention**
  A) Patient is asked to begin with 100 and count backwards by 7. Provider stops test after 5 subtractions. Score the correct subtractions.
  B) Provider asks the patient to spell the word "WORLD" backwards. The score is the number of letters in correct position.
- **Delayed Verbal Recall**
  Provider asks the patient to recall the 3 words previously asked of him to remember.
- **Naming**
  Provider shows the patient a wristwatch and asks him/her what it is. Repeat for pencil.
- **Repetition**
  Provider asks the individual to repeat the following:
  "No if, ands, or buts"

PO Box 2308, Woburn, MA 01888-0508, **p:** 781-729-3736, **www.EmbracingCulture.com**
PO Box 6401, Manchester, NH 03108, **p:** 1-888-678-CCCS

- **Stage Command**
  Provider gives patient a plain piece of paper and says, "Take the paper in your hand, fold it in half, and put it on the floor." Patient is scored on each activity separately.
- **Reading**
  Provider holds up a sign reading: "Close your eyes" so the patient can see it clearly. Provider asks him/her to read it and do what it says. This item is scored correctly only if the patient actually closes his/her eyes.
- **Writing**
  Provider gives the patient a piece of paper and asks him/her to write a sentence. It is to be written spontaneously. It must contain a subject and verb and be sensible.
- **Copying**
  Provider gives the individual a piece of paper and asks him/her to copy a design of two intersecting shapes. One point is awarded for correctly copying the shapes. All angles on both figures must be present, and the figures must have one overlapping angle.
- **Other things a provider will look for in a mental status examination include:**

  General Behavior: Is this person well groomed? Connected? Showed appropriate eye contact? Is her/his affect (demeanor) congruent with what is being said?

  Speech: Refers to the patient's style of talking. Is it too fast, slow, and mumbling?

  Emotional state: An evaluation of the patient's emotions expressed verbally and through body language.

  Thought processes: This involves at least two aspects of a patients' thinking, the form (how someone thinks) and the content (what someone thinks). In most cases, there is logic to someone's thinking but in the cases of a thought form disorder, one can observe a patient going on and on with ideas that seem to lack an order, confusing the listener. A thought content disorder refers to the patient's understanding of reality. This is when a clinician may need to clarify information, assess suicidal ideation, delusional or hallucinatory thinking.

  Sensorium and mental capacities: When a clinician checks for recall of long, short and immediate memory, and ability to concentrate. (Includes mini mental status exam, plus proverb interpretation to check intelligence, associations, abstraction.)

  Insight and judgment: Insight is the patient's ability to understand the roots of his or her own feelings and actions. Judgment refers to his/her ability to make appropriate decisions about life circumstances.

Mental Health Glossary for Medical Interpreters

WORD	MEANING
Abstinence Model	When the person stops taking all substances and remains drug free. Model used by AA meetings and other forms of treatment.
Addiction	An illness that results when a person takes a drug for a certain time and the body gets used to having this drug.
Adjustment Disorders	The development of emotional or behavioral symptoms in response to an identifiable stressor (such as immigrating to a new country, marriage, life changes and more), occurring within three months of the onset of the stressor(s).
Affective Disorder	A mental health category also known as mood disorder, characterized by problems that include depressive disorders. An individual may feel too down or overly elated, happy.
Agoraphobia	Fear of the outside space, or an anxiety disorder related to the fear of having a panic attack when one is in an open space.
Anorexia Nervosa	An eating disorder also called anorexia. An individual develops a distorted image of his/her body. Shows an intense preoccupation with gaining weight and most likely is 85% underweight.
Asperger's Disorder	One type of pervasive developmental disorder that is characterized by severe and sustained impairment in social interaction and the development of restricted, repetitive patterns of behavior, interests, and activities.
Attention-Deficit/ Hyperactivity Disorder (ADHD)	A behavior disorder, usually first diagnosed in childhood, which is characterized by inattention, impulsivity, and, in some cases, hyperactivity.
Attention Deficit Disorder (ADD)	A syndrome consisting of inattention, excessive motor activity, and impulsivity. ADHD: Attention Deficit Disorder with Hyperactivity.
Autistic Disorder	A neurological and developmental disorder known as autism. It usually appears during the first three years of life. A child with autism appears to live in his/her own world and appears unattached to others, avoiding eye and physical contact with others. Repeating occurred behaviors, at times making undeciphered sounds, showing little interest in others, and showing no or poor social awareness.
Binge Eating Disorder	A disorder that is similar to bulimia nervosa. It is defined by episodes of uncontrolled eating. It differs from bulimia, however, because the individual does not purge the body of the excess food via vomiting, laxative abuse, or diuretic abuse.

continued

PO Box 2308, Woburn, MA 01888-0508, **p:** 781-729-3736, **www.EmbracingCulture.com**
PO Box 6401, Manchester, NH 03108, **p:** 1-888-678-CCCS

Mental Health Glossary *(continued)*

WORD	MEANING
Bipolar Disorder	A mental illness that causes extreme mood swings, also known as manic depressive disorder. An individual may feel very happy, over friendly, with a tendency to overspend or overexpose the body. Soon after, the individual may feel depressed, unable to get up in the morning, with suicidal thoughts or behaviors.
Blackout	A loss of memory when drinking alcohol.
Blood Alcohol Level (BAL) or Blood Alcohol Content (BAC)	The percentage of alcohol in a person's blood. A person with a .01% is considered legally intoxicated. This level has gone down to .08% in many states.
Co-dependency	When a family member, a friend or a co-worker keeps supporting substance abuse by protecting the substance abuser by covering up for his or her behaviors through lies or by giving the abuser money.
Central Nervous System	The parts of the brain that are responsible for intellectual development, body activity and the ability to concentrate.
Conduct Disorders	(Behavior disorders) A group of childhood/adolescent disturbances of repetitive and persistent antisocial activities that violate the rights of others.
Delirium Tremens	The shakes and the confusion that occurs with some patients who stop taking the substance they are abusing.
Delusions	A perception that is thought to be true by the person experiencing it, although the perception is wrong. A constructed belief system that is not based on reality. "I am the president of the United States," this is called a grandiose delusion. A persecutory one is: "I know the FBI is after me." There are many different types of delusions.
Depression	A mood disorder characterized by extreme feelings of sadness, lack of self-worth, and an inability to cope with daily activities, such as self grooming, feeding, work and social activities, sleep disorder and more.
Detoxification (Detox)	When a person is physically addicted to a substance and stops it and needs to go through a process that is medically watched due to potential withdrawal symptoms
Dyslexia	A learning disability or reading and or writing disorder characterized by an individual's inability to sort out a series of sequential images in the brain. For example, an individual may have difficulty with the spelling or reading of the letters b, d, and p, by inverting them or by mixing up their pronunciation. There is no correlation with low intelligence; in fact, many famous people in the world suffer from dyslexia. There is a possibility that it passes from generation to generation, more common among males. Individuals who overcome this challenge end up learning how to decode their language such as with inversion of the order of letters and sounds.

continued

Mental Health Glossary *(continued)*

WORD	MEANING
Dementia	Deterioration of intellectual functioning and personality changes due to physical causes as in Alzheimer's and Parkinson's disease.
Dissociative Disorders	A group of disorders characterized by alterations, typically sudden in onset and of temporary duration, of the normally integrated functions of consciousness or identity. Individuals who have suffered intense abuse, may develop this disorder as their way to cope with the abuse. For example, often therapists hear the stories of children who, at the moment of being abused, look up at the ceiling and imagine one of their favorite TV shows. This dissociation is a defense mechanism that becomes more permanent.
Dyskinesia	An involuntary and rhythmic muscular activity. Often patients who suffer from a psychotic disorder and are treated for it, may develop these involuntary movements with almost a chewing-like affect in their mouths, a passing back and forth and other involuntary movements.
	Difficulty in swallowing.
Dysphagia Dysthymia	A type of an affective disorder or mood disorder that may be less severe, but yet more chronic than the clinical depression. Individual with dysthymia may also experience major depressive episodes at times.
Eating Disorders	A group of disorders in which there are significant disturbances in eating. Two common examples are Anorexia Nervosa, a refusal to maintain an acceptable body weight for one's age and height; and Bulimia Nervosa, uncontrollable binge eating which may be followed by purging or forced throwing up of the food. Individuals may induce vomiting or take laxatives or diuretics.
Enabling	To create and support an avenue, most often unconsciously, for the substance abuser to continue with the abuse.
Endorphins	Chemicals in the brain that are responsible for positive moods. Chocolate is known for having great amount of endorphins.
Euphoria	A feeling of elation, of being too happy, that is not based on reality and is commonly exaggerated.
Generalized Anxiety Disorder (GAD)	A mental disorder characterized by chronic, excessive worry and fear that seems to have no real cause. Children or adolescents with generalized anxiety disorder often worry a lot about things such as future events, past behaviors, social acceptance, family matters, their personal abilities, and/or school performance. For example, a child might not want to go to school for fear of losing his mother or being hit by a car.

continued

PO Box 2308, Woburn, MA 01888-0508, **p:** 781-729-3736, **www.EmbracingCulture.com**
PO Box 6401, Manchester, NH 03108, **p:** 1-888-678-CCCS

Mental Health Glossary *(continued)*

WORD	MEANING
Hallucinations	A strong perception of an event or object when no such situation is present; may occur in any of the senses (i.e., visual, auditory, gustatory, olfactory, or tactile). A false sensory perception without a concrete external stimulus. For example, an individual hears voices telling him that he needs to "take a shower."
Identity	Self -knowledge about one's characteristics or personality; a sense of self.
Ingestion	To swallow in
Illusion	False perception and misinterpretation of an actual sensory stimulus. Individually, as part of and involving the family unit, and/or in a group setting.
Insight	Conscious awareness and understanding of an individual's own psychodynamic. An example is an individual that after complaining of serious headaches arrives to the conclusion that his/her headaches are a way for him/her to stop a stressful relationship with a boss who is abusive.
Insomnia	A pathological inability to sleep.
Learning Disorder	Learning disorders are characterized by difficulties in an academic area, either reading, mathematics, or written expression, such that the child's ability to achieve in the specific academic area is below what is expected for the child's age, schooling, and level of intelligence.
Major Depression	Classified as a type of affective disorder (or mood disorder), that goes beyond the day's ordinary ups and downs, and has become a serious medical condition and important health concern in this country. A person notices major changes in their sleep, eating, work and social habits. A lack of "gusto" for life.
Mania	A mood disorder that may be characterized by extreme elation, impulsivity, irritability, rapid speech, nervousness, distractibility, and/or poor judgment.
Obsessive-compulsive disorder (OCD)	An anxiety disorder in which a person has an unreasonable thought, fear, or worry that s/he tries to manage through a ritualized activity to reduce the anxiety. Frequently occurring disturbing thoughts or images are called obsessions, and the rituals performed to try to prevent or dispel them are called compulsions. A common obsessive disorder is the need to wash hands more often than normal.
Panic Disorder	Chronic, repeated, and unexpected panic attacks, bouts of overwhelming fear of being in danger when there is no specific cause for the fear. In between panic attacks, persons with panic disorder worry excessively about when and where the next attack may occur.

continued

Mental Health Glossary *(continued)*

WORD	MEANING
Personality Disorders	Refers to habitual ways of seeing and relating to self and the environment that are so fixed and rigid as to cause a significant degree of personal distress, and limits the individual's ability to effectively cope with the day-to-day demands of life's situations.
Phobia	An uncontrollable, irrational, and persistent fear of a specific object, situation, or activity.
Polydrug Use	When one is taking more than one drug at the time.
Post-Traumatic Stress Disorder (PTSD)	A flashback, feeling, image, or experience that was dormant (a terrifying physical or emotional event or trauma causing the person who survived the event to have persistent, frightening thoughts and memories) in one's conscious; that is awakened and characterized by an intense anxiety. Persons with PTSD often feel chronically emotionally numb. It's a common feeling among people who were exposed to a violent incident.
Relapse	When one resumes taking drugs.
Remission	When one has not taken drugs for a long period of time.
Schizophrenia Disorders	A group of mental illnesses characterized by delusions (bizarre, somatic, grandiose, persecutory), hallucinations (imagined voices), and thinking disturbances (incoherence, markedly illogical thinking). Schizophrenia is not the same as "split" or Dissociative Personality Disorder. Schizophrenia is one of the most complex of all mental health disorders, characterized by distorted thinking, strange feelings, and unusual behavior and use of language; involves a severe, chronic, and disabling disturbance of the brain.
Sedative	A drug taken for a calming effect.
Selective Mutism	The inability to speak in specific social situations in a child or adolescent who can and does speak in other situations.
Self-Esteem	Feelings about one's self or one's worth.
Self-Medication	When a person takes drugs (self-prescribes) to help an underlying illness such as depression or mania.
Stimulan	Adrug that increases energy and activity levels.
Suicidal Behavior	Actions taken by one who is considering or preparing to cause his/her own death.
Suicidal Ideation	Thoughts of suicide or wanting to take one's own life.
Suicide	The intentional taking of one's own life.
Tolerance	The body's ability to accept large quantities of drugs or substances without noticeable side effects.

continued

PO Box 2308, Woburn, MA 01888-0508, **p:** 781-729-3736, **www.EmbracingCulture.com**
PO Box 6401, Manchester, NH 03108, **p:** 1-888-678-CCCS

Mental Health Glossary *(continued)*

WORD	MEANING
Tourette's syndrome (TS)	A tic disorder characterized by repeated involuntary movements and uncontrollable vocal sounds. This disorder usually begins during childhood or early adolescence. It is common for some patients to swear out loud, making the people around them uncomfortable.
Transference	Unconscious event or experience in which the feelings, attitudes and wishes that were experienced in an individual's early life are now projected onto others. The transference can be of a positive or negative nature. For example: you had a teacher that was not very respectful of you, thus invoking feelings of anger. Now, as an adult, you meet someone that reminds you of that teacher, or you are in a similar dynamic and you begin to have negative feelings towards the person.
Withdrawal	When one stops taking drugs and during this stage one may have physical and psychological changes that need to be medically watched.

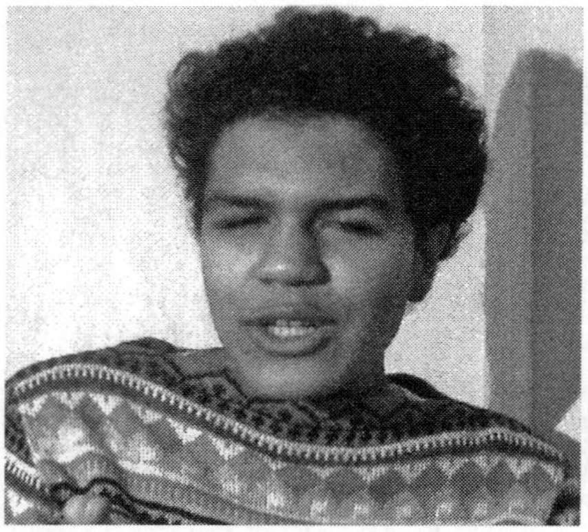
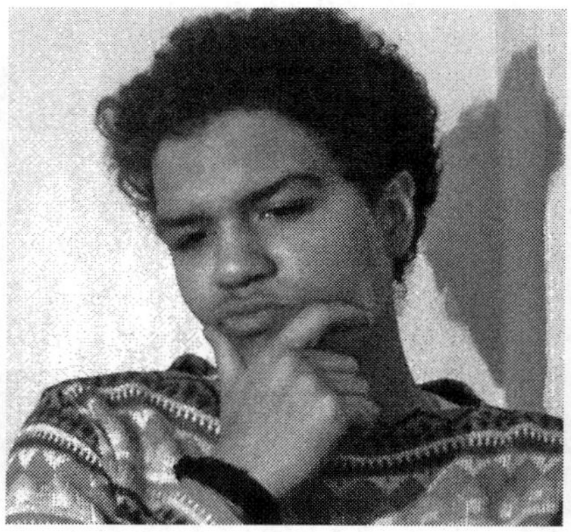
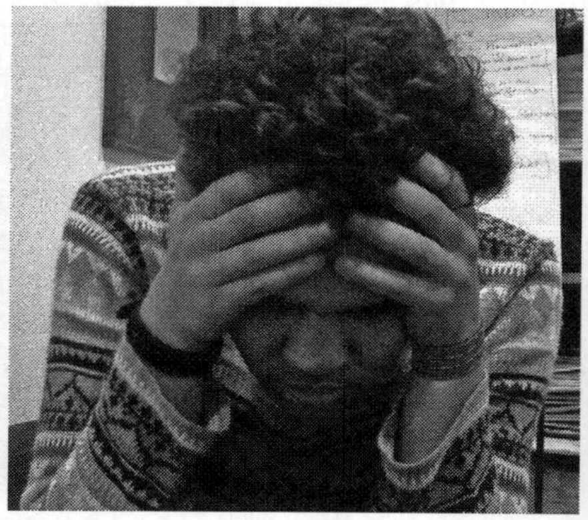

Lesson Thirteen: Homework
Interpreting in Mental Health Encounters

1. Go over your notes for today's lesson and read section "Additional Resources"
2. Read and practice all role-plays for this lesson and add words to your glossary
3. Translate the following words from the Mental Health Glossary for medical interpreters:

Word	Target Language
1. Adjustment disorders	
2. Agoraphobia	
3. Attention-deficit disorder	
4. Attention-deficit hyperactivity disorder	
5. Bipolar disorder	
6. Blackout	
7. Conduct disorders	
8. Delirium tremens	
9. Dyslexia	
10. Dementia	
11. Dissociative disorders	
12. Dyskinesia	
13. Hallucinations	
14. Learning disorder	
15. Major depression	
16. Post-traumatic stress disorder	
17. Self-esteem	
18. Suicidal behavior	
19. Suicidal ideation	
20. Suicide	

PO Box 2308, Woburn, MA 01888-0508, **p:** 781-729-3736, **www.EmbracingCulture.com**
PO Box 6401, Manchester, NH 03108, **p:** 1-888-678-CCCS

4. Translate the following proverbs into your TL:

English	Target Language
People who live in glass houses should not throw stones.	
A stitch in time saves nine.	
A watched pot never boils.	
Never judge a book by its cover.	
Better be safe than sorry.	
Rolling stone gather no moss.	

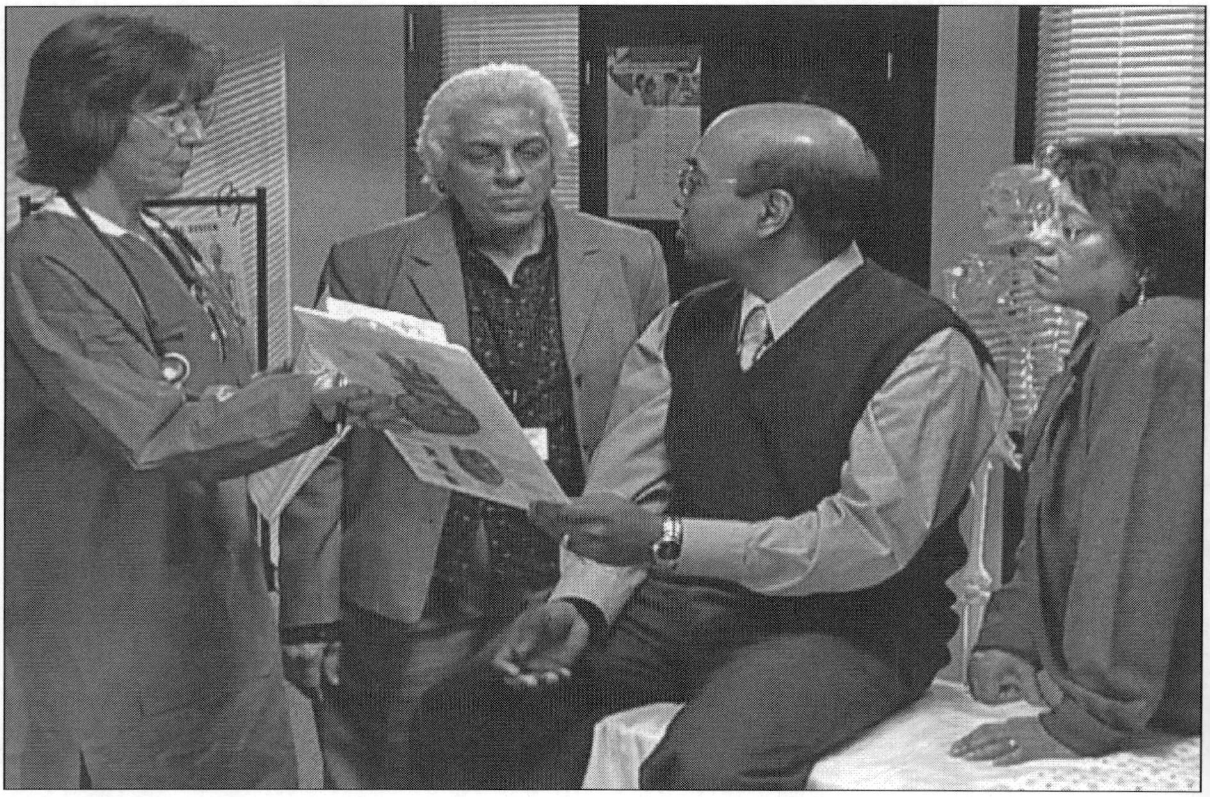

Lesson Thirteen: Role-Plays
Insight how providers communicate with each other about a patient

Work individually at first:

- Read the entire role-play
- Get a general sense of its meaning
- Circle the most challenging medical terms
- Apply the Samurai! technique to those terms
- Read the role-play again for a deeper understanding
- Find an accurate equivalent in the target language

Work in a language-specific group of friends, fellow students or colleagues:

- Share your doubts
- Ask for other ways of expressing the same meaning
- Develop a glossary
- Check the dictionary
- Practice the role-plays remember to do CIFE for all your role-plays
- Have your colleagues observe you and provide feedback on your accuracy and register.
- These colleagues can keep track of any omissions, additions, mistakes or distortions in your interpreting and point these out to you in a follow-up discussion.

Student Interpreter Evaluation

Student Name ______ Date ______

Language ______

Mode of Interpreting (check one): ☐ Consecutive ☐ Simultaneous

Role-Play/System ______

Areas Observed ______

Accuracy

Register ______

Omissions ______

Additions ______

Distortions ______

Pronunciation ______

Speaker's emotions conveyed? ______

Explain ______

Technique

General flow ______

Flow when requesting clarification ______

Speed ______

Eye Contact ______

Distracting Habits ______

Ethical Issues

Answered questions for patient? ______

Advised patient? ______

Vocabulary Expansion Recommendations

______

______

Other Recommendations

______

______

Language Coach Signature ______ Date ______

PO Box 2308, Woburn, MA 01888-0508, **p:** 781-729-3736, **www.EmbracingCulture.com**
PO Box 6401, Manchester, NH 03108, **p:** 1-888-678-CCCS

Role-Play 89: The young man who thought he had an anxiety attack

Jim Towers is a 27-year-old single new car salesman who lives with two roommates in an apartment in the city. His lifestyle is one in which he works hard, makes a lot of money and spends a lot of money eating out, going to clubs and using alcohol and cocaine on the weekends (which he sees no problem in). On Sunday morning he felt some tightness in his chest and a rapid heart beat. He felt warm and lightheaded. One of his roommates took him to the local emergency room where medically, he checked out fine but they were concerned that he might have been having a panic attack so they referred him back to his primary care provider to follow-up. Since Mr. Towers had not been seen before, he was assigned to the Emergency Doctor who saw him the next morning.

	Pronunciation	Additions	Omissions	Mistakes
Dr. J: Good morning Mr. Towers, how are you today?				
Mr. T: A lot better than yesterday.				
Dr. J: Can you tell me what happened to you to get you into the ER?				
Mr. T: Sure. I had woken up Sunday morning and I felt terrible! I was all sweaty and sick to my stomach and my heart was pounding like crazy.				
Dr. J: Had you ever felt this way before?				
Mr. T: Not really. I mean, I've felt hung over before but not like this.				
Dr. J: So, I'm guessing that on Saturday nights you go out and have a pretty good time?				
Mr. T: I would say that's true. My friends and I usually go out, and have some drinks and look for girls.				
Dr. J: And was last Saturday night pretty typical for you guys?				
Mr. T: Pretty much.				
Dr. J: Just so I get a good sense of what was happening, could you go through the night for me?				
Mr. T: Sure. We started off about 8:00 at Charlie's, where we all had a mixed drink or two. Then we went over the Kitchen, on first and Broadway, and started looking for women. There was nothing really happening there so we went over to Second Street to see if we could find any action.				
Dr. J: Did you drink at the Kitchen?				
Mr. T: Yea, we each had another mixed drink or two.				
Dr. J: Do they make those drinks pretty strong?				

continued

Role-Play 89 *(continued)*

	Pronunciation	Additions	Omissions	Mistakes
Mr. T: Oh yea! They know us so they serve us well. So, over on Second Street we ran into a couple of guys who we've run into before and bought a gram of cocaine.				
Dr. J: Is cocaine usually part of your Saturday nights?				
Mr. T: Well, yea, usually we share the gram and it keeps us going.				
Dr. J: You snort it?				
Mr. T: We never smoke it, if that's what you mean.				
Dr. J: Well, I'm glad to hear that but then after you snort the coke you're back out going to clubs for the rest of the night?				
Mr. T: yep!				
Dr. J: How long would you go for?				
Mr. T: Until about 2:00 or sometimes 3:00 am.				
Dr. J: And how many drinks would you say you buy throughout the night?				
Mr. T: Impossible to say. We never count them.				
Dr. J: So, if you go to a club every hour, from 8:00 to 2:00, that's six clubs. And if you have two strong drinks in every club that's 12 drinks and if some of the drinks are double strength you could end up having about 18 servings of alcohol, plus cocaine. And you do that every Saturday night?				
Mr. T: Well, last weekend, we hit it up a bit harder. We got two grams of cocaine instead of the usual one and I think I pretty much snorted a gram by myself.				
Dr. J: And do you eat anything or drink any non-alcoholic fluids throughout the night?				
Mr. T: Nope, just alcohol and cocaine.				
Dr. J: Jim, I've got to tell you that, as a doctor, I'm really concerned about what you're doing to yourself on the weekends. Between all the alcohol and cocaine you're using, I think you're going to start causing some serious medical damage to yourself. I sure hope you don't have a history of high blood pressure or heart disease in your family.				
Mr. T: I'm really not sure.				
Dr. J: You may want to find out before you spend another Saturday night pushing your body like that.				
Mr. T: You think that's bad?				

continued

PO Box 2308, Woburn, MA 01888-0508, **p:** 781-729-3736, **www.EmbracingCulture.com**
PO Box 6401, Manchester, NH 03108, **p:** 1-888-678-CCCS

	Pronunciation	Additions	Omissions	Mistakes
Dr. J: Actually, I do. And I think that's what caused your reaction on Sunday morning. I imagine that was pretty scary for you.				
Mr. T: It really was!				
Dr. J: Well, if you don't want to feel that way again I suggest you cut back on your alcohol and your cocaine use and make sure you have something to eat before you go out.				
Mr. T: OK.				
Dr. J: You may also want to make sure you drink non-alcoholic fluids during the evening as well, so you don't get yourself dehydrated.				
Mr. T: So you think that's what it was?				
Dr. J: I do, and if you don't follow my advice, I believe it will get worse.				
Mr. T: Whoa…				
Dr. J: By the way, if you find you have a problem cutting back, we have counselors here who could talk to your more in depth about what the alcohol and cocaine are doing to you.				
Mr. T: Well, I'll give it a try.				
Dr. J: Great! Why don't you give me a call next week, and let's see how you do.				
Break It Down	☐	☐	☐	☐

☐ **CIFE with patient** ☐ **CIFE with provider** ☐ **FLOW** ☐ **REGISTER**

Role-Play 89: Glossary

continued

1. Pathology (diseases, conditions)

2. Laboratory Tests and Diagnostic Procedures

3. Treatment Procedures

4. Idiomatic Expressions (if any)

5. Other (vocabulary in this particular role-play that you feel is important/relevant or that you anticipate problems with)

PO Box 2308, Woburn, MA 01888-0508, **p:** 781-729-3736, **www.EmbracingCulture.com**
PO Box 6401, Manchester, NH 03108, **p:** 1-888-678-CCCS

Role-Play 90: The man who still used Heroin

Mr. R, a 50 year old divorced man, with two grown children, and on disability (for depression), comes in wishing to discuss his need to stop using heroin. He is self-referred and is in generally good physical health (on high blood pressure medication) but finds he has gotten himself re-addicted to heroin again.

	Pronunciation	Additions	Omissions	Mistakes
Dr. L: Good morning Mr. R, how can I help you today?				
Mr. R: Well, doc, I got back into heroin again and I need to get myself off.				
Dr. L: You say "again." Does that mean you've been drug free before?				
Mr. R: Yea, I was clean for about 7 months before I started using again.				
Dr. L: When was that?				
Mr. R: About three or four months ago.				
Dr. L: How did you get started again?				
Mr. R: Same old story. I was feeling lonely and sorry for myself so I bought a bag and shot up and that started the whole thing going again.				
Dr. L: And has this happened to you before?				
Mr. R: Many, many times.				
Dr. L: You've been in treatment before?				
Mr. R: I've been in detoxes, rehabs, halfway houses…you name it and I've been in it.				
Dr. L: So, this is not something new to you?				
Mr. R: Nope. This is something I've been through a million times.				
Dr. L: So, Mr. R, you've been in plenty of treatment so I'm not sure how I can be helpful to you today.				
Mr. R: I need to detox again.				
Dr. L: Yea…				
Mr. R: But I don't want to go back into another hospital so I thought maybe you could give me something to help me stop using.				
Dr. L: Did you have something particular in mind?				
Mr. R: Well, I heard about this new thing that people are talking about called Suboxone.				
Dr. L: And how did you hear about it?				
Mr. R: You know how guys on the street will talk and they say this is pretty good for stopping withdrawal.				

continued

Role-Play 90 *(continued)*

	Pronunciation	Additions	Omissions	Mistakes
Dr. L: Do you know anything else about it?				
Mr. R: Only that docs can prescribe it in their offices and you don't have to go to a clinic to get it, like Methadone.				
Dr. L: Have you been on Methadone before?				
Mr. R: Oh sure. I've tried Methadone a few times.				
Dr. L: What ends up happening?				
Mr. R: I usually go back to heroin and they kick me off the clinic.				
Dr. L: Weren't they dosing you high enough?				
Mr. R: No, they were giving me plenty of Methadone. I just missed getting high.				
Dr. L: They don't usually kick you off of clinics for getting high once, do they?				
Mr. R: Oh, they give you a bunch of chances. It's just when I get back to heroin I'm gone.				
Dr. L: What ends up happening that makes you want to stop?				
Mr. R: I usually just get sick and tired of using so I clean up my act for a while.				
Dr. L: How long is it that you usually stay clean for?				
Mr. R: I don't know…5 or 6 months, or so.				
Dr. L: How do you get the money for all this?				
Mr. R: Well, that's another problem. I don't have the money to keep a habit going for very long so that's when I have to detox.				
Dr. L: So, by now I'm assuming you know all there is to know about being addicted to heroin and how that affects your health and other medications you might be taking.				
Mr. R: By now, I know more about heroin addiction than most addiction counselors I run into.				
Dr. L: And you know how it affects your anti-depressant and your blood pressure medication?				
Mr. R: Doc, I know it's no good for me and that I shouldn't be using it but I can't help myself.				
Dr. L: So, you're here basically for the Suboxone.				
Mr. R: Correct.				

continued

PO Box 2308, Woburn, MA 01888-0508, **p:** 781-729-3736, **www.EmbracingCulture.com**
PO Box 6401, Manchester, NH 03108, **p:** 1-888-678-CCCS

Role-Play 90 *(continued)*

	Pronunciation	Additions	Omissions	Mistakes
Dr. L: Well, Mr. R, the thing that I know about Suboxone is that in order to be able to prescribe it, a doctor has to go through a special training, which I have not gone through.				
Mr. R: So you can't prescribe it?				
Dr. L: That's true and as I understand it, most doctors who can prescribe it are usually not willing to unless their patient is in a program of some sort.				
Mr. R: What about all those stories I've hard about guys just getting as much suboxone as they wanted from different doctors?				
Dr. L: I can't answer that but I can tell you the doctors I know who can prescribe it insist on additional treatment.				
Mr. R: Oh. Well. I guess I won't be getting any Suboxone from you then.				
Dr. L: That's correct. You may want to consider trying methadone again. But you may want to make sure you're on a high enough dose so you don't need to keep using heroin.				
Mr. R: Yea. Well, I was hoping I wouldn't have to go back on a clinic. You don't know what a pain it is. They make you come in everyday and then you have to go to groups and meet with a counselor. I just wanted the drug. I really don't want to do the rest of the stuff that goes along with it.				
Dr. L: Sorry I can't help you.				
Mr. R: Yea, me too. Well, thanks for your time doc.				
Dr. L: Good luck.				
Break It Down	☐	☐	☐	☐

☐ **CIFE with patient** ☐ **CIFE with provider** ☐ **FLOW** ☐ **REGISTER**

Role-Play 82: Glossary

continued

1. Pathology (diseases, conditions)

2. Laboratory Tests and Diagnostic Procedures

3. Treatment Procedures

4. Idiomatic Expressions (if any)

5. Other (vocabulary in this particular role-play that you feel is important/relevant or that you anticipate problems with)

Role-Play 91: The man who couldn't stop smoking pot

Mr. Rivers is a 42-year-old man who lives with his wife of 15 years and their 10-year-old son and 6-year-old daughter. They currently rent an apartment in the city. Mr. Rivers works in construction. Over the years, Mrs. Rivers has complained about her husband's regular use of marijuana. Mr. Rivers has not considered it to be a problem so he has not stopped smoking. Lately, he and his wife have been having arguments over money and his lack of help around the house. They have come as a couple to speak to Dr A, Mr. River's primary care physician for some guidance:

	Pronunciation	Additions	Omissions	Mistakes
Dr. A: Good morning Mr. and Mrs. Rivers, how can I help you today?				
Mrs. R: Doctor, I have been getting very frustrated with my husband's lack of interest in either helping with the children or with jobs around the house. He comes home and sits in front of the TV, smokes his marijuana and does nothing around the house. I am tired of it.				
Dr. A: Is this true Mr. Rivers?				
Mr. R: Doctor, I work hard all day. I'm in construction and it's very physical work. I sometimes work 10 to 12 hour days so when I come home I just want to relax. I don't want to be bothered with anything. I just want everyone to leave me alone.				
Dr. A: And what about the marijuana use?				
Mr. R: You know, I find that marijuana relaxes me. It takes the edge off, you know? I can come home all tense and aggravated and have a few hits and then everything is fine.				
Mrs. R: Yes, it's fine for you but not for the rest of us. Doctor, I work too. And after a hard day of work, I'd love to be able to come home and sit down and relax but I can't. I have two children who need to be taken care of. There's a lot to do and I don't have the luxury of sitting around getting high!				
Mr. R: Listen, I don't know what the big deal is. I don't gamble. I don't run around with other women…				
Mrs. R: Of course not! You're so high every night you couldn't get yourself out of your chair if the house was on fire.				
Dr. A: Let me see if I understand what the situation is. Mrs. Rivers, you come home from work and make supper and get the kids fed and homework started and things like that. Is that so?				

Role-Play 91 *(continued)*

	Pronunciation	Additions	Omissions	Mistakes
Mrs. R: Yes.				
Dr. A: Mr. Rivers, you come home from work, eat supper, I assume?				
Mr. R: Yes.				
Dr. A: And then you head for the TV and spend the rest of the night high on marijuana watching TV?				
Mr. R: Well, basically, yes.				
Dr. A: Now, your wife sees this as a problem but you don't. Is that correct?				
Mr. R: Yes, that's so.				
Dr. A: So, have you been doing this for a while?				
Mrs. R: Doctor, he's been doing this for as long as I've known him.				
Dr. A: So, what's different now? After all these years, why is this now a problem?				
Mrs. R: First of all, our oldest boy is getting to the point where he knows what his father is doing. They teach drug abuse in school so he caught his father getting high last week. I was furious. And, I just got a promotion at work and it's a lot more money and I'm not so afraid to face a life without my husband.				
Dr. A: So, Mr. R, what do you think about your son seeing you smoking marijuana?				
Mr. R: Well, to be honest, it did concern me. I didn't want him to find out I was smoking.				
Dr. A: Do you think he would try it, seeing how his dad thinks it's ok?				
Mrs. R: I do! And if that boy starts using drugs because his father is using drugs I don't know what I'd do.				
Dr. A: Mr. Rivers, it sounds to me like there's more of a problem here than you originally thought. Even if you don't believe marijuana is doing you any harm, it does seem to be causing a lot of conflict between you and your wife plus the risk of giving a message to your son that drug use is OK. What do you think?				
Mr. R: Yea, well, I guess what you say is true.				

continued

Role-Play 91 *(continued)*

Dr. A: You know, there is a person here in our center who could give you a lot more information about this. He's our local substance abuse expert and works with people with these issues all the time. What if I set up a time for you two to meet with him and then you can decide what makes the most sense. How does that sound?				
Mrs. R: That sounds good to me.				
Mr. R: I'd go.				
Dr. A: Good! Nancy at the front desk will set that up for you and then why don't you give me a call and let me know how it goes?				
Break It Down	☐	☐	☐	☐

☐ **CIFE with patient** ☐ **CIFE with provider** ☐ **FLOW** ☐ **REGISTER**

Role-Play 91: Glossary

continued

1. Pathology (diseases, conditions)

2. Laboratory Tests and Diagnostic Procedures

3. Treatment Procedures

4. Idiomatic Expressions (if any)

5. Other (vocabulary in this particular role-play that you feel is important/relevant or that you anticipate problems with)

PO Box 2308, Woburn, MA 01888-0508, **p:** 781-729-3736, **www.EmbracingCulture.com**
PO Box 6401, Manchester, NH 03108, **p:** 1-888-678-CCCS

Lesson Thirteen: Additional Resources Interpreting in Mental Health Encounters

A Mental Health Clinician's Perspective When Working with an Interpreter

By Zarita Araújo-Lane, LICSW

I am a clinician who has worked with interpreters. I am also an interpreter who has worked with clinicians. Trainers often educate interpreters from an interpreter's perspective. In an attempt to introduce a different viewpoint, which I like to call the clinician's lens, this article outlines a case study in an outpatient community mental health clinic with an explanation of the clinical intervention. The interpreter's role is examined closely and tips for a successful interpretation in mental health treatment settings are offered.

Each clinician is an individual and each mental health profession utilizes a different approach to clinical work, but all use the same type of thinking when evaluating and diagnosing a client. The presence of an interpreter is a mixed blessing to the majority o clinicians. These are thankful for the opportunity to communicate with their clients, bu are soon beset by an onslaught of worries, like "Is my message being interpreted accurately?," or "How am I going to work with a third person who is not a family member or a co-therapist?" The presence of a third person in a mental health session changes the clinical dynamic. Interpreters and providers need to share a common understanding of their respective roles and expectations before they meet with the clie

In group therapy, clinicians generally avoid having three clients in any given session since invariably one will be left out. In the triadic encounter with an interpreter, the or "left out" will be either the therapist or the patient. The interpreter has the gift of speaking both languages and likely shares both cultures, so the tendency for the interpreter to ally, consciously or unconsciously, with one party against the other is strong.

The following is a real life clinical case detailing a volatile situation encountered in a mental health session in which a clinician worked with an interpreter. This interprete was experienced and highly regarded. Most of her work involved interpreting for the medication clinic and in family meetings where children spoke English but their pare did not. Her job description also included handling over-the-phone intakes when clie called the clinic.

Background Case Information: Presenting Problem

The clinician was called by a local school to handle a case involving a colleagues' client. Early that morning, the client, a boy, had spoken of wanting to burn someone with diesel, but he had not specified a target, date or time. Upon further questioning, he revealed that he had no access to the fuel and that his comments were born of a generalized anger. In short, the boy was presenting homicidal ideation with a vague plan, serious enough to warrant an immediate call to the clinic.

Today, in the aftermath of Columbine and subsequent school massacres, the clinical intervention would have followed a different pattern. For example, the police would have been contacted right away. But years ago, intervention methods were different. The clinician drove to the school to evaluate the child. Although the boy denied feeling homicidal or suicidal, or having any weapons or even the money to buy fuel, his situation posed a threat and his parents had to be called in.

Prior Treatment History

A year prior to the clinician's involvement in this emergency, she had done the initial evaluation of this case. At that time, the youngster appeared to be suffering from a reactive depression due his immigration and to difficulties with his parents. He subsequently developed an appropriate rapport with the assigned therapist and even looked forward to his weekly sessions. The therapist became the liaison between the school, the clinic and the child and his family.

The boy's parents did not speak English, and interpreter services were utilized each month at the family meeting. The parents had a difficult time empathizing with their son's need to socialize with his peers. This youngster was always well groomed but showed poor eye contact and seemed disengaged from life. Treatment goals were behavior-oriented so that his lack of self-esteem and anger were addressed. However, his parents refused a consult with the clinic's psychiatrist.

Mental Status: Day of the Intervention

On the day of the emergency call, the clinician noticed some changes in the youngster. This information was gathered through meeting with the child and the school staff and reviewing the individual treatment notes left by the child's therapist. In the month prior to the incident, new academic issues had arisen, such as incomplete homework and a drop in grade average. The child had also stopped seeking out his favorite teacher to express his frustrations as he had done so often in the past. He seemed to be withdrawing from his peers and from the authority figures he cared for.

The boy's affect was flat. He described waking up in the middle of the night, losing the desire to socialize with friends, and experiencing bursts of anger that at times scared even him. He had made the remark about burning someone in an impulsive response to teasing by a schoolmate. In the clinical interview, he emphasized that he really did not want to hurt anyone. However, he spoke of some past incidents in which he had grabbed a peer by the shirt after being teased about his clothing. But he showed remorse for this impulsive behavior.

PO Box 2308, Woburn, MA 01888-0508, **p:** 781-729-3736, **www.EmbracingCulture.com**
PO Box 6401, Manchester, NH 03108, **p:** 1-888-678-CCCS

The youngster was oriented in time, place and person. He denied having delusions or hallucinations. His thoughts seemed congruent with his affect. He showed appropriate judgment when reflecting on the seriousness of his threat. He denied experimenting with drugs. He also denied being a victim of any form of abuse by peers, family members or teachers.

In the absence of actual suicidal or homicidal planning, where there is just a feeling or ideation, the client may be able to contract not to act on those feelings. The therapist can then develop with the client a set of concrete steps detailing what to do and whom to call when the feelings resurface. Inversely, if homicidal ideation is towards a specific person, the clinician may have to report it to that person and to the proper authorities in accordance with state and federal guidelines.

Questions to Rule Out Depression and Suicidal/Homicidal Ideation

1. Tell me more about how you have been feeling.
2. How long have you been feeling this way?
3. Any changes in your life or health?
4. When do you feel like hurting yourself or others?
5. What do you do about it?
6. Do you have a plan?
7. Who knows about these feelings?
8. Have you ever acted on them?
9. What has stopped you from doing it?
10. Are you hearing voices?
11. What would you do about these feelings?
12. Did you feel like this before?
13. What did you do?
14. What are you going to do when you leave this session?

Homicidal and Suicidal Ideation: How Serious?

The school was about to close and the clinician was not comfortable sending the patient home without having him evaluated in a hospital. The clinician contacted the interpreter and during a three-way phone conversation informed the parents that their son was feeling very sad and that he would have to be seen by the hospital as soon as possible. The parents asked that the son be taken to the clinic instead of to the hospital, and gave the clinician permission to transport him.

After bringing the boy to the clinic, the clinician again went over safety issues. The youngster denied having homicidal or suicidal ideation. The clinician went over some safe rules, assuring the boy that if, when meeting with the clinician and his family, he did not feel safe, he could ask to leave the room and another clinician would then stay with him, but that he was not allowed to run out of the clinic or to hurt anyone in the process. He agreed and his affect changed. He seemed relieved.

The clinician and client then went over sleep disturbances and the boy suddenly disclosed that at times he would wake up and want to kill his father. The clinician told the boy that he needed help and that together they would have to inform his parents of both his sadness and his homicidal ideation towards his father. The youngster asked that the clinician start the conversation with the father.

Pre-Session with the Interpreter Alone

The father arrived alone, since the mother could not leave work. The clinician met with the interpreter before the session, informing her of the client's homicidal ideation. The interpreter was told that the meeting with the father had the purpose of convincing him to authorize a voluntary hospitalization for his son at a local hospital. If the father refused to support a hospitalization, the clinician might have to involve a psychiatrist and ask for a pink slip, or involuntary hospitalization.

The clinician also told the interpreter that they would first meet with the father and only bring the son into the session if it felt like a safe move for everyone. The clinician did not discuss safety issues and seating arrangements with the interpreter, and the interpreter ended up seated in a corner with the father, next to the door.

Triadic Encounter: Meeting with the Father

The clinician informed the father that his son seemed very sad and as a result was having thoughts of hurting others. She then paused, the interpreter relayed the information in the consecutive mode, and both waited for the father's reaction. The clinician continued by sharing the boy's recent disclosure of being afraid of hurting his father. She paused, the interpreter again interpreted, and clinician started again by letting the father know that his son had shared thoughts of wanting to kill him in the middle of the night. The clinician paused and the interpreter continued.

The father smiled and said that his wife was not able to come in and that he would rather have his son go to a hospital outside the community to preserve the family's confidentiality. As a standard procedure, the clinician told the father that when the son entered the room, she would go over this

PO Box 2308, Woburn, MA 01888-0508, **p:** 781-729-3736, **www.EmbracingCulture.com**
PO Box 6401, Manchester, NH 03108, **p:** 1-888-678-CCCS

information again with both of them. She reminded the father that although he might feel upset, he was not allowed to hurt his son or anyone else in the clinic.

The clinician asked if the father was concerned. He replied that his son wanted to go out with friends and that this was the reason he was acting out. The clinician responded that young people can have bursts of anger as expressions of major depression and that this was an opportunity to help his son and the family. The clinician asked the father how he felt about this news. He answered that he did not believe his son could hurt him but that if the therapist felt the boy needed help he would agree to the hospitalization.

A Group Encounter: Client, Father, Clinician and Interpreter

The son sat right next to the clinician, across from the father. The interpreter used the simultaneous mode to interpret to the father the conversation between the clinician and the boy. The clinician started the session by thanking the father and son for agreeing to meet and by acknowledging that this may be a difficult time for both of them. She told them that at times people ask for help in different ways and that the youngster was doing this now. She reassured them that the clinic's staff was there to support them.

As the clinician started to introduce the client's homicidal ideation and desire to hurt his father, the father suddenly got up from his chair, challenging the son to "do it now" as he crossed the room and started to hit the son on the head. In a heartbeat, the boy got up and hid behind the clinician.

The clinician firmly instructed the father to leave the room, but the father kept coming towards the son and hitting him. The clinician turned around to ask the child to leave the room. His eyes were changed. He looked like an animal, foaming at the mouth. Suddenly, he had a knife on the clinician's neck.

The interpreter, worried for the clinician's safety, inserted herself between the therapist and the boy, and got stuck there. Now both women were trapped in between the client and his father. Finally, the clinician was able to get the interpreter out of this sandwich and instructed her to call the police and ask for help from other colleagues.

Maintaining eye contact with the client, the clinician told him that he was going to be safe but that he could not hurt her and that he needed to drop the knife on the file cabinet right next to them. The therapist was able to take the boy out of the room while holding on to his hand. The boy was still gripping the knife, and the therapist locked herself in a room with him so that the father could not reach them.

After police questioning, it became evident that the father had indeed been abusing the son. The boy needed to be hospitalized. The Department of Social Services became involved and began to investigate removing the boy from the home.

Looking Back

When the case was initially reviewed, the clinic examined the clinical intervention and judged it to be solid. At the time, the interpretation was not questioned. Looking back, it is clear that this volatile situation was not the interpreter's fault. But could the interpreter have inadvertently contributed to the escalation of violence by misunderstanding the meaning of the clinician's pauses between each message? And could the clinician have done more to make the interpreter aware of this intended meaning?

Each of the clinician's pauses had the dual purpose of soliciting a reaction from the father and allowing him to assimilate all the information. However, in the above mentioned session, the clinical pauses, which would have equaled moments of silence in a monolingual session, were filled by the interpreter's rendition of the original message.

Were the clinician fully aware of the import of this dynamic, she would have paused for effect after the interpreter's rendition of each message. The importance of clinical pauses would have been discussed in the pre-session. The clinician and interpreter might even have agreed on a simple hand signal or gesture indicating the need for a pause.

Understanding Tools for Clinical Intervention

Echoing

In order to develop clinical rapport, the clinician first empathizes with the situation or the individual by repeating words or phrases used by the client. This echoing allows the client to feel that he or she is being heard. It also allows clients to hear their own thoughts repeated back to them through another voice, as if the clinician were the client's mirror. The clinician can then evaluate the client's insight and ability to reflect on and question his or her own thinking.

The interpreter's omission of the clinician's assuring words like "good" or "I see," or the interpreter's failure to convey the clinician's repetition of the client's last words, may interfere with development of the therapeutic alliance between patient and clinician. It may also cause the clinician to perceive the client as a poor listener.

Silence

Clinicians are more active with their questioning when assessing an emergency situation. However, a client's comfort level will increase in an environment where trust is built. This is essential when a patient is about to disclose intimate information. Thus, during an on-going treatment session, the clinicians are less active with questioning, and pause more often. Interpreters should respect and replicate these moments of silence in their target language rendition of the message.

PO Box 2308, Woburn, MA 01888-0508, **p:** 781-729-3736, **www.EmbracingCulture.com**
PO Box 6401, Manchester, NH 03108, **p:** 1-888-678-CCCS

Repetition

During an emergency intervention for cases of homicidal ideation, astute clinicians predict behaviors and reactions of family members and provide them with alternatives and safe avenues, as did this clinician. Clinicians will repeat these options several times during the session, first with the client and then with the family or group. But, is this repetition always interpreted? Or do interpreters omit the clinician's repetitions, perhaps feeling that once or twice is enough?

Tone

Clinicians working with emergencies maintain clear, precise communication in a calm and firm manner. As physical violence erupted in the above-mentioned session, was the interpreter interpreting firmly with the same tone of voice that the therapist used? Would this have made a difference?

Seating

Where should an interpreter sit in the session: in a corner next to the door or in an open space? If the father were the one sitting in the corner, would he have felt boxed in and reacted with greater violence towards his son? These are all questions that clinicians and interpreters must consider in pre-session meetings.

Cooperation

During the violence, should the interpreter have left the room? Was she right to get in the middle of the skirmish? This issue is often addressed among clinicians doing co-therapy with potentially violent families. Most clinical literature refers to just one leader in times of crisis, and this leader should be the primary therapist in the session. So, if the therapist tells the interpreter to leave the room, the interpreter should follow this direction - no questions asked.

In Summary

Every day, we learn something new. Perhaps what we can learn from this case is that clinicians and interpreters need to communicate at different levels. We can see the importance of clinical thinking and a clinician's intervention. We know now that the way a clinician's message is relayed can affect the client's reaction, for better or for worse.

The Mode of Interpreting

Although the consecutive mode would have been appropriate for some parts of this session, perhaps the interpreter should have been interpreting simultaneously when the clinician was speaking in short sentences with pauses, and also when the physical confrontation erupted. In times like these, words and timing are crucial and should be conveyed as quickly as possible.

References:

American Psychiatric Association. 1994. Diagnostic and Statistical Manual of Mental Disorders Fourth Edition. DSM-IV.

World Health Organization. 1993. The ICD-10 Classification of Mental and Behavioral Disorders: Diagnostic criteria for research.

CCCS Substance Abuse Manual (insert credits)

CAGE Questionnaire (adapted from http://pubs.niaaa.nih.gov/publications/Assesing%20Alcohol/InstrumentPDFs/16_CAGE.pdf, the website of the National Institute on Alcohol Abuse and Alcoholism)

List of Antidepressants (copied and/or adapted from http://www.antidepressants.ws/list-of-antidepressants.html)

Mini Mental Status Exam (copied and/or adapted from http://www.nmaging.state.nm.us/pdf_files/Mini_Mental_Status_Exam.pdf, the website of the New Mexico Aging and Long-term Services Department)

Medline Plus Medical Encyclopedia http://www.nlm.nih.gov/medlineplus/encyclopedia.html

Interpreting Names of Medications

Interpreting names of medications can be dangerous for the interpreter, and it is best to use the English names when interpreting the provider's words to the patient. Do not try to match American medications with those in your country, as the chemical composition is often different. Below, we provide you with a list of common medications so you become familiar with their names as you hear these from the provider.

When in doubt, ask the provider to write down the name of the medication, and always take note of dosages in your notebook, as it is important to get this right when interpreting the provider's treatment instructions. Some psychotropic medications can kill a patient if taken in an improper dosage, so repeat the instructions back to the provider to be sure that you have accurately transmitted them to the patient.

Per the following table, we have divided a list of antidepressants into four main categories:
1-antidepressants (SSSRI'S), 2-antidepressants (MOAI's), 3- antidepressants (TCA).
4- antidepressants (others).

PO Box 2308, Woburn, MA 01888-0508, **p:** 781-729-3736, **www.EmbracingCulture.com**
PO Box 6401, Manchester, NH 03108, **p:** 1-888-678-CCCS

List of Antidepressants: SSRI's (selective serotonin reuptake inhibitors)
Paxil (paroxetine) Prozac (fluoxetine) Zoloft (sertraline) Celexa (citalopram) Lexapro (escitalopram oxalate) Luvox (fluvoxamine) Nardil (phenelzine) Parnate (tranylcypromine)
Antidepressants: MOAI's (monoamine oxidase inhibitors)
Adapin (doxepin) Anafranil (clomipramine) Elavil (amitriptyline) Endep (amitriptyline) Ludiomil (maprotiline) Norpramin (desipramine)
Antidepressants:TCA's (tricyclic antidepressants)
Pamelor(nortryptyline) Pertofrane(desipramin Sinequan (doxepin) Surmontil(trimipramine) Tofranil (imipramine) Vivactil (protriptyline)
Antidepressant Drug List: Others (Effexor is one of the "newer" antidepressants. SSRI's have fewer side effects than TCA's or MOAI's (not as sedating, fewer anticholinergic side effects, safe in overdose)
Effexor (venlafaxine) Cymbalta (duloxetine) Desyrel (trazodone) Buspar (buspirone) Edronax,Vestra (reboxetine) Remeron (mirtazapine) Serzone (nefazodone) Wellbutrin (bupropion)

Copied/adapted from http://www.antidepressants.ws/list-of-antidepressants.html

Lesson Fourteen: Professionalism in Medical Interpretation

Understanding Goals

Students will be able to:

- review learned concepts about the professional interpreter
- understand key aspects of the interpreter screening and hiring process
- understand appropriate dress code
- assess learning growth and plan for future professional development
- understand the interpreter movement towards certification

Key concepts:

- Professional interpreter
- Professional Attire
- Time management/business administration
- Conflict resolution
- Professional development

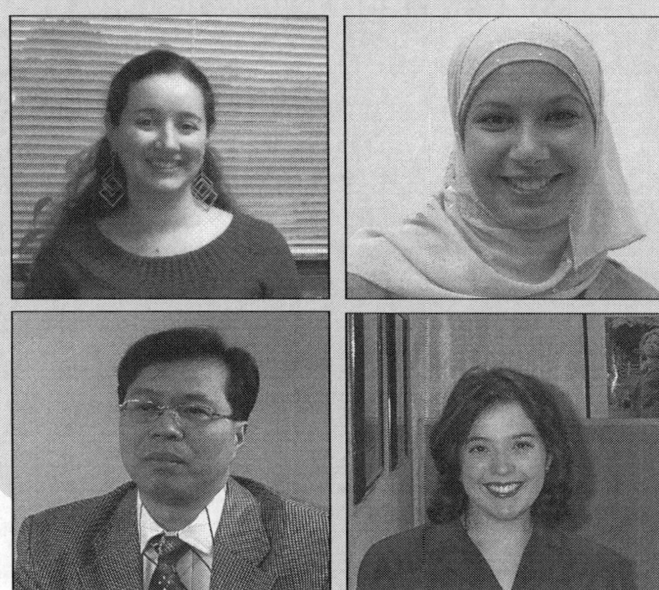

PO Box 2308, Woburn, MA 01888-0508, **p:** 781-729-3736, **www.EmbracingCulture.com**
PO Box 6401, Manchester, NH 03108, **p:** 1-888-678-CCCS

Quiz

THE ART OF MEDICAL INTERPRETATION®

Lesson Fourteen: Quiz
Professionalism in Medical Interpretation

Mark each item "True" or "False."

1. Professional interpreters' skills are formally tested just once at the beginning of their careers.
   O True O False
2. Interpreters who call themselves "certified interpreters" have all been tested according to the same standards.
   O True O False
3. Before going to an interview, it is a good idea to jot down a few key questions you have about the organization's mission or function.
   O True O False
4. In a job interview, it is okay to make negative comments about a former employer.
   O True O False
5. Successful freelance interpreters keep a calendar in which they make note of their appointments and any commitments that may affect their interpreting work.
   O True O False
6. Interpreters who consistently fail to submit documentation after assignments are eventually terminated from service within their organizations.
   O True O False
7. A medical interpreter trained only in the consecutive mode should likely not accept a simultaneous conference interpreting assignment.
   O True O False
8. Prolonged job stress can lead to poor physical and/or mental health.
   O True O False
9. Once you graduate from an interpreter's program, you will not need to attend additional workshops, seminars or certificate programs.
   O True O False
10. Due to a lack of public awareness of the interpreter's professional standards, it is still common for interpreters to be judged based on the outcome of an encounter, rather than on actual skills or performance.
    O True O False
11. Interpreters should not independently persuade a provider or patient to accept the position or counsel of the other party.
    O True O False
12. One of the keys to successful conflict resolution is to "say no while saying yes."
    O True O False
13. The proper dress code for medical interpreters is "casual."
    O True O False
14. Freelance interpreters, as independent contractors, are responsible for paying local, state and federal taxes where applicable.
    O True O False
15. Interpreters possess a fixed skill set and cannot develop new expertise over time.
    O True O False

Lesson Fourteen: Class Activities
Professionalism in Medical Interpretation

Getting to Know Yourself as an Interpreter

REFLECT

Go back into your notes from lesson 1 where you described your understanding of what constitutes a "professional interpreter."

- **Add new information to the diagram**
- As you are completing this training and getting ready to market yourself as an interpreter, list below your areas of strengths, as well as areas that need improvement:

Strengths	Needs improvement

As you are getting ready to find jobs, there are two important and distinctive aspects of an interpreter, which we call **internal skills** (understanding the interpreting profession at a cognitive level) and **external skills** (being able to demonstrate skills through use of projection, terminology, overall demeanor, grooming, time management and professional boundaries).

THINK

List below skills and behaviors that employers will look for in the following two areas:

Internal skills	External skills

PO Box 2308, Woburn, MA 01888-0508, **p:** 781-729-3736, **www.EmbracingCulture.com**
PO Box 6401, Manchester, NH 03108, **p:** 1-888-678-CCCS

Copy the list above into the table below. As you complete this list, check the areas where you will need improvement and establish a deadline for when you will be addressing and completing each checked need:

Internal skills	Deadline	External skills	Deadline

The Hiring Process

THINK

Showing Professionalism in a Medical Interpreter Interview:

Have you ever stopped to think about how you will carry yourself as a professional interpreter?

____

____

How would you dress for the interview?

____

____

Not only will your behavior impact your income, it will also reflect upon the profession in general. In the absence of national certification, there are many determining factors to whether an interpreter is "qualified" or not.

What are your strengths as an interpreter?

____

____

Job interviews will vary depending on the type of position and medical setting for which you are applying. For example, hospitals with an international patient component may require a higher register in both English and target language as patients in general are very familiar with their illnesses and target language medical terminology around diagnoses, testing, and treatments.

What are your weaknesses?

____

____

What are you going to do about them? How can you address your weaknesses?

____

____

PO Box 2308, Woburn, MA 01888-0508, **p:** 781-729-3736, **www.EmbracingCulture.com**
PO Box 6401, Manchester, NH 03108, **p:** 1-888-678-CCCS

The Hiring Process

There are four stages in the hiring process:

1. **Pre-Interview** (resume, research job openings, communication, follow-up)
2. **Interview** (dress code, time management, strengths and weaknesses)
3. **Follow-up** to the interview (keep your promises, communication, review policies and standards)
4. **Short and long-term goals**

ACTIVITY

Brainstorm what you need to do for each of these stages

Pre-Interview	**Interview**
Follow-up	**Short and Long-Term Goals**

Many active interpreters entered the profession at the recommendation of informal acquaintances who considered them to have done a "good job" interpreting for friends or family. Ten years ago, if you had a high school diploma and spoke passable English, you could get yourself hired for an interpreter position. Although the standards for professional interpreter services have since improved, the mentality of the "back door" recommendation is still alive and does influence the selection of the interpreter workforce.

Daily, we read email and listserv postings regarding interpreting assignments. Typically, they read, "(company) looking for (name of language) interpreter for (date and time) assignment in (city). If interested, contact (telephone number)." End of story. No mention of screening or training requirements.

Individuals with varying degrees of language fluency and training have listed themselves as "interpreters" or "certified interpreters" in interpreter association databases, regardless of how they have been tested, and despite the fact that national certification does not yet exist. These listings generate potentially lucrative business opportunities as agencies and organizations work their way down an alphabetical interpreter listing, offering assignments to just about anyone who will accept them. Often, these so-called "interpreters" accept assignments they know little about or already realize are far beyond their levels of expertise. The behaviors exhibited by these agencies, healthcare institutions and freelance interpreters are destructive and do not promote the advancement of the profession. When you hire an interpreter with no questions asked, or accept a case without a formal interview and screening, you are working against your own reputation and this will inevitably change the public's perception of our profession as a whole.

An informed hiring organization will test the language skills of its interpreter applicants prior to proceeding with the hiring process. Some interpreters have expressed consternation at the idea of being tested. Others who have attended certificate programs seem to feel that their one completed course has transformed them into professionals with no need for additional testing.

It's funny, this resistance towards evaluation. Even medical doctors who have undergone six or more years of specialized training in their field still undergo formal screening and peer evaluation. Why would interpreters cleave to a standard lower than that of other health professions? Let's take a look at a true professional's approach to the hiring process, evaluation and ongoing professional development.

Embrace the pre-hire screening process

A reputable healthcare organization or agency, while requiring proof of successful completion of an interpreter-training program, will also evaluate your written and oral conversion ability in both the source and target languages. Embrace the pre-hire screening process as an exercise of your previously developed language and interpretation skills, and an opportunity for complimentary evaluation.

After the initial screening is complete and your skills have passed examination, you may be asked to interview for a freelance or staff position. Prepare yourself for this interview. In a professional portfolio, pack two copies of your resume, two letters of recommendation, copies of your training certificates and your immunization records.

Two days prior to the interview, visit the organization's website. Review the information presented and jot down a few key questions you have about the organization's mission or function. During the interview, the hiring agent will want to see if you are a critical thinker. Be prepared to share a few short stories that illustrate your problem-solving skills (strengths), as well as examples in which you articulate lessons learned from a past mistake. When presenting these examples, never divulge names of people or organizations. Do not make negative comments about a competitor or former employer. Keep your focus on the positive.

Once you have been hired, you may be asked to undergo additional testing or training. Some hospitals take new interpreters "out on the floor" for a period of shadowing, in which they are evaluated by an experienced interpreter. Other organizations mandate that new employees attend HIPAA (Health Insurance Portability and Accountability Act) training, or complete an infectious disease prevention program.

PO Box 2308, Woburn, MA 01888-0508, **p:** 781-729-3736, **www.EmbracingCulture.com**
PO Box 6401, Manchester, NH 03108, **p:** 1-888-678-CCCS

Dress Code

Class exercise: In small groups, discuss which of these four individuals you believe are dressed appropriately for a medical interpreting assignment. Explain why.

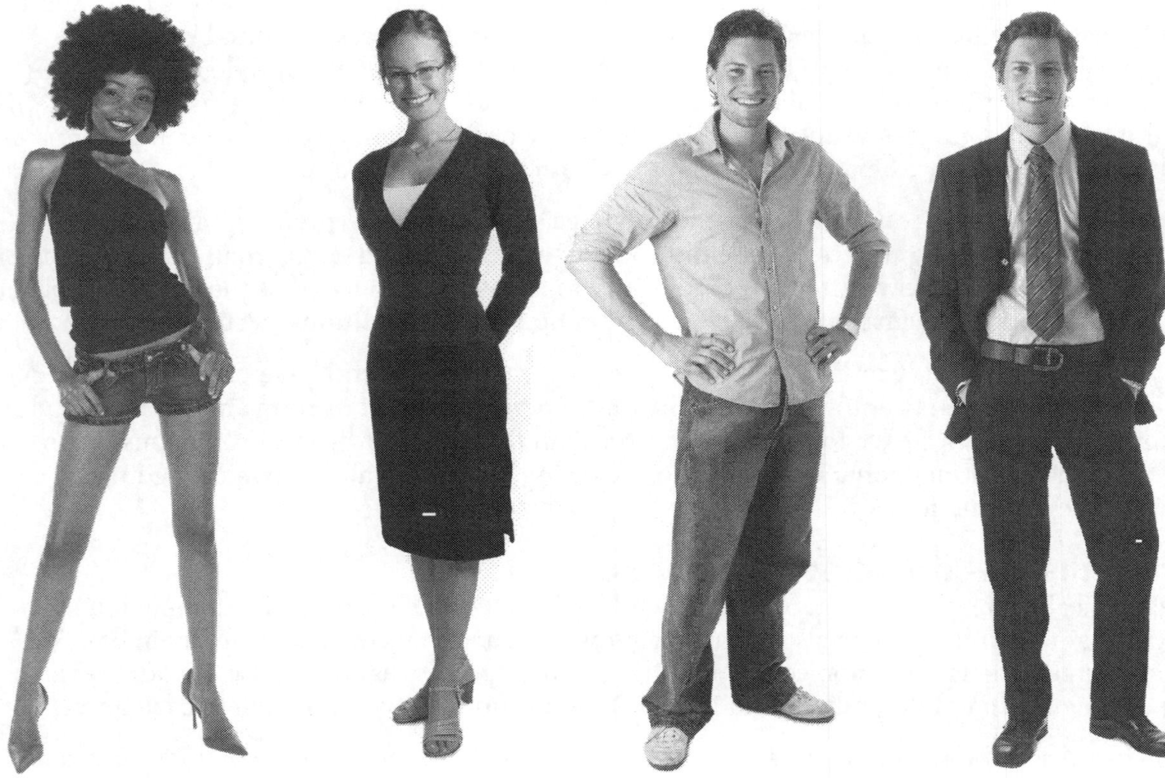

Investing in Your Career

The purchase of proper attire can be considered an investment in your medical interpreting career. The dress code for medical interpreters in most organizations varies between "business attire" and "business casual." The following are some examples of dress and grooming that are expressly prohibited in many hospitals and healthcare organizations:

- Miniskirts
- Jeans
- Sneakers
- Low-cuts
- See-through material
- Spaghetti straps or halter tops
- Sandals and open-toe shoes
- Shorts
- Hats (except when worn to fulfill a religious requirement)
- Perfume

Once you have secured the job or contract, continue to invest in your career. A freelance interpreter will need a beeper, cell phone, fax and email address. One or two quality bilingual medical dictionaries are also a must.

To set up a home office, many freelancers take out a small loan from a family member, local bank or credit union. Of course, technology is only beneficial to the extent that the user implements it. Simply put, a phone is no good unless you answer it, and voicemail and email are meant to be replied to. As a freelancer, you are in business for yourself, so be prompt about following up on possible assignment or job offers.

Serious freelancers also purchase an "Errors and Omissions"-type policy to protect themselves from liability in cases where the quality of their interpretation is called into question. An excellent resource for information on liability insurance is the American Translators Association (see www.atanet.org).

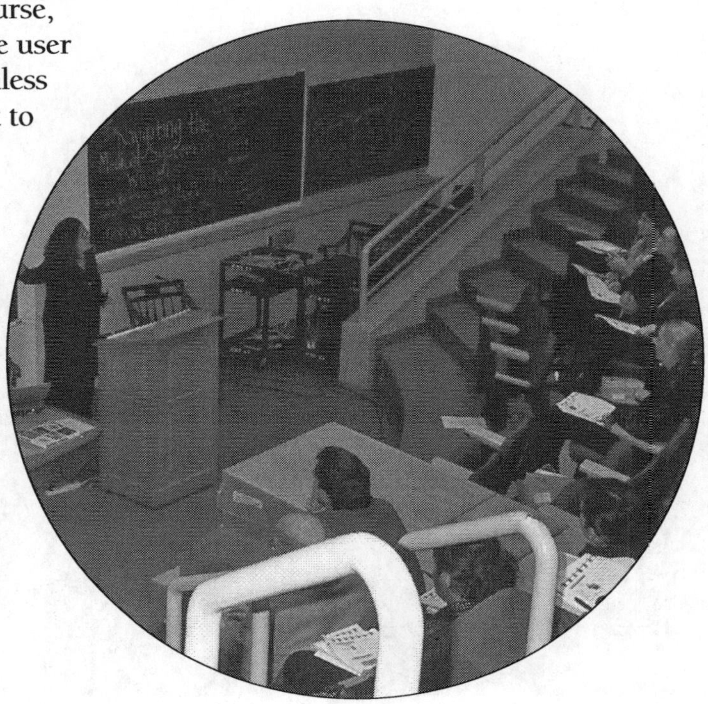

PO Box 2308, Woburn, MA 01888-0508, **p:** 781-729-3736, **www.EmbracingCulture.com**
PO Box 6401, Manchester, NH 03108, **p:** 1-888-678-CCCS

How to prepare for a job interview:

In order for you to stay calm during the interview it is important that you prepare for the interview beforehand:

- Do your homework – research about the company you are applying to, so that you have some understanding of what the company does
- Try to anticipate the questions you are going to be asked
- The night before, get your interview clothes and important documentation ready. You want to anticipate any possible delays by leaving early and allowing extra travel time.

ACTIVITY

A Mock Interview

Divide into groups of twos. Take turns interviewing and giving each other feedback. Act the part as if you were in a real job interview. Come prepared with the tools you find important for the interview.

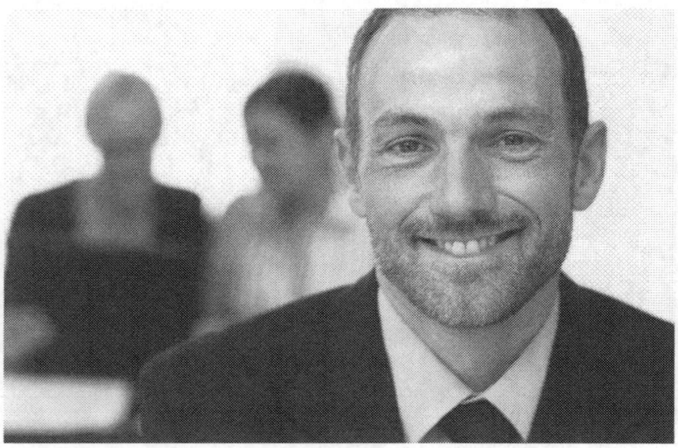

Mock Interview:

Instructions:
- Interviewer and applicant decide on the healthcare setting
- Interviewer decides on Code of Ethics based on NCIHC code.
- Grade answer by level of content (information) and presentation (format):

1 not appropriate / 10 very appropriate.

1. I am looking at your resume, and it looks like you have finished your interpreter training at…..?
   Answer: ___

   ○1 ○2 ○3 ○4 ○5 ○6 ○7 ○8 ○9 ○10
2. Can you tell me more about your interpreter training?
   Answer: ___

   ○1 ○2 ○3 ○4 ○5 ○6 ○7 ○8 ○9 ○10
3. I see that you worked at some jobs for 2 years, and at other jobs for 6 months. Can you tell me more about this?
   Answer: ___

   ○1 ○2 ○3 ○4 ○5 ○6 ○7 ○8 ○9 ○10
4. What is the most important accomplishment, achievement or innovation you brought to your present/past job?
   Answer: ___

   ○1 ○2 ○3 ○4 ○5 ○6 ○7 ○8 ○9 ○10
5. Exactly what were you responsible for in your last job?
   Answer: ___

   ○1 ○2 ○3 ○4 ○5 ○6 ○7 ○8 ○9 ○10
6. What do you want to be doing 5 years from now?
   Answer: ___

   ○1 ○2 ○3 ○4 ○5 ○6 ○7 ○8 ○9 ○10
7. What was the most difficult work problem you have ever encountered and how did you solve it?
   Answer: ___

   ○1 ○2 ○3 ○4 ○5 ○6 ○7 ○8 ○9 ○10

PO Box 2308, Woburn, MA 01888-0508, **p:** 781-729-3736, **www.EmbracingCulture.com**
PO Box 6401, Manchester, NH 03108, **p:** 1-888-678-CCCS

8. What do you feel are your outstanding qualities?
   Answer:

   ○1 ○2 ○3 ○4 ○5 ○6 ○7 ○8 ○9 ○10
9. What characteristics might differentiate you from other candidates?
   Answer:

   ○1 ○2 ○3 ○4 ○5 ○6 ○7 ○8 ○9 ○10
10. Why do you want to be an interpreter?
    Answer:

    ○1 ○2 ○3 ○4 ○5 ○6 ○7 ○8 ○9 ○10
11. What do you hope to gain from an organization like ours?
    Answer:

    ○1 ○2 ○3 ○4 ○5 ○6 ○7 ○8 ○9 ○10
12. Which languages do you speak fluently? In which languages have you been tested as an interpreter?
    Answer:

    ○1 ○2 ○3 ○4 ○5 ○6 ○7 ○8 ○9 ○10
13. Are you familiar with language regionalisms? Can you give me an example?
    Answer:

    ○1 ○2 ○3 ○4 ○5 ○6 ○7 ○8 ○9 ○10
14. Are you certified? Where did you get your certification from?
    Answer:

    ○1 ○2 ○3 ○4 ○5 ○6 ○7 ○8 ○9 ○10
15. Tell me about your philosophy on interpreting. What are your core values?
    Answer:

    ○1 ○2 ○3 ○4 ○5 ○6 ○7 ○8 ○9 ○10
16. How would you feel interpreting for a patient who has beliefs that are different than yours?
    Answer:

    ○1 ○2 ○3 ○4 ○5 ○6 ○7 ○8 ○9 ○10

17. How would you feel about interpreting for a patient who discloses that he or she has been sexually abused?

Answer: __________

○1 ○2 ○3 ○4 ○5 ○6 ○7 ○8 ○9 ○10

18. How would you handle a patient who asks you to keep a secret?

Answer: __________

○1 ○2 ○3 ○4 ○5 ○6 ○7 ○8 ○9 ○10

19. Which interpreting mode are you most comfortable using?

Answer: __________

○1 ○2 ○3 ○4 ○5 ○6 ○7 ○8 ○9 ○10

20. What is your availability?

Answer: __________

○1 ○2 ○3 ○4 ○5 ○6 ○7 ○8 ○9 ○10

21. If you were asked to interpret a consent form and sign as a witness, what would you do?

Answer: __________

○1 ○2 ○3 ○4 ○5 ○6 ○7 ○8 ○9 ○10

22. Imagine that you were in the ER interpreting for a patient who just got into a car crash. The police come in and demand that you interpret for this patient so that he can be served the Miranda Rights. What would you do?

Answer: __________

○1 ○2 ○3 ○4 ○5 ○6 ○7 ○8 ○9 ○10

23. Where can I reach you in the next week?

Answer: __________

○1 ○2 ○3 ○4 ○5 ○6 ○7 ○8 ○9 ○10

PO Box 2308, Woburn, MA 01888-0508, **p:** 781-729-3736, **www.EmbracingCulture.com**
PO Box 6401, Manchester, NH 03108, **p:** 1-888-678-CCCS

Be aware of what you say in the interview.

Which of these comments were made by interpreter applicants during an interview?

1	I am sorry I was late for this interview – your assistant gave me the wrong floor.	
2	I understand how important it is to speak English clearly because my mother's doctor is from India and I cannot understand him.	
3	I love the work I do. See, I carry this photo (showing cell phone with a picture of a mother holding a baby) of the baby born during the first labor and delivery assignment I interpreted for.	
4	I would love to work with you! I did not expect you to be so nice.	
5	Latinos like us understand these things. (Interviewer is not Latina but has a Spanish last name from her husband).	
6	I love to be a "translator" and to help those less fortunate than me!	
7	During a test, the interpreter does not understand a statement pronounced by the tester, and comments, "You speak in a funny way dear!"	
8	Due to my religious beliefs, I have to decline certain assignments such as birth control and anything to do with abortion.	

How would you reframe any of these statements if you felt compelled to make them?

1. ____________________
2. ____________________
3. ____________________
4. ____________________
5. ____________________
6. ____________________
7. ____________________
8. ____________________

9 ____________________

10. ____________________

Congratulations! You have been hired. Now, what?

Up to now, you have proved that you are a qualified interpreter. You completed your training, got your certification, researched the job market, prepared for the interview, and you have finally landed the job of your dreams. After going through this ordeal, many interpreters minimize the importance of keeping their profissional promises in regards to being a reliable interpreter, and end up losing their jobs.
Aside from language conversion skills and ethical practice, the single most important quality of the professional interpreter is **reliability**.

Here are some statements and behaviors "full of white lies" based on real life situations by interpreters who were not able to manage their time and showed up late for their appointments:

1	I am not feeling well today so I cannot cover for the case.
2	I arrived on time yet I was parking my car at the time of the appointment.
3	I can not cover the shift today because there was a bad storm where I was staying for the weekend. *Supervisor googled weather and it was a sunny day!*
4	I arrived on time but I had to use the bathroom.
5	Interpreter called the clinic: "The patient stated that he can only get to the appointment ten minutes later." *Supervisor found out that in fact the interpreter asked patient to arrive late because the interpreter was late.*
6	My car broke down, I cannot make it on time to the appointment.
7	Authorized signature on the Service Confirmation form was misspelled – Who really signed it?
8	I was late because "my people" are always late.

So what defines a white lie?

____

____

What happens to the work place when one is caught with a white lie?

____

____

Is there a thin line between an excuse and a white lie?

____

____

PO Box 2308, Woburn, MA 01888-0508, **p:** 781-729-3736, **www.EmbracingCulture.com**
PO Box 6401, Manchester, NH 03108, **p:** 1-888-678-CCCS

Managing Your Schedule

Free-lance Contractors/Independent Contractors

Please pay special attention to the following tips on managing your schedule:

- If contacted by your organization or agency while driving a vehicle, do not accept the assignment. Park your vehicle safely, and then return the call.
- Return all calls, even if you cannot accept the assignment in question.
- When calling to confirm an assignment, state your name and the date, time, location and language of the assignment in question.
- When accepting an assignment, record the details in your assignment book. You will need to record the date, time, location, language and patient name, if available. Keep your assignment book in a safe place accessible only to you.
- Allow yourself sufficient travel and parking time between assignments. You are expected to be at your assignment at least 15 minutes prior to the scheduled assignment.
- Do not make it a habit to cancel cases. Only accept cases you are sure you can cover. If you face an emergency situation and need to cancel an assignment, contact your organization/agency immediately.
- Check your voicemail on a regular basis. Your organization/agency might leave notices of any cancellations on your voice mail. Often, cases cancelled twenty-four hours prior to scheduled assignments are not paid.

Interpreters who practice poor schedule management are at risk of not receiving assignments .

Part-time, Full-time or Per-diem Interpreters

Part-time, full-time or per-diem interpreters normally get a set schedule from the organization they work for. Try to avoid:

- being late
- calling in sick at the last minute
- forgetting to carry your beeper or cell phone
- forgetting your I.D.

Ethical Challenges

1. **How would you "say no while saying yes," staying within professional boundaries, in the following situations? Write your ideas in the lines below.**

   A. A patient asks you on a date.

   B. A provider asks you to convince a patient to accept a treatment plan.

   C. A husband stops you in the lobby to ask what his wife's diagnosis is.

   D. A patient asks you to hold her child while she undresses on the other side of a curtain.

   E. A provider asks you to not interpret certain information to a patient.

2. **With the help of your classmates, act out each situation, taking turns being the interpreter and practicing "saying no while saying yes."**

PO Box 2308, Woburn, MA 01888-0508, **p:** 781-729-3736, **www.EmbracingCulture.com**
PO Box 6401, Manchester, NH 03108, **p:** 1-888-678-CCCS

Ethical Challenges When Conducting Business With On-Site Interpretation

The following situations occurred with interpreters who are independent contractors with CCCS, Inc.™

Case # 1

An interpreter arrived 15 minutes late for her appointment, however, on her Service Verification Form, she stated that she arrived on time. When questioned about the discrepancy, the interpreter insisted that she was in the building on time but that it took a few minutes to wait for the elevator. It happens that the customer, a local hospital, has a security camera that records activity in the main lobby and according to the camera's clock the interpreter did, in fact, arrive 15 minutes late.

Case #2

An interpreter forgot to ask for the authorized contact signature on the Service Verification Form. The interpreter took it upon himself and printed the provider's name. CCCS, Inc.™ staff noticed the difference in the provider's signature. When questioned by CCCS, Inc.™, the interpreter stated this had not violated any ethics because he hand-printed (and did not actually "sign") the provider's name.

Case # 3

A patient is crying uncontrollably during a session. She has suffered severe physical loss of three fingers in a work-related accident. The interpreter asks the patient not be so loud for the sake of not upsetting other patients.

Case #4

A patient arrives nervously for her first appointment with a psychologist. At the beginning of the session the three parties, psychologist, patient, and interpreter, are being seated and the interpreter takes the initiative to make the patient comfortable by offering Kleenex and showing the patient where to place her coat and purse.

Case # 5

The interpreter is asked to help the patient complete the initial medical history questionnaire. The patient cannot read, and the interpreter helps to fill out the form. Every time the patient does not understand the meaning of a medical question, the interpreter explains the meaning. For example, the form asks about a history of hepatitis, and the interpreter explains that hepatitis is an inflammation of the liver.

Case # 6

An interpreter is asked to interpret a consent form for a simple procedure. The provider is reading the information and the interpreter is interpreting it into the target language. After completion, the provider asks the interpreter to sign the form as a witness.

Ethical Questions and Application of CCCS, Inc.™ Policies and Guidelines to the Above Mentioned Case Studies.

Case #1

Q: Is it OK for an interpreter to take the risk of not telling the truth about arrival time?

A: No, this behavior breaks trust between CCCS, Inc.™, our customer and the interpreter. It questions the integrity of the interpreter and raises a red flag about this interpreter's lack of professionalism.

Case #2

Q: Is it OK for an interpreter to handprint the provider's name, in lieu of his signature, on the Service Verification form?

A: No, the provider, or the duly authorized representative of the provider, must sign the Service Verification form. This action by the interpreter is considered fraud and interpreters can be held accountable for fraudulent behavior in a court of law.

Case # 3

Q: Is it OK for an interpreter to add information in a session or to give their own instructions to a patient, even if it is for the good of other patients?

A: No, interpreters are only the accurate bridge, or language facilitators, of all information spoken between the patient and the provider.

Case # 4

Q: Should the role of an interpreter be that of personal assistant to the patient/provider?

A: Be careful! An interpreter's first reaction may be to make a patient feel comfortable, perhaps helping with his coat or providing tissues; but these natural actions may interfere with the provider's assessment, totally disarming the provider and, can be misconstrued as taking over the provider's role. Interpreters need to be patient, understanding that the provider may not take the same route as the interpreter when greeting a patient, particularly in some mental health settings. Interpreters may discuss these issues in a post-session with the provider. Interpreters must accurately interpret all information and, if certain elements of greeting were not conveyed by the provider, interpreters should not add them in.

Case # 5

Q: Should an interpreter explain any medical information when helping fill out a patient history questionnaire or any other type of form?

A: No, helping patients complete medical history questionnaires is only acceptable if the interpreter informs the patient that any questionable section will be circled and brought to the attention of the provider, who is qualified to give explanations to the patient.

Case # 6

Q: Should an interpreter be a witness of her/his own work?

A: No, interpreters can only sign consent forms as interpreters and the target language should be indicated. The provider will need another person to sign the form as a witness.

PO Box 2308, Woburn, MA 01888-0508, **p:** 781-729-3736, **www.EmbracingCulture.com**
PO Box 6401, Manchester, NH 03108, **p:** 1-888-678-CCCS

Your Interpreting Career

Interpreters, whether staff or freelance, work primarily alone. There are many ways, though, to avoid a sense of isolation and stay connected to the professional community.

CCCS, Inc.™ encourages its interpreters to join a professional interpreter association, attend ongoing skill development workshops and trainings, and form study groups with colleagues.

Another essential practice for professional interpreters is regular home study. Set aside some time each week for reading about recent developments in medical interpretation. The *Communicator Express*, our monthly newsletter for interpreters, administrators, providers and trainers, is an excellent source of new information.

CCCS, Inc.™ also recommends two key reports made available by The California Endowment at www.calendow.org:

Language Services Resource Guide for Health Care Providers - This guide, developed by the National Health Law Program, aids providers, administrators, interpreters, and others in improving language access and improving healthcare for their patients.

Certifying Health Care Interpreters - This report provides an overview of certification issues for healthcare interpreters in the United States, examines specific programs currently in existence, and explores the potential for the development of a national certification process for spoken-language healthcare interpreters.

Ongoing Self-Assessment

Regular honest self-assessment is vital to your growth as a professional interpreter. After each session, ask yourself questions like these:

- Did I help client/patient with registration?
- Did I explain CIFE to both client/patient and provider?
- Did I handle the waiting period appropriately?
- Did I maintain appropriate eye contact with both parties?
- Did I handle side comments from client/patient or provider in an appropriate manner?
- Did I stay alone in the room with the client/patient?
- Did I select the best mode of interpretation?
- Was my interpretation accurate and complete?
- Did I check in to see that the client/patient understood the message?
- How did I handle cultural issues in the interpreting session?
- Did I assist client/patient with follow-up activities?

Note: Laws change from state to state. Every organization has its own requirements , applicants must become familiar with the hiring and contracting protocol for each organization

Lesson Fourteen: Homework
Professionalism in Medical Interpretation

After you have successfully completed your training you can still stay engaged in your professional development. Start the process now!

- Write your resume
- Develop your business card
- Get a phone and fax
- Record a professional greeting in your voice mail
- Get an e-mail account with an appropriate address (avoid email addresses that could give an employer the wrong impression, e.g. hotlips71@juno.com or hellboy63@gmail.com, etc.)
- Build a professional wardrobe
- Check professional association web pages for updated information
- Check on certification status and take necessary steps to get prepared

Earlier in the chapter, it was mentioned that each interpreter would do well to set aside time at least once a month to review the National Interpreter Code of Ethics and Standards of Practice (available online at www.ncihc.org), and perform a self-assessment. Imagine that you are entering the field now. **Use the Code of Ethics and Standards to assess your potential readiness as an interpreter, answering the following questions:**

1. Is there a standard that I do not agree with? Explain.

____

____

____

____

2. Is there a standard that I feel I might have trouble following? Explain.

____

____

____

____

PO Box 2308, Woburn, MA 01888-0508, **p:** 781-729-3736, **www.EmbracingCulture.com**
PO Box 6401, Manchester, NH 03108, **p:** 1-888-678-CCCS

3. Is there a standard that I believe I will excel in applying? Explain.

4. Have I seen a professional interpreter violate one of these standards? Explain, and outline how you will avoid making the same mistake.

If you find that you fall short of certain standards, make a conscious effort to improve. Yes, you yourself can raise the bar and take medical interpretation to a higher level!

- Register with as many professional associations as possible
- Be an active listserv participant
- Look for on-going trainings and workshops
- Write about topics that are dear to you and have them published in professional magazines
- Attend at least one professional conference per year
- Research medical vocabulary and medical topics
- Develop a bilingual glossary with regionalisms
- Be an ambassador to our profession. Keep your promises!!!

Lesson Fourteen: Additional Resources
Professionalism in Medical Interpretation

Possible REQUIREMENTS when contracting for freelance interpreters

Initial Requirements

In keeping with our commitment to provide quality interpreter services to a diverse customer base, CCCS, Inc.™ has developed and maintained a Four Step Application Process that includes:

1. **Initial Resume Review/Phone Screening**
   CCCS, Inc.™ representatives conduct a preliminary 20-30 minute information gathering and screening process. Applicants who have not undergone interpreter training, and others, may be encouraged to reapply after completion of a training program.

2. **Preliminary Application Process**
   Applicants whose qualifications meet CCCS, Inc.™ requirements receive the Independent Contractor Interpreter Application Package. This package contains the:
   - Independent Contractor Application
   - Business Associate Agreement (HIPAA-based confidentiality agreement)
   - Medical Terminology Exam (to be completed by applicant)
   - Request for current Immunization Records
   - Request for Work Eligibility Documentation
   - Proof of Interpreter Training

   CCCS, Inc.™ reserves the right to request a Criminal Offender Record Check (CORI) for interpreters residing in Massachusetts, and a Criminal Record Release Authorization Form for interpreters residing in New Hampshire.

3. **Application Package Review**
   Upon receipt of a complete Independent Contractor Interpreter Application Package, the Medical Terminology Exam is reviewed by a senior interpreter. When applicable, a senior interpreter telephones the applicant, verifying information through conversation in the target language.

PO Box 2308, Woburn, MA 01888-0508, **p:** 781-729-3736, **www.EmbracingCulture.com**
PO Box 6401, Manchester, NH 03108, **p:** 1-888-678-CCCS

4. Applicant Interview

Applicants who meet CCCS, Inc.™ standards are invited to a face-to-face interview, during which a CCCS, Inc.™ representative explains interpreter guidelines and policies.

All new CCCS, Inc.™ interpreters are required to attend an 8-hour Medical Interpreter Assessment Training at our Massachusetts or New Hampshire offices. This manual is a summary of topics covered in this full-day workshop. Assessment Training attendees are required to complete pre-test, post-test and final evaluation prior to receiving photo-identification badges for their assignments from CCCS, Inc.™.

Applicants are reminded that CCCS, Inc.™ reserves the right to discontinue the application process at any time.

Yearly Renewal Requirements

All CCCS, Inc.™ interpreters are required to submit proof of current MMR vaccination and PPD (TB) tests as a pre-requisite to yearly renewal. In addition, interpreters are strongly encouraged to undergo vaccination against other communicable diseases, including Hepatitis B. Ask your medical provider about other vaccines that may be applicable to your work as an interpreter. Interpreters who do not comply with vaccination and test requirements will no longer receive assignments from CCCS, Inc.™.

CCCS, Inc.™ interpreters must supply proof of current work eligibility each year on the anniversary date of their initial contract with CCCS, Inc.™. Interpreters must present original documents for CCCS, Inc.™ verification and a new Interpreter ID Badge photo will be taken at the time of this assignment.

CCCS, Inc.™ interpreters are also asked to submit proof of ongoing education, which may include copies of training certificates.

Dress Requirements

Dress and grooming are important to the professional interpreter. When you interpret, you are a representative of CCCS, Inc.™. You are also the "face" from which providers, support staff and patients will form impressions, both of you as a person and of the medical interpreting profession at large. For this reason, your dress and grooming should reflect a professionalism and dignity appropriate to the medical setting.

Attire deemed unprofessional and prohibited in CCCS, Inc.™ assignments include:

- Shorts, jeans or leggings
- Low-cut or see-through tops
- Sneakers, open-toe shoes, and flip flops

Perfume is also prohibited, as many patients have severe allergies to scented oils and sprays. Interpreters are also asked to be moderate in their use of jewelry and make-up.

Interpreters must wear their CCCS, Inc.™ Interpreter ID Badge to all assignments. (Note that CCCS, Inc.™ badges cannot be worn outside of CCCS, Inc.™ assignments.)

Preparing For An Assignment

1. Calling a Client/Patient

The Service Verification Form, or other forms provided to you by your organization/agency, might have special requests. Pay special attention to those "specific requests."

Telephone messages should be discrete. Do not leave the name of the provider or the type of assignment on a client/patient's voice mail. If someone other than the client/patient offers to take a message, never share specific assignment information. Do not leave messages at a client/patient's place of employment unless requested by your organization/agency. Check with your organization/agency in regard to their policies.

If the number provided is not in service, or a client/patient tells you they cancelled the appointment, inform your organization/agency immediately. Unless your organization/agency officially cancels the assignment, you are expected to keep the assignment.

Interpreters are not allowed to contact patients if not asked to do so by their organization/agency. Interpreters will be immediately barred from assignments if it is determined that they maintain an outside contact with patients. This also means not soliciting work from or hiring clients/patients.

2. "Brushing Up" on Terminology

Often, the Service Verification Form or Invoice will provide a clue as to the content of the interpretation you will perform. For example, you might see "Neurology" or "Pediatrics" in the "Department" category. Plan ahead by reviewing a glossary or reading an article related to the specialty of each department to which you are assigned as an interpreter. Some interpreters set aside study time each night during which they prepare for the next day's appointments. Interpreters who use public transportation often find that time spent in transit is perfect for a last minute "brush-up" on medical terminology.

Develop your own glossary. Pay particular attention to linguistic and cultural variations in the different countries representing your target language group(s).

Memorize one or two culturally appropriate proverbs and be ready to cite them when interpreting during a mental status evaluation.

3. Planning your Trip

There are many sites that provide free driving directions, such as www.mapquest.com. Often, it is best to consult more than one internet site for directions, and to compare the suggested routes and estimated driving times. Be sure to print the directions and carry them with you as you head to the assignment.

Early each morning, check the internet or listen to the radio for weather and traffic conditions. Continue to check media sources throughout the day. Be prepared for any

PO Box 2308, Woburn, MA 01888-0508, **p:** 781-729-3736, **www.EmbracingCulture.com**
PO Box 6401, Manchester, NH 03108, **p:** 1-888-678-CCCS

possible delays. Check your voice mail periodically for any cancellations or last minute changes concerning your assignment.

Interpreters must be on time. "On time" for a CCCS interpreter means arriving 15 minutes prior to the scheduled assignment.

Confidentiality

Federal and State Laws prohibit the disclosure of information concerning a client/patient in treatment. This information is protected by Federal Confidentiality Rules, 42 CFR Part 2. Criminal penalties may be imposed on persons who violate any provision of the Federal Confidentiality Laws and Regulations.

The U.S. Department of Health and Human Services has issued the Privacy Rule to complement the Health Insurance Portability and Accountability Act of 1996 (also known as "HIPAA"). The Privacy Rule addresses the use and disclosure of individuals' health information. (See www.hhs.gov for more information).

The Privacy Rule protects all "individually identifiable health information", whether electronic, paper, or oral. This includes any information related to a patient's past, present or future physical or mental health that can be used to identify the individual, for example, information on a patient's medical record or conversations between medical team members about a patient's care.

Thus, medical interpreters must respect confidentiality rules. For example, CCCS requires that all documentation related to interpreting assignments be stored in a sealed envelope labeled "Confidential", in a place accessible only to the interpreter. When making patient reminder calls from your home or cell phone, do so in a manner that you will not be overheard by family members, housemates or anyone else who is not a member of the medical team assigned to the care of that patient.

Avoid discussing the content of your assignments with anyone other than your supervisor. If you must discuss an assignment, share stories in a way in which the client/patient cannot be identified. Never use client/patient names or other identifying information when discussing an assignment.

Information shared in a session cannot be carried into other sessions with other providers, nor can it be shared in the community. For example: You are interpreting for a client who is diagnosed in a session, but in a different session with different provider, this client decides not to mention the previous diagnosis. The interpreter is not allowed to disclose this information to the second provider.

Remember, though, that a session starts with the first contact between interpreter and client/patient, often in a waiting room or reception area, and that there are "no secrets" between client/patient, interpreter, and provider. For example: You are waiting with a patient who tells you something and asks you not to share the information with the provider. You must reiterate "CIFE" (everything must be interpreted), and encourage the patient to volunteer this information to the provider. If the patient does not share the information with the provider, you are required to do so.

Interpreters must immediately report to the provider or to a clinical supervisor any information that could be considered life-threatening. For example:

- A client has chest pain while waiting for the provider.
- A client says that he/she is going to kill him/herself or others.
- An interpreter witnesses spousal, child or elder abuse.

Another note on confidentiality: Some interpreters use notes as memory aids. If you need to take notes during the session in order to interpret accurately, please inform client/patient beforehand and discard the information in front of the client/patient right after the session.

General Safety

- Do not enter a client/patient's home unless in the presence of a provider. Arrange for a safe place to meet the provider before the session. Enter and leave with the provider.
- Follow the safety instructions given by the provider.
- Only meet with the client when a provider is present in the room. If the provider leaves the room, step into the hallway until the provider returns. Always keep the door open if a provider is not present.
- Do not give your phone number, email or address to client or provider.
- Do not offer rides to, or accept rides from, a client/patient or provider.
- Turn your cell phone off during a session, and keep your pager on "silent" mode.

Check with your organization/agency in regard to its Safety policies.

Health Safety

The US Occupational Safety and Health Administration (OSHA) reports that healthcare workers are at risk for exposure to infectious organisms and can then become infected and/or become carriers, spreading the infection to other staff and patients. (See www.osha.gov)

According to OSHA, hand washing is the single most important procedure for preventing infections. Good hand washing involves using an adequate amount of soap, rubbing the hands together to create some friction, and rinsing under running water. Dry your hands thoroughly with an air dryer or clean paper towel.

Washing hands between patient contacts and after contact with blood, body fluids, secretions, excretions, and equipment or articles contaminated by them is an important component of infection control and isolation precautions.

Treat all blood and other potentially infectious materials with appropriate precautions. For example, use gloves, masks, and gowns if blood or body fluid exposure is anticipated. As a rule of thumb, if the medical staff is wearing protective gear, such as masks or gowns, the interpreter should ask for similar protection.

Respect biohazard and patient quarantine signage and procedures. If in doubt, ask a clinical supervisor for guidance. Always follow provider and hospital staff instructions for safety.

PO Box 2308, Woburn, MA 01888-0508, **p:** 781-729-3736, **www.EmbracingCulture.com**
PO Box 6401, Manchester, NH 03108, **p:** 1-888-678-CCCS

Reporting Critical Incidents

Not every organization has a Critical Incident site team. However, interpreters should inquire with their organization/agency about what to do when faced with a critical incident.

At CCCS, Inc.™ a Critical Incident is any out of the ordinary behavior or event that takes place during an assignment. Most Critical Incidents must be reported within 24 hours of the assignment. However, other Critical Incidents are urgent and call for immediate action.

Interpreters must use good judgment in deciding when and how to report a Critical Incident. For example, if you are sitting with a patient in a clinic waiting room, and the patient tells you they are experiencing chest pain, you would immediately notify clinic staff.

The following are examples of different types of critical incidents:

- You were late for an assignment
- A provider asked you not to interpret
- You realized you made a mistake
- You were exposed to a contagious disease
- If a customer asked to hire you independently from CCCS, Inc.™
- A patient insisted that you provide your telephone number
- A patient got your number from their caller ID machine and contacted you
- Threats of violence or other personal safety concerns

To report a Critical Incident, call your institution. If no one is available, leave your name, number, and a detailed message, including the date, time, location and language of the assignment, and a brief description of the persons involved (no names of clients/patients, specify only provider's names).

Not every Critical Incident will be considered your fault; often there are situations in which you have little control.

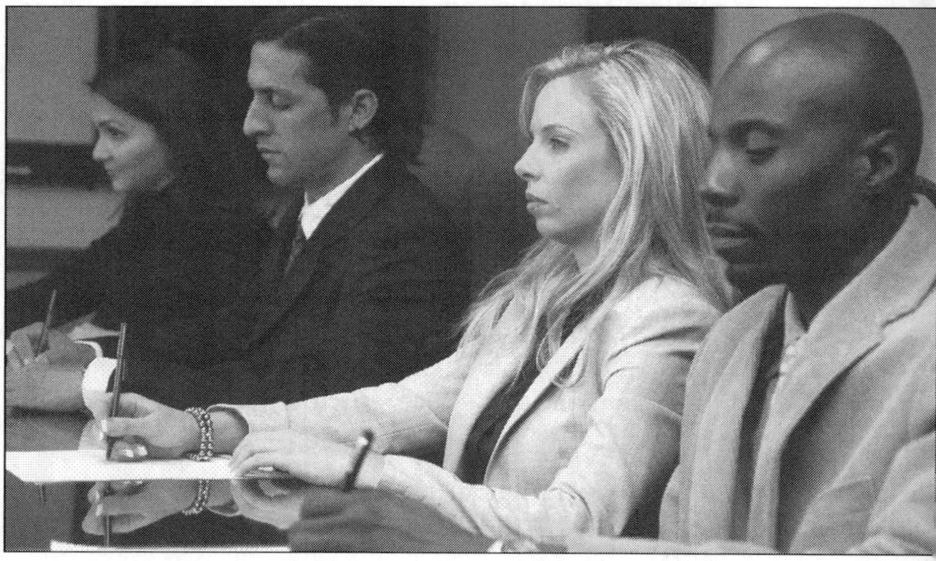

Take your assignments seriously

If you are an independent contractor or a per diem interpreter, you may receive assignments by phone, fax or email. If accepting an assignment over the phone, make sure that you write down the information correctly. Repeat key information back to the speaker as a means of verification. Stay safe, and do not put others in danger by accepting assignments while driving.

Managing your schedule is not a difficult task, but it does require an initial investment of time and money, as well as regular upkeep. All successful independent contractors keep a calendar in which they make note of their appointments and any commitments that may affect their interpreting work. Some interpreters prefer a traditional appointment book, while others make use of electronic scheduling tools. Whatever the tool, it will only be of use to the interpreter if all assignments and all commitments are recorded within.

Interpreters must be careful not to double book their time slots. Nothing is more frustrating to a client organization than an interpreter who fails to report to assignments due to overbooking. Another scheduling consideration is travel-the independent contractor must estimate and block out a generous amount of time for driving, traffic and parking.

Most interpreting agencies and hospitals that hire independent contractors provide some sort of service verification form that must be completed by the interpreter after each assignment. Often, there is a window of time (hours or days) during which the interpreter must submit appropriate documentation to the contracting organization for purposes of billing and payment.

If the interpreter fails to submit the required documentation, the contracting organization can neither bill the requestor of services nor pay the interpreter. Interpreter service coordinators have commented that interpreters who consistently fail to submit documentation after assignments are eventually terminated from service within their organizations.

Freelance interpreters, as independent contractors, are responsible for keeping their own financial records and for paying local, state and federal taxes where applicable. Many professional interpreters who work with accounting software, such as Quicken or QuickBooks, report that this method allows them to avoid mathematical errors and easily match accounts received to specific assignments. By taking charge of their own business records, these interpreters cut down on unnecessary calls to their clients' accounting offices. Check your local computer or office supply store for the latest in home and small business accounting software.

United States Spoken-Language Healthcare Interpreters Need State Regulation

As an owner of an interpreting company and a nationwide trainer of medical interpreters, I have been faced with ethical issues regarding the supervision of interpreter services. At our company, we have a team of staff members that oversees any critical incidents reported by interpreters, customers or office staff. "Critical incidents" are defined as out-of-the-ordinary situations, events or behaviors. A sampling of recent critical incidents includes an interpreter who was late, a provider who was rude, an interpreter who walked out of an appointment and left the patient without language services, and an interpreter who sent a relative to cover an assignment without permission from our company.

Although critical incidents constitute less than 1% of our caseload, we take each and every incident quite seriously. We interview to uncover both sides of the story and within one business day, we issue a recommendation. Recommendations vary. They can be as simple as assisting an interpreter to manage his or her schedule, or as complex as addressing an irate provider who clearly carries anti immigrant sentiment.

None of these critical incidents are taken lightly and some of them require an immediate termination of services with a freelancer or with a provider who refuses to follow professional protocol. The issue is that even if we take a drastic measure, the interpreter (or the provider) will most likely continue with their behavior because in this country there is no board that oversees disciplinary matters related to interpreter services.

As a licensed social worker, I always knew that my colleagues in mental health could contact the state that licensed me, or even the National Association of Social Workers (NASW), and report any concerns regarding my professional actions, behaviors, or clinical thinking. Although several of our great interpreter associations have done an excellent job developing standards and opening a professional path for all healthcare interpreters, I believe that we now need to take a step forward and ask that each state develop its own interpreter review board and invite to the table representatives of professional interpreter associations as well as of organizations that hire interpreters.

A first step for an interpreter review board would be to set the standards that will serve as a backbone for recommendations of disciplinary actions for providers of interpreter services, both companies and individuals. Right now, any information on companies and interpreters is based on "rumors", and is often poorly represented. Often, directors of interpreter programs informally counsel others to refrain from hiring a certain interpreter, for whatever reason. For example, one director of interpreter services was told by another director to watch out for a certain interpreter's "lack of boundaries." It happened that this interpreter was engaged to a provider, and her supervisor had perceived this as a "lack of boundaries." In truth, this interpreter had not carried on any inappropriate behavior, but she was thus "blacklisted" and never got the chance to present her side of the story.

On another occasion, a company found out that a freelance interpreter was conducting a side business by sending her friends on assignments she had personally accepted from the company. Although her services were terminated with this company, she is still active as an interpreter with another agency. Whether she continues to engage in this illegal practice is unknown, and legally the company that terminated her services cannot warn the second agency about her behavior.

At a training a few years ago, I heard of an interpreter who had impregnated two of his female patients. Apparently, he continued to serve as interpreter to both women during their pregnancies. It appears that this interpreter had first met the patients while interpreting for them and had pursued inappropriate relationships with them. As far as I know, he is still working as an interpreter and has not been disciplined.

At the same organization that hosted this training, I also heard from providers who did not want to be perceived as "politically incorrect", but were concerned with the fact that the interpreters at their organization would freely start the medical interview without waiting for the provider to speak. When the providers confronted the interpreters about this problem, the interpreters accused them of discrimination.

On the flip side, translators and interpreters are now posting complaints on websites geared towards identifying companies and agencies that do not pay their freelancers on time. However, there is no room on these sites for a rebuttal. While abuse of freelancers does occur and should be addressed, there is the possibility that an unjust posting on such a site could forever tarnish the name of a company. Could it be that the company had not paid because the interpreter had not provided the service? We may never know, since all we hear (or read) is one side of the story.

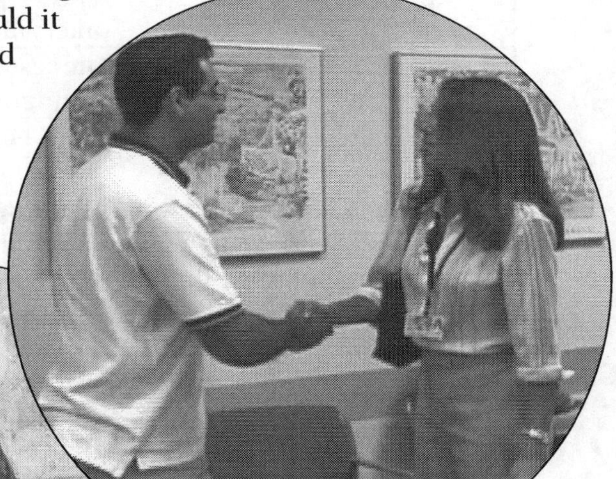

All the cases mentioned above, no matter how horrible they sound, deserve a dual process, a representation of both sides of the story. As professional healthcare interpreters of spoken language, we have two choices: isolate ourselves and pretend there is not an issue; or begin to push for the guidance and supervision of an interpreter review board. While this task may sound daunting, we are not obligated to reinvent the wheel. Why not begin to look at the culture of ASL interpreter regulation and see what we can learn?

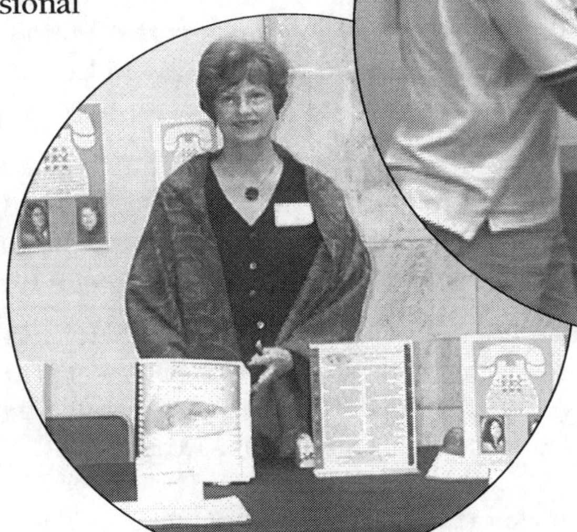

PO Box 2308, Woburn, MA 01888-0508, **p:** 781-729-3736, **www.EmbracingCulture.com**
PO Box 6401, Manchester, NH 03108, **p:** 1-888-678-CCCS

Surviving Job Stress in Freelance Interpretation

Many folks dream of running their own businesses-they imagine a life of freedom from the demands of a supervisor or boss. The reality of the freelance interpreter, though, is that each client organization plays the role of 'boss'. It can be said, then, that the stresses of freelance interpreting are potentially many times greater than those of a regular salaried employee.

Job stress can be defined as the harmful physical and emotional responses that occur when the requirements of the job do not match the capabilities, resources, or needs of the worker. Anyone who has at some point made a living in freelance interpreting can identify with the challenges of maintaining a reasonable schedule while earning what is necessary to 'pay the bills'.

Most successful freelance interpreters contract with several organizations. At times, the demands of these clients overlap, and the interpreter may begin to feel 'pulled' in different directions as, in an attempt to keep everyone happy, s/he takes on more assignments than humanly manageable.

Consider a day in the life of an interpreter we'll call Stella. Stella works with three client organizations. Stella's calendar reflects the following medical interpreting assignments, each with a two-hour minimum:

Daily Calendar

THURSDAY	
9:00 a.m.	Somerville, MA (Client A)
11:30 a.m.	Dorchester, MA (Client B)
1:45 p.m.	Reading, MA (Client A)
6:30 p.m.	Salem, NH (Client C)

Can you spot the overbooking? Although Stella has blocked out a two-hour minimum for each assignment, she has not allotted a proper amount of time for driving from one appointment to the next. Despite knowing that it is impossible to make the 40-minute trip from Dorchester to Reading in just 15 minutes, Stella will speed down the highway in the false hope of arriving on time for the 1:45 assignment.

The effects of Stella's overbooking are far-reaching. A quick glance at her appointment book reveals that in addition to jeopardizing road safety and client satisfaction, Stella has not set aside time in her 12-hour work day to rest or eat. During the last assignment of the day, she begins to feel faint and a bit dizzy from this dangerous combination of stress and hunger.

Interestingly, the US Department of Health and Human Services reports that four studies which focused on effects during extended shifts reported that the 9th to 12th hours of work were associated with feelings of decreased alertness and increased fatigue, lower cognitive function, declines in vigilance on task measures, and increased injuries.

Differences in individual characteristics such as personality and coping style are important in predicting whether certain job conditions will result in stress. Examples of individual and situational factors that can help to reduce the effects of stressful working conditions include:

- Balance between work and personal life
- A support network of friends and coworkers
- A relaxed and positive outlook

How can an interpreter know if s/he is suffering from stress? It is important to take action at a personal level and to review your lifestyle to see if you can identify any contributing factors. A simple checklist might include:

- Do I often eat 'on the run' or in a disorganized manner?
- Am I always rushing, trying to be available to everyone?
- Do I often exceed the speed limit when traveling from one assignment to the next?
- Do I usually miss breaks?
- Do I regularly schedule time for exercise and relaxation?
- Do I allow myself adequate time for sleep (a minimum of 7-8 hours)?
- Am I smoking or drinking excessively?
- Are my clients less and less satisfied due to my tardiness or rushed performance?
- Have I lost jobs because of unsatisfactory performance?

In many cases, prolonged stress can lead to poor physical and/or mental health. If you think you are currently experiencing stress-related ill health, you may benefit from a discussion with your primary care provider.

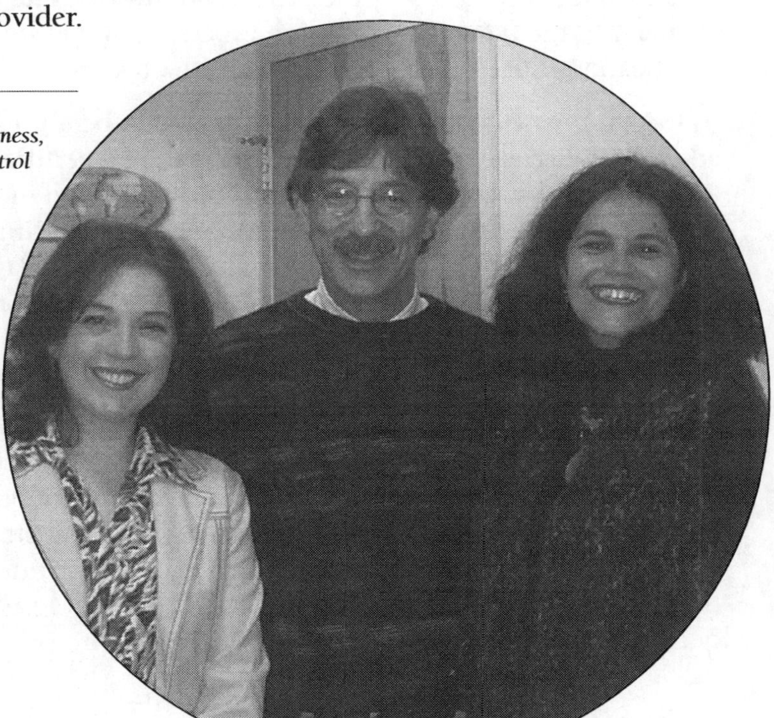

Our sources:

"Overtime and Extended Work Shifts: Recent Findings on Illness, Injuries, and Health Behaviors", Centers for Disease Control and Prevention, National Institute for Occupational Safety and Health. DHHS (NIOSH) Publication No. 2004-143.

"Stress...At Work", US Department of Health and Human Services, Centers for Disease Control and Prevention, National Institute for Occupational Safety and Health.

PO Box 2308, Woburn, MA 01888-0508, **p:** 781-729-3736, **www.EmbracingCulture.com**
PO Box 6401, Manchester, NH 03108, **p:** 1-888-678-CCCS

Interpreter Certification:

Recently there have been many questions and discussions regarding a formal certification process for healthcare interpreters. While there are not many clear answers how this process will affect interpreters in the field, I have summarized information to give you some of the background of what has precipitated this move towards a certification process at this time.

In November 2003, a pilot project was developed with several partnering organizations. The Massachusetts Medical Interpreters Association (MMIA now IMIA) hosted the project with volunteer representatives from CHIA (California Health Care Interpreting Association) the National Council on Interpreting in Health Care (NCIHC) Committee of Standards, Training and Certification as well as Healthy House of Merced. This coalition created the MIAC (Medical Interpreting Assessment for Certification) group.

The MMIA is an interpreter organization founded in 1986 and became an official non-profit in 1992 known as MMIA. They developed the first Standards of Practice. In 2007, the MMIA officially became the International Medical Interpreters Association, IMIA. Since 1997, the IMIA has held annual conferences providing educational and informative opportunities to the profession.

During the certification pilot in November 2003, two of the representatives from the partnering organizations (MMIA, NCIHC) signed a "Memorandum of Understanding (MOA)."The MOA signed and agreed to by MMIA and NCIHC, stated that the intellectual property in the certification process piloted project was the property of MMIA. The MOA essentially protected the intellectual property of the piloted certification process. For additional information on the MOA and the certification process, see the IMIA website on Certification http://www.imiaweb.org/certification. [1]

In the summer of 2006, during an annual membership meeting, the NCIHC continued with additional discussions with respect to a national certification process as a response to its members. A consensus was reached to continue with open and inclusive dialogues resulting in several national forums being held by NCIHC Standards, Training and Certification Committee (STC) around the country. A total of 11 forums were held on the topic of a national certification culminating in a published report. The report, "Are we ready for National Certification of Health Care Interpreters? A summary of NCIHC Open Forums" authored by Maria-Paz Beltran Avery, Ph.D. was released in October 2007, by the NCIHC. To see the full report, go to www.ncihc.org.

The report summarized many of the questions, concerns and direction of the national certification process by those participating in the forums. This report came to the conclusion that although "there was a general sense of urgency to create a national certification process, the forum highlighted the need to ensure a well thought-out, systematic and systemic process of development that addresses not only the creation of a testing instrument of high technical quality but also fosters the conditions that would make the certification of healthcare interpreters a valued element of high quality." [2]

In December of 2007 NCIHC "convened a meeting to discuss forming a coalition to move the healthcare certification process forward."[3] Several representatives from national organizations (NCIHC, IMIA, CHIA and ATA) met to bring the process to a more formal and inclusive way by inviting additional national stakeholder to the table as well as forming a group specifically for the process. For additional information on who is on the committee, go to www.ncihc.org.

Bi-monthly meetings continued to be held with all the representatives from all four organizations (NCIHC, CHIA, IMIA, ATA).The four organizations formed a coordinating committee to move the process of interpreter certification forward. The first official meeting of the coordinating committee was scheduled to be held in the spring 2008 partially funded by the California Endowment. [4]

In March 2008, representatives from the four organizations met and officially formed a national coalition to work towards developing "a national certification for healthcare interpreters." The coordinating committee officially became the National Coalition on Health Care Interpreter Certification Coordinating Committee (NCC). The official coalition, NCC began the process of inviting national stakeholders to join the coalition. In June 2008, applications from national stakeholders were reviewed and 14 organizations were accepted to become part of the coalition. See National Council on Interpreting in Health Care Latest Updates on Certification page at www.ncihc.org.

A second meeting was held in September 2008, in Minnesota, with all the participating invited organizations and the original members of the initial coalition, as well as two representatives from the California Endowment. The purpose of the meeting was to discuss the structure to move the process forward. During this meeting, however, the focus of the NCC moved the process from that of "developing a national certification process" to "developing standards for a national certification process."[5]

Concurrently the IMIA decided to work on a separate and independent Certification for interpreters. The separate certification for interpreters is independent of the NCC project. IMIA has continued to meet and recently partnered with a for profit organization to continue the formal certification process. Recently the IMIA issued two press releases explaining the status of their work and their partnership. For additional information on this topic go to **http://www.imiaweb.org/certification**.The IMIA site explains the certification background as well as "The Purposes of the Certification", "Criterion referenced" and much more.[5]

On January 28, 2009, the National Coalition on Health Care Interpreter Certification group (NCC) released a letter summarizing the result of a two day meeting held on January 22-23 in California. During this meeting, plans were developed to continue "pursuing work on certification development, certification for languages of lesser diffusion and the legal aspects of certification, beginning with the development of objective standards for the pre-qualification, training and

PO Box 2308, Woburn, MA 01888-0508, **p:** 781-729-3736, **www.EmbracingCulture.com**
PO Box 6401, Manchester, NH 03108, **p:** 1-888-678-CCCS

testing, and continuing education of healthcare interpreters." The NCC committee will also be inviting more stakeholders to continue with the certification process. (6)

This summary is only intended as an informational piece and a glimpse of the process and may not include all the details and discussions which have culminated in where the certification is today. We hope you take the time to review all the available materials with respect to the certification process and we encourage you to visit the various sites for more information and clarification and to identify any possible corrections to this summary. It is only through discussion and direct information that your questions will be answered.

(1) *IMIA website on Certification http://www.imiaweb.org/certification.*
(2) *Are we ready for National Certification of Health Care Interpreters? A summary of NCIHC Open Forums" authored by Maria-Paz Beltran Avery, Ph.D. was released in October 2007, by the NCIHC.*
(3) *NCIHC website, www.ncihc.org.*
(4) *NCIHC website, www.ncihc.org.*
(5) *IMIA website on Certification http://www.imiaweb.org/certification.*
(6) *NCC letter dated January 28, 2009, "National Coalition Surges Ahead with National Healthcare Interpreter Certification."*

Writing an Interpreter Resume

Any newcomer to the interpreting profession will need to update his/her resume, customizing it in a way that will present him/her as an attractive candidate for an interpreting position.

Some students of interpretation are not familiar with basic resume writing guidelines, while others possess a professional resume that needs some customization.

For basic resume-writing guidelines, see "The Resume Guide", a publication of the Massachusetts Department of Workforce Development. This 40-page guide walks the job seeker through the process of writing an effective resume, and includes sample resumes and helpful hints for special situations, such as job hopping, employment gaps, and changing careers. See

http://www.mass.gov/?pageID=elwdsubtopic&L=4&L0=Home&L1=Government&L2=EOLWD+Publications&L3=Publications+for+Job+Seekers&sid=Elwd or http://www.mass.gov/Elwd/docs/dcs/1865_508.pdf.

For tips on customizing your resume for a medical interpreting position, the IMIA lists nine tips for new interpreters at http://www.imiaweb.org/members/samplecv.asp.

We wish you the best in your job search and invite you to share your experiences with us!

Interpreter's Associations by State

Interested in contacting your local interpreter association? Both the NCIHC and IMIA websites contain links to state and regional interpreter associations. These include:

Alabama .... Interpreter Association of Alabama (IAA)

Arizona .... Arizona Interpreter and Translators Association (AITA)

California .... California Healthcare Interpreter Association (CHIA)

Colorado .... Colorado Association of Professional Interpreters (CAPI)

Connecticut .... Medical Interpreting Association of Connecticut (MIAC)

Georgia .... Medical Interpreter Network of Georgia (MING)

Idaho .... Treasure Valley Interpreters Association (TVIA)

Illinois .... Illinois Association of Healthcare Interpreters (IAHI)

Indiana .... Northern Indiana Medical Interpreter Association (NIMIA)

Iowa .... Iowa Interpreter and Translator Association (IITA)

Kentucky .... Kentucky Translator and Interpreter Association (KTIA)

Massachusetts .... International Medical Interpreters Association (IMIA)

Michigan .... Michigan Translators/Interpreters Network (MiTIN)

Midwest .... Midwest Association of Translators and Interpreters (MATI)

Minnesota .... Upper Midwest Translators and Interpreters Association (UMTIA)

Nebraska .... Nebraska Association for Translators and Interpreters (NATI)

New England .... New England Translators Association (NETA)

New Hampshire .... New England Trained Interpreters Association (NETIA)

New York .... Multicultural Association of Medical Interpreters of Central New York (MAMI),
New York Association of Medical Interpreters (NYAMI)
Association of Medical Interpreters of New York (AMINY)

North Carolina .... North Carolina Professional Interpreters Association (NCPIA)

Ohio .... Community and Court Interpreters of the Ohio Valley (CCIO)

Oregon .... Oregon Association of Interpreters (OIA)

South Carolina .... South Carolina Healthcare Interpreter Association (SCHIA)

PO Box 2308, Woburn, MA 01888-0508, **p:** 781-729-3736, **www.EmbracingCulture.com**
PO Box 6401, Manchester, NH 03108, **p:** 1-888-678-CCCS

Tennessee..................Tennessee Association of Medical Interpreters and Translators (TAMIT)
Tennessee Association of Professional Interpreters and Translators (TAPIT)

Texas...........................Austin Area Translators and Interpreters Association (AATIA)
Houston Interpreters and Translators Association (HITA)
Texas Association of Healthcare Interpreters and Translators (TAHIT)

Virginia......................Mid Atlantic Interpreters Association (MAIA)

Washington...............Northwest Translators and Interpreters Society (NOTIS)

This information on local and regional associations was copied from www.ncihc.org. See website for links and other updated information.

Other Websites That Contain Information For Interpreters:

1. **DiversityRx:** Promoting language and cultural competence to improve the quality of healthcare for minority, immigrant, and ethnically diverse communities.

   www.diversityrx.org/

2. **National Health Law Program**

   The National Health Law Program Works for Justice in Health Care for Low-Income People.

   www.healthlaw.org

3. **The Interpreters Division of ATA**

   A chapter of the American Translators Association for the interpreting industry. Tips and Resources.

   www.ata-divisions.org

4. **The Joint Commission** exists to make a difference in people's lives. From patients to family members to caregivers—real improvement in real time. www.jointcommission.org

5. **The Office of Minority Health** advises the Secretary and the OPHS on public health issues affecting American Indians, and Alaska Natives, Asian Americans, etc. www.omhrc.gov

6. **Office for Civil Rights**

   Jun 11, 2007 ... Home page and access point for the Office of Civil Rights (OCR) website. www.ed.gov/about/offices/list/ocr/index.html

The Joint Commission Standards in Support of Hospital Provisions for Language and Cultural Services

The Joint Commission is a non-profit independent body providing voluntary accreditation standards to hospitals. The Joint Commission's mission is to..."continuously improve the safety and quality of care provided to the public through the provision of healthcare accreditation and related services that support performance improvement in healthcare organizations.."[(1)]

Between 2005 and 2006, The Joint Commission conducted a study of 60 hospitals on the topic of **"addressing issues related to culture and language in the populations they serve."** Recognizing the need for a more inclusive system of care and to improve patient safety given the changing demographics in the United States, the study was designed to identify best practices, concerns and challenges of providing healthcare services to a linguistic and culturally diverse population. The resulting report of the study by The Joint Commission, *"Hospitals, Culture and Language: A Snapshot of the Nation, Exploring Cultural and Linguistic Services in the Nation's Hospitals: A Report of Findings,"* by Amy Wilson-Stronks and Erica Galvez, highlights the study and recommendations for including provisions of language services. These recommendations include written policies that specifically address among others, working with trained healthcare interpreters, ensuring that stringent requirements for interpreting are in place and that organizations do not use family members as interpreters, specifically minors. The Joint Commission recognizes that working with trained interpreters is associated with improved healthcare encounters and outcomes and improves safety and quality. [(2)]

In April 2008, a second report was released entitled *"One Size Does Not Fit All: Meeting the Health Care Needs of Diverse Populations."* The report builds on the study of the 60 hospitals and subsequent report *"Hospitals, Culture and Language: A snapshot of the nation..."* The framework of the April 2008 report expands on the recommendations addressing hospital policies of including provisions for "culturally and linguistically appropriate services." One of the recommendations provided in the report, "Integrating Cultural Competence into Patient Care" suggests that organizations identify appropriate language services such as **interpreting and translation services.** [(3)]

Additionally, current Joint Commission standards RI.2.100 now RI.01.01.01, EP 5 under *Requirements Related to the Provision of Cultural and Linguistically Appropriate Health Care*, states that "The hospital respects the patient's right to and need for effective communication." Also, standard RI.01.01.03 states that "The hospital respects the patient's right to receive information in a manner he or she understands," under which there is EP 2 requiring organizations to "provide interpreting and translation services, as necessary. [(4)]

In a February 2008 article *"Promoting Effective Communication,"* several of the recommendations made addressing working with interpreters, were summarized specifically under *"How to Address Language Barriers?"*[(5)]

PO Box 2308, Woburn, MA 01888-0508, **p:** 781-729-3736, **www.EmbracingCulture.com**
PO Box 6401, Manchester, NH 03108, **p:** 1-888-678-CCCS

These recommendations include:

- Working with trained interpreters vs. ad hoc interpreters.
- Organizations should not rely on family members and in particular minors except during an emergency.
- While working with telephone interpreters can provide quick access, it is not recommended for certain types of interpreting; such as end-of-life situations.
- Suggests working with trained interpreters who are skilled in understanding privacy issues under Health Insurance Portability and Accountability Act of 1996 better know as the HIPAA law as well as ethical standards.

To provide effective communication with culturally and linguistically diverse population, The Joint Commission standards acknowledges that to improve healthcare encounters, outcomes and improve safety and quality, hospitals should work with **trained interpreters who are an important factor in provider-patient relationships**. For more information on The Joint Commission, visit www.jointcomission.org.

The information has been collected, edited and adapted from The Joint Commission, www.jointcomission.org, and the following references.

(1) *http://www.jointcommission.org/AboutUS.*

(2) *Amy Wilson-Stronks and Erica Galvez, "Hospitals, Language and Culture: A Snapshot of the Nation: Exploring Cultural and Linguistic Services in the Nation's Hospitals," A report of Findings, c. 2007, funded by the California Endowment.*

(3) *"One Size Does Not Fit All: Meeting the Health Care Needs of Diverse Populations." http://www.jointcommision.org/PatientSafety/HLC/one_size_meeting_need_of_diverse-population_htm*

(4) *The Joint Commission 2008 Requirements Related to the Provision of Cultural and Linguistically Appropriate Health Care, April 2008 - www.jointcommission.org/NR/rdonlyres/1401C2EF-62F0-4715-B28A*

(5) *"Promoting Effective Communication" Joint Commission Perspectives. Feb. 2008, Volume 28, Issue 2*

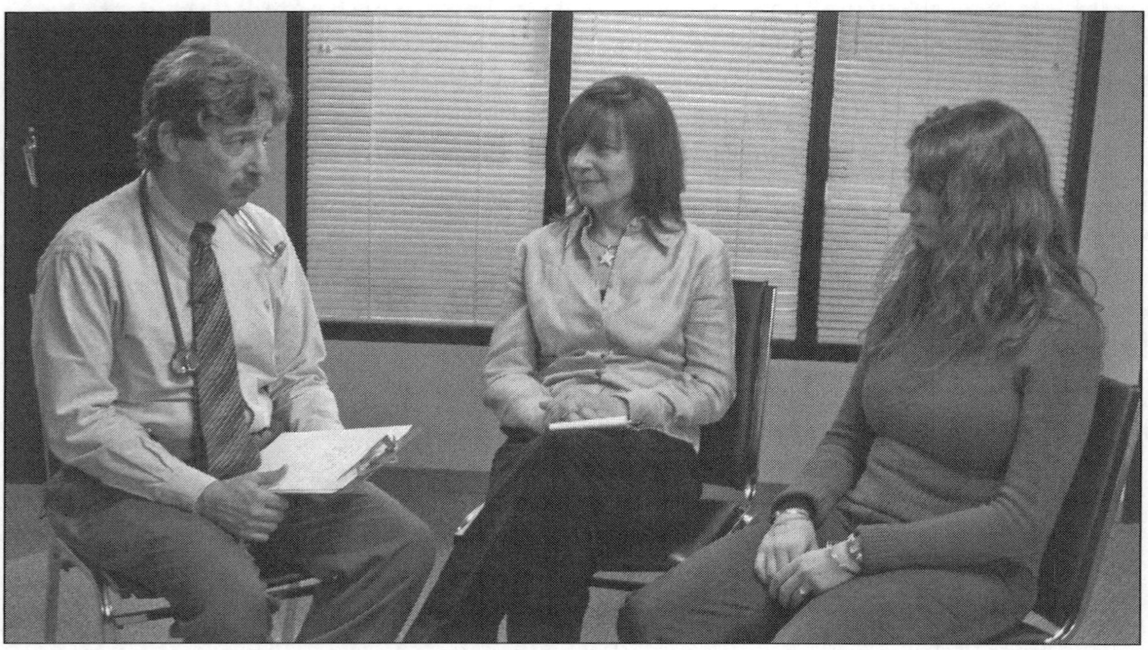

HEALTH CARE INTERPRETERS: Are They Mandatory Reporters of Child Abuse?[1]

I. Introduction

As the nation continues to diversify and more healthcare providers are using interpreters to communicate with their patients, one issue that arises is whether interpreters are covered by mandatory child abuse reporting laws. Members of some professions are mandated by state law to report known and suspected cases of child abuse seen within the course of their employment.[2] While most states require healthcare workers to report child abuse, the laws are not clear if interpreters in healthcare settings fall within the parameters of the healthcare profession. It is important that interpreters know whether or not they fall within a state's mandatory reporter category, as they could be liable for not reporting cases of child abuse. Failure to report cases of abuse is a misdemeanor in many states.

II. Are Health Care Interpreters Mandatory Reporters?

Individuals who are required to report usually have direct contact with children. Some state statutes are very explicit in how they define healthcare workers, while others are not. Depending on the wording and interpretation of a statute, an interpreter may or may not fall into this designation and be a mandatory reporter. Although interpreters generally work in clinical settings with a practitioner who is usually required to report, interpreters cannot assume that the practitioner will report a child abuse case. The wording of a mandatory reporting statute may independently require the interpreter to report.

Whether an interpreter has a duty to report suspected or known child abuse depends on the laws of a particular state. Those who must report pursuant to state reporting laws generally fit into four categories. The state breakdown is as follows:[3]

- Four states[4] require "any person" or "every person" to report
- Thirty-three states[5] require healthcare workers or "hospital personnel" to report
- Thirteen states[6] require "any person" or "every person" and healthcare workers to report[7]
- Texas requires "any person" or "every person" and "professionals" to report[8]

Ten states (including those with the highest LEP populations) were examined to ascertain whether interpreters are required to report child abuse observed in healthcare settings.[9] None of the reporting statutes in those states specifically requires interpreters to report. However, three states have adopted statutes that require all persons to report suspected abuse regardless of their profession. Four states require "hospital personnel" to report, which may sometimes include interpreters (see below). Two of the ten states have adopted both the catchall "any person" provision, and a specific healthcare worker provision. One state has an "any person" as well as a "professional" provision. Only one state clearly did not require healthcare interpreters to report child abuse.

PO Box 2308, Woburn, MA 01888-0508, **p:** 781-729-3736, **www.EmbracingCulture.com**
PO Box 6401, Manchester, NH 03108, **p:** 1-888-678-CCCS

a. The "Any Person" or "Every Person" Requirement

Three of the ten states we examined require "any person" or "every person" to report suspected cases of child abuse. These states are Florida, New Jersey, and North Carolina. For example, in New Jersey, the statute states that "any person having reasonable cause to believe that a child has been subjected to child abuse or acts of child abuse shall report…."[10] Thus, a healthcare interpreter would be required to report child abuse, regardless of the context within which she learned of the abuse.

Although Florida has an "any person" requirement, the state additionally requires healthcare workers to give their name when making a report of child abuse. Individuals who are not healthcare workers (or members of certain other professions listed in the statute) are allowed to report anonymously.[11]

b. The "Healthcare Worker" Requirement

Of the ten states we examined, California, Illinois, Massachusetts, and New York require some categories of healthcare workers to report suspected cases of child abuse.

New York requires "hospital personnel engaged in the admission, examination, care or treatment of persons" to report child abuse and neglect.12 Thus, whether or not healthcare interpreters fall into this category depends on whether (1) they are hospital "personnel;" and (2) they are engaged in the "admission, examination, care or treatment of persons." For example, a full time interpreter employed by a hospital would likely be considered hospital "personnel," while an interpreter who independently contracted with a hospital might not be. If interpreters are hospital personnel, the second question is whether they are engaged in "admission, examination, care or treatment." If an interpreter is used to communicate with LEP patients in the hospital admissions process, they are likely to be considered mandatory reporters.

Illinois and Massachusetts have statutory language that requires reporting from similar personnel, with the only difference being that hospital personnel engaged in admissions are not included.[13]

California exhaustively lists every profession that is required to report, but does not list interpreters or include a category as broad as "healthcare worker," as do the three states above.[14] While California's statute also requires child abuse reporting by persons who are currently licensed under a section of the Business and Professions Code;[15] interpreters are not among those so licensed. Therefore, healthcare interpreters are not mandated to report child abuse.

c. The "Any Person" and a "Health Care Worker" Requirement

A state with an "any" or "every" person mandatory reporting provision obviously requires all interpreters to report child abuse because they definitely fall within the catch-all "any"/"every" person. Of the states examined, New Mexico and Maryland have adopted the "any person" requirement, augmented by a specific requirement for certain types of healthcare workers to report child abuse. While Maryland has also adopted the "any person" requirement, it also has a separate requirement for health practitioners.[16] Maryland's statutory definition of health practitioner does not encompass interpreters, yet the "any person" requirement obligates interpreters to report cases of child abuse. New Mexico's healthcare worker provision is limited to physicians, residents and interns, although interpreters would be included under the "every person" provision.[17]

d. The "Any Person" and "Professional" Requirement

Like the states above which have a healthcare worker requirement in addition to an "any person" requirement, Texas requires "any person" as well as "professionals" to report child abuse.[18] In Texas, interpreters are obligated to report any suspected case of child abuse under the "any person" requirement.

Other states may use "professional" instead of "healthcare worker" and thus an examination of the Texas requirement may be helpful. The Texas statute defines a professional as "an individual who is licensed or certified by the state or who is an employee of a facility licensed, certified, or operated by the state and who, in the normal course of official duties or duties for which a license or certification is required, has direct contact with children."[19] Currently, Texas has no licensure or certification requirement for interpreters; however, an interpreter falls into this category if they are employed by a hospital or other licensed facility. The question will therefore be the meaning of "employee" and it is likely independent contractors would be excluded under this provision.

III. Other Important Components of Mandatory Reporting Laws

There are several other important components regarding failure to report and protections for good faith reporting. Interpreters need to know these requirements because a failure to report can have negative repercussions.

Failure to report a suspected case is a misdemeanor in six of the states we examined –California, Florida, Illinois, New Mexico, New York and Texas.[20] In Illinois, a first violation is a misdemeanor and any subsequent failure to report is considered a felony.[21] Massachusetts fines non-reporters up to $1000.[22] In New Jersey, a person is deemed a "disorderly person" for failing to report child abuse.[23] North Carolina and Maryland have no punishment for non-reporting.

Finally, most states give immunity from civil and criminal liability to mandatory reporters who report in good faith. If a healthcare interpreter suspects child abuse and reports it, but later the child abuse charge is determined to be unfounded, the interpreter cannot be held liable for reporting what he/she believed to be abuse. All ten states examined here give this immunity.

PO Box 2308, Woburn, MA 01888-0508, **p:** 781-729-3736, **www.EmbracingCulture.com**
PO Box 6401, Manchester, NH 03108, **p:** 1-888-678-CCCS

IV. Conclusion

To determine whether healthcare interpreters are required to report child abuse in a state, one should examine the state's child abuse and neglect statute regarding mandatory reporting. The National Clearinghouse on Child Abuse and Neglect Information has produced a chart with citations to every state's child abuse laws. The chart is also useful as a quick guide for the individuals and/or professions who must report child abuse and neglect.[24]

---

1 *© 2003 by the National Health Law Program. This report was made possible through the generous support of The California Endowment.*

2 *There may be a similar reporting requirement for elder abuse, but that is beyond the scope of this paper.*

3 *For a breakdown of all states, see National Clearinghouse on Child Abuse and Neglect Information, Statutes At-a-Glance, Mandatory Reporters of Child Abuse and Neglect (Feb. 2002), available at http://www.calib.com/nccanch/pubs/sag/manda.pdf.*

4 *Florida, New Jersey, North Carolina and Wyoming. See http://www.calib.com/nccanch/pubs/sag/manda.pdf.*

5 *Alabama, Alaska, Arizona, Arkansas, California, Colorado, Connecticut, District of Columbia, Georgia, Hawaii, Illinois, Iowa, Kansas, Louisiana, Maine, Massachusetts, Michigan, Minnesota, Missouri, Montana, Nevada, New York, North Dakota, Ohio, Oregon, Pennsylvania, South Carolina, South Dakota, Vermont, Virginia, Washington, West Virginia, and Wisconsin. See http://www.calib.com/nccanch/pubs/sag/manda.pdf.*

6 *Delaware, Idaho, Indiana, Kentucky, Maryland, Mississippi, Nebraska, New Hampshire, New Mexico, Oklahoma, Rhode Island, Tennessee, and Utah. See http://www.calib.com/nccanch/pubs/sag/manda.pdf.*

7 *Although it may seem redundant and illogical, many state statutes contain a provision requiring healthcare workers or professionals to report child abuse in addition to having a provision requiring "any" or "every" person to do so. Why this is so and how it originated is beyond the scope of this paper.*

8 *Other states from the thirteen that have an "any" or "every" person and healthcare worker requirement may fit into this category, but that is beyond the scope of this paper and not available from the chart cited above.*

9 *The chosen states were California, Florida, Illinois, Maryland, Massachusetts, New Jersey, New Mexico, New York, North Carolina, and Texas.*

10 *N.J. STAT. ANN. § 9:6-8.10 (West 2002).*

11 *FLA. STAT. ANN. §39.201(1) (b) (West 2003).*

12 *N.Y. SOC. SERV. LAW § 413(1) (McKinney 2003).*

13 *325 ILL. COMP. STAT. 5/4 (2001 & Supp. 2003); MASS. ANN. LAWS ch. 119, § 51A (Law. Co-op 2003).*

14 *CAL. PENAL CODE § 11165.7 (West 2003).*

15 *CAL. PENAL CODE § 11165.7(21) (West 2003).*

16 *MD. CODE ANN., FAM. LAW §§5-704-705 (2002).*

17 *N.M. STAT. ANN. § 32A-4-3(A) (Michie 2002).*

18 *TEX. FAM. CODE ANN. § 261.101 (Vernon 2002).*

19 *TEX. FAM. CODE ANN. § 261.101(a)-(b) (Vernon 2002).*

20 *See CAL. PENAL CODE § 11166(b) (West 2003); FLA. STAT. ANN. § 39.205 (West 2003); 325 ILL. COMP. STAT. 5/4 (2001 & Supp. 2003); N.M. STAT. ANN. § 32A-4-3(F) (Michie 2002); N.Y. SOC. SERV. LAW § 420 (McKinney 2003); TEX. FAM. CODE ANN. § 261.109 (Vernon 2002).*

21 *325 ILL. COMP. STAT. 5/4 (2001 & Supp. 2003).*

22 *MASS. ANN. LAWS ch. 119, § 51A (Law. Co-op 2003).*

23 *N.J. STAT. ANN. § 9:6-8.14 (West 2002). A disorderly persons offense is a petty offense and is not a crime. N.J. STAT. ANN. § 2C:1-4 (West 2003).*

24 *National Clearinghouse on Child Abuse and Neglect Information, Statutes At-a-Glance, Mandatory Reporters of Child Abuse and Neglect (Feb. 2002), available at http://www.calib.com/nccanch/pubs/sag/manda.pdf.*

Checklist:

What to look for in a state mandatory reporting statute:

- **Is there an "any person" requirement clause?**

  If yes, then all healthcare interpreters have a mandatory reporting duty, and you need not go any further.

  If no, check if another provision may apply to interpreters
- **Is there a healthcare worker, health personnel or hospital personnel requirement clause?**

  If yes, then look to see if a healthcare interpreter would fit within such a profession. If the terms are not defined within the clause, look for a definitions provision, usually in an earlier subsection of the statute or in cases decided by the courts in your state.
- **Is the interpreter considered a hospital "employee" or "personnel," as opposed to an independent contractor or an employee of an interpreter service?**

  If yes, the interpreter must report

  If no, check if another provision may apply to interpreters

  If no, check if another provision may apply to interpreters
- **Is the interpreter engaged in the activities covered by the statute – e.g. admission, examination, care or treatment of patients?**

  If yes, the interpreter must report

  If no, check if another provision may apply to interpreters
- Look for other relevant provisions:

  Is there punishment for non-reporting?

  Is there immunity for good faith reporting?

Notes

General Vocabulary

	VOCABULARY	TARGET
A	Abdomen	
	Abdominal cramps	
	Abdominal pain	
	Abnormalities	
	Abstinence model	
	Accutane	
	Ace wraps	venda elástica
	Acid	
	Acid indigestion	
	Acne	
	Active	
	Addiction	
	Adjustment disorders	trastorno de adaptación
	Admit (to)	
	Adolescents	
	Adults	
	Adverse drug reaction	
	Affective disorder	
	Agoraphobia	
	Air-conditioned	
	Alcohol consumption	
	Alcohol hand swabs	
	Alcohol withdrawal	
	Alcoholic	
	Alcoholism	
	Allergic reactions	
	Allergies	
	Allergist	
	Allergy clinic	
	Amenorrhea	
	Amniocentesis	
	Amputation	
	Anaphylaxis	
	Androgens	
	Anemia	
	Anesthesia	
	Aneurism	
	Angina	
	Angioplasty	
	Ankle	tobillo
	Anorexia nervosa	
	Anterior	
	Anterior wall	
	Antibiotics	
	Antibodies	
	Anti-depressant	
	Anti-inflammatory pills	
	Anti-malarial drug	
	Anti-nuclear antibody	
	Appear (to)	
	Appendectomy	
	Appendicitis	
	Appendix	
	Appetite	
	Arms	
	Arrange (to)	
	Arrythmia	
	Arteries	
	Arthritis	
	Arthrocentesis	
	Arthrography	
	Arthroscopic surgery	
	Arthroscopy	
	Asleep	
	Aspirin	
	Assure (to)	

General Vocabulary *(continued)*

VOCABULARY	TARGET
Asthma	
Asthma cancer	
At risk (to be)	
Attack	
Attention-deficit/ hyperactivity disorder	
Autistic disorder	
Autoimmune activity	
Autoimmune disorder	
B Bacteria	
Bad luck	
Balanitis	
Barely	
Barium enema test	
Barrel-shaped chest	
Barrier methods	
Baseline (a)	
Bath	
BCG vaccine Bacillus Calmette-Guérin	vacuna contra la tuberculosis
Beans	
Bear weight (to)	
Beating	
Become (to)	
Behavior	
Belly	
Bend (to)	
Bend down (to)	
Bend it back (to)	
Bend up (to)	
Bent over	
Benzoyl Peroxide	
Biliary tract	

VOCABULARY	TARGET
Binge eating disorder	
Biopsy	
Bipolar disorder	
Birth control	
Birth defects	
Bit too much (a)	
Bit touched (a)	
Bite (to)	
Blackout lapso memoria	desmayo pérdida conciencia
Bladder	vegiga
Bleeding	
Blindness	
Blisters	
Bloated	hinchado
Blockage	
Blood clot	
Blood in the stool	
Blood pressure	
Blood test	
Blood thinners	anticoagulante
Blood transfusions	
Blood work	
Bloodstream	torrente sanguíneo
Bloody phlegm	
Blurred vision	visión borrosa
Blurry	
Bodes well	
Bone cancer	
Bone scan	
Bony spurs	espolones
Booster	
Boot	
Bother (to)	

General Vocabulary *(continued)*

VOCABULARY	TARGET
Bowel	
Bowel habits	
Brace (a)	
Brain	
Brain edema	
Break up (to)	
Breakthrough bleeding	
Breast	
Breast cancer	
Breast tenderness	
Breathe (to)	
Breathing problems	
Breathlessness	
Bronchitis	
Bronchoscopy	
Bronchus	
Bruises	
Bruising	
Brunch	
Buckle (to)	
Bumps	golpes
Burning pain	
Burning sensation	
Bursitis	
Burst (to)	
Bushes	
Buttocks	nalgas
By mouth	
C CABG-Coronary artery	
bypass surgery	
Calf	
Calmer	

VOCABULARY	TARGET
Cane	
Canker sores	úlceras bucales
Cardiac enzyme	
Cardiologist	
Careful	
Carotids	
Carpenter's knee	
Carry (to)	
Cartilage	
Cast	
Casting	
Cataracts	
Catheter	
Catheterization	
Cauterization	
Ceiling	
Cells	
Cervical cap	capuchón cervical
Cervical mucous	
Cervical spinal film	
Cervicitis	
Cervix	
Cervix uterus	
Chamber	
Chart	
Check (to)	
Cheek	
Chemicals	
Chest	
Chest CT scan	
Chest pain	
Chest tightness	
Chest X-ray	

PO Box 2308, Woburn, MA 01888-0508, **p:** 781-729-3736, **www.EmbracingCulture.com**
PO Box 6401, Manchester, NH 03108, **p:** 1-888-678-CCCS

General Vocabulary *(continued)*

VOCABULARY	TARGET
Chicken pox	varicela
Chief concern	
Childbearing	
Childhood	
Children	
Children's Panadol (Tylenol)	
Chills	
Chin	
Chlamydia	
Choices	
Cholera	
Chronic sore	
Circulation	
Circumcision	
Climb (to)	
Close off (to)	
Closed reduction of fractures	
Clot	
Clubbing hipocratismo digital	dedos en palillo de tambor
Cold	
Cold sores	
Cold symptoms	
Colon	
Colon cancer	
Colonoscopy	
Colposcopy	
Coma	
Common procedure	
Communicable tuberculosis	
Complain (to)	
Compound fracture	
Concussions	
Condom	

VOCABULARY	TARGET
Congestive heart failure	
Conjunctivitis	
Consent form	
Constipation	estreñimiento
Contagious	
Contributing	
Control (to)	
Contusions	
Coolness	
Cosmetics	
Cotton swab	
Cough	
Coughing up	
Coumadin	
Counselors	
Court stenographer	
Covering	
Crabby	malhumorado hosco
Crabs (pubic lice)	
Crackles	
Cramp	
Craziness	
Croup	
Crushing pain	
Crutches	
Cryptorchism/ Cryptorchidism	
CT Scan	
Culture	
Cut (to)	
Cut back on something (to)	
Cute	

General Vocabulary *(continued)*

VOCABULARY	TARGET
CVA (Cerebrovascular Accident)	
CXR (Chest x-Ray)	
D.P.T vaccine	tos ferina ← Difteria Pertussis Tetanus
Dangerous	
Dawn	
Daytime	
Deafness	
Death	
Decongestants	
Decreased	
Deep breath	
Deep venous structures	
DEET	
Defect	
Deformed	
Delicacy	
Delirium	
Delirium tremens	
Delusions	
Dementia	
Department of Public Health	
Depression	
DES	
Describe (to)	
Detox (to)	
Detoxification	
Diabetes	
Diabetic keto-acidosis	
Diaper rash	
Diaphragm	
Diarrhea	

VOCABULARY	TARGET
Diet	
Dietary suggestions	
Difficulty breathing	
Digest (to)	
Dinner	
Diphtheria	
Disability	
Disability insurance	
Discharge (a)	
Disease	
Disease-carrying organisms	
Disinfect (to)	
Displaced (to be)	
Dissociative disorders	
Distal end of the fibula	
Distal radial bone	
Distal ulna	
Distal wrist dysfunction	
Dizziness	
Dizzy	
Dodge a bullet (to)	
Dollies	
Doppler ultrasound	
Dormant	
Dose	
Draw (to)	
DRE	
Dressing	
Droplets	
Dropping	
Drops	
Drowsiness	
Drug store	

PO Box 2308, Woburn, MA 01888-0508, **p:** 781-729-3736, **www.EmbracingCulture.com**
PO Box 6401, Manchester, NH 03108, **p:** 1-888-678-CCCS

General Vocabulary *(continued)*

VOCABULARY	TARGET
DT	
DTaP	
Dusk	
Dust diseases	
Dye	
Dyskinesia	
Dyslexia	
Dysmenorrheal	
Dysphasia	
E Ear	
Ear congestion	
Earache	
Ease the pain (to)	
Eating disorders	
EC emergency contraception	
Echocardiogram	
Ectopic Pregnancy	
Edema	
Effective	
Effusion	
EKG (Electrocardiogram)	
Elastic bandage	
Electrocardiogram	
Elevated	
Emphysema	
Endocarditis	
Endometriosis	
Endometritis	
Endoscopy	
Endotracheal intubation	
Endurance	
Enlarged	

VOCABULARY	TARGET
Enroll (to)	
Epidural	
EpiPen	
Episodes	
Epithelial tissue	
ER	
Esophageal reflux	
Esophagus	
Estrogen	
Euphoria	
Examine (to)	
Exercise	
Exercise-induced asthma	
Exert (to)	
Exposed	
Exposure	
Extend (to)	
F Face	
Faintness	
Fallopian tubes	
Family planning counselor	
Family therapist	
Family's health history	
Fat	
Fatal	
Fatigue	
Fatty foods	
Feeling ill	
Femur	
Fever	
Fiber optic tube	
Fibroids	

General Vocabulary *(continued)*

VOCABULARY	TARGET
Fingers	
Flat cells	
Flex (to)	
Flu	
Flu shot	
Fluids	
Flu-like illness	
Flying insects	
FOBT-fecal occult blood test	
Follicles	
Follow (to)	
Follow up	
Food poisoning	
Food pyramid	
Foreign-born	
Fractured (to be)	
Fractures	
Frostbite	
Full blown disease	
G Gain (to)	
Gall bladder	
Gall bladder surgery	
Gallstones	
Gargle (to)	
Gastritis	
Gastrointestinal tract	
Gel	
General anesthesia	
Genes	
Genital herpes	
German measles	

VOCABULARY	TARGET
Germs	
Gestational Diabetes	
Get better (to)	
Get worse (to)	
GI specialist	
Give way (to)	
Glands	
Glaucoma	
Gloves	
Glucose	
Godmother	
Gonorrhea	
Good-sized	
Gout	
Gowns	
Grab (to)	
Grabbing	
Gray	
Greasy foods	
Green	
Groin	
Gross	
Group therapy	
Grow a thick skin (to)	
Growth (a)	
Gut	
Gynecological exam	
H Halfway houses	
Hallucinations	
Hand tremors	
Harm	
Hay fever	

PO Box 2308, Woburn, MA 01888-0508, **p:** 781-729-3736, **www.EmbracingCulture.com**
PO Box 6401, Manchester, NH 03108, **p:** 1-888-678-CCCS

General Vocabulary *(continued)*

VOCABULARY	TARGET
Headache	
Health insurance	
Health proxy	
Heart	
Heart attack	
Heart defects	
Heart disease	
Heart failure	
Heart muscle	
Heart problems	
Heart rate	
Heart's arteries	
Heartburn	
Hematoma	
Hemoccult cards	
Hemoccults	
Hemoptysis	
Hemorrhoids	
Hepatitis A vaccine series	
Hepatitis B vaccine series	
Hereditary tendency	
Heredity	
Heroin	
Herpes progenitalis	
Herpes zoster	
Hide-and-seek	
High blood pressure	
High school age	
Hip	
HIV positive	
Hives	
Hoarse	
Hoarseness	

VOCABULARY	TARGET
Hole	
Hormonal changes	
Hormonal methods	
Hormone	
Hospitalized	
Hot	
Housekeeper's knee	
HPV (Human Papilloma Virus)	
HPV vaccine series	
HSV	
Huge	
Human being	
Human body	
Hungry	
Hurt	
Hyper	
Hypersensitivity tests	
Hypertension	
Hyrodrocholorthiazide	
Hystagmus	
Hysterectomy	
I	
Ice packs	
Ice the knee (to)	
Icing	
Illness	
Immune system	
Immunity	
Immunization history	
Immunizations	
Immunizing agent	
Impact (to)	

General Vocabulary *(continued)*

VOCABULARY	TARGET
Impotence	
Improve (to)	
In between pregnancies	
Incontinence	
Infant	
Infantile paralysis	
Infected	
Infection	
Infectious disease	
Inferior pubic ramus	
Infertile	
Inflamed	
Inflammation	
Influenza vaccine	
Informed consent form	
Inhaler	
Inject (to)	
Injection site	
Injections	
Injury	
INR	
Insect repellent	
Insert (to)	
Insomnia	
Insulin	
Insulin drip	
Insurance	
Intercourse	
Interstitial disease	
Intoxication	
Intra-uterine device	
Invade (to)	

VOCABULARY	TARGET
IPV (Inactivated Polio Vaccine)	
Irreversible	
Isolate (to)	
Isolated	
Itching	
IV	
IV drip	
IV Morphine	
J Jaundice	
Jaw	
Johnny	
Joints	
Jungle disease	
K Keep (to)	
Kid	
Kidney disease	
Kidney failure	
Kidney function	
Kidney stones	
Kidneys	
Knee	
Kneeling	
Known function	
Knuckles	
L Labored breathing	
Laminectomy	
Laparoscope	
Large	
Laryngitis	
Laryngoscopy	

PO Box 2308, Woburn, MA 01888-0508, **p:** 781-729-3736, **www.EmbracingCulture.com**
PO Box 6401, Manchester, NH 03108, **p:** 1-888-678-CCCS

General Vocabulary *(continued)*

VOCABULARY	TARGET
Latent	
Lateral malleolus	
Lead (to)	
Learning disorder	
Left upper long	
Leg pain	
Lenses	
Let go (to)	
Lift (to)	
Ligaments	
Limbs	
Lime disease	
Limp (to)	
Lips	
Liver	
Liver cells	
Liver damage	
Lobe	
Long- lasting	
Long pants	
Long term	
Lose (to)	
Lose consciousness (to)	
Lotion	
Lovenox	
Low grade fever	
Lower right side	
Lump	
Lunch	
Lung cancer	
Lung carcinoma	
Lungs	
Lymph nodes	

M

VOCABULARY	TARGET
Make me better (to)	
Make up	
Malaria	
Malaria risk area	
Malaria-infected mosquito	
Malarone	
Males	
Malignant squamous cells	
Mammogram	
Mammography	
Manage the pain (to)	
Mania	
Masks	
Massage therapy	
Maternal grandfather	
MD	
Meals	
Measles	
Measles-Mumps-Rubella (MMR) vaccine series	
Measure (to)	
Medial joint line	
Medial meniscus	
Medical attention	
Medical Directive	
Medical history	
Medical records	
Medication	
Medicine	
Memory impairment	
Meningococcal vaccine	
Menorrhagia	
Menstrual cramps	

General Vocabulary *(continued)*

VOCABULARY	TARGET
Menstrual cycle	
Menstrual flow	
Mental health	
Mental retardation	
Mesh	
Metamucil	
Micro tools	
Mild	
Mild small airway disease	
Miracle drug (a)	
Miscarriage	
Mist humidifier	
MMR vaccine	
Monilial vagintis	
Monkey business	
Mononucleosis	
Mood changes	
Mosquito bed net	
Mosquitoes	
Mouth	
Move my bowels (to)	
MRI	
Mucus	
Mumps	
Muscle	
Muscle ache	
Myelography	
Myocardial infarction	
Myocarditis	
Myomectomy	
N Nail	
Napping	

VOCABULARY	TARGET
Narcotic	
Narcotic pain medicine	
Nasal congestion	
Nasty bite	
Nationwide	
Nausea	
Nausea vomiting	
Nauseated	
Navel	
Neck	
Neck film	
Nerve	
Nervous system	
Neuropraxia	
Neurological exam	
Neutralize (to)	
Night owl (a)	
Nitroglycerin	
Nodule	
Non-invasive tests	
Non-smoking programs	
Non-steroidal anti-inflammatory medicine	
Non-steroidals	
Normal pregnancies	
Numb	
Numbness	
Nurse practitioner	
Nutrition	
O Oatmeal	
Oatmeal bath	
Obsessive-compulsive disorder	

PO Box 2308, Woburn, MA 01888-0508, **p:** 781-729-3736, **www.EmbracingCulture.com**
PO Box 6401, Manchester, NH 03108, **p:** 1-888-678-CCCS

General Vocabulary *(continued)*

VOCABULARY	TARGET
Obstructing clot	
Occupational therapy	
Odd	
Oil	
Ointment	
Older children	
Once in a while	
Open reduction of fractures	
Open-heart surgery	
Open-heart surgical repair	
Operating room	
OPV (Oral Polio Vaccine)	
Oral sex	
Orchidectomy	
Orchiopexy	
Orchitis	
Organ	
Ortho clinic	
Orthopedic doctor	
Orthopedic physician's assistant	
Osteoarthritis	
Osteomalacia	
Osteoporosis	
Outbreak	
Outcome	
Outpatient clinic	
Ovarian cancer	
Ovaries	
Ovary	
Overdose	
Over-the-counter medications	
Ovulation	

VOCABULARY	TARGET
Oxygen	
P	
Paget's disease	
Pain	
Pain in the limbs	
Pain killers	
Painful	
Painful joints	
Pale	
Paleness	
Palpitation	
Panadol	
Panic disorder	
Pap smear	
Paralysis	
Paralyzed	
Paraphimosis	
Parasite	
Park bench	
Parotid salivary glands	
Pass it along (to)	
Passing out	
Passive	
Patch	
Patella	
Paternal grandmother	
Peak flow	
Pelvic bone	
Pelvic exam	
Pelvic inflammatory disease	
Pelvic rami fracture	
Pelvicultrasopography	
Pelvis	

General Vocabulary *(continued)*

VOCABULARY	TARGET
Penis	
Pepto Bismol	
Periods	
Peritoneal inflammation	
Peritonitis	
Pertussis	
PFTS-Pulmonary Function Tests	
Pharyngitis	
Phimotic foreskin	
Phlegm	
Phobia	
Physical	
Physical therapist	
Physical therapy	
Pill	
Pimples	
Pinch (to)	
Pinching	
Pit of the stomach	
Placebo pill	
Placement	
Plain films	
Plasmodium	
Plasmodium species	
Playground	
Plugged oil ducts	
PMS	
Pneumococcal polysaccharide (PPV) vaccine	
Pneumonectomy	
Pneumonia	
Pneumothorax	
Polio	

VOCABULARY	TARGET
Polio vaccine	
Polio vaccine series	
Poliomyelitis	
Polydrug use	
Polyps	
Pop out (to)	
Pork	
Portions	
Position	
Positive reaction	
Post-traumatic disorder	
Potassium	
Pound	
Pounding heartbeat	
PPD skin test	
PPD test	
Precautionary measure	
Pregnancy	
Pregnancy test	
Preoperative evaluation	
Pre-patellar bursitis	
Prescription	
Prescription drug	
Press (to)	
Pressure	
Pressure pain	
Pressure system	
Pretty good	
Pretty healthy	
Prevent (to)	
Primary care doctor	
Primary Care Physician	
Procedure	

PO Box 2308, Woburn, MA 01888-0508, **p:** 781-729-3736, **www.EmbracingCulture.com**
PO Box 6401, Manchester, NH 03108, **p:** 1-888-678-CCCS

General Vocabulary *(continued)*

VOCABULARY	TARGET
Produce (to)	
Progestin	
Prostate	
Prostatectomy	
Prostatic carcinoma	
Prostatitis	
Protected intercourse	
Protective clothes	
Protective gear	
Proteins	
Psychiatric problems	
Puberty	
Public health	
Public health issue	
Puffs	
Pull (to)	
Pull them apart (to)	
Pulmonary angiography	
Pulmonary embolism	
Pulmonary fibrosis	
Pulse	
Pump (to)	
Pumping fully	
Push away (to)	
Push it down (to)	
Put off (to)	
Put out (to)	
Q	
Q-tip	
R	
Rabies	
Rabies immune globulin	
Radiologist	

VOCABULARY	TARGET
Ragweed	
Rales	
Rash	
Rate	
Realize (to)	
Reasonable	
Rebound type	
Re-check	
Recovery room	
Rectum	
Recuperate (to)	
Red blood	
Red blood cells	
Red blotches	
Red spots	
Redness	
Referral	
Refill (a)	
Reflexes	
Regular	
Rehab	
Relapse	
Release (to)	
Relieved (to be)	
Religious beliefs	
Rely (to)	
Remedies	
Remission	
Repeat EKG	
Resolve (to)	
Rest (to)	
Rheumatoid arthritis	
Rheumatoid factor	

General Vocabulary *(continued)*

VOCABULARY	TARGET
Rhythm method	
Rib cage	
Rice	
Right flank	
Right upper quadrant	
Ringing in the ears	
Rise (to)	
Risk area	
Rubbing sensation	
Rubella	
Run test (to)	
Running a fever	
Runny nose	
Runny poops	
Rupture	
Rusty	
S	
Safety	
Salad	
Saliva	
Salivary glands	
Salpingectomy	
Sample	
SARS (Severe Acute Respiratory Syndrome)	
Scale	
Scar	
Scarred	
Schizophrenia	
Scratch (to)	
Scratchy throat	
Screened	
Screening	

VOCABULARY	TARGET
Screening test	
Sedative	
Seizures	
Self-esteem	
Self-medication	
Semen analysis	
Sequestrectomy	
Severe	
Severe illnesses	
Sexual abstinence	
Sexual intercourse	
Sexually transmitted diseases	
Shaking chills	
Shaky	
Sharp pain	
Shift	
Shingles	
Shock	
Shortness of breath	
Shot area	
Shots	
Shoulder	
Shrug (to)	
Siblings	
Sick time	
Sickness	
Side effects	
Sigmoidoscopy	
Sign	
Significant illnesses	
Sinusitis	
Skin eruptions	
Skin rash	

PO Box 2308, Woburn, MA 01888-0508, **p:** 781-729-3736, **www.EmbracingCulture.com**
PO Box 6401, Manchester, NH 03108, **p:** 1-888-678-CCCS

General Vocabulary *(continued)*

VOCABULARY	TARGET
Skin test	
Skunk	
Sleeping pill	
Sleeves	
Slide	
Slight	
Slightly	
Slow	
Slurred speech	
Sneeze (to)	
Snort (to)	
SOB	
Social worker	
Solids	
Soothing	
Sore	
Sore arm	
Sore throat	
Soreness	
Soreness of the skin	
Sores	
Sound (to)	
Speculum	
Speech	
Speedy recovery	
Sperm	
Sperm count	
Spermicide	
Spinal tap	
Spine	
Spiral CAT Scan	
Spirometer	
Spirometry	

VOCABULARY	TARGET
Spit (to)	
Spitting up	
Spleen	
Splint	
Splinting	
Spores	
Spotting	
Sprains	
Spray	
Spread (to)	
Sputum	
Sputum test	
Squeeze (to)	
Stamina	
Starving	
Stent	
Step on (to)	
Stew	
Stick (to)	
Stick to it (to)	
Stiff neck	
Stiffness	
Stiffness in the neck	
Still	
Stimulant	
Sting (to)	
Stinging	
Stirrups	
Stomach	
Stomatitis	
Stones	
Stool card	
Stool sample	

General Vocabulary *(continued)*

VOCABULARY	TARGET
Stools	
Straighten (to)	
Strain (to)	
Strength	
Strep	
Strep throat	
Streptococcus	
Stretcher	
Stroke	
Stuffy	
Stuffy nose	
Stupor	
Sub acute rehabilitation center	
Subcutaneous nodules	
Substance abuse	
Substance dependency	
Substance use	
Substitute	
Sudafed	
Suicidal behavior	
Suicide	
Summersault	
Support stockings	
Surgeon	
Surgery	
Surgical mask	
Surgical resection	
Surgicenter	
Swab (to)	
Swallowing	
Swamps	
Sweat (to)	
Sweating	

VOCABULARY	TARGET
Sweats	
Sweaty	
Swell (to)	
Swelling	
Swollen	
Swollen patches	
Symptoms	
Syphilis	
T Take the edge off (to)	
Taking a breath	
Tarry	
TB infection	
TB skin test	
TB test	
TB vaccine	
Td	
Tdap	
Teary eyes	
Teenage girl	
Temperature	
Tempra	
Tender	
Tenderness	
Tendinitis	
Test	
Testicles	
Testicular carcinoma	
Tetanus	
Tetanus shots	
Thalidomide	
The pill	
The runs	

PO Box 2308, Woburn, MA 01888-0508, **p:** 781-729-3736, **www.EmbracingCulture.com**
PO Box 6401, Manchester, NH 03108, **p:** 1-888-678-CCCS

General Vocabulary *(continued)*

VOCABULARY	TARGET
Thermometer	
Thick	
Thin (to)	
Third wheel (a)	
Thoracic surgeon	
Thoracotomy	
Throat	
Thyroid	
Thyroid disease	
Tibia	
Tick	
Tightness in the chest	
Tilt (to)	
Tingling	
Tiny	
Tips	
Tiredness	
Toes	
Tolerance	
Tolerated	
Tongue	
Tonsillitis	
Torn (to)	
Touch (to)	
Tough	
Toward	
Tox screen	
Toxins	
Tracheostomy	
Traction	
Transaminases	
Transesophageal	
Transesophageal echo	

VOCABULARY	TARGET
Transient ischemic attack	
Traumatic brain injury	
Traumatized	
Travel (to)	
Treated	
Tretinoin	
Trichomoniasis	
Trigger (to)	
Tropical climate	
Troponin	
Trunk	
TSH	
Tubal ligation	
Tuberculin test	
Tuberculosis	
Tummy	
TURP	
Twice a day	
Twist (to)	
Tylenol	
U Ulcer	
Ultimately	
Ultrasound	
Uncommon	
Uncoordinated	
Unsteady gait	
Unusual headaches	
Upper arm	
Upper eyelid	
Upset stomach	
Urethritis	
Urinary tract infection	

General Vocabulary *(continued)*

	VOCABULARY	TARGET
	Urinating	
	Urine sample	
	Urine tests	
	Urologist	
	Uterine lining	
	Uterus	
V	Vaccines	
	Vaginal Candidiasis (yeast infection)	
	Vaginal ring	
	Vaginitis	
	Vaporizer	
	Varicella (chickenpox) vaccine series	
	Vasectomy	
	Venereal disease	
	Ventricule	
	Via	
	Viral hepatitis	
	Viral infection	
	Virus	
	Vital signs	
	Vitamin deficiency	
	Vitamins	
	Vomiting	
	Vulnerable	
W	Wake me up (to)	
	Walker (a)	
	Walk-in patient	
	Walking cast	
	Warm	

	VOCABULARY	TARGET
	Warm soaks	
	Watchful	
	Watery diarrhea	
	Weak	
	Weather	
	Weigh the pros and cons (to)	
	Weight	
	Weight gain	
	Wheeze	
	Wheezing	
	White blood cells	
	Whooping cough	
	Widely used	
	Wiernicke's encephalopathy	
	Wiggle one's toes (to)	
	Withdrawal	
	Womb	
	Wooden spatula	
	Workman's compensation	
	Worse	
	Wound	
	Wrist	
X	X-rays	
Y	Yeast	
	Yikes	
	You're in luck	
	Young adult	
	Yucky	
Z	Zantac	

PO Box 2308, Woburn, MA 01888-0508, **p:** 781-729-3736, **www.EmbracingCulture.com**
PO Box 6401, Manchester, NH 03108, **p:** 1-888-678-CCCS

Body Parts/Organs Vocabulary

	VOCABULARY	TARGET
A	Abdomen	
	Ankle	
	Antibodies	
	Appendix	
	Arms	
	Arteries	
B	Belly	
	Biliary tract	
	Bladder	
	Bloodstream	
	Bowel	
	Brain	
	Breast	
	Bronchus	
	Buttocks	
C	Calf	
	Cardiac enzyme	
	Carotids	
	Cartilage	
	Cervical mucous	
	Cervix	
	Cervix uterus	
	Cheek	
	Chest	
	Chin	
	Circulation	
	Colon	
D	Deep venous structures	
	Diaphragm	
	Distal end of the fibula	

	VOCABULARY	TARGET
	Distal radial bone	
	Distal ulna	
E	Ear	
	Epithelial tissue	
	Esophagus	
	Estrogen	
F	Face	
	Fallopian tubes	
	Femur	
	Fingers	
	Flat cells	
	Follicles	
G	Gall bladder	
	Gastrointestinal tract	
	Genes	
	Glands	
	Glucose	
	Groin	
	Gut	
H	Heart	
	Heart muscle	
	Heart's arteries	
	Hip	
	Hormonal changes	
	Hormone	
I	Immune system	
	Inferior pubic ramus	

Body Parts/Organs Vocabulary *(continued)*

	VOCABULARY	TARGET
J	Jaw	
	Joints	
K	Kidneys	
	Knee	
	Knuckles	
L	Lateral malleolus	
	Left upper long	
	Lenses	
	Ligaments	
	Limbs	
	Lips	
	Liver	
	Liver cells	
	Lobe	
	Lungs	
M	Medial joint line	
	Medial meniscus	
	Menstrual cycle	
	Menstrual flow	
	Mouth	
	Muscle	
N	Nail	
	Navel	
	Neck	
	Nerve	
	Nervous system	
O	Organ	
	Ovaries	

	VOCABULARY	TARGET
	Ovary	
	Ovulation	
P	Parotid salivary glands	
	Patella	
	Pelvic bone	
	Pelvis	
	Penis	
	Periods	
	Pit of the stomach	
	Prostate	
R	Rectum	
	Red blood	
	Red blood cells	
	Rib cage	
S	Saliva	
	Salivary glands	
	Shoulder	
	Sperm	
	Spine	
	Spleen	
	Stirrups	
	Stomach	
	Stools	
T	Testicles	
	Throat	
	Thyroid	
	Tibia	
	Toes	
	Tongue	

PO Box 2308, Woburn, MA 01888-0508, **p:** 781-729-3736, **www.EmbracingCulture.com**
PO Box 6401, Manchester, NH 03108, **p:** 1-888-678-CCCS

Body Parts/Organs Vocabulary *(continued)*

	VOCABULARY	TARGET
T	Tummy	
U	Upper arm	
	Upper eyelid	
	Uterine lining	
	Uterus	

	VOCABULARY	TARGET
V	Ventricule	
W	White blood cells	
	Womb	
	Wrist	

Pathology/Symptoms/Conditions Vocabulary

	VOCABULARY	TARGET
A	Abdominal cramps	
	Abdominal pain	
	Acid indigestion	
	Acne	
	Addiction	
	Adjustment disorders	
	Affective disorder	
	Agoraphobia	
	Alcohol withdrawal	
	Alcoholism	
	Allergic reactions	
	Allergies	
	Amenorrhea	
	Anaphylaxis	
	Anemia	
	Aneurism	
	Angina	
	Anorexia nervosa	
	Appendicitis	
	Arrythmia	
	Arthritis	
	Asthma	

	VOCABULARY	TARGET
	Asthma cancer	
	Attack	
	Attention-deficit/	
	hyperactivity disorder	
	Autistic disorder	
	Autoimmune disorder	
B	Balanitis	
	Barrel-shaped chest	
	Binge eating disorder	
	Bipolar disorder	
	Birth defects	
	Blackout	
	Bleeding	
	Blindness	
	Blisters	
	Bloated	
	Blockage	
	Blood clot	
	Blood in the stool	
	Blood pressure	
	Bloody phlegm	
	Blurred vision	

Pathology/Symptoms/Conditions Vocabulary *(continued)*

VOCABULARY	TARGET
Bone cancer	
Bony spurs	
Brain edema	
Breakthrough bleeding	
Breast cancer	
Breast tenderness	
Breathing problems	
Breathlessness	
Bronchitis	
Bruises	
Bruising	
Bumps	
Burning pain	
Burning sensation	
Bursitis	
C Canker sores	
Carpenter's knee	
Cataracts	
Cells	
Cervicitis	
Chest pain	
Chest tightness	
Chicken pox	
Chills	
Chlamydia	
Cholera	
Chronic sore	
Clot	
Clubbing	
Cold	
Cold sores	
Cold symptoms	

VOCABULARY	TARGET
Colon cancer	
Coma	
Communicable tuberculosis	
Compound fracture	
Concussions	
Congestive heart failure	
Conjunctivitis	
Constipation	
Contusions	
Coolness	
Cough	
Coughing up	
Crabs (pubic lice)	
Crackles	
Cramp	
Craziness	
Croup	
Crushing pain	
Cryptorchism/Cryptorchidism	
CVA (Cerebrovascular Accident)	
D Deafness	
Defect	
Deformed	
Delirium	
Delirium tremens	
Delusions	
Dementia	
Depression	
Diabetes	
Diabetic keto-acidosis	
Diaper rash	

PO Box 2308, Woburn, MA 01888-0508, **p:** 781-729-3736, **www.EmbracingCulture.com**
PO Box 6401, Manchester, NH 03108, **p:** 1-888-678-CCCS

Pathology/Symptoms/Conditions Vocabulary *(continued)*

VOCABULARY	TARGET
Diarrhea	
Difficulty breathing	
Diphtheria	
Disability	
Displaced (to be)	
Dissociative disorders	
Distal wrist dysfunction	
Dizziness	
Dizzy	
Drowsiness	
DT	
Dust diseases	
Dyskinesia	
Dyslexia	
Dysmenorrheal	
Dysphasia	
E Ear congestion	
Earache	
Eating disorders	
Ectopic Pregnancy	
Edema	
Effusion	
Emphysema	
Endocarditis	
Endometriosis	
Endometritis	
Episodes	
Esophageal reflux	
Euphoria	
Exercise-induced asthma	
F Faintness	

VOCABULARY	TARGET
Fatigue	
Feeling ill	
Fever	
Fibroids	
Flu	
Flu-like illness	
FOBT-fecal occult blood test	
Food poisoning	
Fractured (to be)	
Fractures	
Frostbite	
G Gallstones	
Gastritis	
Genital herpes	
German measles	
Germs	
Gestational Diabetes	
Glaucoma	
Gonorrhea	
Gout	
Growth (a)	
H Hallucinations	
Hand tremors	
Hay fever	
Headache	
Heart attack	
Heart defects	
Heart disease	
Heart failure	
Heart problems	
Heartburn	

Pathology/Symptoms/Conditions Vocabulary *(continued)*

	VOCABULARY	TARGET
	Hematoma	
	Hemoptysis	
	Hemorrhoids	
	Herpes progenitalis	
	Herpes zoster	
	High blood pressure	
	HIV positive	
	Hives	
	Hoarse	
	Hoarseness	
	Housekeeper's knee	
	HPV (Human Papilloma Virus)	
	HSV	
	Hypertension	
	Hystagmus	
I	Impotence	
	Incontinence	
	Infantile paralysis	
	Infertile	
	Inflamed	
	Inflammation	
	Insomnia	
	Interstitial disease	
	Intoxication	
	Itching	
J	Jaundice	
	Jungle disease	
K	Kidney disease	
	Kidney failure	
	Kidney stones	

	VOCABULARY	TARGET
L	Laryngitis	
	Learning disorder	
	Leg pain	
	Lime disease	
	Liver damage	
	Lose consciousness (to)	
	Low grade fever	
	Lump	
	Lung cancer	
	Lung carcinoma	
	Lymph nodes	
M	Malaria	
	Malignant squamous cells	
	Mania	
	Measles	
	Measles-Mumps-Rubella (MMR) vaccine series	
	Memory impairment	
	Menorrhagia	
	Menstrual cramps	
	Mental retardation	
	Mesh	
	Mild small airway disease	
	Miscarriage	
	Monilial vagintis	
	Mononucleosis	
	Mood changes	
	Mucus	
	Mumps	
	Muscle ache	
	Myocardial infarction	
	Myocarditis	

O Box 2308, Woburn, MA 01888-0508, **p:** 781-729-3736, **www.EmbracingCulture.com**
O Box 6401, Manchester, NH 03108, **p:** 1-888-678-CCCS

Pathology/Symptoms/Conditions Vocabulary *(continued)*

	VOCABULARY	TARGET
N	Nasal congestion	
	Nausea	
	Nausea vomiting	
	Nauseated	
	Neuropraxia	
	Nodule	
	Numb	
	Numbness	
O	Obsessive-compulsive disorder	
	Obstructing clot	
	Orchitis	
	Osteoarthritis	
	Osteomalacia	
	Osteoporosis	
	Ovarian cancer	
P	Paget's disease	
	Pain	
	Pain in the limbs	
	Painful	
	Painful joints	
	Pale	
	Paleness	
	Palpitation	
	Panic disorder	
	Paralysis	
	Paraphimosis	
	Parasite	
	Passing out	
	Pelvic inflammatory disease	
	Pelvic rami fracture	

	VOCABULARY	TARGET
	Peritoneal inflammation	
	Peritonitis	
	Pertussis	
	Pharyngitis	
	Phimotic foreskin	
	Phlegm	
	Phobia	
	Pimples	
	Plugged oil ducts	
	PMS	
	Pneumonia	
	Polio	
	Poliomyelitis	
	Polyps	
	Post-traumatic disorder	
	Pounding heartbeat	
	Pregnancy	
	Pre-patellar bursitis	
	Pressure pain	
	Prostatic carcinoma	
	Prostatitis	
	Psychiatric problems	
	Pulmonary embolism	
	Pulmonary fibrosis	
R	Rabies	
	Rash	
	Red spots	
	Redness	
	Rheumatoid arthritis	
	Ringing in the ears	
	Rubbing sensation	
	Rubella	
	Running a fever	

Pathology/Symptoms/Conditions Vocabulary *(continued)*

VOCABULARY	TARGET
Runny nose	
Runny poops	
Rupture	
S SARS Severe Acute Respiratory Syndrome	
Schizophrenia	
Scratchy throat	
Seizures	
Sexually transmitted diseases	
Shaking chills	
Shaky	
Sharp pain	
Shingles	
Sinusitis	
Skin eruptions	
Skin rash	
Slurred speech	
Sneeze (to)	
Snort (to)	
SOB	
Sore arm	
Sore throat	
Soreness	
Soreness of the skin	
Sores	
Stiff neck	
Stiffness	
Stiffness in the neck	
Stomatitis	
Stones	
Strain (to)	
Strep	

VOCABULARY	TARGET
Strep throat	
Streptococcus	
Stroke	
Stuffy	
Stuffy nose	
Stupor	
Subcutaneous nodules	
Substance abuse	
Substance dependency	
Substance use	
Suicidal behavior	
Syphilis	
T TB infection	
Teary eyes	
Temperature	
Tender	
Tenderness	
Tendinitis	
Testicular carcinoma	
Tetanus	
Thyroid disease	
Tightness in the chest	
Tingling	
Tiredness	
Tonsillitis	
Transient ischemic attack	
Traumatic brain injury	
Traumatized	
Trichomoniasis	
Tuberculosis	
U Ulcer	
Unsteady gait	

O Box 2308, Woburn, MA 01888-0508, **p:** 781-729-3736, **www.EmbracingCulture.com**
O Box 6401, Manchester, NH 03108, **p:** 1-888-678-CCCS

Pathology/Symptoms/Conditions Vocabulary *(continued)*

	VOCABULARY	TARGET
	Unusual headaches	
	Upset stomach	
	Urethritis	
	Urinary tract infection	
V	Vaginal Candidiasis (yeast infection)	
	Vaginal ring	
	Vaginitis	
	Varicella (chickenpox) vaccine series	
	Venereal disease	
	Viral hepatitis	
	Viral infection	
	Vitamin deficiency	
	Vomiting	
W	Watery diarrhea	
	Wheeze	
	Wheezing	
	Whooping cough	
	Wiernicke's encephalopathy	
	Withdrawal	
Y	Yeast	

Laboratory Tests and Diagnostic Procedures Vocabulary

	VOCABULARY	TARGET
A	Amniocentesis	
	Anti-nuclear antibody	
	Arthrography	
	Arthroscopy	
B	Barium enema test	
	Biopsy	
	Blood test	
	Blood work	
	Bone scan	
	Bronchoscopy	
C	Cervical spinal film	
	Chest CT scan	
	Chest X-ray	
	Colonoscopy	
	Colposcopy	
	CT Scan	
	Culture	
	CXR (Chest x-Ray)	
D	Doppler ultrasound	
E	Echocardiogram	
	EKG	
	EKG (Electrocardiogram)	
	Electrocardiogram	
	Endoscopy	
F	Fiber optic tube	
G	Gynecological exam	

Laboratory Tests and Diagnostic Procedures Vocabulary *(continued)*

	VOCABULARY	TARGET
H	Hemoccults	
	Hemoccult cards	
	Hypersensitivity tests	
I	INR	
L	Laryngoscopy	
M	Mammogram	
	Mammography	
	MRI	
	Myelography	
N	Neck film	
	Non-invasive tests	
	Neurological exam	
P	Pap smear	
	Peak flow	
	Pelvicultrasopography	
	Pelvic exam	
	PFTS-Pulmonary Function Tests	
	Physical	
	PPD skin test	
	PPD test	
	Pregnancy test	
	Preoperative evaluation	
	Pulmonary angiography	
R	Repeat EKG	

	VOCABULARY	TARGET
S	Screening test	
	Semen analysis	
	Sigmoidoscopy	
	Skin test	
	Sperm count	
	Spinal tap	
	Spiral CAT Scan	
	Spirometer	
	Spirometry	
	Sputum test	
	Stool card	
	Stool sample	
T	Troponin	
	Tox screen	
	TB skin test	
	TB test	
	Test	
	Transesophageal echo	
	Tuberculin test	
U	Ultrasound	
	Urine tests	
X	X-rays	

PO Box 2308, Woburn, MA 01888-0508, **p:** 781-729-3736, **www.EmbracingCulture.com**
PO Box 6401, Manchester, NH 03108, **p:** 1-888-678-CCCS

Idiomatic Expressions Vocabulary

	VOCABULARY	TARGET
B	Bit too much (a)	
	Bit touched (a)	
	Bodes well	
C	Crabby	
D	Dodge a bullet (to)	
G	Grow a thick skin (to)	
M	Monkey business	
	Move my vowels (to)	
N	Night owl (a)	
T	Take the edge off (to)	
	The runs	
	Third wheel (a)	
W	Weigh the pros and cons (to)	
Y	You're in luck	

Treatment Procedures Vocabulary

	VOCABULARY	TARGET
A	Amputation	
	Angioplasty	
	Appendectomy	
	Arthrocentesis	
	Arthroscopic surgery	
B	Blood transfusions	
	Boot	
	Brace (a)	
C	CABG-Coronary artery bypass surgery	
	Cast	
	Catheterization	
	Cauterization	
	Circumcision	
	Closed reduction of fractures	
D	Detox (to)	
	Detoxification	
	Disinfect (to)	
E	Endotracheal intubation	
G	Gall bladder surgery	
	Gargle (to)	
	Gargle (to)	
	Group therapy	
H	Hysterectomy	
I	Inhaler	
	Inhalers	
L	Laminectomy	
	Laparoscope	

Treatment Procedures Vocabulary *(continued)*

	VOCABULARY	TARGET
M	Manage the pain (to)	
	Massage therapy	
	Mist humidifier	
	Myomectomy	
O	Open reduction of fractures	
	Open-heart surgery	
	Open-heart surgical repair	
	Orchidectomy	
	Orchiopexy	
P	Physical therapy	
	Pneumonectomy	
	Prostatectomy	

	VOCABULARY	TARGET
S	Salpingectomy	
	Sequestrectomy	
T	Thoracotomy	
	Tracheostomy	
	Tubal ligation	
	TURP	
V	Vaporizer	
	Vasectomy	

Medications Vocabulary

	VOCABULARY	TARGET
A	Accutane	
	Adverse drug reaction	
	Anesthesia	
	Antibiotics	
	Anti-depressant	
	Anti-inflammatory pills	
	Anti-malarial drug	
	Aspirin	
B	Barrier methods	
	BCG vaccine	
	Benzoyl Peroxide	
	Birth control	
	Blood thinners	
	Booster	

	VOCABULARY	TARGET
C	Chemicals	
	Children's Panadol	
	Condom	
	Coumadin	
D	D.P.T vaccine	
	Decongestants	
	DEET	
	Dose	
	DTaP	
	Dye	
E	EC emergency contraception	
	Epidural	
	EpiPen	

PO Box 2308, Woburn, MA 01888-0508, **p:** 781-729-3736, **www.EmbracingCulture.com**
PO Box 6401, Manchester, NH 03108, **p:** 1-888-678-CCCS

Medications Vocabulary *(continued)*

	VOCABULARY	TARGET
F	Flu shot	
G	Gel	
	General anesthesia	
H	Hepatitis A vaccine series	
	Hepatitis B vaccine series	
	Heroin	
	Hormonal methods	
	HPV vaccine series	
	Hyrodrocholorthiazide	
I	Immunizations	
	Influenza vaccine	
	Insect repellent	
	Insulin	
	Insulin drip	
	Intra-uterine device	
	IPV (Inactivated Polio Vaccine)	
	IV	
	IV drip	
	IV Morphine	
L	Lotion	
	Lovenox	
M	Malarone	
	Medication	
	Medicine	
	Meningococcal vaccine	
	Metamucil	
	MMR vaccine	
	Mosquito bed net	

	VOCABULARY	TARGET
N	Narcotic	
	Narcotic pain medicine	
	Nitroglycerin	
	Non-steroidal anti-inflammatory medicine	
	Non-steroidals	
O	Ointment	
	OPV (Oral Polio Vaccine)	
P	Pain killers	
	Panadol	
	Pepto Bismol	
	Pill	
	Placebo pill	
	Pneumococcal polysaccharide (PPV) vaccine	
	Polio vaccine	
	Polio vaccine series	
	Potassium	
	Progestin	
R	Rabies immune globulin	
	Rhythm method	
S	Sedative	
	Shots	
	Sleeping pill	
	Spermicide	
	Stimulant	
	Sudafed	
T	TB vaccine	

Medications *(continued)*

VOCABULARY	TARGET
Td	
Tdap	
Tempra	
Tetanus shots	
Thalidomide	
Tretinoin	

	VOCABULARY	TARGET
	Tylenol	
	Vaccines	
	Vitamins	
Z	Zantac	

Medical Supplies Vocabulary

	VOCABULARY	TARGET
A	Adhesive	
	Antiseptics	
	Arch Supports	
	Armslings	
	Aural Speculum	
B	Bariatric Bath Benches	
	Basin	
	Bassinets	
	Blade	
	Blind(n)	
	Blood Glucose Meter	
C	Cabinet	
	Cane	
	Canister	
	Cast	
	Chapel	
	Clamp	
	Commode	
	Crutch	
	Cuff	
	Curette	

	VOCABULARY	TARGET
D	Decongestant	
	Defibrillator	
	Diabetes Test Strips	
	Dilator	
	Disinfectants	
	Dressing	
E	Elbow Strap	
	Elbow Support	
	Electrode	
	Eye drops	
F	Face Shield	
	Feeding Tube	
	Forceps	
G	Gauze Pads	
	Gauze Sponges	
	Gel	
	Glass Slide	
	Glove Dispenser	
	Gurney	

'O Box 2308, Woburn, MA 01888-0508, **p:** 781-729-3736, **www.EmbracingCulture.com**
'O Box 6401, Manchester, NH 03108, **p:** 1-888-678-CCCS

Medical Supplies Vocabulary *(continued)*

	VOCABULARY	TARGET
H	Hammer	
	Hamper	impedir / interferir
	Hand Sanitizer	
	Heat Pack	
	Humidifier	
I	Inhaler	
	IV	
K	Kinesio Tape	
	Knee Brace	
L	Lancet	
	Lumbar Support	
M	Mask	
	Medical record	
	Medicine Samples	
	Microscope	
	Monitor	
	Mouthpiece	
N	Nebulizers	
	Neck Immobilizer	
	Nippers	pinzas
O	Oximeter	
	Oxygen Flow Meter	
	Oxygen Tank	
P	Paramedic	
	PH Test Strips	
	Pliers	tenazas / alicates

	VOCABULARY	TARGET
	Pneumatic Armband	
	Power Lift Chair	
R	Respirator	
	Retractor	
S	Scale	
	Scalpel	
	Scissors	
	Shoehorns	
	Sitz Bath	
	Splint	tablilla
	Sterile Pad	
	Sterilizer	
	Stethoscope	
	Suction Cups	
	Surgical Rasp	
	Suture	
	Swab Dispenser	
T	Tongs	tenazas
	Tourniquet	
	Trays	
	Treadmill	caminador / cinta rodante
	Tweezers	pinzas
V	Ventilator	

Other Vocabulary

	VOCABULARY	TARGET
A	Abnormalities	
	Adolescents	
	Adults	
	Air-conditioned	
	Alcohol consumption	
	Alcohol hand swabs	
	Allergist	
	Allergy clinic	
	Androgens	
	Anterior	
	Anterior wall	
	Appear (to)	
	Appetite	
	Arrange (to)	
	Asleep	
	Assure (to)	
	At risk (to be)	
	Autoimmune activity	
B	Bacteria	
	Bad luck	
	Barely	
	Baseline (a)	
	Bath	
	Beans	
	Bear weight (to)	
	Beating	
	Become (to)	
	Behavior	
	Bend (to)	
	Bend down (to)	
	Bend it back (to)	
	Bend up (to)	

	VOCABULARY	TARGET
	Bent over	
	Bite (to)	
	Blurry	
	Bother (to)	
	Bowel habits	
	Break up (to)	
	Breathe (to)	
	Brunch	
	Buckle (to)	
	Burst (to)	
	Bushes	
	By mouth	
C	Calmer	
	Cane	
	Cardiologist	
	Careful	
	Carry (to)	
	Casting	
	Catheter	
	Ceiling	
	Chamber	
	Chart	
	Check (to)	
	Chief concern	
	Childbearing	
	Childhood	
	Children	
	Choices	
	Climb (to)	
	Close off (to)	
	Common procedure	
	Complain (to)	

PO Box 2308, Woburn, MA 01888-0508, p: 781-729-3736, www.EmbracingCulture.com
PO Box 6401, Manchester, NH 03108, p: 1-888-678-CCCS

Other Vocabulary *(continued)*

VOCABULARY	TARGET
Consent form	
Contagious	
Contributing	
Control (to)	
Cosmetics	
Cotton swab	
Counselors	
Court stenographer	
Covering	
Crutches	
Cut (to)	
Cut back on something (to)	
Cute	
D Dangerous	
Dawn	
Daytime	
Death	
Decreased	
Deep breath	
Delicacy	
Department of Public Health	
Describe (to)	
Diet	
Dietary suggestions	
Digest (to)	
Dinner	
Disability insurance	
Discharge (a)	
Disease	
Disease-carrying organisms	
Dollies	
Dormant	

VOCABULARY	TARGET
Draw (to)	
Dressing	
Droplets	
Dropping	
Drops	
Drug store	
Dusk	
E Ease the pain (to)	
Effective	
Elastic bandage	
Elevated	
Endurance	
Enlarged	
Enroll (to)	
ER	
Examine (to)	
Exercise	
Exert (to)	
Exposed	
Exposure	
Extend (to)	
F Family planning counselor	
Family therapist	
Family's health history	
Fat	
Fatal	
Fatty foods	
Flex (to)	
Fluids	
Flying insects	
Follow (to)	

Other Vocabulary *(continued)*

VOCABULARY	TARGET
Follow up	
Food pyramid	
Foreign-born	
French fries	
Full blown disease	
G Gain (to)	
Get better (to)	
Get worse (to)	
GI specialist	
Give way (to)	
Gloves	
Godmother	
Good-sized	
Gowns	
Grab (to)	
Grabbing	
Gray	
Greasy foods	
Green	
Gross	
H Halfway houses	
Harm	
Health insurance	
Health proxy	
Heart rate	
Hereditary tendency	
Heredity	
Hide-and-seek	
High school age	
Hole	
Hospitalized	

VOCABULARY	TARGET
Hot	
Huge	
Human being	
Human body	
Hungry	
Hurt	
Hyper	
I Ice packs	
Ice the knee (to)	
Icing	
Illness	
Immunity	
Immunization history	
Immunizing agent	
Impact (to)	
Improve (to)	
In between pregnancies	
Infant	
Infected	
Infection	
Infectious disease	
Informed consent form	
Inject (to)	
Injection site	
Injections	
Injury	
Insert (to)	
Insurance	
Intercourse	
Invade (to)	
Irreversible	
Isolate (to)	
Isolated	

PO Box 2308, Woburn, MA 01888-0508, **p:** 781-729-3736, **www.EmbracingCulture.com**
PO Box 6401, Manchester, NH 03108, **p:** 1-888-678-CCCS

Other Vocabulary *(continued)*

	VOCABULARY	TARGET
J	Johnny	
K	Keep (to)	
	Kid	
	Kidney function	
	Kneeling	
	Known function	
L	Labored breathing	
	Large	
	Latent	
	Lead (to)	
	Let go (to)	
	Lift (to)	
	Limp (to)	
	Long- lasting	
	Long pants	
	Long term	
	Lose (to)	
	Lower right side	
	Lunch	
M	Make me better (to)	
	Makeup	
	Malaria risk area	
	Malaria-infected mosquito	
	Males	
	Masks	
	Maternal grandfather	
	MD	
	Meals	
	Measure (to)	
	Medical attention	

	VOCABULARY	TARGET
	Medical Directive	
	Medical history	
	Medical records	
	Mental health	
	Micro tools	
	Mild	
	Miracle drug (a)	
	Mosquitoes	
N	Napping	
	Nasty bite	
	Nationwide	
	Neutralize (to)	
	Non-smoking programs	
	Normal pregnancies	
	Nurse practitioner	
	Nutrition	
O	Oatmeal	
	Oatmeal bath	
	Occupational therapy	
	Odd	
	Oil	
	Older children	
	Once in a while	
	Operating room	
	Oral sex	
	Ortho clinic	
	Orthopedic doctor	
	Orthopedic physician's assistant	
	Outbreak	
	Outcome	
	Outpatient clinic	

Other Vocabulary *(continued)*

VOCABULARY	TARGET
Overdose	
Over-the-counter medications	
Oxygen	
P Paralyzed	
Park bench	
Pass it along (to)	
Passive	
Patch	
Paternal grandmother	
Physical therapist	
Pinch (to)	
Pinching	
Placement	
Plain films	
Plasmodium	
Plasmodium species	
Playground	
Polydrug use	
Pop out (to)	
Pork	
Portions	
Position	
Positive reaction	
Pound	
Precautionary measure	
Prescription	
Prescription drug	
Press (to)	
Pressure	
Pressure system	
Pretty good	
Pretty healthy	

VOCABULARY	TARGET
Prevent (to)	
Primary care doctor	
Primary Care Physician	
Procedure	
Produce (to)	
Protected intercourse	
Protective clothes	
Protective gear	
Puberty	
Public health	
Public health issue	
Puffs	
Pull (to)	
Pull them apart (to)	
Pulse	
Pump (to)	
Pumping fully	
Push away (to)	
Push it down (to)	
Put off (to)	
Put out (to)	
Q Q-tip	
R Radiologist	
Ragweed	
Rate	
Realize (to)	
Reasonable	
Rebound type	
Re-check	
Recovery room	
Recuperate (to)	

0 Box 2308, Woburn, MA 01888-0508, **p:** 781-729-3736, **www.EmbracingCulture.com**
0 Box 6401, Manchester, NH 03108, **p:** 1-888-678-CCCS

Other Vocabulary *(continued)*

VOCABULARY	TARGET
Referral	
Refill (a)	
Reflexes	
Regular	
Rehab	
Relapse	
Release (to)	
Relieved (to be)	
Religious beliefs	
Rely (to)	
Remedies	
Remission	
Resolve (to)	
Rest (to)	
Rice	
Right flank	
Right upper quadrant	
Rise (to)	
Risk area	
Run test (to)	
Rusty	

S

VOCABULARY	TARGET
Safety	
Salad	
Sample	
Scale	
Scar	
Scarred	
Scratch (to)	
Screened	
Screening	
Self-esteem	
Self-medication	

VOCABULARY	TARGET
Severe	
Severe illnesses	
Sexual abstinence	
Sexual intercourse	
Shift	
Shock	
Shortness of breath	
Shot area	
Shrug (to)	
Siblings	
Sick time	
Sickness	
Side effects	
Sign	
Significant illnesses	
Skunk	
Sleeves	
Slide	
Slight	
Slightly	
Slow	
Social worker	
Solids	
Soothing	
Sore	
Sound (to)	
Speculum	
Speech	
Speedy recovery	
Spit (to)	
Spitting up	
Splint	
Splinting	

Vocabulary *(continued)*

VOCABULARY	TARGET
Spores	
Spotting	
Spray	
Spread (to)	
Sputum	
Squeeze (to)	
Stamina	
Starving	
Stent	
Step on (to)	
Stew	
Stick (to)	
Stick to it (to)	
Still	
Sting (to)	
Stinging	
Straighten (to)	
Strength	
Stretcher	
Sub acute rehabilitation center	
Substitute	
Suicide	
Summersault	
Support stockings	
Surgeon	
Surgery	
Surgical mask	
Surgical resection	
Surgicenter	
Swab (to)	
Swallowing	
Swamps	
Sweat (to)	

VOCABULARY	TARGET
Sweating	
Sweats	
Sweaty	
Swell (to)	
Swelling	
Swollen	
Swollen patches	
Symptoms	
T Taking a breath	
Tarry	
Teenage girl	
The pill	
Thermometer	
Thick	
Thin (to)	
Thoracic surgeon	
Tick	
Tilt (to)	
Tiny	
Tips	
Tolerance	
Tolerated	
Torn (to)	
Touch (to)	
Tough	
Toward	
Toxins	
Traction	
Transaminases	
Transesophageal	
Travel (to)	
Treated	

PO Box 2308, Woburn, MA 01888-0508, **p:** 781-729-3736, **www.EmbracingCulture.com**
PO Box 6401, Manchester, NH 03108, **p:** 1-888-678-CCCS

Other Vocabulary *(continued)*

	VOCABULARY	TARGET
	Trigger (to)	provocar/desencadenar
	Tropical climate	
	Trunk	
	TSH	
	Twice a day	
	Twist (to)	
U	Ultimately	
	Uncommon	
	Uncoordinated	
	Urinating	
	Urine sample	
	Urologist	
V	Via	
	Virus	
	Vital signs	
	Vulnerable	
W	Wake me up (to)	
	Walker (a)	
	Walk-in patient	

	VOCABULARY	TARGET
	Walking cast	
	Warm	
	Warm soaks	
	Watchful	
	Weak	
	Weather	
	Weight	
	Weight gain	
	Widely used	
	Wiggle one's toes (to)	
	Wooden spatula	
	Workman's compensation	
	Worse	
	Wound	
Y	Yikes	
	Young adult	
	Younger than	
	Yucky	

The Art of Medical Interpretation®, A Chronology of Editions

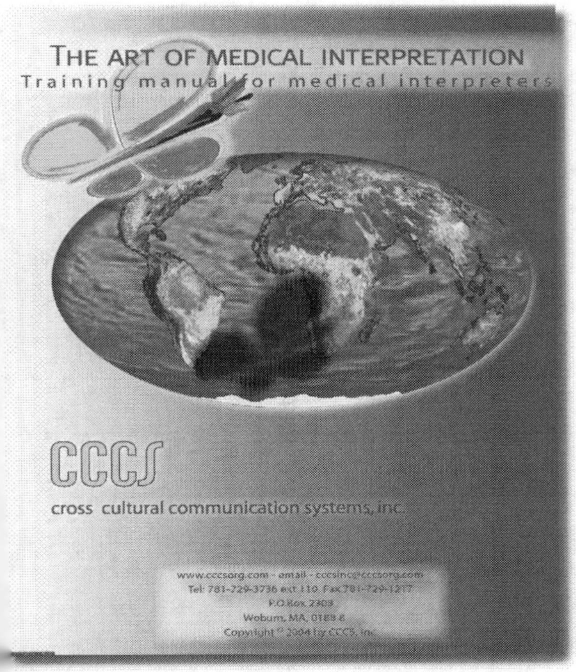

March 2002 - First Edition

The Art of Medical Interpretation®, First Edition was completed in March 2002. In their introductory message for students of interpretation, the editors stated, "Although the trade you have chosen requires many technical skills, it is more an art form than an occupation...How is medical interpretation an art? Perhaps the best way to answer that is by explaining where we're coming from and why we've spent the last twenty-three years studying, practicing and teaching this art form."

"The strength of this manual lies in the fact that its writers have professionally interpreted as well as taught in the field of medicine for over twenty-three years. In 1979 and 1980, Dr. Richard Lane and I taught the first trainings for medical interpreters while we were both working at The Cambridge Hospital in Cambridge, Massachusetts. Perhaps the different perspectives we've brought to trainings ever since then, Dr. Lane's perspective as a medical provider and my perspective as a mental health provider, have helped us connect to people in a way we would never have been able to alone."

"For this manual we have contributed ideas and experiences for the sample clinical cases, prepared many additional tools, done extensive research and compiled a library of educational texts and videos that compliment our interactive teaching style. And what would a classroom be without skeletons, charts and an assortment of body part models you can get your hands on? Touching is believing, seeing is believing, practicing and asking questions is believing."

"Whether you're signed up for a twenty or fifty-four hour training, this manual should keep you active and stimulated, even long after the course has ended. In designing this manual we have provided space for you to take notes, to write your thoughts, to scribble questions or to draw diagrams. So please do so! This text should be alive, but only you can make it yours. It is a working tool, just as you are a working interpreter."

0 Box 2308, Woburn, MA 01888-0508, **p:** 781-729-3736, **www.EmbracingCulture.com**
0 Box 6401, Manchester, NH 03108, **p:** 1-888-678-CCCS

"The first step is learning how we learn. There are three general non-linear learning steps: denial, acceptance, and finally the integration of new knowledge. To help each other grow as people and as professional medical interpreters, we ask students (and ourselves) which stage we think we're in. Are we ready to put aside our pre-conceived notions and fully embrace other cultures, classes and idioms? Are we ready to acknowledge the biases of our own culture? One of the most difficult challenges for faculty is the loop between the learning stages of acceptance to integration, but it is a journey we'll make together through the course of the training."

June 2004 - Second Edition

The Art of Medical Interpretation®, Second Edition was completed in June 2004. In their introductory message for students of interpretation, the editors stated, "In March 2002, a team of extremely dedicated staff and volunteers at Cross Cultural Communication Systems, Inc.™ put together a wonderful manual for you, the interpreter and the trainer. In just two years, we have sold manuals to individuals, institutions and faculty responsible for the training of medical interpreters. Some were bought at book shows at interpreting conferences; others were purchased as part of a CCCS, Inc.™ training package."

"CCCS, Inc.™ has made several updates to The Art of Medical Interpretation® manual. New information is listed under highlighted subtitles in our Table of Contents. We have added…new graphics of body parts and organs. We thank MegaSystems for the use of their illustrations, you may visit their website at www.megasystemsUSA.com. We also added exciting new role-plays and elaborated on the ethics of interpretation. Updates were made on the importance of a pre-session and on the CIFE acronym, a mnemonic created by CCCS, Inc.™ to help interpreters remember the four main points to be addressed during interpreter, patient and provider introductions. New information on the ethics of interpreting in alternative treatment cases is also included…We hope that this manual is the seeding for increased learning. We welcome feedback, including suggestions on content and format, at any time."

Bibliography

Across Cultures Newsletter. 1998. January. Pages 3-5. Washington: CCHP

Alvarez, Julia. 2001. *In the Name of Salome.* New York: A Plume Book.

Alves, E. 1997. *Dicionario Medico.* São Paulo: Atheneu.

Almeida, G. 1996. *Estórias de Dentro de Casa.* Lisboa: Editorial Caminho

Alvord, Lori Arviso. M.D. and Van Pelt, Elizabeth Cohen. 2000. *The Scalpel and the Silver Bear.* New York: Bantam Books.

American Heart Association Web Page

American Psychiatric Association. 1994. Diagnostic and Statistical Manual of Mental Health Fourth Edition. DSM-IV

Andrews, Margaret and Boyle, Joyceen S. 1999. *Transcultural Concepts in Nursing and Adolescents, Assessment, Diagnosis and Treatment.* New York: Guilford Press.

Angelelli, Claudia, V. 2005. *Medical Interpreting and Cross Cultural Communication*, Cambridge, United Kingdom, Cambridge University Press.

Araujo, Z. 1996. **Portuguese Families. Ethnicity & Family Therapy, Second Edition**, pp. 583-594.

Araujo-Lane, Z. October 2003. *Erros in Interpretation: Aiming for 100% Accuracy.* The Cross Cultural Communication Vol. 6. Cross Cultural Communication Systems, Inc.

Araujo-Lane, Z. Phillips,V. September 2003. *Ethics anda Medical Interpretation: The Value of a Pre-Session.* Chronicle. American Translators Association.

Araujo-Lane, Z. Phillips, V. November 2003. *Understanding the Power of a Medical Interpreter.* Proceedings of the 44th Annual Conference of the American Translators Association. American Translators Association.

Araujo-Lane, Z. Ready, B. Lane, R. November 2002. *The Art of Medical Interpretation: An Inclusive Approach to Teaching.* Proceedings of the 43rd Annual Conference of the American Translators Association. American Translators Association.

PO Box 2308, Woburn, MA 01888-0508, **p:** 781-729-3736, **www.EmbracingCulture.com**
PO Box 6401, Manchester, NH 03108, **p:** 1-888-678-CCCS

Ávila, Ermelindo. 1996. *Emigrados, Imigrantes*. Ponta Delgada, Azores: Gráfica Açoriana, Lta.

Awake! January 8th. 2000. *Bloodless Medicine and Surgery*. The Growing Demand.

Baggaley, A., Freeman, S. 2001. *Human Body. An Illustrated Guide to Every Part of the Human Body and How it Works*. England: Dorling Kindersley.

Bander, R. *Using Your Brain – for a Change, Neuro-Linguistic Programming*. 1985 Real People Press. Utah.

Barron's. 2001. *Essential Atlas of Anatomy*. New York: Barron's Educational Series, Inc.

Battle, M. *General Guidelines for Providers in Cross-Cultural Settings*. Pages 44-50. Massachusetts General Hospital.

Berkow, R., Beers, M., Fletcher, A. 1997. *The Merck Manual of Medical Information*. Home Edtion. New Jersey: Merck Research Laboratories.

Bonder, B., Martin, L., Miracle, A. 2002. *Culture in Clinical Care*. New Jersey: Slack Inc.

Buzan, T. *Use Both Sides of Your Brain. Third Edition*. 1989. Plume. New York.

Bragdon, Allen & Gamon, David, PHD. *Brains that work a little bit differently*. 2000. The Brainwavers Center, Cape Cod and San Francisco.

Buckman, Robert. 1992. *How to Break Bad News*. Maryland: Baltimore. The Johns Hopkins University Press.

Bughwald, D., Caralis, P., Gany, F., Hardt, E., Muecke, M., Putschlll, R. 1993. *The Medical Interview Across Cultures*. Pages 141-166. Patient Care.

Burns, A., Lovich, R., Maxwell, J., Shapiro, K. 1997. *Where Women Have No Doctor*. A Health Guide for Women. California: Hesperian Foundation.

Buchwald, Dedra, MD et all. 1993. *The Medical Interview Across Cultures*. Patient Care. April 15, pp. 141-166.

Burke, Garance. November 2. 2005. *California Seeks to Ban Interpreters*. The Associated Press.

Cabrera,Yvette, 2005. *Two Chilfren Translators, Two Views on Measure*. Register Columnist. (ycarera@ocregister,com)

Canino, Ian, M.D and Jean Spurlock, M.D. *Culturally Diverse Children and Adolescents, Assessment Diagnosis and Treatment*. New York: Guilford Press.

Campbell, Robert, M.D. *Psychiatric Dictionary.* 1996. Oxford University Press, New York.

Carr-Ruffino, Norma. 1999. *Diversity Success Strategies*. Boston, MA: Butterworth Heinnemann.

Carrillo, J. Emilio, Green, Alexander R. and Betancourt, Joseph R. *Cross- Cultural Primary Care: A Patient-Based Approach.* May 1999. Annals of Internal Medicine, Volume 130, Issue 10. American College of Physicians.

Commonwealth of Massachusetts. Executive Office of Health and Human Services Massachusetts Department of Public Health, 2001. *Best Practice Recommendations For Hospitals-Based Interpreter Services.*

Chabner, D. 1991. *The Language of Medicine. Fourth Edtion.* Pennsylvania: W.B. Saunders Co.

Chan, Paul, D., MD and Winkle, Peter, J., MD. 2001-2002. *History and Physical Examination.* Laguna Hills, CA. Current Clinical Strategies Publishing.

Clayman, C. 1995. *The Human Body. An Illustrated Guide to it's Structure. Function, and Disorders.* England: Dorling Kindersley.

Clever, S., Edwards, K. Feudtner, C., Braddock, C. 2001. *Ethics and Communication.* Volume 16. Pages 559-562. JGIM.

Cross Cultural Communication Systems, Inc. 2002. *The Art of Medical Interpretation: Training Manual for Medical Interpreters.* Winchester, MA

Cross Cultural Health Care Program. 1996. *Bridging the Gap. A Basic Training for Medical Interpreters Handbook.* Washington: CCHCP.

Daniel Tatum, B. 1992. *Taking About Race, Learning About Racism: The Application of Racial Identity Development Theory in the Classroom.* Harvard Educational Review. Vol. 62, No. 1, pp. 1-24.

Daniels, H. 1983. *Famous Last Words: The American Language Crisis Reconsidered.* Illinois: Southern Illinois University Press.

O Box 2308, Woburn, MA 01888-0508, **p:** 781-729-3736, **www.EmbracingCulture.com**
O Box 6401, Manchester, NH 03108, **p:** 1-888-678-CCCS

Danticat, Edwidge. 2001. *The Butterfly's Way. Voices from the Haitian Dyaspora in the United States.* New York: SOHO Press

Danticat, Edwidge. 1991. *Krik? Krak!* New York: Vintage Contemporaries, Vintage Books, A division of Random House, Inc.

Danticat, Edwidge. 1994. *Breath, Eyes, Memory. A Novel.* New York: Vintage Contemporaries, Vintage Books, A division of Random House, Inc.

Delvecchio Good, M., Brodwin, P., Good, B,. Keinman, A. 1992. *Pain as Human Experience. An Antrhopological Perspective.* California: University of California Press.

Deska Pagana, K., Pagana, T. 2002. *Mosby Manual of Diagnostic and Laboratory Test.* Second Edition. Missouri: Mosby Inc.

Desmond, Joanne and Copeland, Lanny, R., M.D. 2000. *Communicating with Today's Patient. Essentials to Save Time, Decrease Risk and Increase Patient Compliance.* San Francisco, CA: Josey-Bass Publisher.

Dickson, M. 1983. *Where There is No Dentist.* California: Hesperian Foundation.

Dixon, Lowell, M.D. 1988. *Blood: Whose Choice And Whose Conscience?* Journal of Medicine, New York State.

Drachaman, D. 1995. *Immigration Statuses and Their Influence on Service Provision, Access and Use.* Social Work, 40(2): 188-197.

Goleman, Daniel. *Emotional Intelligence. Why it can matter more than IQ.* 1995. Bantam Books. New York.

Fadiman, Anne. 1997. *The Spirit Catches You and You Fall Down – A Hmong Child, Her American Doctors, and the Collision of Two Cultures.* New York: Farrar, Straus and Giroux

Flores, Glenn, et all. 2004. *Error in Medical Interpretation and their Potential Clinical Consequences in Pediatric Encounters. American Academy of Pediatrics.* October 22. Pp: 6-15.

Freedman, Alfred M., MD; Harold I. Kaplan, MD; Benjamin J. Sadock, MD. *Modern Synopsis of Psychiatry II.* Maryland: The Williams & Williams Co. 1976.

Frishberg, Nancy. *Interpreting: An Introduction, 3rd printing.* 1996. RID Publications, Silver Spring, Maryland.

Galanti, Geri-Ann. 1997. *Caring for Patients from Different Cultures. Case Studies from American Hospitals. Second Edition.* Philadelphia, PA: University of Pennsylvania Press.

Garland, James A., Jones, Hubert E., Kolodny, Ralph L., "A Model For Stages of Development in Social Work Groups" in Bernstein, Saul (ed.). *Explorations In Group Work.* Boston: Milford House, Inc. 1973.

Gaspar, F. 1999. *Leaving Pico. A Novel.* Hanover, NH. University Press of New England.

Gaw, Albert. M.D. 1993. *Culture, Ethnicity and Mental Illness.* Washington DC: American Psychiatric Press.

Hall, Edward, T. 1973. *The Silent Language.* New York: Anchor Books.

Hall, Edward, T. 1977. *Beyond Culture.* New York: Anchor Books.

Hanchack, Nicholas, MD., et. all. 1996. *Patient Misunderstanding of Dosing Instructions.* JGIM. June-Volume 11

Hatton, Diane, C., DNS, RN, CS. 1992. *Information Transmission in Bilingual Bicultural Contexts.* Journal of Community Helath Nursing, 9(1), pp:53-59.

Harkness and Charles M. Super 1996. *Parent's Belief Systems. Their Origins, Expressions and Consequences.* New York: Guilford Press.

Hardwood, Alan. 1981. *Ethnicity & Medical Care.* Cambridge, MA: Harvard University Press.

Heller, Jean. 1972. *Syphillis Victims in the U.S.* Study Went Wrong. July. Associate Press. Washington Star.

Him, Chanrithy. 2000. *Growing Up Under the Khmer Rouge. When Broken Glass Floats.* New York: W.W. Norton & Company, Inc.

Hoffman, E. 1963. *Lost in Translation.* New Your, Penguin Books USA, Inc.

Ioward, David. 2000. *Dominican Republic.* New York: Interlink Books.

Katan, D. 1999. *Translating Cultures. An Introduction for Translators, Interpreters and Mediators.* United Kingdom: St. Jerome Publishing.

Kato, P. and Mann, T. 1996. *Handbook of Diversity Issues in Health Psychology.* New York: Plenum Press.

Katz, L. and Manning, R. *Keep Your Brain Active.* 1999. Workman Publishing Company. New York.

Kaufer, Joseph, M. and Putsh, Robert, W. *Communication through Interpreters in Healthcare: Ethical Dilemmas Arising from Differences in Class, Culture, Language, and Power.* The Journal of Clinical Ethics, Vol. 8, Number 1. Pp: 71-87.

Klein, S. 1995. *A Book for Midwives. A Manual for Traditional Birth Attendants and Community Midwives.* California: Hesperian Foundation.

Kleinman, A.M.D., et al. February 1978. *Clinical Lessons from Anthropologic And Cross-Cultural Research.* Annals of Internal Medicine Vol. 88: No. 2

Kleinman, Arthur, M.D., et all. 1978. *Culture, Illness, and Care.* Annals of Internal Medicine 88:251. American College of Physicians. Pp:251-258.

Kleinman, A. 1995. *Writing at the Margin. Discourse Between Anthropology and Medicine.* California: University of California Press.

Kleinman, A. 1980. *Patients and Healers in the Context of Culture; An Exploration of the Bordeland between Anthropology, Medicine, and Psychiatry.* California: University Press.

Klessig, Jill, MD. September 1992. *Cross-Cultural Medicine A Decade Later.* West J Med. 157. Pp: 316-3222.

Kovner, A., Jonas, S. 1999. *Health Care Delivery in the United States. Sixth Editon.* New York: Springer Publishing Company.

Kubler-Ross,E., 1973. On *Death and Dying,* Routledge

Lapp, D. *Don't Forget! Easy Exercises for a Better Memory;* 1987. Perseus Books. Massachusetts.

Leonard, P. 1995. *Quick & Easy Medical Terminology, Second Edtion.* Pennsylvania: W. B. Saunders Co.

Lott, B. and Maluso, D. 1995. *The Social Psychology of Interpersonal Discrimination.* New York: Guilford Press.

Luckman, Joan. RN, MA 1999. *Transcultural Communication in Nursing.* Boston, MA: Delmar Publishers Lyons, R.Ph, 9/96 Vital Signs Bulletin.

McCabe, Marsha L. and Thomas, J. D. (ed.) 1998. *Portuguese Spinner – An American Story.* New Bedford: Spinner Publications, Inc.

McElroy, A., Townsend, P. 1996. *Medical Anthropology in Ecological Perspective.* Third Edtition. Colorado: Westview Press.

McGoldrick, M., Giordano, J., and Pearce, J. 1983. *Ethnicity & Family Therapy.* First Edition. New York: Guilford Press.

McGoldrick, M., et all. 1996. *Ethinicity & Family Therapy.* Second Edition. New York: Guilford Press.

McGoldrick, et all. 2005. *Ethnicity & Family Therapy.* Third Edition. New York: Guilford Press.

McKenzie-Pollock, Lorna, MSW. 1996. *Cambodian Families.* **McGoldrick, M., et all.** 1996. *Ethnicity & Family Therapy.* Second Edition. New York: Guilford Press. Pp: 307-323.

McIntire, M. 1986. *Interpreting: The Art of Cross Cultural Mediation. Proceedings of the Ninth National Convention of the Registry of Interpreters for the Deaf.* Maryland: RID Publications.

Maduro, Renaldo, PhD. December 1983. *Curanderismo and Latino Views of Disease and Curing.* The Western Medicine Journal of Medicine, pages: 868-874.

Manuila, L. Manuila, A., Lewalle P. and Nicoulin M. 1999. *Dicionário Médico.* Lisboa, Portugal: Climepsi.

Margolis, Maxine L. 1994. *Litlle Brazil. An Ethnography of Brazilian Immigrants in New York City.* New York Princeton University Press.

Mass. Medical Interpreters Assoc. 1995. *Medical Interpreting Standards of Practice.* Massachusetts: MMIA.

Massachusetts Department of Public Health, 2000. *Public Health Sheet, Adult Immunization*, Jamaica Plain, MA

O Box 2308, Woburn, MA 01888-0508, **p:** 781-729-3736, **www.EmbracingCulture.com**
O Box 6401, Manchester, NH 03108, **p:** 1-888-678-CCCS

Medscape, 2002. *Health Literacy: A review from Pharmacotheraphy. Pharmacptherapy* 2293):282-3002, Pharmacotherapy Publications

Millman, J. 1997 *"Typicalness: Massachustts and Minas Gerais." The Other Americans. How Immigrant Renew Our Country, Our Econony and Our Values*. New York: Vicking Penguin.

Minninger, J. *Total Recall. How to Maximize your Memory Power.* 1984, MJF Books. New York.

Mira, M. 1998. *The Forgotten Portuguese. The Melungeons And Other Groups. The Portuguese And Other Groups. The Portuguese Making of America.* North Carolina: Franklin.

National Heart, Lung and Blood Institute. *Heart Disease and Women: Be Physically Active.*

New England Journal of Medicine. 1989. *Sounding Board.* Pages 53-56. Vol. 320, No. 1

New England Journal of Medicine. 2001. Editorials. Pages 133-138. *Sounding Office for Civil Rights*. 1999. Federal Civil Rights Laws.

NHLBI, www.nhlbi.nih.gov/health

Nickens, W. Herbert, MD, MA. 1991. *The Health Status of Minority Populations in The United States*. West J medicine. July: 155: pp. 27-32.

Noon Parsons, G, Kinsman, S., Bosk, C., Sankar, P., Ubel, P. 2001. *Between Two Worlds*. Vol. 16. Pages 544-588. JGIM.

Office of Civil Rights. 1999. *Federal Rights Laws.*

Olohan, M. 2000. *Intercultural Faultlines. Research Models in Translation Studies 1 Textual and Cognitive Aspects*. United Kingdom: St. Jerome Publishing.

Opaku, Samuel, O. 1998. *Clinical Methods in Transcultural Psychiatry.* American Psychiatric Association, Washington, DC.

Pap, L. 1992. *The Portuguese-American*. Boston, Massachusetts: Twayne Publishers.

Pavão, J. A. 1981. *Aspectos Populares Micaelenses*. Angra do Heroísmo, Azores: S.R.E.C.

Pepetela. 1979. *Mayombe (Romance)*. Lisbon, Portugal: Edições 70.

Pinderhughes, E. 1989. *Understanding Race, Ethnicity and Power: The Key to Clinical Efficacy.* New York: Free Press.

Phillips, V. *Alternative Treatment Beliefs and the Medical Interpreter.* August 2002. ATA Chronicle. American Translators Association.

Poneterotto, J.G. Casa, J.M., Suzuki, L A. & Alexander, C.M. (Eds.) 1995. *Handbook of Multicultural Counseling*. New York: Sage.

Prendergast, A., Fulton, Frances. 1997. *Medical Terminology.* Text Workbook. Fourth Edition. California: Addison Wesley Longman, Inc.

Putsch, Robert W. December 1985. Cross-Cultural Communication. *The Special Case of Interpreters in Health Care.* JAMA-Vol. 254. No. 2. Pp: 3344-3348.

Puenell and Betty J. Paulanka.F.A. 1998. *Transcultural Health Care. A Culturally Competent Approach.* Philadelphia, PA F.A. Davis Company.

Rothenberg, P. 1995. *Race, Class, and Gender in the United States. An Integrated Study.* Third Edition. New York: St. Martin's Press.

Roter, Debra, L. and Hall, Judith, A. 1993. *Doctors Talking with Patients, Improving Communication in Medical Visits. Patients Talking to Doctors.* Westport, Connecticut: Auburn House.

Santiago, Esmeralda. 1994. *When I Was Puerto Rican.* New York: First Vintage Books.

Santiago, Esmeralda. 1998. *Almost a Woman.* New York: First Vintage Books.

Salopek, J. *Train Your Brain.* Pages 313-320.

Sleskovitch, D. 1978. *Interpreting for Internation Conferences.* Washington, D.C.: Pen and Booth.

Seleskovitch, D. *Interpreting for International Conference.* 1978. Pena and Booth. Washington, DC.

Seleskobithc, D. & Lederer Marianne. *A Systematic Approach to Teaching Interpretation.* 1978. Pen and Booth. Washington, DC.

Sleskovitch, D., Lederer, M. 1995. *A Systematic Approach to Teaching Interpretation.* Registry of Interpreters for the Deaf.

PO Box 2308, Woburn, MA 01888-0508, **p:** 781-729-3736, **www.EmbracingCulture.com**
PO Box 6401, Manchester, NH 03108, **p:** 1-888-678-CCCS

Serpa, C. 1996. *Guiomar: Boston, Massachusetts: Portuguese Continental Union.*

Singer, L. 1994. *Setting Disputes: Conflict Resolution in Business, Families, and the Legal System.* Colorado: Westview Press.

Slomski, Anita. May 24,1993. *Making Sure Your Case Doesn't Get lost in Translation.* Medical Economics, pp.122-134

Sluzki, C. 1979. *Migration and Family Conflict. Family Process.* Vol. 18, Number-4, December 1979, pp. 379-385.

Sotomayer, M. 1977. *Language, Culture, and Ethnicity in Developing Self-Concept.* Pages 321-327.

State of New Hampshire Department of Health and Human Services, 2000. *Childhood Immunization, Vaccines are FREE in New Hampshire.*

Stedman, T. L. 1996. *Dicionário Médico.* Rio de Janeiro: Editora Guanabara Koogan S. A.

Stavans, Ilan. 2005. *Dic.tion.ary|days [< a defining passion>]* Saint Paul Minnesota: Graywolf Press.

Stein, Howard. 1985. *The Psychodynamics of Medical Practice. Unconscious Factors In Patient Care.* Berkley, CA: University of California Press.

Stoeckle, J.M.D. 1987. *Encounters Between Patients and Doctors. An Anthology.* Cambridge: MIT Press.

Stoeckle, John, D., et all. 2002. *Doctoring Together, a physician's guide to manners, duties and communication in the shared care of patients.* Boston, MA: Massachusetts General Hospital Primary Care Division, Harvard Medical School.

Sue, Derald, Wing and Sue, David. 2003. *Counseling the Culturally Diverse. Theory and Practice.* 4th Edition John Willey & Sons, Inc. New York.

Suzuki, Lisa, A., et al. 2001. *Handbook of Multicultural Assessment. Clinical, Psychological and Educational Applications.* Second Edition. Jossey-Bass, San Francisco, CA.

The Communicator Express Vol. 2. 2003. Cross Cultural Communication Systems, Inc.

The Portuguese – American Historical Research Foundation, Inc. (P.A.H.R.F, Inc.). New England Journal of Medicine. 1989. *Sounding Board.* Pages 53-56. Volume 320, No. 1.

Thernstrom, S., Orlov, A., Handlin, O. 1980. *Harvard Encyclopedia of American Ethnic Groups.* Massachusetts: The Belknap Press of Harvard University Press.

Thomas, D. and Wetlaufer, S. 1997. *A Question of Color: A Debate on Race in the U.S. Workplace.* Harvard Bussiness Review, September 1997. Pp. 118-132.

Travis, T. 1998. *Psychiatry, Solving Patient Problems. Pattern Recognition Process. Case Studies.* Massachusetts: Blackwell Science, Inc.

Uba, Laura, PhD. September-October 1992. *Cultural Barriers to Health Care for Southeast Asian Refugees.* Public Health Reports. Vol. 107, No. 5 pp. 542-547.

Ung, Loung. 2000. *First They Killed My Father.* New York: Perenial.

Urdang, S. 1977. *Fighting Two Colonialisms.* New York: Monthly review Press.

U. S. Department of Health & Human Services, Measles, Mumps and Rubella. *What You Need to Know.* Public Health Centers for Disease Control, Atlanta Georgia 30333

Vaz, K. 1994. *Saudade: A Novel.* New York: St. Martin's Press.

Voeks, Robert A. 1997. *Sacred Magic, Medicine, and Religion in Brazil.* Austin, Texas: University of Texas Press.

Wadensj, Cecilia. 1998. *Interpreting as Interaction.* London and New York: Longman.

Wafer, Jim. 1991. *The Taste of Blood.* Philadelphia: University of Pennsylvania Press.

Werner, D., Thuman, C., Maxwell, J. 1999. *Where There is No Doctor. A Village Health Care Handbook.* California: Hesperian Foundation.

Woloshin, Steven, MD, et al. March 1995. *Language Barriers in Medicine in the United States.* Special Communication. JAMA. Vol. 273. No. 9. Pp: 724-728.

Websites Consulted

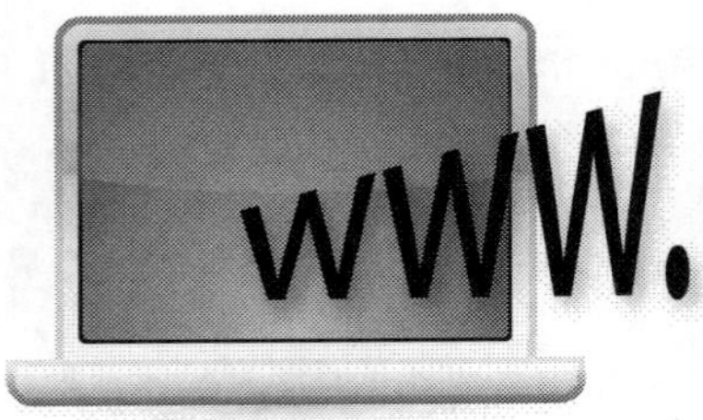

American Family Physician – **www.aafp.org**

Brain Injury Association – **www.biausa.org**

Center for Disease Control and Prevention – **www.bt.cdc.gov**

Department of Human Services – **www.hna.ffh.vic.gov.au.phb.hprot/food/fhpp/fpi.html**

Dr./Reddys Pediatric Office – **www.drready.com**

Jehovahs Witnesses Official Website – **www.watchtower.org**

KidSource – **www.kidsource.com**

Leesburg Orthopaedics and Sports Medicine – **http://leesburgortho.com/brokenbones.htm**

Listen Here – **www.yourhealth.com**

Massachusetts Public Health Department – **www.state.ma.us/dph.htm**

National Health Law Program – **www.howstuffworks.com**

Southern Illinois University School of Medicine – **www.siumed.edu**

http://www.whitehouse.gov/omb/

http://www.healthlaw.org/

http://www.healthlink.com/home.asp

http://www.dhhs.state.nc.us/

http://cdc.gov/

http://www.hhs.gov/

http://mmia.org/

http://www.chia.ws/

http://www.ncihc.org

http://www.diversityrx.org

http://www.ama.org

http://www.cirp.org

http://www.freemedicineprogram.com

http://www.thehealthpages.com

http://www.mass.gov/legis/laws/seslaw00/sl000066.htm

http://www.health.state.ny.us

http://www.nscardiology.com

http://www.nimh.nih.gov

http://www.acob.org

http://www.ncrel.org/sdrs/areas/issues/envrnmnt/css/cs3lk1.htm

http://www.hhs.gov/acr/hipaa/

http://www.usa.gov

http://cancernet.nci.nih.gov/

Media Resources

Lesson 1:

- *The Professional Interpreter.* Vancouver Community College and Surrey Delta Immigrant Services Society (1998).

- *The Healthcare Interpreter's Tools for Successful Communication in the Triadic Encounter,* volume one: CIFE and the Pre-Session (DVD-2006) http://cccsorg.com/training/tools_videos.html or call (781) 729 3736 x110

Lesson 2:

- *Mental Health Interpreting: A Mentored Curriculum* (Orders should be sent to Dr. Robert Pollard, URMC Department of Psychiatry, 300 Crittenden Boulevard, Rochester, NY 14642 (Robert_Pollard@urmc.rochester.edu) , or contact the Deaf Wellness Center at 585-275-6785 or via fax at 585-273-1117.

Lesson 3:

- *Consecutive Interpreting Theory & Consecutive Note Taking, ACEBO* http://acebo.com/order.htm or call (831) 455-1507

Lesson 4:

- *Consecutive Interpreting Theory & Consecutive Note Taking, ACEBO* http://acebo.com/order.htm or call (831) 455-1507

- *The Healthcare Interpreter's Tools for Successful Communication in the Triadic Encounter,* volume three: Clinical Insight in Medical Interpretation (DVD-2005) http://cccsorg.com/training/tools_videos.html or call (781) 729 3736 x110

Lesson 5:

- *Patient Diversity: Beyond the Vital Signs* http://www.crmlearning.com/

Lesson 6:

- *Body Story – The Beast Within & Crash* (DVD-2003) ASIN: B000JOVN6W

Lesson 7:

- *Body Story – Out of Control. Spreading Menace & Teen Dreams* (DVD-2003) ASIN: B000JOU390

PO Box 2308, Woburn, MA 01888-0508, **p:** 781-729-3736, **www.EmbracingCulture.com**
PO Box 6401, Manchester, NH 03108, **p:** 1-888-678-CCCS

Lesson 8:

- *Body Story – Body Snatchers & Breaking Down* (DVD-2003) ASIN: B000JOS7KW

Lesson 10:

- *Body Story – Body Snatchers & Breaking Down* (DVD-2003) ASIN: B000JOS7KW

Lesson 11:

- *Body Story – Body Snatchers & Breaking Down* (DVD-2003) ASIN: B000JOS7KW

Lesson 12:

- *The Healthcare Interpreter's Tools for Successful Communication in the Triadic Encounter,* volume two: Interpreting for Sensitive Topics (DVD-2006) http://cccsorg.com/training/tools_videos.html or call (781) 729 3736 x110

Lesson 13:

- *The Healthcare Interpreter's Tools for Mental Health Interpreting,* volume 2: Mental Status Exams for Patients with Early Dementia (DVD/CD 2007) http://cccsorg.com/training/tools_videos.html or call (781) 729 3736 x110